CW01263825

Physical Principles
of Medical Ultrasonics

Physical Principles of Medical Ultrasonics

Second Edition

Editors

C. R. Hill
J. C. Bamber
G. R. ter Haar

Physics Department, Institute of Cancer Research,
Royal Marsden Hospital, Sutton, Surrey, UK

John Wiley & Sons, Ltd

First Edition published in 1986 by Ellis Horwood Limited, Chichester, West Sussex
Copyright © 2004   John Wiley & Sons Ltd, The Atrium, Southern Gate, Chichester,
West Sussex PO19 8SQ, England

Telephone (+44) 1243 779777

Email (for orders and customer service enquiries): cs-books@wiley.co.uk
Visit our Home Page on www.wileyeurope.com or www.wiley.com

This publication is designed to provide accurate and authoritative information in regard to
the subject matter covered. It is sold on the understanding that the Publisher is not engaged
in rendering professional services. If professional advice or other expert assistance is
required, the services of a competent professional should be sought.

Other Wiley Editorial Offices

John Wiley & Sons Inc., 111 River Street, Hoboken, NJ 07030, USA

Jossey-Bass, 989 Market Street, San Francisco, CA 94103-1741, USA

Wiley-VCH Verlag GmbH, Boschstr. 12, D-69469 Weinheim, Germany

John Wiley & Sons Australia Ltd, 33 Park Road, Milton, Queensland 4064, Australia

John Wiley & Sons (Asia) Pte Ltd, 2 Clementi Loop #02-01, Jin Xing Distripark, Singapore 129809

John Wiley & Sons Canada Ltd, 22 Worcester Road, Etobicoke, Ontario, Canada M9W 1L1

Wiley also publishes its books in a variety of electronic formats. Some content that appears
in print may not be available in electronic books.

British Library Cataloguing in Publication Data
A catalogue record for this book is available from the British Library

ISBN 0 471 97002 6

Typeset in 9/11pt Times by Dobbie Typesetting Ltd, Tavistock, Devon
Printed and bound in Great Britain by CPI Antony Rowe, Eastbourne
This book is printed on acid-free paper responsibly manufactured from sustainable forestry
in which at least two trees are planted for each one used for paper production.

To Dr John Wild

– Who had the vision –

'My Dear Strutt,

I am glad you are writing a book on Acoustics....You speak modestly of a want of Sound books in English. In what language are there such, except Helmholtz, who is sound not because he is German but because he is Helmholtz....'

> (Letter from James Clerk Maxwell to John William Strutt, Lord Rayleigh, 20th May 1873, referring to Rayleigh's *Theory of Sound*, which he had started writing earlier that year whilst on a honeymoon trip up the river Nile)

'Compound utterances addressed themselves to their senses, and it was possible to view by ear the features of the neighbourhood. Acoustic pictures were returned from the darkened scenery;...'

> (From *The Return of the Native*, 1878, Thomas Hardy)

Contents

List of Contributors xi

Preface xiii

Chapter 1   Basic Acoustic Theory   1
S. J. Leeman
    1.1   Introduction   1
    1.2   The Canonical Inhomogeneous Wave Equation
         of Linear Acoustics.   2
    1.3   Acoustic Wave Variables   7
    1.4   Some Special Solutions   9
    1.5   Green's Function and Rayleigh's Integral 13
    1.6   Transducer Fields 15
    1.7   Propagation Across Planar Boundaries 26
    1.8   Finite Amplitude Waves. 34
         References 39

Chapter 2   Generation and Structure of Acoustic Fields 41
C. R. Hill
    2.1   Introduction 41
    2.2   Piezoelectric Devices 42
    2.3   The Fields of 'Simple', CW Excited Sources. 46
    2.4   The Pulsed Acoustic Field 48
    2.5   Focused Fields 48
    2.6   Effects of the Human Body on Beam Propagation 56
    2.7   Beam Formation by Transducer Arrays. 56
    2.8   The Field of the Toronto Hybrid 59
    2.9   Generation of Therapy Fields. 59
    2.10 Magnitudes of Acoustic Field Variables. 62
         References 63

Chapter 3   Detection and Measurement of Acoustic Fields 69
C. R. Hill
    3.1   Introduction 69
    3.2   Piezoelectric Devices 70
    3.3   Displacement Detectors 77

	3.4	Radiation Force Measurements	78
	3.5	Calorimetry.	83
	3.6	Optical Diffraction Methods.	84
	3.7	Miscellaneous Methods and Techniques	86
	3.8	Measurement of Biologically Effective Exposure and Dose	86
		References	88

Chapter 4 **Attenuation and Absorption.** 93
J. C. Bamber

	4.1	Introduction	93
	4.2	Tissue–Ultrasound Interaction Cross-Sections	94
	4.3	Theory of Mechanisms for the Absorption of Ultrasonic Longitudinal Waves.	96
	4.4	Measurement of Attenuation and Absorption Coefficients in Tissue	119
	4.5	Published Data on Attenuation and Absorption Coefficients	143
	4.6	Conclusion	155
		References	156

Chapter 5 **Speed of Sound** 167
J. C. Bamber

	5.1	Introduction	167
	5.2	Measurement of the Speed of Ultrasound in Tissues.	167
	5.3	Published Data for Speed of Sound Values	176
	5.4	Finite Amplitude ('Non-Linear') Propagation.	183
	5.5	Conclusion	185
		References	186

Chapter 6 **Reflection and Scattering** 191
R. J. Dickinson and D. K. Nassiri

	6.1	Introduction	191
	6.2	Scattering Theory	193
	6.3	Scattering Measurements	204
	6.4	Models.	211
	6.5	Scattering and the B-Mode Image.	215
	6.6	Concluding Remarks	219
		References.	220

Chapter 7 **Physical Chemistry of the Ultrasound–Tissue Interaction** 223
A. P. Sarvazyan and C. R. Hill

	7.1	Introduction	223
	7.2	Acoustic Properties Reflecting Different Levels of Tissue Organisation.	223
	7.3	Molecular Aspects of Soft Tissue Mechanics	225
	7.4	Relationship Between Ultrasonic Parameters and Fundamental Thermodynamic Potentials of a Medium.	228
	7.5	Structural Contribution to Bulk and Shear Acoustic Properties of Tissues.	232
	7.6	Relevance to Tissue Characterisation.	233
		References	234

Chapter 8   Ultrasonic Images and the Eye of the Observer   237
            C. R. Hill
            8.1 Introduction   237
            8.2 Quantitative Measures of Imaging and Perception   238
            8.3 Images and Human Visual Perception   239
            8.4 The Place of Ultrasound in Medical Imaging   248
            8.5 The Systematics of Image Interpretation   249
                 References   252

Chapter 9   Methodology for Clinical Investigation   255
            C. R. Hill and J. C. Bamber
            9.1 Introduction   255
            9.2 Imaging and Measurement: State of the Pulse–Echo Art   256
            9.3 A Broader Look: Performance Criteria   284
            9.4 Further Prospects for Ultrasonology and Image Parameterisation .   288
            9.5 Summary and Conclusions   295
                 References   296

Chapter 10 Methodology for Imaging Time-Dependent Phenomena   303
            R. J. Eckersley and J. C. Bamber
            10.1 Introduction   303
            10.2 The Principles of Ultrasound Motion Detection   304
            10.3 Techniques for Measuring Target Velocity   305
            10.4 Phase Fluctuation (Doppler) Methods   305
            10.5 Envelope Fluctuation Methods   320
            10.6 Phase Tracking Methods   321
            10.7 Envelope Tracking Techniques   325
            10.8 Considerations Specific to Colour Flow Imaging   326
            10.9 Angle-Independent Velocity Motion Imaging   326
            10.10 Tissue Elasticity and Echo Strain Imaging   328
            10.11 Performance Criteria   329
            10.12 Use of Contrast Media   330
            10.13 Concluding Remarks   332
                  References   333

Chapter 11 The Wider Context of Sonography   337
            C. R. Hill
            11.1 Introduction   337
            11.2 Macroscopic Techniques   337
            11.3 Acoustic Microscopy   341
                  References   346

Chapter 12 Ultrasonic Biophysics   349
            Gail R. ter Haar
            12.1 Introduction   349
            12.2 Thermal Mechanisms   350
            12.3 Cavitation   358
            12.4 Radiation Pressure, Acoustic Streaming and 'Other' Non-Thermal
                  Mechanisms   378
            12.5 Non-Cavitational Sources of Shear Stress   389

12.6   Evidence for Non-Thermal Effects in Structured Tissues   390
12.7   Thermal and Mechanical Indices   396
12.8   Conclusion   398
       References   398

Chapter 13   Therapeutic and Surgical Applications   407
Gail R. ter Haar
13.1   Introduction   407
13.2   Physiological Basis for Ultrasound Therapy   407
13.3   Physiotherapy   413
13.4   Ultrasound in Tumour Control   422
13.5   Surgery   428
       References   443

Chapter 14   Assessment of Possible Hazard in Use   457
Gail R. ter Haar
14.1   Introduction   457
14.2   Exposure Practice and Levels   457
14.3   Studies of Isolated Cells   459
14.4   Studies on Multicellular Organisms   462
14.5   Human Fetal Studies   471
14.6   Summary of Recommendations and Guidelines for Exposure. . .   475
14.7   Conclusion   479
       References   480

Chapter 15   Epilogue: Historical Perspectives   487
C. R. Hill
       References   489

List of Symbols   491

Index   497

List of Contributors

J. C. Bamber — Physics Department, Institute of Cancer Research, Royal Marsden Hospital, Sutton, Surrey, UK

R. J. Dickinson — Department of Bioengineering, Imperial College, London, UK

R. J. Eckersley — Imaging Science Department, Imperial College School of Medicine, London, UK

G. R. ter Haar — Physics Department, Institute of Cancer Research, Royal Marsden Hospital, Sutton, Surrey, UK

C. R. Hill — Physics Department, Institute of Cancer Research, Royal Marsden Hospital, Sutton, Surrey, UK

S. J. Leeman — Medical Engineering & Physics Department, King's College Hospital Medical School, London, UK

D. K. Nassiri — Department of Medical Physics and Bioengineering, St George's Hospital, London, UK

A. P. Sarvazyan — Artann Laboratories, NJ, USA

Preface

Ancient Hebrew and Christian tradition relates that the universe was created in six days, following which there was a day of rest. What the old chronicles never recorded was that, on the eighth day, the Creator must have dropped back into the lab to do some tidying up. Only then, coming across his rough notes for Maxwell's and the acoustic wave equations, did the thought occur that the creation of light and sound could be logically extrapolated to x-rays and ultrasound. The practical outcome of this realisation took some time to materialise but eventually, in the twentieth century, it led to a revolution in the practice of medicine. This book is concerned with one strand of that revolution, and attempts to explore its foundations in basic mathematical and scientific principles.

Within the past 30 years the clinical application of ultrasound imaging has grown from being a rare oddity to the point that it now accounts for well over 20% of all medical imaging procedures world-wide; second only to plain X-rays, and still growing. In addition, the longer-established therapeutic uses of ultrasound have continued to develop and are now being joined by methods employing strongly focused beams of ultrasound for minimally invasive surgical destruction of deep tissue structures.

Technologically, much of this development has been empirical; often without benefit of any systematic knowledge of the physics and biophysics underlying the essential phenomena. Valuable though much of this development has been, when viewed with the benefit of hindsight it can be seen that many opportunities were missed and much time and effort was spent travelling up blind alleys. The first edition of this book was therefore written in the hope that it might contribute to deeper and more general understanding in this field of applied science, and thus perhaps point the way to further, more scientifically based practical developments and clinical applications.

That first edition was published in 1986, has now sold out, but remains unique of its kind. In the meantime scientific knowledge has advanced and so also, with much help from constructively critical readers, have our ideas on what now seems to be needed in a book of this sort. Thus, much of the material in this edition has been completely rewritten, often by new authors. The rest we have thoroughly revised and brought up to date. As before, the book is aimed, broadly, at graduate students in the Physical Sciences and Engineering. It should also, however, have plenty to offer, for example, to undergraduates specialising in Physics-Applied-to-Medicine, and also to that increasingly common breed: physics-literate physicians.

The book is divided, somewhat arbitrarily, into four parts: *theory*, *basics*, *investigation*, and *intervention*.

Acoustics – the branch of Physics to which this subject belongs – has a well-developed theoretical background, that provides the essential basis for a proper understanding of the experimentally observed phenomena and their interrelationships. Chapter 1 therefore attempts to outline those aspects of theoretical acoustics that underlie the principal phenomena that are encountered in medical ultrasonics, and which will be addressed individually later in the book.

The following six chapters take up various practical manifestations of ultrasonic physics that have relevance in both the investigative and interventional contexts of clinical application. Flowing closely from theoretical descriptions are the formation and structure of ultrasonic fields (or 'beams') and this is coupled, in Chapter 2, with the practicalities of their generation. The counterpart to this, in Chapter 3, is the principles and methods for detecting and measuring such fields.

An important simplifying assumption, stated and used in the theoretical discussion of Chapter 1 – as indeed it is in all other such 'first order' treatments – is that the media of interest are homogeneous and non-attenuating. Chapters 4 to 7 are concerned with the reasons for, and implications of, the departures from this condition that arise in actual, living tissue. The phenomena concerned are the attenuation of ultrasound by tissues, differences in speed of sound propagation as between different tissues, implications of the departure from a linear stress-strain relationship in acoustic propagation, and the particular behaviour of tissues as acoustic scatterers. Finally in this section, Chapter 7 discusses those aspects of the physical chemistry of tissue constituents that seem to determine their acoustic behaviour, and that may provide clues for novel ways of exploiting such behaviour in clinical use.

Section 3 addresses the principles and methods of application of ultrasound to the investigation of human pathology and physiology. This is a subject that is commonly referred to as *imaging* or *sonography* and, although, as will be seen, its scope is considerably wider than such terms imply, much of it is concerned with the formation of images that are to be presented to a human observer, whose characteristics often turn out to be crucial to the overall performance of an investigative process. Thus Chapter 8 examines the way in which human visual physiology handles the rather peculiar nature of ultrasonic images.

By far the most commonly used approach to sonography is via the pulse-echo method, and Chapter 9 opens with an account of the principles and practice involved. This approach is, however, to some extent arbitrary and, at least for the solution of certain clinical problems, there may exist other options that offer attractive prospects for *tissue characterisation* or, perhaps better, *parametric imaging*. Discussion of these leads, in turn, to considerations of how best, and by what *performance criteria* to choose methods to address particular clinical problems. In the past it has been common practice in ultrasound texts to deal separately with *pulse-echo* and *Doppler* methods. It is now well recognised, however, that the Doppler phenomenon is no more than an optional tool (albeit one that tends to be very simple and cheap to implement) among several that are available for extracting time-domain information from ultrasonic data sets. Thus, although here for reasons of convenience we devote a separate chapter to the investigation of tissue movement, it will be seen that Chapter 10 is logically a somewhat seamless extension of its predecessor. Finally in this section we describe briefly, in Chapter 11, a miscellaneous set of imaging techniques, and in particular those of *acoustic microscopy*, that seem to be of potential interest in biomedicine but that, at present at least, have not found substantial clinical application.

The final section of the book is concerned with the *interventional* manifestations of ultrasound, whether deliberate or otherwise. It has been known since the pioneering observations of Langevin, in about 1917, that ultrasound can affect, and sometimes damage or destroy, living organisms; the reasons why such changes happen have, however, turned out to be complex, and it is only recently that something approaching systematic understanding has been achieved in this field. In Chapter 12 we describe what is now known of the biophysics of ultrasound: the mechanisms that lead from physical exposure to an acoustic stress and thus through to observable biological change. The exploitation of such changes for therapeutic and surgical purposes, some already well established in the clinic and others still under development, is discussed in Chapter 13. Another implication of the occurrence of such changes, however, is that there might be some hazard to patients or operators in various medical procedures based on ultrasound, and the final chapter examines the various possibilities that exist here.

The writing of this book has been a collaborative effort to which many people have contributed, consciously or otherwise, and not least through thoughtful and constructive criticism of the first edition. To a considerable extent the book reflects the interests of our own research group over the past 40 years and we are very grateful for the contributions that have been made during this period by a wide circle of colleagues, students, visitors and other collaborators, not all of whom may have been adequately acknowledged in the text. The opportunity to take up and carry through work in this field was provided for us by the Institute of Cancer Research and the Royal Marsden Hospital and their funding agencies, particularly the UK Medical Research Council and Cancer Research UK, and for this also we are most grateful. Finally, we are indebted to a number of individuals and publishers for permission to use illustrative material, the sources of which are indicated in the text.

Kit Hill
Jeff Bamber
Gail ter Haar

1

Basic Acoustic Theory

S. J. LEEMAN

Institute of Cancer Research, Royal Marsden Hospital, UK

1.1   INTRODUCTION

No true understanding of medical ultrasound methods is possible without an appreciation of the physics of ultrasound, and, for most applications, that essentially entails a good grasp of the principles of the propagation of ultrasound waves in tissue-like media. Many treatments of the subject emphasise continuous waves, but it is the transient (pulsed) wave that is utilised in the vast majority of cases. This chapter therefore aims to avoid the simplifying assumption of harmonic waves, except to introduce it as a case of special interest, or where it significantly reduces the complexity of the analysis.

A study of pulse propagation requires the specification of a wave equation, which, in the case of interest here, rests heavily on the ability to specify a model of the (mechanical) behaviour of tissue-like media. At present, such a model still eludes the medical ultrasound community, but it will be seen below that some moderately uncomplicated assumptions go a long way towards achieving that goal. However, 'uncomplicated' does not mean 'insignificant', and a substantial degree of simplification is achieved at the cost of neglecting absorption. It must be firmly stated that this is unrealistic; indeed, absorption of the ultrasound waves used medically is an easily – sometimes despairingly – noted feature in most applications. But it is possible to add absorption to a lossless model, and this is one justification for not attempting to include it at this stage. Another justification is that the topic is dealt with in some depth in later chapters.

A second easily observed phenomenon (one without which most medical ultrasound imaging techniques would be useless) is that tissues scatter ultrasound waves. The model developed below embodies scattering processes, probably in a realistic way, but these are temporarily dropped, to be taken up in a later chapter. Because most scattering theories require the non-scattered wave (i.e., the wave that would exist in the absence of scattering interactions) as a necessary initial input, scattering can also be regarded as a refinement to be added later to the more simple model discussed in this chapter.

Thus, the theory developed below relates primarily to ultrasound pulses in a lossless homogeneous medium, and to investigation of the phenomena to be observed when the wave passes from one such medium to another, with different 'acoustic' properties. For wave frequencies that are employed in medical applications, shear waves are so heavily absorbed in soft tissues that they can reasonably be neglected in propagation models, and included, if necessary, in theories of absorption processes. Shear wave propagation is not necessarily

Physical Principles of Medical Ultrasonics, Second Edition. Edited by C. R. Hill, J. C. Bamber and G. R. ter Haar.
© 2004 John Wiley & Sons, Ltd: ISBN 0 471 97002 6

negligible in hard tissues, such as bone, and the treatment below must be seen as ultimately pertaining to soft tissues only, for waves in the 'medical' frequency range. The neglect of shear effects has another bonus: ultrasound waves can be regarded as being described by a pressure (scalar) field only.

Ultrasound waves are intrinsically non-linear, but, for many purposes, an assumption of linearity appears to be reasonable. However, there is a growing awareness that features of non-linear propagation should not be disregarded; indeed, they are already beginning to be commercially exploited for medical imaging. Non-linear theory is complicated, and much remains to be clarified; the necessary brief and limited treatment presented below is consequently restricted to one-dimensional harmonic waves only.

1.2   THE CANONICAL INHOMOGENEOUS WAVE EQUATION OF LINEAR ACOUSTICS

Numerous texts consider the derivation of an acoustic wave equation, but the standard, if slightly ageing, reference is still the book by Morse and Ingard (1968).

In order to arrive at a tractable equation which governs the propagation of a pressure wave inside a medium as complicated as soft tissue, some simplifications will clearly have to be made. Foremost among these is the specification of the physical nature of the medium itself. One of the simplest, but nonetheless realistic, starting points is that the medium can be considered to be stationary, with a spatially varying density $\varrho_0(\mathbf{r})$, where $\mathbf{r}$ denotes the location vector with Cartesian components written as (x, y, z). In order to avoid the full complexities of a three-dimensional treatment, it is common, in practice, to consider the one-dimensional situation first, and then to extend the result to higher dimensions at a later stage. Bearing this in mind, the medium may thus tentatively be considered to be specified by its constant pressure, p_0, and by its varying density, $\varrho_0(x)$.

The static state of the medium will be perturbed in the presence of a propagating pressure wave, and, under such circumstances, the total (time-varying) pressure, p_T, at location x will be denoted by:

$$p_T(x, t) = p_0 + p(x, t) \tag{1.1}$$

where t denotes time and p, the pressure perturbation caused by the wave, is called the 'acoustic pressure'. In addition, the density of the medium will also be disturbed by the wave, and the total, time-varying, density can be written, in an analogous notation, as:

$$\varrho_T(x, t) = \varrho_0(x) + \varrho(x, t) \tag{1.2}$$

A passing ultrasound wave not only modifies the density and pressure of the supporting medium, but also sets it into local motion, displacing small elements of the medium and imparting them with a 'particle velocity', $u(x, t)$. It is important to be clear about the meaning of the functional notation: $u(x, t)$ denotes the velocity of whatever 'particle' (defined as a small element of the medium which reacts as a whole to the forces on it, over which the pressure and density may be considered to have single values, and which can be designated as having a single velocity, at any instant) happens to be located at position x at time t, and is not the time-dependent velocity of a *particular* particle. Such a description, whereby field variables are expressed with respect to a coordinate system fixed in space, rather than with respect to the individual elements of the medium, is referred to as the Euler formalism. This is the descriptive framework that is adopted here.

Associated with the particle velocity is the notion of 'particle displacement', designated $\xi(x, t)$. Conventionally, this is introduced as the displacement, at time t, of the particle that was located at x at some reference time, conveniently chosen as $t = 0$. This is clearly not an Eulerian description, and constitutes what has become known as the Lagrange formalism. It is, however, not too difficult to uncover a link between physical variables expressed in the two formalisms. Consider, for example, some variable which is written as q^E in the Eulerian, and q^L in the Lagrangian, formalism. It is apparent that

$$q^E(x, t) = q^L(x - \xi(x_0, t), t) \tag{1.3}$$

with x_0 denoting the value of x at time $t = 0$. The Lagrangian variable can be expanded, to give

$$q^E(x, t) = q^L(x, t) - \xi(x_0, t)\frac{\partial q^L}{\partial x}\bigg|_{x_0} + \text{higher order terms} \tag{1.4}$$

and it follows that, in particular, the Eulerian variable

$$u(x, t) = \frac{\partial \xi}{\partial t} \tag{1.5}$$

only in the limit that the amplitude of the particle displacement is very small, so that only the first term in the expansion in equation (1.4) is significant.

1.2.1 THE EQUATION OF MOTION

As in any dynamical problem, a first line of approach is to specify the forces acting on the system: in the present case, it is assumed that it is the (scalar) pressure, only, that maintains the motion. The force acting on any element of the continuous medium then depends on the pressure gradient, and Newton's second law may be written as (Beranek 1986):

$$-\frac{\partial p_T}{\partial x} = \varrho_T \frac{Du}{Dt} \tag{1.6}$$

The unexpected notation for the time derivative (D/Dt) is introduced because Newton's law, as stated, applies only to a particular particle, with fixed mass, and with its acceleration given as it moves in space in response to the local forces acting on it. Such a situation is most naturally described in the Lagrange formalism, but the convention has already been adopted that all variables (except ξ) are to be expressed as Eulerian. The time derivative introduced above has its conventional meaning of total rate of change with time, $viz.$:

$$\frac{D}{Dt}[u(x, t)] \equiv \lim_{\Delta t \to 0} \frac{u(x + \Delta x, t + \Delta t) - u(x, t)}{\Delta t} \tag{1.7}$$

where $x + \Delta x$ indicates the new spatial position that the particle originally located at x, at time t, has moved to during the time interval Δt. Clearly,

$$\Delta x = u(x, t)\Delta t \tag{1.8}$$

and a liberal application of Taylor's expansion theorem results in:

$$\frac{D}{Dt}[u(x, t)] = \frac{\partial u}{\partial t} + u\frac{\partial u}{\partial x} \tag{1.9}$$

D/Dt is termed the 'material' or 'convective' derivative, and is required when calculating the rate of change, in Eulerian terms, of a quantity, when it is more appropriate to use the Lagrangian description.

Equation (1.6) reduces to

$$-\frac{\partial p_T}{\partial x} = \varrho_T \frac{\partial u}{\partial t} + \varrho_T u \frac{\partial u}{\partial x} \tag{1.10}$$

In this (or equivalent) form, the equation of motion is more commonly known as Euler's equation. In order to make the equation more manageable, it is convenient to assume that the action of the wave is such that only very small perturbations of the medium are generated:

$$|p/p_0| \ll 1; \quad |\varrho/\varrho_0| \ll 1 \tag{1.11}$$

It is assumed that these conditions are ensured if the particle displacement and its derivatives are small. If only the dominant terms, i.e. no higher than first order in small quantities, are retained (a procedure commonly referred to as 'linearisation'), then the equation of motion may be expressed as:

$$-\frac{\partial p}{\partial x} = \varrho_0 \frac{\partial u}{\partial t} \tag{1.12}$$

1.2.2 THE CONTINUITY EQUATION

Another principle to be invoked is the conservation of mass. In the present situation, it implies that any local change in the density of the medium must be the result of exchange of mass between the surroundings and the location under consideration. Since the mass flux across a plane fixed in space, at location x, is given by $\varrho_T(x, t)u(x, t)$, the 'continuity equation', for mass conservation, may be written as:

$$-\frac{\partial \varrho_T}{\partial t} = \frac{\partial}{\partial x}[\varrho_T u] \tag{1.13}$$

Linearisation then results in:

$$-\frac{\partial \varrho}{\partial t} = \varrho_0 \frac{\partial u}{\partial x} \tag{1.14}$$

Note that, in this case, the Euler formalism is the natural way in which to write the equations.

1.2.3 THE CONSTITUTIVE EQUATION

The particle velocity may be eliminated from equations (1.12) and (1.14) to give a relationship between p and ϱ. However, to obtain a wave equation in p alone, which is the goal of the present discussion, an additional condition relating these two variables is required. The precise relationship depends on the nature of the medium itself, and, in general terms, is characterised by the class of material to which the medium belongs. One particularly simple 'constitutive equation', as the sought-for relationship is termed, is to demand that any change in the local density induced by the wave is some function, F, of the acoustic pressure only, i.e.

$$\varrho = F(p) \tag{1.15}$$

Clearly, $F(0) = 0$, and, bearing in mind that we are concerned only with small acoustic pressure excursions, a Taylor expansion gives:

$$F(p) = \left[\frac{dF}{dp}\right]_{p=0} p + \text{negligible terms of higher order in } p \qquad (1.16)$$

Approximating the function F in this way, and dropping higher order terms, allows a linearised constitutive equation to be written as

$$\varrho = \left[\frac{d\varrho}{dp}\right]_{p=0} p \equiv \varrho_0 \beta_0 p \qquad (1.17)$$

where β_0, the (adiabatic) compressibility of the medium, is given by

$$\beta_0 \equiv -\frac{1}{V}\left[\frac{\partial V}{\partial p}\right]_{ad} = \frac{1}{\varrho_0}\left[\frac{\partial \varrho}{\partial p}\right]_{ad} \qquad (1.18)$$

with V denoting the volume of a region of the unperturbed medium which contains a fixed mass of material, and which is small enough for the density to be regarded as effectively constant throughout. General thermodynamic considerations require that the density of a material is uniquely fixed by specifying two thermodynamic variables, such as the pressure and temperature (say). The thermodynamic pathway along which the partial derivatives in equation (1.18) are to be taken requires, therefore, to be specified: the subscript indicates that adiabatic conditions are intended.

The compressibility is the reciprocal of the (perhaps better known and more commonly tabulated) bulk modulus of the medium, and is, for the inhomogeneous medium presently under consideration, a function of position. The choice of adiabatic conditions for its evaluation should, at this stage, be seen as an assumption, and it is by no means clear that it is a valid one, but it has been seen to be consistent with observation (Kinsler *et al.* 1982). The assumption of adiabaticity is consistent with, and can be regarded as underpinning, the validity of equation (1.15). There can be little doubt, though, that the pressure wave also, in general, induces temperature changes in the medium, particularly at the ultrasound frequencies utilised in medical applications. However, the proper inclusion of temperature into the theory would require more detailed thermodynamic arguments – resulting in a degree of complexity that is best avoided at this stage in the development of a crude tissue model.

1.2.4 A WAVE EQUATION

Equations (1.12), (1.14) and (1.17) may now be combined to give a wave equation for the pressure,

$$\frac{\partial^2 p}{\partial x^2} - \frac{1}{C_0^2}\frac{\partial^2 p}{\partial t^2} = \left(\frac{\partial}{\partial x}\ln \varrho_0\right)\frac{\partial p}{\partial x} \qquad (1.19)$$

with $C_0^2(x) \equiv (\varrho_0 \beta_0)^{-1}$. Equation (1.19) may be converted into a rather more physically transparent, canonical, form by introducing density and compressibility 'fluctuation' terms $\tilde{\varrho}$ and $\tilde{\beta}$ respectively, defined as follows:

$$\tilde{\varrho} \equiv \frac{\varrho_0 - \bar{\varrho}}{\varrho_0} \qquad (1.20)$$

$$\tilde{\beta} \equiv \frac{\beta_0 - \bar{\beta}}{\bar{\beta}} \qquad (1.21)$$

Here, $\bar{\varrho}$ and $\bar{\beta}$ denote the spatial mean values of the density and compressibility. Some fairly tedious algebraic manipulations will transform the inhomogenous wave equation into

$$\frac{\partial^2 p}{\partial x^2} - \frac{1}{\bar{C}^2}\frac{\partial^2 p}{\partial t^2} = \frac{1}{\bar{C}^2}\tilde{\beta}\frac{\partial^2 p}{\partial t^2} + \frac{\partial}{\partial x}\left[\tilde{\varrho}\frac{\partial p}{\partial x}\right] \tag{1.22}$$

where $\bar{C} \equiv 1/\sqrt{\bar{\varrho},\bar{\kappa}}$, and which has a constant positive value, dependent only on the (mean) physical properties of the medium.

The three-dimensional form of equation (1.22) is readily seen to be

$$\nabla^2 p - \frac{1}{\bar{C}^2}\frac{\partial^2 p}{\partial t^2} = \frac{1}{\bar{C}^2}\tilde{\beta}\frac{\partial^2 p}{\partial t^2} + \nabla\cdot[\tilde{\varrho}\nabla p] \tag{1.23}$$

where p now denotes a function of the three-dimensional position vector, $\mathbf{r}$, and the time, t. ∇ is the well-known (vector) gradient operator, with $\nabla^2(\equiv \nabla\cdot\nabla)$ commonly referred to as the 'Laplacian' operator. The important feature of equation (1.23) is that the spatially varying terms, $\tilde{\varrho}$ and $\tilde{\beta}$, appear only on the right-hand side. It will be made clear, in Chapter 6, that such fluctuations represent the properties of the medium that give rise to wave scattering. If these terms should vanish, as would occur for a medium with uniformly constant density and compressibility, then the wave propagation is described by the homogeneous equation

$$\nabla^2 p - \frac{1}{C^2}\frac{\partial^2 p}{\partial t^2} = 0 \tag{1.24}$$

where, for notational convenience, $\bar{C}$ has been replaced by $C \equiv 1/\sqrt{\varrho_0\beta_0}$, with ϱ_0 and β_0 now obviously regarded as constant. Because scattering is not observed when a wave traverses a uniform medium, and because scattering by an inhomogeneity requires the presence of the wave at that location in the medium, the two terms on the right-hand side of equation (1.23) are referred to as *scattering* 'source terms' (*viz.*, they contain *both* the fluctuations *and p*). This neat separation, of the scattering and uniform propagational aspects of the wave behaviour, is perhaps the most compelling reason for writing the wave equation in its canonical form, and is the starting point for a number of theoretical descriptions of wave scattering. The focus of this chapter, however, is to describe some of the solutions of the homogeneous wave equation, equation (1.24), and to investigate them in order to acquire an understanding of the acoustic fields utilised in medical applications of ultrasound. Despite the fact that the vast majority of soft tissues are clearly inhomogeneous, the solutions of the homogeneous wave equation are nonetheless of great interest not only because they provide an approximate, but fundamental, understanding of the quite complex behaviour of ultrasound fields, even in less simple media, but also because they are the primary input to many scattering theories. Moreover, they accurately describe the ultrasound fields measured in the ubiquitous water tank in calibration and research laboratories.

1.2.5 HARMONIC WAVES

A case of particular interest is that of the harmonic wave, *viz.* one which can be written, in complex form, as

$$p(\mathbf{r},\ t) = p_\omega(\mathbf{r})e^{-i\omega t} \tag{1.25}$$

where

$$\omega \equiv 2\pi f \tag{1.26}$$

and f is the frequency of the wave. It is readily established that, in a homogeneous medium, the wave amplitude $p_\omega(\mathbf{r})$ satisfies the so-called 'Helmholtz equation':

$$\nabla^2 p_\omega + \frac{\omega^2}{C^2} p_\omega = 0 \tag{1.27}$$

The harmonic wave approximation is not as restrictive as it appears at first sight. Indeed, in most cases, the types of fields employed for ultrasound therapeutic purposes consist of such long pulses that they are very appropriately represented in this way. Moreover, even more general fields may be expressed in terms of harmonic waves via a Fourier representation, which may be written as:

$$p(\mathbf{r}, t) = \int_{-\infty}^{\infty} p_\omega(\mathbf{r}) e^{-i\omega t} d\omega \tag{1.28}$$

In general, p_ω may be complex, in which case it carries information about the phase of the wave, and is then called the 'complex amplitude'.

1.3 ACOUSTIC WAVE VARIABLES

The description of the ultrasound field in terms of the pressure is, for most measurement purposes, the most direct and convenient, since pressure is the primary physical variable that is detected by most of the hydrophones and receiving transducers in general use. However, the space–time behaviour of a number of other wave variables may be used to describe the field, and one of these may be deemed to be more appropriate than the pressure, in particular applications. Of course, relationships exist between these other wave variables and the pressure, so that a knowledge of any one may be used to establish, in principle, the space–time behaviour of any other. In this section, the argument is developed for pressure waves in homogeneous media (so that ϱ_0 and β_0 are constant), in the linear approximation.

The 'particle acceleration',

$$\mathbf{a} \equiv \frac{\partial \mathbf{u}}{\partial t} \tag{1.29}$$

with $\mathbf{u}(\mathbf{r}, t)$ the particle velocity vector at location $\mathbf{r}$ in three-dimensional space. The particle acceleration is readily seen from equation (1.12) to be expressible as

$$\mathbf{a} = -\frac{1}{\varrho_0} \nabla p \tag{1.30}$$

The 'condensation',

$$s = \frac{\varrho}{\varrho_0} \tag{1.31}$$

may be shown, directly from equation (1.17), to be given by

$$s = \frac{p(\mathbf{r}, t)}{\varrho_0 C^2} \tag{1.32}$$

Other wave variables are less conveniently expressed in terms of the pressure. For example, equation (1.12) shows that, in general, a first-order differential equation would have to be solved in order to establish the behaviour of the particle velocity field, $\mathbf{u}(\mathbf{r}, t)$, from the (gradient of the) pressure wave. Specifying $\xi(\mathbf{r}, t)$ would require a second-order differential equation to be solved. One way round this difficulty is to note that imposing the condition

$$\mathbf{u} = -\nabla\phi \tag{1.33}$$

is fully compatible with the above derivation of the wave equation for p. The new field, $\phi(\mathbf{r}, t)$, introduced in equation (1.33) is called the 'velocity potential' and has its origins in theoretical fluid mechanics. It is readily shown that:

$$s = \frac{1}{C^2}\frac{\partial}{\partial t}\phi(\mathbf{r}, t) \tag{1.34}$$

and

$$p = \varrho_0\frac{\partial}{\partial t}\phi(\mathbf{r}, t) \tag{1.35}$$

Some simple algebra shows that ϕ also satisfies equation (1.24), and, boundary conditions permitting, calculating the velocity potential presents no more computational difficulty than calculating the pressure field. Since it provides a more rapid access to the particle velocity field, it may be considered that it is more appropriate to frame theories (as many authors do) in terms of the velocity potential. But it should be borne in mind that the velocity potential has no straightforward physical interpretation, that it is not directly measurable, and that further calculation would be required in order to obtain some observable entities, such as s and p. Moreover, a differential equation would nonetheless have to be solved if the particle displacement field were required. For these reasons, it is deemed preferable here to formulate the theory in terms of the pressure field.

It is almost self-evident that a travelling acoustic wave transports energy, and the rate at which this is transported may be derived. If the scalar ('dot') product of $\mathbf{u}$ with both sides of equation (1.12) is carried out, it is straightforward to show that

$$\nabla \cdot (p\mathbf{u}) - p\nabla \cdot \mathbf{u} = -\tfrac{1}{2}\varrho_0\frac{\partial u^2}{\partial t} \tag{1.36}$$

with $u(\mathbf{r}, t) \equiv \mathbf{u}(\mathbf{r}, t) \cdot \mathbf{n}$, where $\mathbf{n}(\mathbf{r})$ is a unit vector that may be identified as the local direction of propagation of the field. Invoking equations (1.14) and (1.17) leads to

$$\nabla \cdot (p\mathbf{u}) + \frac{p}{\varrho_0 C^2}\frac{\partial p}{\partial t} = -\tfrac{1}{2}\varrho_0\frac{\partial u^2}{\partial t} \tag{1.37}$$

and it follows that

$$\nabla \cdot \mathbf{Q} + \frac{\partial E}{\partial t} = 0 \tag{1.38}$$

with

$$\mathbf{Q} \equiv p\mathbf{u} \tag{1.39}$$

$$E \equiv \tfrac{1}{2}\varrho_0 u^2 + \tfrac{1}{2}\frac{p^2}{\varrho_0 C^2} \tag{1.40}$$

The entity, E, is readily interpreted as the energy density (per unit volume of medium): the first term in its definition is patently the (acoustic) kinetic energy density, while the second term can be shown to be the (acoustic) potential energy density ($= -\int p\, ds$, the work done by the field per unit volume of medium). Note that, even though a linearised theory has been used, the expression for the energy density is of second order in the acoustical variables. Strictly, the contribution to E of the second-order terms that have been dropped in the derivation of the linear wave equation should be explicitly investigated, but this is rarely done, probably because the form of equation (1.40) is so intuitively reasonable.

Equation (1.38) has the classic form of a conservation equation, so that Q can be interpreted as the energy density flux vector, sometimes referred to as the 'instantaneous intensity' or, perhaps more reasonably, the 'density of energy flow'. It is conventional to remove a possibly rapid time variation in Q by performing a time average, and the (acoustic) intensity of the field is defined by

$$\mathbf{I}(t) \equiv \frac{1}{\tau} \int_{t}^{t+\tau} \boldsymbol{Q}dt' \tag{1.41}$$

Note that the way in which the intensity has been introduced here implies that it is to be regarded as a vector quantity. The choice of the averaging time may be somewhat arbitrary when dealing with pulsed fields, but is usually chosen so that the intensity vector becomes relatively slowly varying in amplitude (compared to Q): choosing τ to be one field cycle in duration appears to be appropriate in a very wide range of circumstances. The local direction of the intensity vector is fixed by the direction of the particle velocity. Thus, a scalar intensity may be defined via

$$I(\mathbf{r},\ t) - \mathbf{I}(\mathbf{r},\ t) \cdot \mathbf{n}(\mathbf{r}) \tag{1.42}$$

I is generally referred to as 'the' intensity of the wave at a particular location, but is frequently further refined by taking its spatial and/or temporal (over times longer than that implicit in its definition) averages.

Another, much used, variable which is introduced when studying wave propagation is the 'specific acoustic impedance', defined as

$$Z = \frac{p}{u} \tag{1.43}$$

Z indicates, in some sense, the resistance of the medium to being disturbed by the wave, and is, in general, location dependent. It reduces to a relatively simple expression for harmonic waves which exhibit simple geometry, as will be seen below.

The above relationships are summarised in Table 1.1.

1.4　SOME SPECIAL SOLUTIONS

The wave equation has some relatively simple solutions when the number of dimensions can be effectively reduced by assuming that some or other symmetry is obeyed. A few special situations are summarised here.

1.4.1 PLANE WAVES

In a Cartesian coordinate system

Table 1.1. Expressions for wave quantities for the simple waveforms discussed

Wave variable	General relationship	Plane wave (forward travelling)	Spherical wave (outgoing)	Cylindrical wave (outgoing; asymptotic = large kr)
Pressure	$p(\mathbf{r}, t)$	$A\exp[i(\omega t - kx)]$	$\dfrac{A}{r}\exp[i(\omega t - kr)]$	$\dfrac{A}{\sqrt{r}}\exp[i(\omega t - kr)]$
Particle velocity	$u = \left[-\dfrac{1}{\varrho_0}\displaystyle\int \nabla p(\mathbf{r}, t')dt' \right] \cdot \mathbf{n}$	$\dfrac{A}{\varrho_0 C}\exp[i(\omega t - kx)]$	$\dfrac{A}{\varrho_0 C}\dfrac{1}{r}\left(1 + \dfrac{1}{k^2 r^2}\right)^{1/2}$ $\times \exp[i(\omega t - kr - \psi)]$	$\dfrac{A}{\varrho_0 C}\dfrac{1}{\sqrt{r}}\left(1 + \dfrac{1}{4k^2 r^2}\right)^{1/2}$ $\times \exp[i(\omega t - kr - \psi)]$
Condensation	$s = p/\varrho_0 C^2$	$\dfrac{A}{\varrho_0 C^2}\exp[i(\omega t - kx)]$	$\dfrac{A}{\varrho_0 C^2}\dfrac{1}{r}\exp[i(\omega t - kr)]$	$\dfrac{A}{\varrho_0 C^2}\dfrac{1}{\sqrt{r}}\exp[i(\omega t - kr)]$
Velocity potential	$\phi = \dfrac{1}{\varrho_0}\displaystyle\int p(\mathbf{r}, t')dt'$	$-\dfrac{iA}{\varrho_0 \omega}\exp[i(\omega t - kx)]$	$\dfrac{-A}{\varrho_0 \omega}\dfrac{1}{r}\exp[i(\omega t - kr + \pi)]$	$\dfrac{A}{\varrho_0 \omega}\dfrac{1}{\sqrt{r}}\exp[i(\omega t - kr + \pi)]$
Specific impedance	$Z = p/u$	$\varrho_0 C$	$\varrho_0 C\left(1 + \dfrac{1}{k^2 r^2}\right)^{-1}\left(1 + \dfrac{i}{kr}\right)$	$\varrho_0 C\left(1 + \dfrac{1}{4k^2 r^2}\right)^{-1}\left(1 + \dfrac{i}{2kr}\right)$
Intensity	$I = \overline{pu}$	$A^2/2\varrho_0 C$	$A^2/2\varrho_0 C r^2$	$A^2/2\varrho_0 C r$
Notes	$\overline{(\cdot)}$ indicates time average		$\tan\psi = 1/kr$	$\tan\psi = 1/2kr$

$$\mathbf{r} = \mathbf{i}x + \mathbf{j}y + \mathbf{k}z \equiv (x, y, z) \tag{1.44}$$

$$\nabla = \mathbf{i}\frac{\partial}{\partial x} + \mathbf{j}\frac{\partial}{\partial y} + \mathbf{k}\frac{\partial}{\partial z} \tag{1.45}$$

$$\nabla^2 = \frac{\partial^2}{\partial x^2} + \frac{\partial^2}{\partial y^2} + \frac{\partial^2}{\partial z^2} \tag{1.46}$$

where $\mathbf{i}$, $\mathbf{j}$ and $\mathbf{k}$ represent unit vectors along the x-, y- and z-axes, respectively. If it is now assumed that the wave depends on only one of the three spatial coordinates (say x), then the three-dimensional homogeneous wave equation, equation (1.24), reduces to

$$\frac{\partial^2 p_x}{\partial x^2} - \frac{1}{C^2}\frac{\partial^2 p_x}{\partial t^2} = 0 \tag{1.47}$$

where p_x denotes the plane wave pressure and C is a material-dependent constant. It may be verified by direct substitution that solutions of equation (1.47) are expressible as

$$p_x(x, t) = g(x - Ct) + q(x + Ct) \tag{1.48}$$

with g and q arbitrary functions, which are readily interpreted as 'plane' waves which travel in the direction of increasing and decreasing x, respectively, without any change of form or amplitude, at constant speed C. Such plane wave solutions are of considerable interest, since much of the elementary theory of ultrasound is often described in terms of such waves.

The relationships between acoustic variables take on particularly simple forms when dealing with harmonic plane wave solutions, *viz.* those of the form:

$$p_{Hx}(x, t) = A\exp\{i(kx - \omega t)\} \tag{1.49}$$

where A is a positive constant (the amplitude of the wave), and

$$k = 2\pi/\lambda = 2\pi f/C = \omega/C \tag{1.50}$$

k is called the 'wave number', and λ denotes the wavelength of the wave. The relationships between the acoustic variables and the harmonic wave's amplitude and frequency are indicated in Table 1.1. Of particular note is that, for a forward travelling wave (in the positive x-direction), the specific acoustic impedance becomes equal to $\varrho_0 C$, i.e., a constant depending only on the nature of the medium, and which is referred to as the 'characteristic acoustic impedance'. Note that for a plane harmonic wave travelling in the opposite direction, the characteristic acoustic impedance is negative, but unchanged in magnitude.

A case of some interest is the sum of two equi-amplitude harmonic plane waves, of the same frequency, travelling in opposite directions:

$$p_{SWx}(x, t) = A\exp\{i(kx - \omega t)\} + A\exp\{-i(kx + \omega t)\} = 2A\cos(kx)\exp(i\omega t) \tag{1.51}$$

This represents a non-travelling wave referred to as a 'standing wave', in which the pressure vanishes at definite locations – the (pressure) 'nodes' – and oscillates maximally, between $\pm 2A$, at other locations – the 'antinodes' – between the nodes. It is straightforward to establish that the particle displacement (ξ) nodes are located at the pressure antinodes, and *vice versa* for the displacement antinodes. Moreover, although such a standing wave has non-zero time-averaged energy density, its time-averaged intensity is identically equal to zero.

1.4.2 SPHERICAL WAVES

In spherical polar coordinates, with $r \equiv |\mathbf{r}|$,

$$\mathbf{r} = (r.\sin\theta.\cos\varphi,\ r.\sin\theta.\sin\varphi,\ r.\cos\varphi) \tag{1.52}$$

where the angles have their usual definitions (Pipes 1958). If only solutions with spherical symmetry (independent of the angles θ and φ) are considered, the wave equation reduces to

$$\frac{\partial^2(rp_r)}{\partial r^2} - \frac{1}{C^2}\frac{\partial^2(rp_r)}{\partial t^2} = 0 \tag{1.53}$$

where p_r denotes the spherical wave pressure function. The similarity between equations (1.47) and (1.53) is striking, and it is immediately apparent that the general solution of the latter is given by

$$p_r(r,\ t) = \frac{1}{r}g(r - Ct) + \frac{1}{r}q(r + Ct) \tag{1.54}$$

Thus, the general solution is a combination of two spherical waves: an outgoing (travelling in the direction of increasing r) and an ingoing wave (travelling in the direction of decreasing r), each propagating without change in form, but, in contrast to planar waves, with appropriate changes in amplitudes.

As before, particular interest focuses on harmonic waves, and an outgoing spherical harmonic wave is given as:

$$p_{Hr}(r,\ t) = \frac{A}{r}\exp\{i(kr - \omega t)\} \tag{1.55}$$

It is clear that the possibility exists for the occurrence of spherical standing waves, but with a decrease in amplitude as r increases. Table 1.1 lists wave variables for an outgoing spherical harmonic wave, and inspection shows that the specific acoustic impedance, in this case, does exhibit a geometric factor, as it will in general. Note also that the phase relationship between the particle displacement (and hence, the particle velocity or acceleration) and the acoustic pressure is not as simple as for a harmonic plane wave. There is an additional complexity, inasmuch as p_{Hr} becomes infinite at the origin, $r = 0$.

1.4.3 CYLINDRICAL WAVES

There is a rather unexpected change in behaviour when cylindrically symmetric waves are considered. With cylindrical polar coordinates,

$$\mathbf{r} = (h\cos\varphi,\ h\sin\varphi,\ z) \tag{1.56}$$

with $h = \sqrt{x^2 + y^2}$. For pressure fields that do not depend on either φ or z, the wave equation reduces to

$$\frac{1}{h}\frac{\partial}{\partial h}\left[h\frac{\partial p_h}{\partial h}\right] - \frac{1}{C^2}\frac{\partial^2 p_h}{\partial t^2} = 0 \tag{1.57}$$

Contrary to the assertion in some texts, there is no simple solution with a dependence on $(h \pm Ct)$, even for harmonic waves. Indeed, for that case, equation (1.57) becomes

$$\frac{\partial^2 p_{Hh}}{\partial h^2} + \frac{1}{h}\frac{\partial p_{Hh}}{\partial h} + k^2 p_{Hh} = 0 \tag{1.58}$$

with p_{Hh} denoting the pressure of a harmonic cylindrical wave. Clearly, a solution involving Bessel functions is indicated. Thus, in contrast to plane and spherical waves, harmonic cylindrical waves do not propagate without shape changes. However, a consideration of the function $q(h) = \sqrt{h}.p_{Hh}(h)$ shows that it satisfies the equation

$$\frac{\partial^2 q}{\partial h^2} + \left(\frac{1}{4h^2} + k^2\right) q = 0 \tag{1.59}$$

Thus, in the asymptotic limit, when $h \to \infty$, the simplified version of equation (1.59) supports solutions of the type $\exp(ikh)$. Outgoing harmonic cylindrical waves described by

$$p_{Hh} = \frac{A}{\sqrt{h}} \exp\{i(kh - \omega t)\} \tag{1.60}$$

exist only for very large h.

1.5　GREEN'S FUNCTION AND RAYLEIGH'S INTEGRAL

An ancillary function, useful in a number of contexts (including scattering theory), may be associated with particular wave equations. The Green's function for equation (1.24) is defined as the solution of

$$\nabla^2 G - \frac{1}{C^2}\frac{\partial^2 G}{\partial t^2} = -4\pi\delta(\mathbf{r} - \mathbf{r}_0)\delta(t - t_0) \tag{1.61}$$

where $G(\mathbf{r}, t; \mathbf{r}_0, t_0)$ denotes the Green's function, and δ represents the Dirac delta function. Boundary and initial conditions have to be specified before the precise form of G can be derived, and it is shown in a number of texts (e.g. Morse & Feshbach 1953) that for an infinite domain, with the so-called Sommerfeld radiation condition (that G drop sufficiently rapidly at large distances from $\mathbf{r}_0$), and applying causality (that G be zero for $t < t_0$), then

$$G_S = \frac{1}{R}\delta(R/C - (t - t_0)) \tag{1.62}$$

with $R = |\mathbf{r} - \mathbf{r}_0|$. G_S, the 'free space Green's function', thus has the form of a spherical outgoing impulsive wave, originating at time t_0 and location $\mathbf{r}_0$ – as can, indeed, be inferred from equation (1.61), which represents a wave equation with an impulsive wave source acting at $(\mathbf{r}_0, t_0)$.

In the context of the present treatment, the main advantage of the Green's function concept is that it allows the wave equation to be solved for a vibrating surface radiating into an unbounded medium, in which equation (1.24) holds. Consider, first, a volume, V, bounded by a closed surface, $\mathbf{S}$. Equation (1.24) holds inside V, but it is required to deduce the field solely from the boundary values (on $\mathbf{S}$) of the pressure and its derivatives. Initial conditions imposed on the pressure field are that both p and its derivative, $\partial p/\partial t$ should vanish at $t = 0$ everywhere within the volume V, but not necessarily on the bounding surface. Multiply equation (1.24) by G, equation (1.61) by p, subtract the two resultants, integrate over time and space within the bounding surface, to obtain

$$\int_0^{t+\varepsilon} dt_0 \int\!\!\int\!\!\int dV_0 \{ G(|\mathbf{r} - \mathbf{r}_0|, t - t_0)\nabla_0^2 p(\mathbf{r}_0, t_0) - p\nabla_0^2 G \} + \cdots$$

$$\int_0^{t+\varepsilon} dt_0 \int\!\!\int\!\!\int dV_0 \frac{1}{C^2}\left(\frac{\partial^2 G}{\partial t_0^2}p - G\frac{\partial^2 p}{\partial t_0^2} \right) = 4\pi p(\mathbf{r}, t) \tag{1.63}$$

where the time integration extends beyond t by an infinitesimal amount, to avoid the possibility of ending the integration on the delta function peak. The subscript on ∇_0^2 indicates that it operates on the integration variable, $\mathbf{r}_0$, and the variables appearing in the functions in the integrand are indicated explicitly only when the functions are first written. Applying Green's theorem, which converts the spatial volume integral into a surface integral (Pipes 1958), to the first term on the left-hand side, and performing integration by parts on the second term, allows some non-trivial integrations to be carried out. Invoking the initial conditions on the pressure field leads to the uncomplicated result

$$\int_0^{t+\varepsilon} dt_0 \int\!\!\int d\mathbf{S}_0 \cdot \{ G(|\mathbf{r} - \mathbf{r}_0|, t - t_0)\nabla_0 p(\mathbf{r}_0, t_0) - p\nabla_0 G \} = p(\mathbf{r}, t) \tag{1.64}$$

In order to proceed further, the boundary conditions (for the pressure field) for the problem in hand have to be stated, and the form of the Green's function, which should satisfy the same boundary conditions, determined. A special case is now considered: let the region being considered be the unbounded half-space, $z > 0$, with the bounding surface considered to be the infinite limit of a hemisphere centred on the origin, plus a plane through the origin. Furthermore, let the planar boundary be idealised as rigid over most of its surface, i.e., the pressure, p, vanishes everywhere on it, except in a finite region, A, where the particle velocity is given as being normal to the boundary. It should be apparent that this situation models a planar transducer located in a planar baffle.

A little thought [invoking the method of images (Morse & Feshbach 1953) widely used in electrostatics] will establish that a suitable form for G is given by:

$$G = \frac{\delta(t_0 - t + R/C)}{R} + \frac{\delta(t_0 - t + R'/C)}{R'} \tag{1.65}$$

with

$$R' \equiv \sqrt{(x_0 - x)^2 + (y_0 - y)^2 + (z_0 + z)^2} \tag{1.66}$$

It is relatively straightforward to show that $(\partial G/\partial z)_{z=0}$, is, indeed, zero for all time. It now follows immediately from equation (1.64) that, in the region $z > 0$, the pressure field is given by

$$p(\mathbf{r}, t) = \frac{\varrho_0}{2\pi} \int\!\!\int dx_0 dy_0 \frac{a_n(x_0, y_0, t - R/C)}{R} \tag{1.67}$$

where a_n denotes the component of the acceleration that is normal to the boundary. Equation (1.67) is the starting point for the evaluation of the transient field emitted by a planar transducer, set in a planar baffle, and is known as Rayleigh's integral. Although the derivation is appropriate only for a planar transducer, the validity of this result for gently curved emitting surfaces (weakly focused transducers) is often assumed (Cathignol & Faure 1996).

1.6 TRANSDUCER FIELDS

A knowledge of the form of the field radiated by a single element transducer is of fundamental importance in medical applications of ultrasound. Although its limitations are apparent in the preceding discussion, Rayleigh's integral is the most convenient basis upon which to build – an approach which is well justified when comparisons can be made between measured fields and those predicted by theory.

It is appropriate to consider the theoretically least complicated case, *viz.* that of a plane, circular, transducer with radius R_T set in a rigid baffle, and radiating into an ideal, lossless medium. The motion of the transducer face is further assumed to be piston-like, i.e., its acceleration a_n is independent of the surface coordinates x_0 and y_0.

1.6.1 THE ON-AXIS FIELD

Initially, only the on-axis field is calculated. Because of the inherent axial symmetry implied, the (cylindrical) coordinate system indicated in Figure 1.1 considerably simplifies the problem.

The Rayleigh integral may now be expressed as

$$p(z,\, t) - \frac{\varrho_0}{2\pi}\, 2\pi \int_0^{R_T} dh.h \frac{a_n\left(t - \sqrt{z^2 + h^2}/C\right)}{\sqrt{z^2 + h^2}} \tag{1.68}$$

On changing the integration variable to $R = \sqrt{z^2 + h^2}$, equation (1.68) transforms to

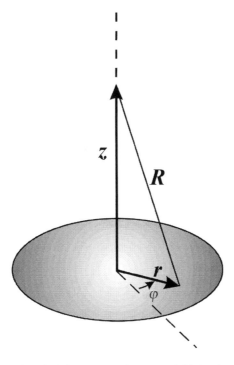

Figure 1.1. Coordinate system for calculating the on-axis pressure field of a planar, disk transducer

$$p(z,\ t) = \varrho_0 \int_{z}^{\sqrt{z^2+R_T^2}} dR.a_n(t - R/C) \tag{1.69}$$

The integration is easily affected by noting that

$$a_n(t - R/C) \equiv \frac{\partial}{\partial t} v_n(t - R/C) = -C\frac{\partial}{\partial R} v_n(t - R/C) \tag{1.70}$$

where v_n denotes the (normal) velocity of the transducer face.

The on-axis field that results is

$$p_A(z,\ t) = \varrho_0 C \left[v_n\left(t - \frac{z}{C}\right) = v_n\left(t - \frac{\sqrt{z^2 + R_T^2}}{C}\right) \right] \tag{1.71}$$

This is, indeed, a remarkable result: it suggests that if the excitation is of sufficiently short duration then, close to the transducer face, the observed on-axis pulse will be observed to be 'split' into two. The first arrival will accurately mimic the time dependence of the transducer face velocity, while the second arrival will be a 'replica pulse' of identical shape to the first, but inverted. While such behaviour is now routinely observed with appropriately pulsed single element transducers (Figure 1.2), it is interesting to note that the first experimental demonstration of pulse splitting in a medical ultrasound context (Gore & Leeman 1977) was some years after the description of the theoretical basis (Tupholme 1969; Stepanishen 1971; Robinson *et al.* 1974) of the effect.

For continuous harmonic excitation, with complex amplitude A_C

$$v_n(t) = A_C \exp(i\omega_0 t) \tag{1.72}$$

The expression for the on-axis field amplitude is readily shown to reduce to

$$|p_{A,\omega_0}(z,\ t)| = 2\varrho_0 C |A_C| \sin\left(\frac{\omega_0}{2C}\left\{\sqrt{z^2 + R_T^2} - z\right\}\right) \tag{1.73}$$

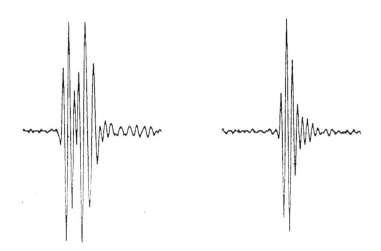

Figure 1.2. On-axis pulse measured near the transducer face (left) and in the far field (right). Pulse splitting is clearly visible in the near field

The on-axis field thus exhibits marked fluctuations in amplitude, with maximal values obtained at

$$z_{\mathrm{max},N} = \frac{R_T^2 - (2N+1)^2\lambda_0^2/4}{(2N+1)\lambda_0} \qquad N = 0, 1, 2, \ldots \tag{1.74}$$

and dropping to zero at

$$z_{\mathrm{min},N} = \frac{R_T^2 - N^2\lambda_0^2}{2N\lambda_0} \qquad N = 1, 2, \ldots \tag{1.75}$$

Remember that the N-sequence terminates when these expressions go negative. Note that the last (i.e., farthest from the transducer face) axial maximum is located at

$$z_{\mathrm{max},0} = (R_T^2 - \lambda_0^2/4)/\lambda_0 \approx R_T^2/\lambda_0 \tag{1.76}$$

The position of the last axial maximum is conventionally taken as the transition point between the 'near' and 'far' fields of the transducer. In the former, the (axial) pressure amplitude may vary quite rapidly between zero and some maximum value. On the other hand, in the far field, the axial field drops monotonically, eventually attaining a $1/z$ behaviour. This diffractive behaviour of a harmonic field is sufficiently well known for it to be regarded as unremarkable, but it gives little indication of the pulse-splitting effects that can arise with sufficiently wide-band fields.

1.6.2 THE OFF-AXIS FIELD

The calculation of the off-axis field is somewhat more complex. Although the basic approach is still the same, the problem is generally treated by introducing the field impulse response, H, as defined below. It is still appropriate to work with cylindrical coordinates, and the relevant variables are defined in Figure 1.3.

Bearing in mind the axial symmetry of the field, the Rayleigh integral is written as

$$p(h, z, t) = \frac{\varrho_0}{2\pi} a_n(t) * \int\int dr d\varphi \, r \frac{\delta(t - R/C)}{R}$$

$$\equiv \varrho_0 a_n(t) * H(h, z, t) = \varrho_0 v_n(t) * \frac{\partial}{\partial t} H(h, z, t) \tag{1.77}$$

In the above equation, $*$ denotes (time-domain) convolution, and $R = \sqrt{h^2 + r^2 + z^2}$. Note that if the pressure field is desired from a knowledge of the piston velocity, rather than from its acceleration, then it is the time derivative of the impulse response that appears in the convolution. The definition of H is a historical convention, relating to its original introduction in the context of the calculation of the velocity potential of the field.

The impulse response represents the pressure field of a circular piston-like transducer with an impulsive acceleration of its face. It is therefore to be understood that the integrand in the definition of H is identically zero whenever the values of r and φ are such that the surface element they designate lies outside the piston face. The integration variables (r, φ) are transformed to (R, θ), with $\theta = \pi - \varphi$, and the impulse response may be written

$$H(h, z, t) = \frac{1}{\pi} \int_{R_1}^{R_2} dR \int_0^{\Theta(R)} d\theta \delta(t - R/C) \tag{1.78}$$

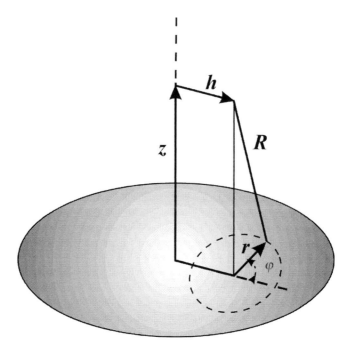

Figure 1.3. Coordinate system for calculating the off-axis field in the geometric shadow of a planar, disk transducer

The integration parameters in equation (1.78) are defined in Figure 1.3, and, given the ease with which the δ-function can be integrated, the result is

$$H(h, z, t) = \frac{C}{\pi} \cdot \Theta(Ct) \cdot H_S(Ct - R_1) \cdot H_S(R_2 - Ct) \tag{1.79}$$

where H_S denotes the Heaviside step function, defined via

$$\begin{aligned} H_S(s) &= 1 \quad \text{for } s \geqslant 0 \\ &= 0 \quad \text{for } s < 0 \end{aligned} \tag{1.80}$$

See Figure 1.4.

The values of R_1, R_2 and Θ depend on the location of the field point, and the final expression for $H(h, z, t)$ may be calculated as:

Region	Time	$H(h, z, t)$
$h < R_T$	$t_2 < t < t_0$	0
	$t_0 < t < t_1$	C
	$t_1 < t < t_2$	$\dfrac{C}{\pi} \cos^{-1} \left(\dfrac{C^2 t^2 + h^2 - z^2 - R_T^2}{2h\sqrt{C^2 t^2 - z^2}} \right)$
$h > R_T$	$t_2 < t < t_1$	0
	$t_1 < t < t_2$	$\dfrac{C}{\pi} \cos^{-1} \left(\dfrac{C^2 t^2 + h^2 - z^2 - R_T^2}{2h\sqrt{C^2 t^2 - z^2}} \right)$

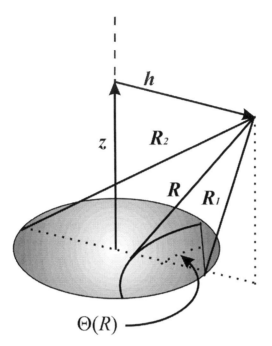

$$\Theta(R)$$

Figure 1.4. Definition of integration parameters used in calculating off-axis field outside the geometric shadow of a planar, disk transducer

Here, $t_0 = z/C$, $t_1 = (1/C)\sqrt{z^2 + (h - R_T)^2}$ and $t_2 = (1/C)\sqrt{z^2 + (h + R_T)^2}$.

At first glance, the structure of the impulse response appears to be quite complex. However, there is a comparatively simple interpretation which follows almost directly when the spatial dependence of $H(h, z, t)$ is plotted at different time instants. This is shown in Figure 1.5, for $\partial H/\partial t \equiv H'$, at two different time instants.

Remember that the pressure field is given by convolution of H' with the face velocity, and it becomes clear from Figure 1.5 that the field structure can be regarded as consisting of two components:

(a) the 'direct wave', which has the same shape and dimensions as the transducer face, and which propagates without any change;

(b) the 'edge wave', which originates at the edge of the transducer face, and which spreads out toroidally as it propagates.

The edge wave is 'attached' to the periphery of the direct wave, and a scrutiny of its phase structure warns against interpreting it as a wave that could exist independently of the other constituents of the field, and which could be generated, on its own, by a 'real' transducer. Since changes in the structure of the pressure field are generated by the continuous evolution of the edge-wave component, it can be argued that the diffractive nature of the field essentially originates in that component. Such a statement is bolstered by the observation that, if the edge wave could be eliminated – a physical impossibility! – then the pressure field would be a plane-wave pulse, of the same dimensions as the transducer face, propagating without any change in shape. Indeed, this understanding is the basis of the technique of apodisation (excitation amplitude shading), which attempts to reduce the edge-wave component in order to ameliorate diffraction effects, as discussed further in Chapter 2.

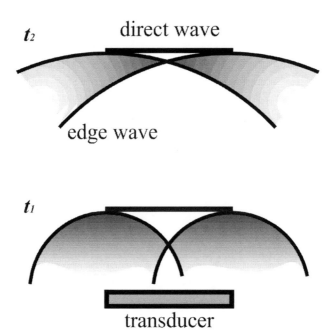

Figure 1.5. Schematic cross-sectional spatial view, in a plane containing the acoustic axis, of the velocity impulse response of a planar, disk transducer, shown at two different time instants. The pressure field is given by the convolution with the transducer face velocity function

1.6.3 THE ANGULAR SPECTRUM APPROACH

In general, the impulse–response technique allows accurate prediction of the pressure field structure only if a detailed knowledge of the transducer excitation and shape is available, and it is only in relatively uncomplicated situations, such as the plane circular piston-like transducer, that analytical calculations can be effected. Another approach to describing the field relies on measurements made in a limited region of the field itself, and using those data to accurately predict the field throughout a region of interest. In that case, reliance must be made on computer calculation (as for the impulse–response technique, in general), but no specific knowledge of the transmitting surface, which can be of arbitrary shape, is required.

The angular spectrum approach was developed to deal with harmonic fields (Goodman 1996), and, although it is not difficult to extend the method to more general pulsed fields, that still remains the major field of application. In general, a (well-behaved) function of the three cartesian spatial coordinates (x, y, z) may be written as

$$f(x, y, z) = \iint\limits_{-\infty}^{\infty} dk_x dk_y F_f(k_x, k_y, z) \exp(-i[k_x x + k_y y]) \tag{1.81}$$

In equation (1.81), the function has been expressed as a Fourier transform, but only over two of its three independent variables. If it is now assumed that the function under consideration is a solution of the Helmholtz equation, equation (1.27), then, by direct substitution, it can be shown that

$$\frac{\partial^2}{\partial z^2} F_f(k_x, k_y, z)_f k_z^2 F_f(k_x, k_y, z) = 0 \tag{1.82}$$

with

$$k_z^2 = k_0^2 - (k_x^2 + k_y^2) \tag{1.83}$$

and where k_0 denotes the quantity ω/C, i.e. the wave number associated with the frequency of the harmonic field. The forward propagating (in the direction of increasing z) solution of equation (1.82) is given by

$$F_f(k_x, k_y, z) = F_f(k_x, k_y, 0)e^{-ik_z z} \equiv A(k_x, k_y)e^{-ik_z z} \tag{1.84}$$

In the above, $F_f(k_x, k_y, z)$ is presumed known on some plane, designated as $z = 0$, and this boundary function is called the angular spectrum, denoted here by A. The terminology derives from the observation that A is, in fact, a function also of the direction cosines of the plane waves constituting the Fourier decomposition of $f(x, y, 0)$.

A general harmonic field can thus be expressed in terms of its angular spectrum via

$$p_{\omega_0}(x, y, z) = \iint\limits_{-\infty}^{\infty} dk_x dk_y A(k_x, k_y) \exp(-i[k_x x + k_y y]) \exp(-ik_z z) \tag{1.85}$$

At first glance this looks like a conventional Fourier transform, but there is a complication in applying the angular spectrum technique: since k_x and k_y may take on any real values in the integral, but the value of k_z is fixed by equation (1.83), the possibility exists that k_z may become a negative (in order to maintain finite behaviour at infinity) purely imaginary quantity. Thus part of the contribution to the angular spectrum decomposition of the field consists of 'evanescent' waves, viz. (spatial) spectral components that are damped in the positive z-direction, even when considering propagation in a lossless medium. In this sense, the evanescent waves may be regarded as unphysical. In general this may not be problematic, but difficulties can arise when attempting to calculate the field in a region anterior to the measurement plane. In that case, the amplitudes of the evanescent components become (exponentially) larger with distance from the measurement plane.

In practice, the two dimensional pressure distribution of the (harmonic) field over a plane (designated $z = 0$) is measured, usually with a point hydrophone, and the angular spectrum computed from this via a standard Fourier transformation. The field distribution on some other z-plane is then computed by applying equation (1.85) – with due account taken of the evanescent waves. Clearly, this procedure may be carried out even when specific information about the transducer shape and excitation function is lacking.

A particularly useful application of the angular spectrum approach is when calculating the (harmonic) pressure amplitude distribution emanating from a planar transducer. The $z = 0$ plane is then assumed to coincide with the plane of the transducer face. The Fourier analyses required in order to predict the radiated field at other planes may be performed relatively straightforwardly and rapidly on a modern desktop computer – and even analytically in a few simple cases. Figure 1.6 shows computed views of the axisymmetric pressure amplitude distributions in planes orthogonal to the propagation axis for the harmonic field from a circular aperture over which the harmonic pressure amplitude remains constant.

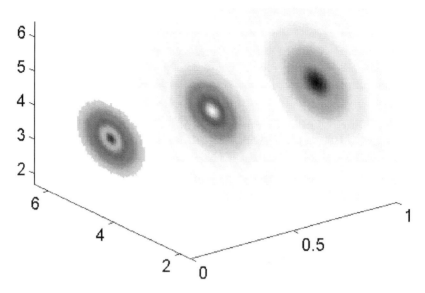

Figure 1.6. Beam cross-sections, calculated by the angular spectrum method, at three different distances from a simulated planar aperture over which the excitation is harmonic, with constant amplitude. Distance from the aperture is normalised with respect to the location of the last axial maximum

1.6.4 THE DIRECTIVITY SPECTRUM APPROACH

The directivity spectrum (Healey *et al.* 1997) is essentially a generalisation of the angular spectrum, and is the basis of a field description and prediction method that handles transient fields with ease, and is not encumbered by evanescent waves. In this case, the starting point is the observation that a general solution of the canonical lossless wave equation may be written as:

$$p(\mathbf{r},\ t) = \iiint\limits_{-\infty}^{\infty} d^3\mathbf{k}\,D(\mathbf{k})\exp(i[\mathbf{k}\cdot\mathbf{r} - Ckt]) \tag{1.86}$$

The formal proof of equation (1.86) is non-trivial, but it may be directly verified by substitution into the wave equation. However, the physical interpretation of the formalism is straightforward: the pressure field $p(\mathbf{r},\ t)$ may be regarded as a superposition of *travelling* harmonic (plane) waves, ranging over all directions and frequencies. The 'directivity spectrum', $D(\mathbf{k})$, expresses the amplitude and relative phase of the plane-wave component with wave vector $\mathbf{k}$. Despite a superficial similarity, equation (1.86) does not represent a conventional Fourier transform of the four ($\mathbf{r}$ and t)-dimensional field, since only a three-dimensional integration is involved. The directivity spectrum may be seen, from equation (1.86), to be the inverse Fourier transform of the spatial extent of the field, at some reference instant in time, which is conveniently regarded as the time origin, $t = 0$. Thus:

$$D(\mathbf{k}) = \frac{1}{(2\pi)^3}\iiint\limits_{\infty}^{\infty} d^3\mathbf{r}\,p(\mathbf{r},\ 0)\exp(-i\mathbf{k}\cdot\mathbf{r}) \tag{1.87}$$

If the directivity spectrum is known, it allows the calculation of the field at any other time instant, via application of equation (1.86). It should be noted that this may be effected even for negative times (i.e., calculation of the spatial distribution of the field at locations anterior to those at which the measurements for evaluation of the directivity spectrum were performed) without the need to introduce troublesome evanescent waves. Unfortunately, this substantial computational advantage appears, at first sight, to be considerably outweighed by the enormous experimental cost implied by the need to measure the three-dimensional pressure distribution of the field at some (initial) time instant. However, the experimental overheads may be considerably reduced by considering the time evolution of the spatial projections of the transient field, as demonstrated below for a special case.

Consider the (two-dimensional) projection of $p(\mathbf{r}, t)$ onto the (z, t) plane:

$$P(z, t) \equiv \iint\limits_{-\infty}^{\infty} dx\, dy\, p(x, y, z, t)$$

$$= \iint\limits_{-\infty}^{\infty} dx\, dy \iiint d^3\mathbf{k}\, D(k_x, k_y, k_z) \exp(i[k_x x + k_y y + k_z z - Ckt]) \tag{1.88}$$

The x and y integrations can be carried out, to give ultimately

$$P(z, t) = \frac{1}{2\pi} \int\limits_{-\infty}^{\infty} dk_z D(0, 0, k_z) \exp(i[k_z z - k_z Ct]) \equiv P(z - Ct) \tag{1.89}$$

Equation (1.89) implies the remarkable result that a spatial projection of the field propagates in the direction perpendicular to the projection plane without change in functional form, much as a true (physically unrealisable) one-dimensional pulse would. The result may be shown to be generally valid, holding for the spatial projection of the field onto *any* plane, and holds for any solution of the canonical wave equation – no matter how spatially varying. Moreover, equation (1.89) shows that the time dependence of the field projection, as measured at a fixed location ($z = 0$, say) is related by Fourier transformation to the values of the directivity spectrum, along a line in $\mathbf{k}$-space, traversing the origin, and oriented in a direction orthogonal to the (spatial) plane of the projection. In this way, the values of the directivity spectrum along as many directions in $\mathbf{k}$-space as are required for its accurate specification may be acquired from measurements of the temporal behaviour of the appropriately oriented projections of the field.

It turns out that the measurement of the field projections may be effected in practice with the aid of a 'large aperture hydrophone', consisting of a thin, uniformly poled and electroded PVDF (polyvinylidene difluoride) membrane, stretched planarly on a suitable supporting framework (Costa & Leeman 1988). A knowledge of the directivity spectrum allows the field to be evaluated for arbitrary $(\mathbf{r}, t)$ values by numerical 'propagation' from the measurement location, via equation (1.86). The theory underlying the technique is strongly associated with the Fourier slice theorem, as utilised for computerised tomography. In common with the angular spectrum approach, all data required are obtained directly from measurements performed only on the field itself, with no details about the transducer needed (in contrast to the impulse–response method), but the directivity spectrum technique is directly applicable to pulsed fields. Figure 1.7 shows the quality of both forward and backward pulse propagation that can be obtained via this method. Such results also confirm that typical single element transducers may perform much in accordance with the assumptions implicit in the direct-edge-wave formalism described above.

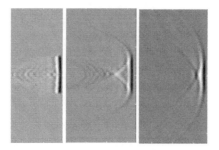

Figure 1.7. Cross-sectional spatial view, in a plane containing the acoustic axis, of the pulse from a commercial wide-band, planar, disk transducer, shown at three different time instants. The pulse is travelling from left to right and the cross-sections were calculated from a directivity spectrum measured at a location between the first and second views. The evolution of the direct and edge waves is clear, and can be seen to be in close accord with the theory developed in the text

1.6.5 THE BEAM PROFILE/AXIAL PULSE DESCRIPTION

Probably the most common, and most traditional, way to describe the pulsed field is to write it as:

$$p(\mathbf{r}, t) \equiv p(h, \phi, z, t) = B(h, \phi)p_A(z - Ct) \tag{1.90}$$

where B designates the beam cross-section and p_A is the 'axial pulse', *viz.* the pulse shape as measured by a point hydrophone located on the acoustic axis. In general, with transducers of the simple geometries that are employed in medical ultrasound applications, it is considered sufficient to determine the variation of the beam cross-section along only a few ϕ values (depending on the assumed symmetry of the field). Such (one-dimensional) functions of the lateral variable, h, are referred to as beam profiles. For the case that the field is close to being cylindrically symmetric about the acoustic axis, an averaged (over a number of ϕ directions) beam profile may be taken. It is conventional to normalise the peak value of the beam profile to unity. Note that the simple propagational properties implied for the axial pulse, or the z-independence of the beam profile, are rarely (if at all) supported by actual measurements of transient fields – except over very restricted ranges.

For axially symmetric fields, the beam profile is represented by a single one-dimensional function, obtained by moving a point hydrophone transversely to the acoustic axis, and plotting the variation of a single feature of the measured pulse (such as the peak value of the detected pulse envelope) as a function of h. For fields with lesser symmetry, more than one such traverse may be deemed necessary: in such cases, the beam profile set is conventionally regarded as the *minimal* set of lateral one-dimensional measurements considered to give adequate information about the beam cross-section. There are no uniformly accepted conventions, or clear guidelines, as to what constitutes such a minimal set, but it is implied that the beam cross-section may be accurately described in terms of it. Note, also, that experimentally determined beam profiles are always quoted as being real and positive quantities, and this restriction may consequently be regarded as being fundamental to the description. However, with pulsed fields, there may be some ambiguity as to how to choose the field feature that is represented in the beam profile: different choices may give different profiles!

The beam profile/axial pulse formalism is alluringly simple, and widely used for describing fields from medical ultrasound transducers; it is appropriate, therefore, to examine its theoretical basis. For general harmonic fields, the close relationship of the beam profile description to the angular spectrum formalism is apparent, but the implied positive-definite character of the former is not guaranteed by the latter. Thus, in this simple case, a knowledge of the beam profile set is not adequate, even in principle, to accurately predict the field at some arbitrary location. Moreover, it should be clear that a field description of the type suggested in equation (1.90) cannot possibly embody all the diffractive subtleties of a general transient field, where the pulse shape will vary – perhaps quite dramatically – as the point hydrophone traverses the lateral direction. Thus, at best, the beam profile/axial pulse formalism can be regarded as a rough approximation, of some utility only in a region where diffractive changes of the field are small enough to be disregarded.

1.6.6 MULTIELEMENT ARRAYS

The transducers in most modern medical ultrasound pulse–echo imaging systems are not of the simple, single element type considered above, but consist of many smaller elements which are activated in groups. Since the elements are generally arranged in some sort of planar array – usually linear arrays – such transducers are referred to as 'multielement arrays' or, depending on how they are activated, as 'phased arrays'. Only a hint of the power and flexibility resulting from the utilisation of such configurations can be suggested here, by considering a linear array that is designed to produce a pulse travelling out at an angle to the geometric axis of the array.

Consider the nth element in the array, located at $\mathbf{r}_n$, and activated at time t_n. The emitted pulse, via equation (1.86), may be written as

$$p_n(\mathbf{r},\, t) = \iiint\limits_{-\infty}^{\infty} d^3\mathbf{k} D_n(\mathbf{k}) \exp(i[\mathbf{k} \cdot (\mathbf{r} - \mathbf{r}_n) - Ck(t - t_n)]) \tag{1.91}$$

where D_n is the directivity spectrum of that element, when located at the coordinate system origin, and activated with zero delay, at $t = 0$. The pulse may be regarded as being emitted from an element with an effective directivity spectrum that can be written as

$$D_{n,\,eff}(\mathbf{k}) = D_n(\mathbf{k}) \exp[-i(\mathbf{k} \cdot \mathbf{r}_n - Ckt_n)] \tag{1.92}$$

In the absence of any interference ('cross-talk') between the elements, then the pulse from the entire array is the sum of the emissions from the individual elements.

A great deal of tedious calculation may be avoided by noting that, if the directivity spectrum of the nth element is peaked about $\mathbf{k}_0$ then the following approximation is valid:

$$D_{n,\,eff}(\mathbf{k}) \approx D_n(\mathbf{k}) \exp[-i(\mathbf{k}_0 \cdot \mathbf{r}_n - Ck_0 t_n)] \tag{1.93}$$

with k_0 denoting the magnitude of $\mathbf{k}_0$. For the case that all the elements are identical, the directivity spectrum for the whole array is then given by

$$D_{array}(\mathbf{k}) \approx D(\mathbf{k}) \sum_n \exp[-i(\mathbf{k}_0 \cdot \mathbf{r}_n - Ck_0 t_n)] \equiv D(\mathbf{k}) \cdot A_F \tag{1.94}$$

where A_F, the array factor, depends on the geometry of the array, as well as on the relative timings of the excitations to the individual elements.

As an example, the array factor for a simple linear array of seven equally spaced identical elements is shown in Figure 1.8. With hindsight, the elements are located at separations of $\lambda_0/2 = \pi C/k_0$ apart (an optimum distance), with the central element placed at the origin. The excitation of the elements is linearly staggered, so that the central element is activated at $t = 0$,

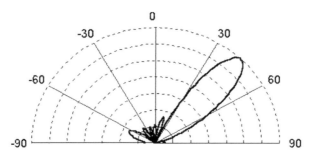

Figure 1.8. Array factor for a seven-element linear array, as described in the text. The delays in the excitations of the elements are linearly staggered and have been chosen to give the array factor a maximum at $\sim 45°$ to the forward-facing axis of the array. The elements are spaced a distance $\lambda_0/2$ apart. There is no apodisation

all the elements to the one side of it activated with progressively longer delays (equal increments), and all the elements to the other side activated progressively earlier (equal increments).

If it can be arranged for the array factor to be strongly peaked in a particular direction (as in Figure 1.8) then the directivity function for the array will generally also be peaked in that direction, so that the emergent pulse travels out at an angle to the forward axis of the linear array. Such 'beam swinging' is achieved by adjusting the excitation delays to the elements and requires no mechanical movement of the transducer array; hence, multielement transducers are an important component in the design of modern real-time imaging devices: the arrangement described above is utilised in the so-called 'sector scanner', although rather more than seven elements will be used in practice.

Multielement transducers may also be utilised in order to focus an emergent beam from a planar emitter: in this case, the focusing from a linear array is implemented by adjusting the element excitations so that they are symmetrically advanced with respect to the central element, and increase as the square, say, of the individual element's distance from the centre. In practice, a host of configurations are possible (see Chapter 3), not only for pulse emission, but also for guiding array sensitivity in reception. Two-dimensional and annular arrays have also been developed.

1.7 PROPAGATION ACROSS PLANAR BOUNDARIES

1.7.1 NORMAL INCIDENCE ON STATIONARY, SHARP BOUNDARY

Consider the case of a one-dimensional pulse entering a uniform lossless medium, with density ϱ_0, which extends for a distance D, where it abruptly changes to a different uniform lossless medium with density ϱ_1. The wave velocities in the two media are different, C_0 and C_1 respectively. The x-axis is set up so that the pulse enters at $x = 0$, and the discontinuity is located at $x = D$. Since the particle velocity also obeys a one-dimensional wave equation of the type indicated in equation (1.47), it follows from equation (1.48) that the following hold:

$$p(x, t) = f_i(x - C_i t) + g_i(x + C_i t) \tag{1.95}$$

That is to say

$$Z_i u(x, t) = f_i(x - C_i t) - g_i(x + C_i t) \tag{1.96}$$

where the subscript i indicates 0 for $0 \leqslant x \leqslant D$ and 1 for $x > D$.

The analysis described below is modelled on the approach described by Gladwell (1993), since it allows pulsed fields to be used directly. It is assumed that there is no ultrasound field present throughout $x > 0$ at time $t = 0$. This implies that

$$f_i(x) = g_i(x) = 0 \tag{1.97}$$

However, for $t > 0$, the arguments of these functions may take on values different to those for which equation (1.97) remains valid. It is only the function g_1 which will remain zero for *all* time. This implies that there is only a forward travelling wave in the region $x > D$.

Continuity conditions apply across the boundary: continuity of pressure is mandated by the requirement that acoustic forces (dependent on the pressure gradient) remain finite, and particle velocity continuity is required if the two media that abut the discontinuity are to remain in close contact. Application of these boundary conditions, at $x = D$, results in

$$f_0(D - C_0 t) + g_0(D + C_0 t) = f_1(D - C_1 t) \tag{1.98}$$

$$f_0(D - C_0 t) - g_0(D + C_0 t) = \frac{Z_0}{Z_1} f_1(D - C_1 t) \tag{1.99}$$

The last two equations may be solved to express g_0 and f_1 in terms of f_0, and, noting the following identities

$$x \pm C_i t = D \pm C_i[t \pm (x - D)/C_i] \tag{1.100}$$

where the $+(-)$ applies when $i = 0$ (1). The following expression for the pressure wave follows:

$$p(x, t) = f_0(x - C_0 t) + \left(\frac{Z_1 - Z_0}{Z_0 + Z_1} \right) f_0(2D - x - C_0 t) \qquad \text{for } 0 \leqslant x \leqslant D \tag{1.101}$$

$$p(x, t) = \frac{2Z_1}{Z_0 + Z_1} f_0 \left(D + \frac{C_0}{C_1}(x - D) - C_0 t \right) \qquad \text{for } x > D \tag{1.102}$$

It is apparent from the above that an incident wave impinging on a discontinuity of the above type gives rise to a reflected wave ('echo'), and that the (amplitude) reflection coefficient, R, is given by

$$R \equiv \frac{\text{Amplitude of reflected wave}}{\text{Amplitude of incident wave}} = \frac{|Z_1 - Z_0|}{Z_0 + Z_1} \tag{1.103}$$

Since R is defined as a ratio of wave amplitudes, it is a positive quantity. When $Z_0 > Z_1$, the factor multiplying the reflected wave in equation (1.101) is negative; this merely means that the echo is 'flipped' (phase shifted though 180°). In a more general model, the reflection coefficient is defined in terms of complex amplitudes, and is thus a complex quantity which indicates both the amplitude and phase of the echo, relative to the incident wave.

Another quantity of interest is the (amplitude) transmission coefficient, T, given by

$$T \equiv \frac{\text{Amplitude of transmitted wave}}{\text{Amplitude of incident wave}} = \frac{2Z_1}{Z_0 + Z_1} \tag{1.104}$$

Note that

$$R^2/Z_0 + T^2/Z_1 = 1/Z_0 \tag{1.105}$$

as conservation of energy requires. The corresponding coefficients of reflection and transmission of intensity are evidently given by $R_E = R^2$ and $T_E = (Z_0/Z_1)T^2$ respectively.

The expression for R is frequently – and incorrectly – interpreted as demonstrating that the amplitude of the echo depends on the difference in the characteristic acoustic impedances of the media across the discontinuity. In fact, it depends uniquely on the *ratio* (rather than the difference) of the two impendances, as a little thought will show. It should also be borne in mind that, despite its ubiquity in interpreting echo amplitudes in medical ultrasound, equation (1.103) results from a particularly simple model. Quite apart from its one-dimensional character, it is doubtful whether all the assumptions of the model are valid in practice. Even the more realistic inclusion of loss in either, or both, of the two adjacent media will modify the result, albeit only weakly for typical tissue values (Livett & Leeman 1983).

An interesting feature demonstrated by the above model is the principle of causality, which, loosely stated, requires that the effect cannot precede the cause. This is made explicit in equation (1.101), where it can be observed that, taking into account equation (1.97), the echo is not generated until the incident wave actually starts to impinge on the discontinuity. If the time taken for the echo to arrive back at $z = 0$ is measured, and if the wave velocity C_0 is known, or can be estimated, then the location of the reflecting interface can be calculated. This is the fundamental basis upon which ultrasound pulse–echo methods for medical imaging are built, and is sometimes, somewhat grandiosely, referred to as the 'pulse–echo principle'.

Clearly the time taken (as measured from the instant of pulse transmission) for the echo from a reflecting interface to return to the transmitting transducer is double that taken for the pulse to reach the interface. Thus, the echo train from two interfaces, separated by distance Δ, shows a delay between the two individual echoes (if they can be resolved) that is given by $2\Delta/C$, where C is the sound speed in the region between the two interfaces. This implies that a pulse–echo ranging technique effectively stretches the distance scale of the structure being probed – a welcome result that boosts the range resolution of pulse–echo devices.

1.7.2 REFLECTION FROM A CONTINUOUSLY VARYING IMPEDANCE PROFILE

A strictly one-dimensional model, as developed in the section above, is not likely to be a realistic representation of echo formation in tissues. One way in which to make the description more attuned to the rather complex situation existing *in vivo* is to relax the condition that the impedance changes in a step-like, discontinuous, manner. Such an approach is suggested by somewhat more formal arguments which suggest that, in the more general three-dimensional situation, the reflected ($\equiv$ backscattered) echo sequence is similar to that from a one-dimensional continuously varying 'effective impedance' given by

$$Z(x) = \int_{-\infty}^{\infty} dy \int_{-\infty}^{\infty} dz\ S(x, y, z)B(y, z) \tag{1.106}$$

where $S(x, y, z)$ is the scattering distribution (see Chapter 6), and $B(y, z)$ is the beam cross-section. Bearing in mind what was indicated earlier about the validity of the axial pulse/beam profile description of ultrasound pulses, it is clear that equation (1.106) must be regarded as an approximation. Note that $Z(x)$ represents a layered (characteristic) impedance distribution that produces the same echo sequence, in a one-dimensional model, as a general, non-layered impedance distribution would in a genuine three-dimensional situation, when probed from a particular direction. It is for that reason referred to as the *effective* impedance.

It is unlikely that the effective impedance would, in general, exhibit sharp discontinuities. A more appropriate model in this context would be to consider an extended interface across which the effective impedance rises continuously from Z_0 to Z_1. This is the analogue of the simple impedance step discussed in the previous section. It is too restrictive to require that the ultrasound wave velocity remain constant throughout the transition zone between the two regions of constant impedance, so it is appropriate to introduce the 'travel time' variable

$$\tau(x) = \int_0^x dx'/C(x') \tag{1.107}$$

The impedance may then be expressed as a function of the travel time. At $\tau = 0$, the impedance has a value Z_0, and it maintains this constant value until τ_0, say, when it commences to rise smoothly to the value Z_1, which it attains at τ_1, after which it stays constant till travel time T (the maximum time of interest). It is not difficult to show, by direct integration, that such an impedance profile can be written, for $0 \leqslant \tau \leqslant T$, as

$$Z(\tau) = Z_0 + \int_{\tau_0}^{\tau_1} d\tau' \frac{dZ(\tau')}{d\tau'} H_S(\tau - \tau') \tag{1.108}$$

The Heaviside step function satisfies

$$\frac{\partial H_S}{\partial \tau'} = -\delta(\tau - \tau') \tag{1.109}$$

and a little manipulation shows that

$$Z(\tau) = Z_0 + \int_{\tau_0}^{\tau_1} d\tau' \left\{ \frac{d}{d\tau'} [\ln Z(\tau')] \right\} \Gamma(\tau; \tau') \tag{1.110}$$

where $\Gamma(\tau; \tau')$ denotes an impedance step, in the τ-domain, located at τ', with the impedance rising from 0 to $Z(\tau')$ across it. Explicitly

$$\Gamma(\tau; \tau') \equiv H_S(\tau - \tau')Z(\tau') \tag{1.111}$$

Consider now a pulse entering the region, and of (temporal) shape $f(t)$ at $\tau = 0$. It is understood that the function $f(t)$ may be considered to be zero when its argument is negative or exceeds T_W, the duration of the pulse. In accordance with the considerations of the previous section, the echo from a particular discontinuity $\Gamma(\tau; \tau')$ is of the form $f(t - 2\tau')$ when it returns back to $\tau = 0$. Provided that the echo from $Z(\tau)$ may be expressed as the sum of the echoes from the individual impedance steps, $\Gamma(\tau; \tau')$, which constitute it, then the complete echo from the continuously varying impedance profile is given by

$$f_Z(t) = \int_{\tau_0}^{\tau_1} d\tau' \left\{ \frac{d}{d\tau'} [\ln Z(\tau')] \right\} f(t - 2\tau') \tag{1.112}$$

Clearly, in this case, $(1/Z)(dZ/d\tau) = d[\ln Z(\tau)]/d\tau$ may be regarded as the reflectivity function.

Note that equation (1.112) satisfies causality: the first arrival of the temporally extended echo appears at $t = 2\tau_0$. Note also that, in contrast to the case of an echo from a single impedance step, the 'shape' (i.e., time dependence) of the echo may have little in common with that of the incident pulse, depending on how rapidly $Z(\tau)$ changes over the extent of the pulse. Clearly, the echo from the extended impedance step is essentially the convolution of the incident pulse shape with a varying 'reflectivity function' given by the logarithmic derivative of the impedance profile (but incorporating the effective distance stretching implicit in pulse–echo measurement techniques).

The approximations made in arriving at equation (1.112) may appear to be somewhat extreme. However, the derivation was made in the spirit of wave-scattering theory (discussed in Chapter 6), and accurately represents a one-dimensional application of the so-called first Born approximation for the field *scattered* (in this case, reflected) from impedance inhomogeneities. The technique may be extended to higher Born approximations (Leeman 1980). It can be established, though, that the first Born approximation is reasonable provided that (in the context of the present example) the product of the maximum absolute value of the reflectivity function with the distance over which it extends (expressed in wavelength units) remains small (Joachain 1983).

1.7.3 TRANSMISSION THROUGH A BARRIER

A case of some interest is where an ultrasound wave penetrates through a barrier, or wall. Again, for simplicity, the analysis is restricted to one dimension, with an incident continuous plane harmonic wave, impinging orthogonally from medium 1, of acoustic impedance Z_1, onto medium 2, of acoustic impedance Z_2, located at $x = 0$. Medium 2 extends to $x = L$, where it changes to medium 3, with acoustic impedance Z_3.

It is clear that there is an incident (amplitude A_I) and reflected wave in medium 1, a transmitted wave (only), with amplitude A_T, in medium 3, and the barrier, for $0 \leqslant x \leqslant L$, contains both a forward- and backward-travelling wave. The situation has been analysed in some detail by Kinsler *et al.* (1982), who show that the intensity transmission coefficient is given by

$$T_E \equiv 4 / \left[2 + \left(\frac{Z_3}{Z_1} + \frac{Z_1}{Z_3} \right) \cos^2 k_2 L + \left(\frac{Z_2^2}{Z_1 Z_3} + \frac{Z_1 Z_3}{Z_2^2} \right) \sin^2 k_2 L \right] \tag{1.113}$$

where k_2 is the value of $2\pi f / C$ in medium 2.

If $k_2 L$ is arranged to take on the value $\pi/2$, then equation (1.113) reduces to

$$T_E = \frac{4 Z_1 Z_3}{\left(Z_2 + \dfrac{Z_1 Z_3}{Z_2} \right)^2} \tag{1.114}$$

so that complete transmission of energy ($T_E = 1$) can occur if $Z_2 = \sqrt{Z_1 Z_3}$. This remarkable result is much utilised in practice, when designing transducers for medical applications, if it is desired to obtain good energy transmission from the high impedance ceramic transducers into the relatively low impedance human tissue: a quarter-wave 'matching layer', of appropriate material, is a ubiquitous feature of such transducers.

Another important result that follows from equation (1.113) is for situations where $Z_2^2 \ll Z_1 Z_3$. Here it will be seen that quite low values of transmission coefficient may arise even when $k_2 L \ll 1$. A case of practical importance, that is avoided in clinical scanning by the use of a coupling gel applied to the skin, is that of a thin film of gas that can be trapped on an 'imperfectly wetted' surface of a transducer.

1.7.4 REFLECTION FROM A PLANAR INTERFACE AT OBLIQUE INCIDENCE

Reflection from an interface oriented orthogonally to the incident pulse is likely to occur only under special circumstances in medical pulse–echo investigations, and it is of some value to

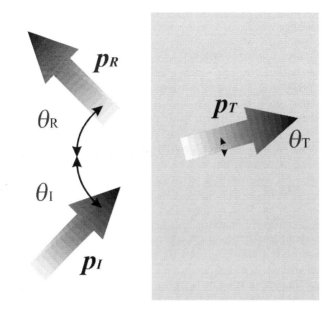

Figure 1.9. Definition of parameters used in calculating reflection from a planar interface, at oblique incidence

examine the case of oblique incidence. The problem cannot be tackled straightforwardly in a one-dimensional model when the incident pulse is spatially bounded, and that case becomes rather more complicated to handle as the dimensionality of the problem rises. For simplicity, therefore, only a two-dimensional situation is described here, with the incident wave taken to be a progressive continuous plane wave, with amplitude A_I and frequency f. The angle of incidence is θ_I and the wave passes from a uniform lossless medium with density ϱ_0 and sound velocity C_0 into a similar medium with acoustic parameters ϱ_1 and C_1. The more general case of a bounded incident pulse may be reconstructed from the plane-wave result, via the directivity spectrum formalism.

It is to be expected that there will be a reflected and transmitted wave, and, given the parameters defined in Figure 1.9, the three waves of interest may be written as:

$$p_J(x, y, t) = A_J \exp\{i\omega[(s_J x \cos \theta_J + y \sin \theta_J)/C_J - t]\} \tag{1.115}$$

where $J = I, R, T$ for the incident, reflected and transmitted waves, respectively, and $s_R = -1$, $s_{I,T} = 1$. The particle velocities associated with the waves can be written as:

$$\mathbf{u}_J(x, y, t) = (A_J/\varrho_J C_J)(\exp\{i\omega[(s_J x \cos \theta_J + y \sin \theta_J)/C_J - t]\})\mathbf{n}_J \tag{1.116}$$

with $\rho_{I,R} = \varrho_0$, $\rho_T = \varrho_1$, and similarly for C_J. $\mathbf{n}_J$ denotes a unit vector in the propagation direction of the appropriate wave:

$$\mathbf{n}_J = \mathbf{i} s_J \cos \theta_J + \mathbf{j} \sin \theta_J \tag{1.117}$$

with $\mathbf{i}$ and $\mathbf{j}$ indicating the unit vectors along the x- and y-axes respectively.

The boundary conditions to be applied are that the (total) pressure and the normal (to the interface) component of the (total) particle velocity remain continuous across the boundary between the two media (i.e., at $x = 0$). After some lengthy algebraic manipulations, the following conditions result:

$$\theta_I = \theta_R \equiv \theta \tag{1.118}$$

$$\frac{\sin \theta}{C_0} = \frac{\sin \theta_T}{C_1} \tag{1.119}$$

$$\frac{A_R}{A_I} \equiv R_\theta = \frac{\varrho_1 C_1 \cos \theta - \varrho_0 \sqrt{C_0^2 - C_1^2 \sin^2 \theta}}{\varrho_1 C_1 \cos \theta + \varrho_0 \sqrt{C_0^2 - C_1^2 \sin^2 \theta}} \tag{1.120}$$

$$\frac{A_T}{A_I} \equiv T_\theta = \frac{2\varrho_1 C_1 \cos \theta}{\varrho_1 C_1 \cos \theta + \varrho_0 \sqrt{C_0^2 - C_1^2 \sin^2 \theta}} \tag{1.121}$$

Equation (1.118) is commonly considered to be the defining characteristic of a 'specular' reflector – a surface which reflects ultrasound as a mirror does light, with the angle of incidence equal to the angle of reflection. In medical applications this property is often ascribed to the reflections from the surfaces of organs (with some justification, although systematic proof appears to be lacking). On the other hand, it is occasionally also attributed to the stronger, presumably scattered, echoes from within an organ – a somewhat more arbitrary assignment. Equation (1.119) states that Snell's law, well known from optics, also governs the refraction of ultrasound waves across interfaces of the type considered here. Again, firm direct evidence for its legitimacy across soft tissue boundaries is lacking, although few doubt its approximate, at least, validity.

The expressions for the (amplitude) reflectivity and transmissivity of an oblique interface, as given by equations (1.120) and (1.121), contain some surprises. It is easily shown that, in this case, R_θ does *not* vanish when the impedances of the two media abutting the interface are equal! Indeed, the condition of zero reflectivity (equivalent to total transmission) can be attained for a whole range of impedance mismatches, provided that the angle of incidence has a value $\hat{\theta}$ given by

$$\tan^2 \hat{\theta} = \frac{Z_1^2 - Z_0^2}{Z_0^2 - \frac{\varrho_0^2}{\varrho_1^2} Z_1^2} \tag{1.122}$$

Note, however, that this equation applies only if the values of the acoustic parameters of the two media are such that $\tan^2 \hat{\theta}$ remains a positive quantity.

Another interesting feature is that total reflectivity ($R_\theta = 1$, equivalent to zero transmission of energy) can be achieved when the angle of incidence is equal to, or larger than, the critical angle, θ_C, given by

$$\sin \theta_C = C_0/C_1 \tag{1.123}$$

Total reflection can occur only if $C_0 \leqslant C_1$. When the angle of incidence is θ_C, Snell's law shows that the angle of refraction is $\pi/2$. This suggests that a refracted wave travels in a direction parallel to the interface, and a more careful analysis shows that there is, in this case, no propagating wave in the second medium. Conservation of energy implies that

$$R_\theta^2 + \frac{\varrho_1}{\varrho_0} \frac{\sqrt{C_0^2 - C_1^2 \sin^2 \theta}}{C_1 \cos \theta} T_\theta^2 = 1 \tag{1.124}$$

The two terms on the left-hand side of equation (1.124) represent the fraction of the incident energy transported by the reflected and refracted waves, respectively. It is clear that under conditions of total reflection, there is no energy transported across the interface.

As foreshadowed in the introduction to this chapter, the above discussion has been conducted exclusively in terms of compressional wave propagation. Whilst this simplifying assumption is generally appropriate in the present context, an important exception occurs for the situation of an interface between soft tissue and a solid, in particular, such as bone. Oblique incidence of a compression mode wave at a soft tissue/bone interface, for example, results in a component of that wave energy being converted to a shear mode in bone, with corresponding inclusion of a shear mode component in the energy reflected back into the soft tissue. Since shear wave absorption coefficients in soft tissue are extremely high at megahertz frequencies, this can result in substantial and very localised heat deposition near the bone surface – an effect whose possible consequences are discussed in Chapter 12.

1.7.5 REFLECTION FROM A MOVING INTERFACE

A situation of considerable interest, and relevance, when ultrasonically probing human tissues by pulse–echo methods is that of reflection from a moving interface. Consider that the interface is moving with constant velocity V in the positive x-direction. At time $t = 0$, the interface is located at $x = D$, and an ultrasound pulse just commences to enter the region, $x \geqslant 0$, which has a wave velocity C. Let the time dependence of the pulse, as measured at $x = 0$, be denoted by $f(t)$, and assume that it is of finite duration, T. For simplicity, assume that the moving interface is a perfect reflector ($R = 1$, with no phase shift).

At time t, the reflector is located at

$$x_R = D + Vt \tag{1.125}$$

and the leading edge of the incident pulse is therefore reflected at time t_L, given by

$$Ct_L = D + Vt_L \tag{1.126}$$

The leading edge of the echo thus arrives back at $x = 0$ at time $2t_L$. The trailing edge of the incident pulse crosses $x = 0$ at $t = CT_W$, and is reflected at time t_T, given by

$$C(t_T - T_W) = D + Vt_T \tag{1.127}$$

The trailing edge of the echo arrives back at $x = 0$ at time $[T_W + 2(t_T - T_W)]$. The duration of the echo, as observed at $x = 0$, is thus

$$T_D = [T_W + 2(t_T - T_W)] - 2t_L = \frac{C + V}{C - V} T_W \tag{1.128}$$

Note that the echo, as measured by a stationary observer at $x = 0$, appears to be stretched, in time, with respect to the outgoing pulse, as measured by that same observer. For a reflecting interface travelling in the opposite direction ($V < 0$), the echo would appear to be compressed in time. This conclusion holds for the time delay between any two distinguishable features of $f(t)$. Thus, the reflection from a moving interface implies a time scaling of the echo (as observed by a stationary observer located at $x = 0$), relative to the incident pulse (as measured by the same stationary observer).

Consider now that the incident wave is a harmonic wave, with period T and frequency f_0. The reflected wave appears to exhibit a period that is related to T in the same way that T_D is related to T_W, and thus the observed frequency, f_R, of the reflected wave is given by

$$f_R = \frac{C - V}{C + V} f_0 \qquad (1.129)$$

The change in frequency derived here embodies the Doppler effect, which states that the observed frequency of a wave depends on the motional states of the wave source and the observer. For interface velocities of physiological relevance, $V/C \ll 1$, equation (1.129) reduces to

$$f_D \equiv f_0 - f_R = 2\frac{V}{C} f_0 \qquad (1.130)$$

This is the famous 'Doppler shift equation' utilised in medical ultrasound applications. It is only at this level of approximation, i.e. $V/C \ll 1$, that the Doppler shift, f_D, depends linearly on the relative velocity between the transducer (wave source) and a moving reflector, and it should be remembered that such a conclusion is not generally valid for acoustic waves reflected from interfaces travelling at higher speeds.

Although the Doppler effect was exploited by some of the first ultrasound devices put to medical use – to estimate blood velocity by measuring the frequency shift in backscattered continuous waves – it has an apparently commanding presence in some of the most recent developments in the field. A unifying feature of these more modern designs is that they utilise pulsed ultrasound fields, thereby being able to inject an element of (moving) scatterer ranging, via the pulse–echo principle. Despite the nomenclature applied to some of these techniques, they are more accurately described as 'moving target indicators', which derive velocity by tracking the rate of change in scatterer location (which is the measured variable), rather than by explicitly measuring the Doppler shift in the returned echo (Thomas & Leeman 1995). It is primarily for this reason that more than one pulse–echo sequence is required before a velocity estimate can be made (see Chapter 10).

1.8   FINITE AMPLITUDE WAVES

Much of the theory developed above was in the so-called linear approximation, as embodied in equation (1.11). Direct measurements of the ultrasound fields used in most medical applications demonstrate that it cannot be assumed that the linearity condition is satisfied, in general. It is of some interest, therefore, to investigate at least some of the features of nonlinear (or 'finite amplitude' as it is commonly referred to) ultrasound wave propagation. This is indeed a vast, and somewhat less well understood, area, and the treatment that follows is only a very small, and simplified, aspect of a complex body of knowledge. Specifically, only one-dimensional waves in lossless, uniform and homogeneous media for which equations (1.10), (1.13) and (1.15) are valid will be considered. It will prove more convenient to write these in a difference guise (Tenkin 1981). The first two equations can be combined to obtain:

$$-\frac{\partial p}{\partial x} = \frac{\partial}{\partial t}(\varrho_T u) + \frac{\partial}{\partial x}(\varrho_T u^2) \qquad (1.131)$$

Another interesting equation can be derived relatively easily from equations (1.10) and (1.13):

$$\frac{\partial^2 p}{\partial t^2} - C^2 \frac{\partial^2 p}{\partial x^2} - \frac{\partial^2}{\partial t^2}(p - \varrho_T C^2) + C^2 \frac{\partial^2}{\partial x^2}(\varrho_T u) \qquad (1.132)$$

Note that, at this stage, no further approximations have been made, so that the last two equations embody the full non-linearity of the Euler and continuity equations.

Also, equation (1.15) may be considered to be inverted, so that p is expressed as a function of ϱ. On expanding in a Taylor series in the condensation, s, the constitutive equation can be expressed in a form that is more conventionally used in the present context, *viz.*

$$p = As + \tfrac{1}{2}Bs^2 + \text{terms of higher order in } s \tag{1.133}$$

with the constants A and B given by

$$A \equiv \varrho_0 \left(\frac{\partial p}{\partial \varrho} \right)_{\varrho=0} = \varrho_0 c^2 \tag{1.134}$$

$$B \equiv \varrho_0^2 \left(\frac{\partial^2 p}{\partial \varrho^2} \right)_{\varrho=0} \tag{1.135}$$

The partial derivatives are understood (as before) to be obtained under adiabatic conditions.

Equation (1.133) obviously reverts to the linear relationship if B, and the coefficients of all the higher order terms vanish. These coefficients depend only on the properties of the medium, and may be expressed, via a sequence of thermodynamic transformations, in terms of measurable entities. It turns out that for many liquids, including water, it is not unreasonable to retain only the first two terms, for excess pressures as high as 10 atmospheres (in the temperature range relevant to the present discussion). The B/A ratio is thus frequently considered indicative of the magnitude of the departure from linearity. However, it should be borne in mind that even if the properties of the medium result in the constitutive equation being essentially linear for a particular pressure range, there may nonetheless be a source of non-linearity from equation (1.131). A distinction may be made between these two different potential sources of non-linearity: that stemming from the constitutive equation is called 'medium non-linearity', while the second cause (which ultimately derives from the use of the convective derivative) is referred to as 'convective non-linearity'. These ideas will be demonstrated more formally below.

1.8.1 RADIATION PRESSURE

Equation (1.131) may be rewritten in a form suggestive of a conservation equation for the momentum density, $\varrho_T u$:

$$\frac{\partial}{\partial x}(p + \varrho_T u^2) + \frac{\partial}{\partial t}(\varrho_T u) = 0 \tag{1.136}$$

Here, analogous to the interpretation of equation (1.38), the entity $p + \varrho_T u^2$ represents a (one-dimensional) momentum density flux vector. Note that its definition incorporates the acoustic pressure, rather than the total pressure; this is because it is assumed, as before, that the static pressure in the medium in the absence of the wave is a constant. Thus a travelling acoustic field, in addition to transporting energy (as shown earlier for the linear case only), also conveys momentum. Time averaging of equation (1.136) reveals that

$$\frac{\partial}{\partial x}\left(\bar{p} + \overline{\varrho_T u^2}\right) = 0 \tag{1.137}$$

where the overbar indicates the time-averaged value

$$\bar{f} \equiv \frac{1}{T} \int_{-T/2}^{T/2} f(t)dt \tag{1.138}$$

For cyclic fields, it is appropriate to consider T to be the wave period; for pulsed fields, it represents the pulse duration. In more general cases, it may be necessary to take the limit as $T \to \infty$. Integration of equation (1.137) leads to

$$\bar{p} + \overline{\varrho_T u^2} = R \tag{1.139}$$

The time-averaged momentum density flux, R, is called the radiation pressure of the field.

A more transparent interpretation of the above results when considering the application of equation (1.139) in the case of a rigid wall fixed in the field. Since $u = 0$ on the surface of the wall, R is the value of the time-averaged pressure exerted by the field on the object. This simple example suggests the suitability of the term 'radiation pressure' for R. Moreover, since the field cannot pass through a rigid wall (so that $\bar{p} = 0$ beyond the wall surface), it also demonstrates that the surface of the object experiences a force. The association of R with the momentum density flux is, of course, consistent with this demonstration of the ability of a field to exert a force on an obstacle. For example, consider an ideally absorbing (non-reflective) wall placed in the beam: all the momentum carried in the field is absorbed by the object, which experiences a force by virtue of Newton's second law which identifies a force with rate of change of momentum.

The measurement of the force exerted by a field on an obstacle ('target') is one of the primary methods for assessing the acoustic output of medical ultrasound devices. However, while the choice of suitable targets may make the relationship between the measured force and the radiation pressure clear, it is by no means a simple matter to extract the field intensity from the measurements. One common approach is to insert the linear approximation for the acoustic variables: if harmonic plane waves are assumed, it is evident that

$$R = \frac{1}{C}I \quad \text{(linear harmonic plane waves)} \tag{1.140}$$

1.8.2 HARMONIC PUMPING

Equation (1.132) is reminiscent of the wave equation with non-linear terms added, but it is no trivial matter to obtain a general solution, as for the linearised case. One approach is adopted whereby the acoustic variables appearing in that equation are expanded as follows:

$$\varrho = \varrho_T - \varrho_0 = \varepsilon\varrho_1 + \varepsilon^2\varrho_2 + \ldots \tag{1.141}$$

$$p = \varepsilon p_1 + \varepsilon^2 p_2 + \ldots \tag{1.142}$$

$$u = \varepsilon u_1 + \varepsilon^2 u_2 + \ldots \tag{1.143}$$

In these approximations, the (dimensionless) parameter $\varepsilon \ll 1$ so that the magnitude of each term in the expansion is approximately a factor ε smaller than its immediate predecessor. At this stage the constitutive equation has not yet been invoked: incorporating equation (1.141), it also reduces to a power series in ε, and the following identification may be made:

$$p_1 = C^2\varrho_1; \quad p_2 = C^2\varrho_2 + \tfrac{1}{2}\beta_N\varrho_1^2 \quad \text{where } \beta_N \equiv \frac{C^2}{\varrho_0}\frac{B}{A} \tag{1.144}$$

The various expansions may be substituted into equation (1.132), and terms of similar orders in ε collected. It may be shown that the collection of terms in each order of ε has to vanish separately, so that a hierarchy of equations requires to be solved. The first-order terms give

$$\frac{\partial^2 p_1}{\partial t^2} - C^2 \frac{\partial^2 p_1}{\partial x^2} = 0 \tag{1.145}$$

The terms of second order in ε lead to

$$\frac{\partial^2 p_2}{\partial t^2} - C^2 \frac{\partial^2 p_2}{\partial x^2} = \tfrac{1}{2} \beta_N \frac{\partial^2 \varrho_1^2}{\partial t^2} + \varrho_0 C^2 \frac{\partial^2 u_1^2}{\partial x^2} \tag{1.146}$$

The propagation of the first-order pressure term, p_1, perhaps not unsurprisingly, proceeds according to the linear wave equation. The structure of the second-order wave equation is somewhat unexpected, but shows a rather satisfying feature: only first-order acoustic variables contribute to the non-linear terms (which have been collected on the right-hand side, and which show their separate 'medium' and 'convective' non-linear origins). Equations corresponding to higher orders in ε all show a similar structure, *viz.* a wave equation linear in a particular p_n, with the source terms of the non-linearity containing only lower order acoustic variables.

Equation (1.146) is not too difficult to solve for the case of a field which starts out as a continuous, linear, harmonic wave. Assume, therefore, a pressure field which has a boundary (at $x = 0$) behaviour described by

$$p(0, t) - A_0 \sin(\omega t) \tag{1.147}$$

Clearly, this implies that

$$p_1(x, t) = A_0 \sin(\omega t - kx) \tag{1.148}$$

Using the linear relationships tabulated in Table 1.1, it becomes possible to write equation (1.147) as

$$\frac{\partial^2 p_2}{\partial t^2} - C^2 \frac{\partial^2 p_2}{\partial x^2} = 2 \frac{(A_0 k)^2}{\varrho_0} \left(1 + \tfrac{1}{2} B/A\right) \cos\{2(\omega t - kx)\} \tag{1.149}$$

This wave equation may be solved by standard methods, subject to the boundary condition equation (1.147), to yield the forward propagating solution

$$p_2 = \tfrac{1}{2} \frac{A_0^2}{\varrho_0 C^2} \left(1 + \tfrac{1}{2} B/A\right) kx \sin\{2(\omega t - kx - \pi/4)\}$$

$$\equiv \frac{A_0^2 \gamma}{\varrho_0 C^2} kx \sin\{2(\omega t - kx - \pi/4)\} \tag{1.150}$$

Some features of this result should be noted. In accord with the imposed boundary conditions, the second-order component vanishes at $x = 0$. Thereafter, its amplitude increases linearly with distance and frequency, and quadratically with the amplitude of the first-order (linear) component. Both the medium and convective non-linearities contribute, but with the former more dominant in a typical liquid such as water ($B/A \approx 5.2$, at 30°C). The amplitudes of the first- and second-order components of the field become equal at a distance

$$x_S = \frac{\varrho_0 C^2}{2A_0\gamma k} \tag{1.151}$$

x_S is called the 'shock-formation distance', and is characteristic of the non-linear processes operating. Although the above treatment is not powerful enough to clearly demonstrate the validity of the nomenclature, a glimpse of its origins may be seen if it is noticed that at this distance the first two terms (as calculated here) in the expansion for the ultrasound field are precisely those that are to be expected in a Fourier series development of a sawtooth wave. It thus represents the distance at which an originally sinusoidal wave becomes discontinuous (shock-like), by virtue of non-linear processes. This conclusion can be valid only in a perfectly lossless medium, and it should also be borne in mind that the theory developed here is, by hypothesis, likely to remain valid only for distances somewhat less than x_S. The second-order component is a harmonic of the (fundamental) linear term. For the initially sinusoidal wave considered here, it turns out that the Nth-order component is a $(N-1)$th harmonic of the fundamental frequency. Since the presence of each harmonic becomes apparent only when its predecessor becomes sufficiently strong, this feature of the non-linear field is picturesquely referred to as 'harmonic pumping' [bearing the interpretation of equation (1.146) in mind].

1.8.3 PRESSURE-DEPENDENT VELOCITY

The treatment above makes it clear that an initially harmonic wave progressively distorts as it travels through a lossless medium, provided that non-linear effects are taken into account. There is a satisfyingly simple physical way to describe this phenomenon, first developed by Riemann (Beyer 1974), which makes it somewhat easier to describe the distortion of even wide-band pulsed fields, and which specifically relies on a constitutive equation that can be written as equation (1.15). In fact, this implies that the particle velocity may also be expressed (in principle) as a function of the pressure only. In this way, equations (1.10) and (1.13) may be rewritten as

$$\frac{\partial u}{\partial t} + u\frac{\partial u}{\partial x} = -\frac{C_N^2}{\varrho_T}\frac{\partial \varrho}{\partial x} \tag{1.152}$$

$$\frac{C_N}{\varrho_T}\frac{\partial \varrho}{\partial t} + \frac{C_N u}{\varrho_T}\frac{\partial \varrho}{\partial x} = -C_N\frac{\partial u}{\partial x} \tag{1.153}$$

with $C_N^2(p) = [\partial p/\partial \varrho]_{ad}$. The last two equations may be added to give

$$dR_I \equiv \frac{\partial R_I}{\partial x}dx + \frac{\partial R_I}{\partial t}dt = \frac{\partial R_I}{\partial x}[dx - (C_N + u)dt] \tag{1.154}$$

where the 'Riemann invariant' for a forward-travelling wave, R_I, is defined as

$$R_I(x,\,t) \equiv u + \int_0^\varrho \frac{C_N}{\varrho_T}d\varrho \tag{1.155}$$

Riemann pointed out that these equations have a very powerful interpretation. Equation (1.155) implies that R_I remains constant (i.e., $dR_I = 0$) in the $(x,\,t)$-plane, along a path given by

$$\frac{dx}{dt} = C_N + u \tag{1.156}$$

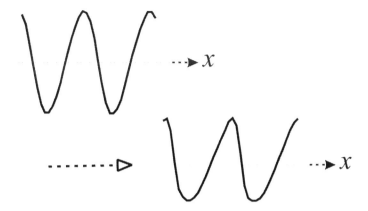

Figure 1.10. Measured harmonic plane wave, showing how non-linear distortion becomes more marked with distance from transducer face

A particular point on the waveform has associated with it a Riemann invariant whose size is fixed, via equation (1.155), by the pressure value at that phase in the cycle. This implies that the phase point under consideration propagates with a (pressure-dependent) velocity determined by equation (1.156). Thus, pressure peaks in the waveform propagate faster than pressure zeros, which, in turn, propagate faster than the pressure troughs. The waveform thus distorts progressively with distance travelled (Figure 1.10) until a shock-like pressure discontinuity is attained. Such a distorted wave would require progressively more higher harmonics in a Fourier decomposition, and this provides the link with the harmonic pumping description. It should be emphasised that the above descriptions break down before a truly discontinuous wave can be achieved, because the effects of absorption cannot then be ignored, and the assumption of adiabaticity is forced, on physics grounds, to break down when the wave approaches such a state. The Riemann approach is intuitively appealing, and allows the non-linear distortion of wide-band pulses to be calculated somewhat more transparently than the harmonic pumping method. It does, however, require the velocities in equation (1.156) to be calculable functions of the pressure.

REFERENCES

Beranek, L.L. (1986). *Acoustics*. AIP, New York.
Beyer, R.T. (1974). *Nonlinear Acoustics*. Dept. of the Navy, Washington, D.C.
Cathignol, D. and Faure, P. (1996). *Acoustical Imaging* **22**, 459.
Costa, E.T. and Leeman, S. (1988). *Acoustical Imaging* **17**, 403.
Gladwell, G.M.L. (1993). *Inverse Problems in Scattering*. Kluwer Academic, Dordrecht.
Goodman, J.W. (1996). *Introduction to Fourier Optics* (2nd edn). McGraw-Hill, New York.
Gore, J.C. and Leeman, S. (1977). *Phys. Med. Biol.* **22**(3), 431.
Healey, A.J., Leeman, S. and Weight, J.P. (1997). *Int. J. Imaging Systems and Technology* **8**, 45.
Joachain, C.J. (1983). *Quantum Collision Theory* (3rd edn). North-Holland, Amsterdam.
Kinsler, L.E., Frey, A.R., Coppens, A.B. and Sanders, J.V. (1982). *Fundamentals of Acoustics* (3rd edn). Wiley, New York.
Leeman, S. (1980). *Acoustical Imaging* **8**, 517.
Livett, A. and Leeman, S. (1983). *Proceedings IEEE 1983 Ultrasonics Symposium*, vol 2, B.R. McAvoy (ed.). IEEE, New York, p. 749.

Morse, P.M. and Feshbach, H. (1953). *Methods of Theoretical Physics*. McGraw-Hill, New York.

Morse, P.M. and Ingard, K.U. (1968). *Theoretical Acoustics*. McGraw-Hill, New York.

Pipes, L.A. (1958). *Applied Mathematics for Engineers and Physicists* (2nd edn). McGraw-Hill, New York.

Robinson, D.A., Lees, S. and Bess, L. (1974). *IEEE Trans. Acoust. Speech & Signal Process.* **22**, 35.

Stepanishen, P.R. (1971). *J. Acoust. Soc. Am.* **49**, 1629.

Temkin, S. (1981). *Elements of Acoustics*. Wiley, New York.

Thomas, N. and Leeman, S. (1995). *Acoustical Imaging* **21**, 543.

Tupholme, G.E. (1969). *Mathematika* **16**, 209.

2

Generation and Structure of Acoustic Fields

C. R. HILL

Institute of Cancer Research, Royal Marsden Hospital, UK

2.1 INTRODUCTION

The various practical applications of ultrasound to medicine arise, almost without exception, from its property of forming directional fields or beams; in other words, its property as a form of radiation. This chapter will have two functions: first, to describe the physical means that are available for generating such acoustic fields; and second, to describe some of the characteristics of the actual fields that can be generated in this way and which, at the same time, can be predicted or modelled by application of some of the analytical results presented in Chapter 1.

In principle there will be an infinite set of solutions to the homogeneous wave equation (1.24). Particular solutions will depend on combinations of factors such as wavelength, size and shape of the acoustically active aperture, and the amplitude and phase distributions of excitation or sensitivity over that aperture. Practical considerations of fabrication and mathematical tractability, however, have tended to limit most discussion to relatively simple conditions; most commonly to circular or rectangular apertures excited by either uniform or Gaussian-shaded distributions of amplitude, and plane or spherical in phase profile. We shall start by following this pattern of presentation and then discuss a number of other conditions that seem to be of inherent interest and practical potential.

Even with such simplification, the subject is large and complex. Some aspects, however, have been well dealt with in recent, readily available reviews, particularly those by Hunt *et al.* (1983) and Lu *et al.* (1994), which are strongly recommended reading. Thus, whilst endeavouring to be comprehensive, we shall pay particular attention to points that seem to have been less well covered elsewhere.

The concept of an acoustic field calls for some further consideration and definition at this stage. In medical ultrasonics, as in other branches of acoustics, practical interest in directional fields derives partly from their property of selectively irradiating or 'insonating' a particular volume of tissue or other material, and partly also from their use in selectively receiving signals from a limited region of space. The general situation is illustrated diagrammatically in Figure 2.1, which suggests that it may be useful to distinguish between three concepts of an acoustic field:

Physical Principles of Medical Ultrasonics, Second Edition. Edited by C. R. Hill, J. C. Bamber and G. R. ter Haar.
© 2004 John Wiley & Sons, Ltd: ISBN 0 471 97002 6

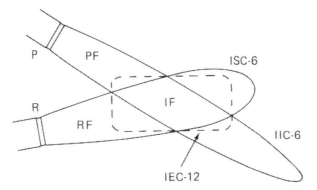

Figure 2.1. Three concepts of an acoustic field: projected field (PF); receptive field (RF); interrogation field (IF). (P: Projector; R: Receiver; IIC-6: 6 dB iso-intensity contour; ISC-6: 6 dB iso-sensitivity contour; IEC-12: 12 dB iso-echo contour)

1. A projected field – the acoustic field in time and space due to energy emitted by a particular device, referred to as a *projector*.
2. A receptive field – the distribution in time and space of phase- and amplitude-sensitivity of some other device, referred to as a *receiver*.
3. An interrogation field – the distribution in time and space of phase- and amplitude-sensitivity for a point target in the interception zone of particular projected and receptive fields.

It will become clear in what follows that the situation will be simplified in the important case of simple 'pulse–echo' diagnostic systems, where the projector and receiver are, to a first approximation, physically identical. It will also appear, however, that the more general situation offers certain practically interesting advantages and, for this, the distinction outlined above will be of value.

   Adoption of the above concepts will imply that the subject of acoustic fields will extend beyond simply the generation of acoustic waves, and that the borderline between this chapter and the next, where we take up particular aspects of acoustic detection, becomes somewhat arbitary.

   In turning now to the physical means that are available for the generation of acoustic fields we shall be concerned, in practical terms, simply with the phenomenon of piezoelectricity. However, if only for completeness, it needs to be remembered that other means exist for generating acoustic waves at ultrasonic frequencies and that, for power generation in the frequency range of approximately 20–100 kHz (encompassing ultrasonic cleaners, cell disintegrators and a number of ultrasonically driven surgical instruments), the magneto-strictive effect may often be used.

2.2 PIEZOELECTRIC DEVICES

The piezoelectric effect is a phenomenon, occurring in certain anisotropic materials, in which mechanical distortion of the material leads to imbalance of distribution of electric charge. Correspondingly, the inverse piezoelectric effect is that in which mechanical distortion of the material results from application of an external electric field. The subject is outlined by Silk (1984), Hunt *et al.* (1983) and Ballato (1995), and is treated in detail in a number of specialised texts (e.g. Berlincourt *et al.* 1964; Jaffe *et al.* 1971).

A variety of types of material can be piezoelectric. One class consists of natural crystals and crystalline materials (including human bone), examples of practical importance in the present context being quartz and lithium niobate. The other important class is the ferroelectrics: amorphous materials such as certain ceramics and plastics which have a microcrystalline structure that can be made permanently piezoelectric by application of a strong electric field ('poling').

Complete description of the electromechanical behaviour of such materials may lead to considerable complexity. In their nature they are anisotropic: their various properties will depend on direction in relation to crystalline and polarisation axes, and interactions between different electrical and mechanical properties will require handling in tensor matrix form. Parameters by which different materials may be characterised will include: electromechanical coupling coefficient (the fraction of dielectric energy that can be extracted as elastic energy, and *vice versa*), piezoelectric constant (electric field per unit strain), dielectric constant, loss factor (a frequency-dependent quantity that expresses the fractional energy lost per cycle), density, elastic compliance, and/or characteristic acoustic impedance. Other factors which will be of importance in particular applications are electrical breakdown field strength, non-linearity (Na & Breazeale 1994), and stability of values of initial parameters in relation to time, temperature and influence of water and chemical action.

Typical values for some of the above parameters, for some important materials, are listed in Table 2.1. For simplicity, and since, in the great majority of applications relevant to biological and medical use, devices are designed for use in thickness-mode operation only, the table merely lists the unidimensional parameter values relevant to that mode. The existence of other, sometimes unwanted, modes should not be neglected, however.

Some practically important differences between the materials will be evident from the table. Quartz, for example, being a pure crystalline material, has very low losses and will thus tend to exhibit sharp resonances. This has the advantage that quartz plates can be used efficiently as both projectors and receivers at a wide set of harmonics in addition to their fundamental frequency. However, having a low electromechanical coupling coefficient, they are rather insensitive off resonance and are thus correspondingly unsatisfactory for broadband operation or in applications as a receiver of detected energy that is not under close frequency control. Thus quartz is used widely for the measurement of material properties (e.g. absorption and sound speed in solutions of biomolecules, and investigation of biological dose–effect relationships) where it is required to carry out accurate observations (quartz has very good

Table 2.1. Typical properties of some piezoelectric materials

	Quartz (x-cut)	PZT-4	PZT-5A	Lead metaniobate	PVDF ('PVF2')
Dielectric constant (relative to free space): $\varepsilon/\varepsilon_0$	5.0	1300	1700	22.5	8
Longitudinal coupling factor: k_{33}	0.1	0.7	0.7	0.38	0.19
Piezoelectric constant: d_{33}	2	290	370	85	17.5
Dissipation (loss) factor: $\tan \delta$	10^{-4}	0.004	0.02	0.01	—
Characteristic acoustic impedance: Z (10^6 Rayl)	15.2	34.5	33.7	20	3.4

stability) over a wide range of spot frequencies, but it is generally unsuitable for diagnostic or dosimetric applications.

The ferroelectric ceramics, such as the lead zirconate-titanates, have relatively high electromechanical coupling coefficients and are appreciably sensitive off resonance, with corresponding potential for at least moderate bandwidth operation. Their high dielectric coefficient implies that even quite small devices can be made without impracticably high values of electrical impedance, and their electromechanical coupling factors (strain per unit applied charge density, or electric field per unit applied stress) can be typically nearly 10 times greater than the corresponding values for quartz. For such reasons, together with their potential for being machined to required shapes, these materials have become very widely used in the generation and detection of acoustic fields of the type used in medical applications (O'Donnell et al. 1981; Kojima 1987; Foster et al. 1991; Ballato 1995). Particular forms of PZT are optimum for different applications: imaging, for example, calls for high sensitivity (e.g. PZT 5), whilst power generation requires low loss material (e.g. PZT 4).

Piezoceramics, nonetheless, have certain limitations, particularly in their extreme acoustical mismatch to human soft tissues and in their unsuitability for truly broadband application, and there is thus considerable interest in a class of piezoelectric plastic materials that exhibit some advantages in these areas. Permanent piezoelectric behaviour can be induced in several synthetic polymers, by means of polarization under high electric fields at elevated temperatures and, among these, polyvinylidene(di-)fluoride ('PVDF' or 'PVF2') is particularly useful (Ohigashi 1976; Swartz & Plummer 1980; Lancee et al. 1985; Lewin & Schafer 1988). An important drawback in the use of PVDF, in comparison with the PZTs, lies, however, in the appreciably lower values of its coupling factors. Thus, whilst it has found considerable use in hydrophone detectors (see Chapter 3), its relatively poor transmission behaviour has hitherto inhibited its widespread use for imaging and related applications. This situation may, however, change with the advent of new developments, an interesting example of which is the complex, multiple sandwich polymer design, described by Zhang and Lewin (1993), which appears to combine the features of high effective coupling with low loss, wide bandwidth and good acoustic impedance matching.

The fact that ferroelectrics can be cut, shaped and combined in a wide variety of ways has led to very flexible and powerful approaches to generation of acoustic fields. Some examples of such approaches will be described later but it will be useful first to discuss some features of one of the simplest and most basic arrangements: that of a single, circular disk transducer element. A typical form for this is shown in Figure 2.2. The disk is here positioned at the interface between two semi-infinite volumes of propagation medium, one of which might be water or a soft tissue and the other an isolation medium, which will commonly be air. Analytical treatments of such a projector are given in Chapter 1 (Section 1.6) for a plane disk and in Section 2.5 for the corresponding focused field.

The disk will inevitably require some means of mechanical support and the nature of this will depend on the intended application. For generation and detection of continuous wave or long pulse (tone burst) fields at a fixed acoustic frequency, a high-Q arrangement will give the most efficient operation and the disk can be supported at its rim only, and thus be 'air backed'. When working with short pulse (broadband) fields, however, a near-uniform frequency response is desirable and it is normal to attempt to damp out any resonance by coupling the disk (e.g. by epoxy casting) to a block of backing material which, ideally, should be matched to it in acoustic impedance. Commonly, an epoxy resin loaded with tungsten powder may be used for this purpose or, alternatively, a block of unpoled but otherwise identical ceramic.

It will be seen later that an important property of the backing should be that it heavily absorbs the backward-generated energy before the wave is reflected or scattered back

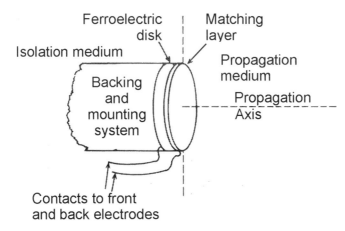

Figure 2.2. Essentials of a disk transducer assembly

(particularly in a coherent manner) to the disk. For this reason the shape and composition of a backing block require careful design.

The acoustic mismatch presented by piezoceramics to water and soft tissues leads to poor coupling of energy to and from the propagation medium (e.g., from Chapter 1, an impedance ratio of 14 will lead to a two-way loss of energy by a factor of 0.062, or −12 dB). To overcome this problem it is common practice to interpose one or more quarter-wave matching layers at the interface (Yamaguchi *et al.* 1986; Richter *et al.* 1987; Inoue *et al.* 1987). Such a matching layer will also serve to provide mechanical protection for the transducer electrode, and it should be made of a material that is adequately wettable, to avoid problems with a trapped air film (Section 1.7.3). Other approaches that have been investigated for solving the impedance matching problem are: to use so-called 'piezoelectric composite materials', which can have Z values much lower than those of simple ceramics (Gururaja *et al.* 1985); and to fabricate a matching layer to incorporate a random, 2D array of step-wedges (Seyed-Bolorforosh 1995).

Piezoelectric devices typically present complex electrical impedances, with multiresonant frequency spectra, for which appropriate equivalent circuits need to be found in order that the devices can be properly connected for drive input and signal extraction. The classical modelling work in this field, on which most subsequent work has been based, is that of Mason (1950), and useful summaries of this and later work have been given by Hunt *et al.* (1983), Capineri *et al.* (1993) and Lockwood and Foster (1994). A problem encountered with some array-configuration transducers (Section 2.7) is the rather high electrical impedance presented by each element, for which a possible solution is a multilayer structure whose components are arranged to operate acoustically in series and electrically in parallel (Goldberg & Smith 1994).

As discussed below, the characteristics of a field due to a particular projector will depend on the form (in time or frequency domain) of the applied electrical drive; with a first-order distinction being between CW and pulsed situations. In its simplest form, pulsed excitation is achieved by means of a very fast step function but, because of the resonant behaviour of the transducer, enhanced acoustic bandwidth can be achieved by the use of multiple electrical excitations, in such a manner as to stop the transducer ringing by adding more electrical signals of proper amplitudes and phases (Krautkramer & Krautkramer 1975).

Apart from the need, already mentioned, to provide proper acoustic backing, a number of special considerations arise in the construction of a transducer mounting. Electrically, the leads and electrodes will need to be capable of carrying high instantaneous currents (good connections, generally by low-temperature soldering will be important), and insulation must be adequate to withstand high applied fields and to be impermeable to water. Transducers intended for pulse–echo and detection use need to be very well screened electrically, since they may be required to handle significant signals at levels of the order of 10^{-12} W, and often to do so in electrically noisy environments. If metal casings are to be used for such electrical screening, however, it will be particularly important to ensure that they are very well acoustically isolated from the transducer element, since otherwise they will tend to function as rather efficient acoustic delay lines. An instructive account of an approach to optimising the design of pulse–echo transducers, and to documenting their performance, has been given by van Kervel and Thijssen (van Kervel & Thijssen 1983; Thijssen *et al.* 1985).

2.3   THE FIELDS OF 'SIMPLE', CW EXCITED SOURCES

As indicated above, and described in detail elsewhere (Lu *et al.* 1994), there exists a substantial hierarchy of directional acoustic fields, and it should be helpful here to start from a relatively simple and basic situation, and work outwards from that.

Simple theoretical treatments (and indeed much of that in Chapter 1) commonly assume that a transducer constructed on the above lines will vibrate as a simple piston, i.e. with uniform motion over the entire surface area of the transducer element. Generally this is a major oversimplification, for at least two reasons: first, a proportion of acoustic energy will appear as radial and flexural modes of vibration; and second, the mechanical mounting configuration may tend to clamp the element peripherally. This latter effect, which constitutes a form of apodisation or shading, may be advantageous since, as will be seen later, it will tend to reduce the proportion of energy that appears in sidelobes of the beam structure. Furthermore, it is not uncommon to find that flaws in manufacture (e.g. in adhesion of a backing or matching layer) can be the cause of markedly anomalous behaviour.

A second major assumption of most simple treatments of acoustic beam formation (although not that taken here, in Chapter 1) is that of continuous wave – CW – excitation. Provided, however, that the implications of this assumption are appreciated, the corresponding theoretical predictions are instructive and are indeed directly relevant to applications in both therapeutic and Doppler diagnostic ultrasound. Some examples of predictions for CW excited fields, due to a circular piston radiator, are shown in Figure 2.3. This indicates the tendency towards increased directionality (but also complexity) as the source aperture in terms of wavelengths (λ) is increased. It also demonstrates the division, somewhat arbitrarily bounded by the axial 'Frèsnel distance', a^2/λ, between the near field, or Frèsnel diffraction zone, with complex structure, and the far field, or Fraunhofer diffraction zone, in which the beam structure becomes simpler and axial intensity proceeds to decrease as the inverse square of distance.

The uniformly excited, plane circular source is a special case, although an important one. The subject of 'focusing' sources (i.e. with phase and/or amplitude variations induced over their aperture) is discussed in Section 2.5, and an illustration of the structure of a field due to a non-circular plane source (uniformly excited) is also shown in Figure 2.3. The important case of the field of a rectangular source is described by Ocheltree and

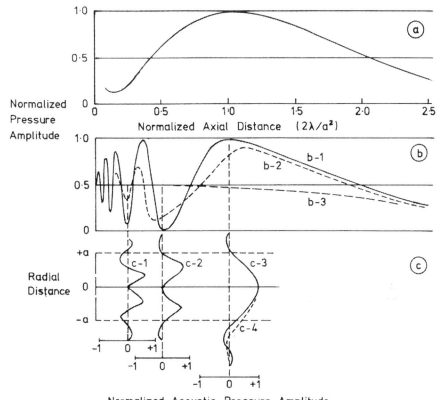

Figure 2.3. Predicted fields due to plane piston radiators
a: axial variation of pressure amplitude for a uniformly excited circular radiator of radius a, for
 which $a/\lambda = 1$
b-1: the same for a circular radiator with $a/\lambda = 5$
b-2: the same for a square radiator of side length s, with $s/2\lambda = 5$
b-3: the same for a circular radiator with $a/\lambda = 5$ and Gaussian apodisation
c: lateral variations of pressure amplitude at the indicated axial distances
 (c-1, c-2, c-3 correspond to curve b-1 and c-4 indicates the effect of some apodisation)

Frizzell (1989). Non-uniform excitation of the source may occur, deliberately or otherwise. In the form of 'apodisation' (excitation amplitude diminishing with increasing radial distance from the axis), this can have the effect of reducing, or even eliminating, side lobes. An interesting technical approach to amplitude apodisation that has been suggested is the manufacture of transducers with non-uniform distribution of piezoelectric coefficient (Chapeau-Blondeau *et al.* 1989).

  A further reason for interest in the structure of fields due to non-uniform sources arises from applications involving compound transducers where, for example, it may be necessary to operate two simple transducers coaxially, with one of them fitted into a hole cut into the centre of the other. Useful predictions of field distributions in such cases have been given by Clarke (1995).

2.4   THE PULSED ACOUSTIC FIELD

For applications involving short pulses, such as those encountered in the pulse–echo diagnostic technique, continuous wave theory fails to give an adequate account of the true situation, and a more general approach needs to be adopted. There are two alternatives. The first is to develop mathematically a single frequency, continuous wave solution for a particular source and then proceed to extend this across an appropriately defined frequency spectrum. The second possibility is to use an impulse response approach (i.e. the solution for an impulse in the time rather than in the frequency domain), from which the pulsed field (or indeed any continuous wave field) may be derived exactly.

This latter, impulse response approach was taken up and discussed in detail in Chapter 1. It will be useful here to recall some aspects of its practical outcome. As illustrated in Figure 1.5, the (in this case plane) source impulse gives rise to two (and sometimes more) separated field impulses: a plane wave that projects perpendicularly from the source shape and that continues undeviated and with constant amplitude to infinity; and a second wave that emerges from the edge or rim of the source, in antiphase with the above plane wave. In general, for interior field points (those within the volume projected by the source), there are three components and, for exterior points, two components, which may interfere depending on their relative positions and lengths (Stepanishen 1971, 1981). The second and third components are sometimes termed 'replica pulses' (Freedman 1970). Penttinen and Luakkala (1976) have extended the analysis to curved bowl sources, whilst Lockwood and Willette (1973) have similarly considered rectangular sources.

For some applications there will be practical advantage in partially suppressing one of these components. Apodising (shading off radially) is used to suppress the edge wave (related to sidelobe structure), whereas annular transducers have been constructed to perform as predominantly edge-wave sources. The interrogation field for a circular pulsed source may consist of three, five or six components (Weight & Hayman 1978).

2.5   FOCUSED FIELDS

The discussion hitherto has been concerned very largely with acoustic fields resulting from 'plane wave' sources: i.e. from sources containing an aperture plane of constant phase. This is, however, in a sense a special case, which happens to be of interest for the somewhat arbitrary reasons: (1) that flat transducers tend to be easy to make (and when quartz is used as the piezoelectric material it is necessary to work with the natural crystal plane); and (2) that analytical theory tends to be more tractable for plane than for curved surfaces. In general, however, the optimum fields for particular applications are often not those that result from uniform plane-wave sources.

Controlled departure from uniformity of either excitation or response over a source aperture – apodisation – has already been mentioned as a method of suppressing edge waves (which may also be manifested as side lobes in a continuous wave beam), thereby modifying the field structure, and in this sense can be considered as a means of achieving a degree of focusing. An extreme example of non-uniform excitation is the 'edge-wave only' (EWO) transducer (see Section 2.5.4), which can achieve useful advantage in spatial resolution at a selected depth, although at some cost in sensitivity and, presumably, in sidelobe level and thus contrast discrimination (Brittain & Weight 1987). Apodisation is an important phenomenon which is often overlooked in this context. Its precise effect on the field will, of course, depend on the particular form used: some illustrative examples have been given in Figure 2.3.

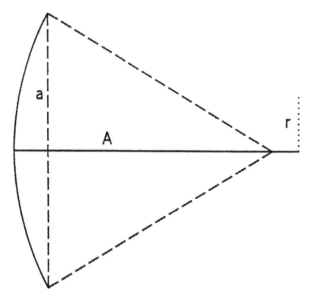

Figure 2.4. Geometry for focusing due to a circular, concave spherically curved projector

A more conventional, if narrower, connotation of focusing is that corresponding to the effects of specific departures from uniform phase over a source aperture. In practice this can be achieved by a number of means: physical shaping of the primary source element (e.g. a piezoceramic or piezoplastic), electrical introduction of appropriate phase shifts between individual elements of a multielement source, acoustic mirrors and acoustic lenses (which will generally introduce additionally a degree of apodisation due to attenuation in the lens material). It will be seen that there are important differences between each of these four approaches.

As in optics, there is a tendency to think of spherical as being the most 'natural' form for an acoustic focusing surface, and it is important to bear in mind that the common use of the spherical surface generally comes about because it can be easier to make, rather than because it is inherently better than alternative surfaces. That being said, however, it is also true that many practical focusing systems have rather modest aperture/wavelength ratios, for which the practical difference between an 'ideal' and a spherical surface becomes unimportant. Exceptions to this occur for some wide-angle focusing systems (e.g. as used in acoustic microscopy – see Chapter 11), in mirror focusing (where, for example, combinations of ellipsoidal and hyperboloidal mirrors may be used, as proposed by Oloffson 1963), and in axicon systems, as described below.

The diffractive field due to a uniformly, harmonically excited, spherically curved circular acoustic radiator has been rigorously calculated by O'Neil (1949), with results that agree well with experimental measurement, under near-linear conditions of propagation. The geometry of the situation is defined by Figure 2.4 and, to an approximation that is good within the region of interest around the focus, O'Neil's results can conveniently be expressed in terms of two dimensionless parameters:

the geometrical aperture $S = a/A$
the wave aperture $K = 2\pi a/\lambda$

His results for radial and axial dependencies of particle pressure amplitude and intensity in the focal region can be summarised as follows.

2.5.1 RADIAL DEPENDENCIES

The variation of particle pressure amplitude, normalised to the on-axis value, in the focal plane is given by:

$$F_0(Z) = 2Z^{-1}J_1(Z) \tag{2.1}$$

where J_1 is a Bessel function and $Z = KR$ where $R = r/A$ (the normalised radial coordinate).

From this it follows, for example, that the commonly used measure of the 'width' of the beam in the focal plane, defined as the distance between the first off-axis intensity minima, is given by:

$$D = 2r_0 = 1.22\lambda A/a \tag{2.2}$$

Also, since from Chapter 1 intensity is proportional to the vector product of particle velocity and pressure, which vectors are co-linear in the focal plane, normalised intensity is simply given by $F_0^2(Z)$.

The forms of $F_0(Z)$ and $F_0^2(Z)$ are shown in Figure 2.5. $F_0(Z)$ is, identically, the directivity function for a plane circular piston at large distance from the piston (*cf.* Figure 2.3, c-3). This result enables the calculation of an intensity gain of such a focusing radiator, relative to the intensity at the Frèsnel distance of a plane circular radiator of the same aperture radius, as:

$$H_F = S^2 K^2/4\pi^2 \tag{2.3}$$

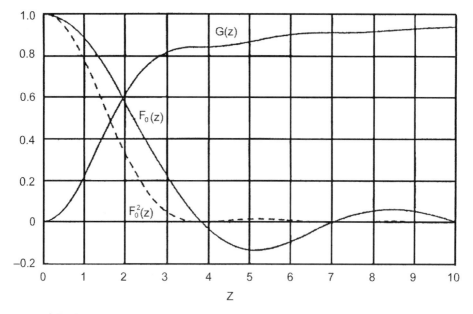

Figure 2.5. Dependence on the parameter Z of the functions $F(Z)$ and $G(Z)$ – see text

O'Neil also derives, as shown in Figure 2.5, the quantity:

$$G(Z) = 1 - J_0^2(Z) - J_1^2(Z) \tag{2.4}$$

which is the fraction of the total acoustic power that traverses that circle in the focal plane defined by the parameter Z.

It follows that we can define an alternative expression for 'intensity gain', in this case relative to intensity at the projector surface, but now with a need to qualify focal intensity, e.g. as spatially averaged within the Z-contour corresponding to a specified $F(Z)$ (e.g. 0.5). Thus:

$$H(F(Z)) = S^2 K^2 G(Z)/Z^2 \tag{2.5}$$

2.5.2 AXIAL DEPENDENCIES

O'Neil expresses variations in the axial value of pressure and intensity as functions of a parameter D, which in turn is a function of normalised axial position. Physically D is a normalised measure of the difference in the path lengths to the transducer surface, from any point on the axis, as between the edge ray and the axial ray, thus being positive within the radius of curvature and negative beyond. Hence, again to a good approximation, the value of pressure amplitude normalised to that at the centre of curvature is given by:

$$P/P_A = 4\{(D + S^2/2)/KSD(1 + D/2)\} \ \sin(KD/2S) \tag{2.6}$$

where the normalised axial distance is:

$$X = 1 - D(1 + D/2)/(D + S^2/2) \tag{2.7}$$

Away from the focal plane the particle pressure and velocity vectors can no longer be assumed to be co-linear and intensity departs by a certain factor, M, from proportionality to the square of pressure. Hence the corresponding normalised intensity is:

$$I/I_A = M(P/P_A)^2 =$$
$$16\{(D + S^2/2)^2 \ \sin^2(KD/2S)\}/\{SK^2 D^2(1 + D/2)^2(S + SD + D^2)\} \tag{2.8}$$

Illustrations of the axial variations of pressure and intensity, and their dependence on the parameters S and K are given in Figures 2.6a,b and 2.6c respectively.

A number of observations may be made at this point:

(a) The process of 'focusing' can only be considered to have clear value and meaning for curvature radii smaller than the Frèsnel distance.
(b) The point of maximum pressure or intensity (one possible candidate for the definition of 'focal length') always falls somewhat inside the radius of curvature.
(c) Some very substantial values of 'intensity gain', however defined, are practically achievable.

O'Neil's treatment, as presented here, has the merit of being analytically tractable and, thus, illustratively useful. Fields of interest in practical application may, however, entail departures from the simple conditions assumed here, and in particular:

(a) Transducers may be required with non-circular apertures.

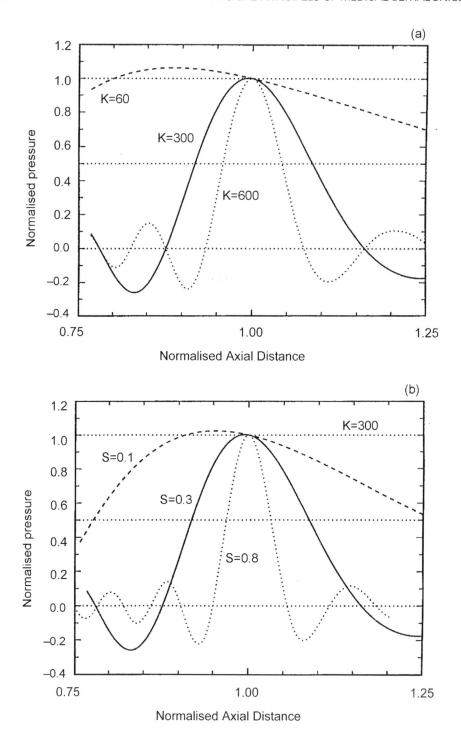

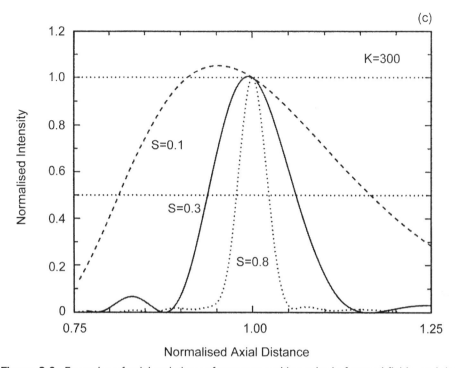

Figure 2.6. Examples of axial variations of pressure and intensity in focused fields, and their dependence on the parameters K and S – see text

(b) Departures from uniform excitation may arise, often deliberately, e.g. through deliberate amplitude apodisation (as previously mentioned), or through a practical need to remove a central portion of a large 'bowl'.

(c) Some form of phase apodisation may be applied.

(d) A special case, combining elements of (b) and (c), is that of lens focusing, which is discussed further in Section 2.4.1. A useful treatment of the fields corresponding to these more general examples of focusing by a circular radiator has been given by Clarke (1995).

(e) In considering the nature of focused fields it becomes very important to take into account the consequences of departure from linearity in propagation (Section 1.8). Rosenberg (1962) considered this topic in a classical paper where he pointed out, *inter alia*, that non-linearity of propagation imposes a finite upper limit to the acoustic power that can be transmitted through a region of high intensity. Lucas and Muir (1982, 1983) extended O'Neil's calculations to take into account second harmonic components and, in so doing, developed a more tractable formulation using a single, rather than double integral. The subject has been discussed more recently by Reilly and Parker (1989) and has also been investigated theoretically, for the important condition of a propagation medium with tissue-like properties, by Swindell (1985), and experimentally by Duck and Starritt (1986), and is further considered in Section 2.7.

(f) Finally, the above analysis only applies directly to continuous wave fields of specific acoustic frequency. In the important case of short pulse excitation there will be modifications to both the radial and axial field distributions, corresponding to the extended frequency bandwidth, with, as a general rule, reduction in the peak amplitudes and in complexity of sidelobe structure (Penttinen & Luakkala 1976; Djelouah *et al.* 1991).

2.5.3 LENS FOCUSING

Conversion from a plane to a converging wave front can be achieved by an acoustic lens. Commonly this is constructed from a solid material that will generally, but not invariably, exhibit a propagation speed higher than that of a water-like loading medium (although liquid lenses, contained between thin curved membranes, have also been used), and may thus have plano-concave form, as shown in Figure 2.7. If the concave surface is spherical, the modified wave front will also be spherical, to an approximation that is good for small apertures. To this extent the situation is equivalent to that described above for fields due to spherically curved transducers if the equivalent radius of curvature is taken as the value derived from ray geometry calculation based on Snell's law, i.e.

$$r_0 = R/(1 - \eta) \tag{2.9}$$

where $\eta = C_2/C_1$, the ratio of sound speed in the loading medium to that in the lens. In practice, however, commonly useful lens materials will exhibit some degree of attenuation, thus leading, for generally concave lenses, to a corresponding degree of apodisation, with consequences indicated above.

   As pointed out in relation to scanning acoustic microscopy systems (Chapter 11), spherical aberration for a given relative aperture reduces as η decreases: an effect that can be understood physically from the consideration that, with increasingly high values of C_1, the wave front transmitted by the lens approximates increasingly to its concave spherical surface (see Fry & Dunn 1962 for a more rigorous discussion of this point). Unfortunately this requirement for a low value of η conflicts with the criterion for minimisation of internal reflections: that of a good acoustic match with the loading medium and thus a correspondingly low density; a combination of properties that seems not to occur in usable materials. The difficulty is partly overcome if the lens material has appreciable attenuation, but this in turn leads to problems either in sensitivity of diagnostic systems or actually in heating and potential distortion or melting of the lens itself in power applications. In practice, cross-linked polystyrene provides a useful compromise as a water-interfaced lens for many applications. Polymethylmethacrylate ('Perspex'/'Plexiglass'), which has a slightly higher sound speed but considerably higher absorption coefficient, is also sometimes used. Fuller accounts of lens focusing have been given by Fry and Dunn (1962), Jones and Kwan (1985) and Beaver *et al.*

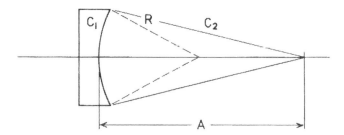

Figure 2.7. Geometrical definition for discussion of acoustic lens focusing

(1977). Weyns (1980a, b) gives an instructive comparative treatment of the fields of pulsed acoustic radiators having various shapes and focusing parameters.

2.5.4 EDGE WAVES AND AXICON FIELDS: LIMITED DIFFRACTION FIELDS

The formation of spherically converging wave fronts is not the only means by which it is possible to achieve strongly directional acoustic beams with desirable properties for particular applications. In the particular case of pulse–echo diagnostics, for example, there is often a need for beams that have a rather uniformly narrow profile over a large depth of focus. A class of beam-forming elements that is of interest here is illustrated in Figure 2.8.

Consider first the thin strip, BB′, of the surface of the truncated cone AC. If this acts as a projector of a short pulse, it will launch a toroidal wave whose circumferential components will combine in phase only along the axis of the cone, from which the echoes may then be recorded by operating the strip as a receiver. Since this device has a large relative aperture over a proportion of the axis comparable to the diameter of the circular strip, its effective field can be expected to have a central peak width comparable to a wavelength over this portion. The properties of such 'edge-wave' transducers (*cf.* Section 2.4) have been investigated by Weight (1984) but tend in practice to lack sensitivity.

We can now, however, consider what is in effect an extension of this device: a transducer extending over the full truncated conical surface AC. If this is used as a projector (or receiver, or both), its field will be built up by a wave front diverging from (or converging to) the cone AC and again combining in phase spatially at the axis, and temporally at that point on the axis for which the distance to the axis along a normal to the conical surface (e.g. DO) corresponds to the propagation time. A good analysis of the fields of such devices is given by Patterson and Foster (1983). The term 'axicon', which was first used in optics, is applied to devices of this kind, and to related 'mirror axicons', in which one or more appropriately shaped mirrors are

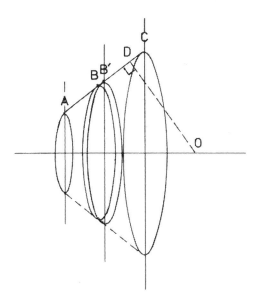

Figure 2.8. Geometrical definition for discussion of edge-wave and axicon fields

used, in combination with a plane or curved transducer, to generate a conical wave front (Burckhardt *et al.* 1973). In general, axicons are found to be able to achieve a diffraction-limited (near one wavelength for large relative aperture) central maximum over a considerable depth of focus although, at least in their simple form, they suffer from predictably high sidelobe levels when compared with spherically focusing systems. The performance of one particularly interesting design of axicon is described in Section 2.8.

Edge-wave and axicon fields can be seen as special case approximations to the more general class of limited diffraction beams, that have been extensively explored by Lu and Greenleaf (Lu & Greenleaf 1994; Lu *et al.* 1994). Such beams are at present largely theoretical concepts, generated from non-spherical, converging wave fronts, and have the property of an approximately unchanged beam shape over a large axial distance. This behaviour is of potential interest in applications requiring rather precise image-data reconstruction, such as transmission reconstruction imaging, and some related forms of tissue characterisation where it is desirable to eliminate the need for diffraction corrections.

2.6   EFFECTS OF THE HUMAN BODY ON BEAM PROPAGATION

One of the beauties of ultrasound as a basis for medical imaging and related technologies is that the perturbation experienced by wave fronts on propagation through much soft tissue anatomy is sufficiently small that refraction and defocusing artefacts can often be neglected. There are, however, situations where these effects may become significant and where, correspondingly, attempts have been made to develop compensatory techniques. Examples of such situations are where propagation takes place through fatty tissues, such as the breast (Hinkelman *et al.* 1995), or through the skin/fat/muscle complex of the abdominal surface (Hinkelman *et al.* 1994). Implementation of such techniques is generally based on transducer array technology and further reference to the topic is made in Chapter 9.

2.7   BEAM FORMATION BY TRANSDUCER ARRAYS

Hitherto the discussion of this chapter has been based on the formation of beams by transducers having a constant pattern of phase exitation (and/or sensitivity) over their surfaces. A considerable increase in flexibility results, however, if it is possible to vary and control the phase relationships over the transducer surface: in practice this can be achieved by physically dividing the surface into a number of separate elements and introducing between them relative phase shifts in the transmitted or received waveforms (or both), in such a way as to give rise to any desired shape in a wave front. A theoretical discussion of this arrangement was presented in Section 1.6.6. Since it is possible to vary very rapidly (e.g. in 10^{-6} s) such electronically determined phase relationships, the beam direction and focusing characteristics can be varied with corresponding speed, e.g. to hold in the receiving focus of a transducer a wave packet that is receding at the speed of sound following projection from the same transducer (Manes *et al.* 1988).

By comparison with the form- and lens-focusing of single element transducers, described above, beam formation by arrays has a further degree of flexibility in that it is not restricted to wave fronts corresponding to simple physical surfaces (e.g. spheres or cones) which are mechanically easy to generate. However, there is also a physical cost (quite apart from a financial cost, which can be considerable), in that the induced phase variations over the wave fronts at the transducer become discontinuous: a factor that generally leads to undesirable modifications in the acoustic field structure (e.g. 'grating lobes'). With this qualification, however, arrays can be seen physically as alternative means of producing aplanar wave fronts, to which much of the above discussion for single element 'focusing' will apply. In discussing particular forms of array, it is convenient to consider three different classes: linear, annular and two-dimensional matrices.

Linear arrays, which are in almost universal use, are typically made up of a series of rectangular elements mounted as an adjacent series (and generally cut from a single block) as indicated in Figure 2.9a. In their simplest application, stepped beam operation, no phase shift is introduced between the elements, and they are simply combined as groups, e.g. elements 1 to k, 2 to $(k + 1)$, ..., $(n + 1 - k)$ to n, thus laterally shifting (by increments of one element spacing) the unfocused beam due to k adjacent elements. In this application the element spacing is determined only by the need to provide adequate spatial sampling frequency in the acoustic field and to suppress the appearance of raster in the image (see Chapter 8).

Achievement of beam steering and focusing by an array imposes more severe constraints on its construction. In this case the directivity of each element must be broad enough (i.e. its width small enough) that the full steering angle (e.g. 40°) can be encompassed within an acceptable gain variation, say 6 dB. At the same time, however, this directivity must be sufficient to provide adequate discrimination against unwanted lobes (Moshfeghi 1987). The design of arrays for this type of operation is a complex topic, of which good accounts have been given by Miller and Thurstone (1977) and Vogel *et al.* (1979). In some respects, the design

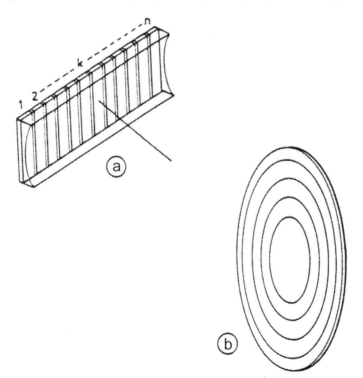

Figure 2.9. Main types of transducer array: (a) linear array (shown with a cylindrical lens, to provide focusing normal to the scan plane); (b) annular array

and construction of transducer arrays may be simplified by the use of piezoelectric polymers (Kimura *et al.* 1985) or, in extending the technology to frequencies of the order of 100 MHz, films incorporating zinc oxide (Ito *et al.* 1995).

Hybrids between the simple stepped array and the fully phase steered and focused system are also becoming common. In these, a degree of focusing is induced by introducing appropriate phase shifts between the elements of a stepped group; additionally, some systems may also introduce a slight degree of beam deflection as a step leading to partial decoherence of the interrogation field.

Strict linear geometry in arrays has proved inconvenient in some clinical applications, particularly in the abdomen, where it may be required to introduce a beam below an acoustic obstacle such as a rib. For this reason, convexly curved 'linear' arrays have been developed, having electronic compensation for the departure from conventional linear geometry.

A potentially valuable feature of array systems is the opportunity that they provide for interactive signal processing. A suggested example of this using linear arrays is the on-line correction of refraction artefacts that arise from propagation through tissue layers (Smith *et al.* 1986).

An obvious limitation of linear arrays is that any beam shaping and steering can only take place in one plane: that normal to the long axes of the elements. Short of going to a 2D array, any out-of-plane focusing must be obtained by means of a lens or, what may be more difficult to implement, by use of appropriately curved elements.

Partly to address this problem, and as a relatively low-cost approach to 2D geometry, there has been some interest in developing annular array transducers (Figure 2.9b). Their principles have been well described in the literature (Melton & Thurstone 1978; Dietz *et al.* 1979; Arditi *et al.* 1982; Foster *et al.* 1989a, b), but they have not found very substantial use. Briefly, an annular transducer consists of a series of concentric annular elements, together forming a surface which may be plane or curved. Introduction of appropriate phase shifts between the projected or received waveforms (or both) from each element can, in principle, give rise to a wave front with circular aperture and any desired shape. In practice, wave fronts are required to be spherical, or nearly so, and optimum design calls for: (a) minimum phase shift over the aperture and hence the use of fixed geometrical focusing (by means of a lens, or shaping of the array itself) to give zero phase shift over the aperture for mid-point focusing, and (b) equal phase shift between adjacent elements, leading to an array in the form of a conventional Frèsnel zone plate, having annuli with relative outer diameters progressing in the series $1:\sqrt{2}:\sqrt{3}:$ . . . etc., and the different annuli all being of equal superficial area. Arditi *et al.* (1982) have shown that arrays designed in this way can generate acoustic fields that correspond well with predictions of diffraction theory as outlined in Chapter 1.

Proposals that have been made for enhancing the performance of simple annular arrays include the use of non-spherical geometry (Song & Park 1989) and a so-called 'non-diffracting' design, achieved by non-uniform excitation of the various array elements (Lu & Greenleaf 1990). The practical benefit of using annular arrays is strongly dependent, however, on use of a large relative aperture. This can be substantially limited by two important factors: the availability of correspondingly large anatomical acoustic windows, giving access to the target region, and the aperture dependence of tissue refraction artefacts (Moshfeghi & Waag 1988; Fishell *et al.* 1990).

More ambitious, and potentially powerful, is the fully two-dimensional array, on which considerable development work has taken place (Turnbull & Foster 1991; Smith *et al.* 1991, 1992). The problem of the high potential cost of such technology may be capable of some alleviation by the judicious use of sparse designs (Davidsen *et al.* 1994). Successful implementation of 2D array technology would clearly offer very interesting potential for interactive signal processing, an example of which is the possibility of automatic compensation for blocked areas of an acoustic access window, for example due to intervening bone or gas: currently a common cause of image degradation (Li & O'Donnell 1994).

2.8   THE FIELD OF THE TORONTO HYBRID

The foregoing has dealt with a variety of aspects of the formation and structure of acoustic fields, and with the role in this of both geometric and electronic shaping of wave fronts. In this section we shall briefly describe a system that, although it has never progressed beyond laboratory experiment, illustrates in an interesting way some of the principles that have been discussed above.

The system, designed in Toronto by Patterson *et al.* (Patterson *et al.* 1982, 1983; Foster *et al.* 1983) was intended for use in imaging the breast: an application where scanning is performed through a water delay path so that the usable depth of focus is about 90% of the minimum working range. The outcome was a hybrid system, as illustrated in Figure 2.10, in which the projector is a spherically prefocused, five-element annular array employing piezoceramic material, and the receiver is an eight-element cone employing piezoplastic. The interrogation field thus exhibits a combination of the features of the two different arrangements and, in particular, the narrow main lobe but high sidelobe level characteristic of the wide aperture axicon focusing of the receiver.

The system, however, offers several interesting approaches to sidelobe reduction. The first of these is electronically to apodise the wave front due to the annular array, by applying different excitation pulse amplitudes to the various annular elements; this is found to be effective, particularly if the number of annular elements is fairly large and the inter-element spacing is small. Another approach is 'antifocusing', in which a composite 'error' signal, due only to sidelobe echoes, is formed by adding in antiphase signals from alternate sectors of the conical receiving array, and is then, following detection, subtracted from the summation signal from all eight sectors. Thirdly, the authors note that the individual signals for the eight cone sectors are very similar for a target on the axis, but change rapidly in shape and arrival time as the target is moved off-centre. In line with this observation they have been able to show considerable reduction in off-axis sensitivity resulting from the process of multiplying together the signals from all eight sectors, and then taking the eighth root to restore linearity.

It will be seen that this system combines, in a novel and illuminating way, most of the major concepts that have been considered in this chapter: apodisation, form focusing in both spherical and aspherical geometry, and beam shaping by electronic control of phase. Additionally, of course, the pulsed nature of the fields generated by such a system is an important factor in determining their calculated and observed behaviour. The discussion here also impinges on themes that will be taken up in more detail in Chapter 9. In particular, it will be seen there that one potential advantage of the segmental receiving arrangement should be in the reduction of the effect of coherent speckle: a form of image noise (see Chapter 8, below, and also Patterson *et al.* 1982). One might also comment here that the sidelobe reduction signal processing procedures appear to be examples of the more general principle of so-called minimum entropy signal processing (Mesdag *et al.* 1982).

2.9   GENERATION OF THERAPY FIELDS

The various, actual and potential, therapeutic uses of ultrasound are dealt with in detail in Chapter 13, where it is shown that the underlying biology and biophysics are often complex,

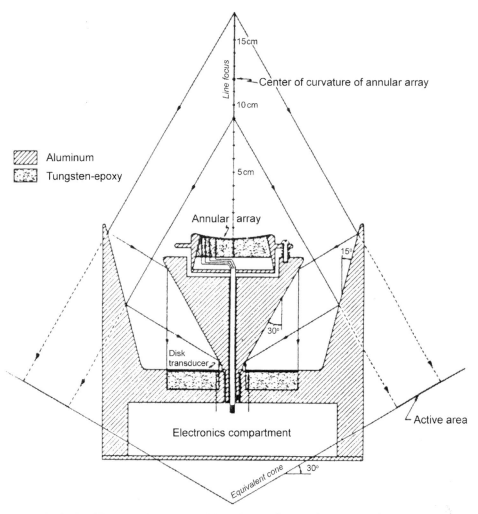

Figure 2.10. The 'Toronto hybrid scanner': lateral view. *Source*: Reproduced from Patterson and Foster (1983), published by Elsevier

and that the precise requirements that may be placed on projected fields intended for use in therapeutic exposure of tissues are still rather incompletely defined.

A considerable variety of therapeutic strategies may exist but many of these are primarily aimed at achieving a specific temperature increase within a target region whilst minimising any corresponding rise elsewhere. Such temperature distributions will be determined by two factors: instantaneous spatial distribution of energy deposition, set predominantly by acoustic beam profiles such as those described in Sections 2.3 and 2.5, and time-dependent redistribution of heat consequent on thermal diffusion and vascular perfusion. In general, such thermal redistribution effects will be of importance only for exposures of more than a few seconds duration (Hill *et al.* 1994). Thus, for strategies employing brief but intense exposures, the peak of the acoustic field will need to conform fairly well to the target tissue volume (e.g. a

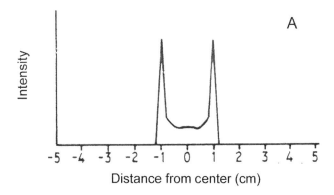

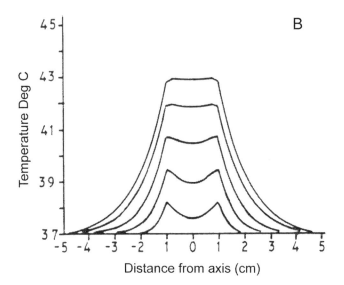

Figure 2.11. Illustration of heat redistribution in human soft tissue: (a) cross-section through a circular intensity distribution calculated to yield a uniform temperature elevation in a plane region of (non-vascularised) muscle 2 cm in diameter, after 30 min of ultrasonic exposure; (b) calculated temperature elevations following exposure as above for successive 2-min. periods; bottom line 2 min. top line 30 min. *Source*: From Hynynen *et al.* (1981), reproduced by permission of Elsevier

tumour), either in a single exposure or by laying down a suitably designed array of exposures. For prolonged exposures, on the other hand, the resulting temperature distribution will be, in effect, a convolution of the acoustic beam profile with a thermal redistribution function. As illustrated in Figure 2.11, this may call for a bimodal distribution of acoustic energy delivery. This, in turn, may be achieved physically either by designing a transducer to produce an appropriate field shape (Hynynen *et al.* 1981; Umemura & Cain 1992; Clarke 1995) or by scanning in time a more conventional beam over an appropriate path, either mechanically

(Lele & Parker 1982) or by means of a phased array transducer (Benkesser *et al.* 1987; Diederich & Hynynen 1991; Yoon & Benkesser 1992; Fan & Hynynen 1996).

As with diagnostic fields (Section 2.6), attenuation and refraction in overlying tissues can, in some circumstances, have an important influence on the *in situ* characteristics of therapeutic fields, both because of wave reflection and refraction at soft tissue interfaces (Fan & Hynynen 1992) and because of forward scattering that results in acoustic energy being transferred from the main lobe of the beam into side lobes (Moros & Hynynen 1992).

A fundamental problem in ultrasound beam therapy (as, of course, it is also in most forms of ionising radiation therapy) is the fall-off in depth with intensity, and thus of energy deposition rate, that occurs owing to attenuation of the incident beam. For tissue volumes whose dimensions lateral to the beam correspond to a few wavelengths, this problem can be overcome by focusing but, where much larger areas are to be treated, and scanning the beam over the treated area thus becomes necessary, this particular advantage of focusing is at least partially negated. Some alleviation of this problem may, however, be obtainable by deliberately creating strongly non-linear propagation conditions in a high-intensity focus, thereby transferring energy locally to higher harmonics with correspondingly higher absorption coefficients. The magnitude of this effect that can be expected under practically interesting conditions has been calculated by Swindell (1985), some of whose predictions are illustrated in Figure 2.12.

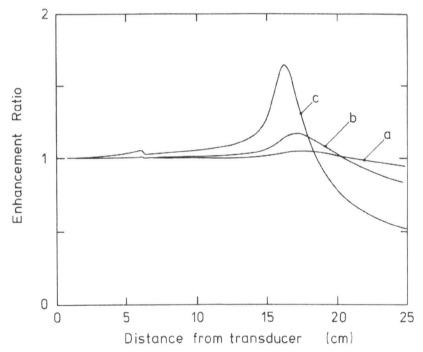

Figure 2.12. Plots of the enhancement in absorbed power density in an ultrasonic beam that results from finite amplitude ('non-linear') propagation, and illustrating the phenomenon of the 'acoustic Bragg peak'. The data are calculated for a 1 MHz spherically focused transducer of aperture diameter 12 cm and radius of curvature 16 cm, transmitting through an initial 6 cm water path into a tissue of absorption coefficient 0.5 dB cm^{-1}. Emitted intensities at the surface of the transducer for the three curves are: (a) 1.0, (b) 3.0 and (c) 10.0 W cm^{-2}

In therapeutic, as indeed in diagnostic, uses of ultrasound, selection of the appropriate acoustic frequency for a particular application is essential for optimum outcome; in general there is a trade-off between strength of ultrasound–tissue interaction at the target site and attenuation in overlying tissues, both of which will be frequency dependent. An analysis of the situation for focused ultrasound surgery has led to the 'rule-of-thumb' that optimum frequency will approximate to that which results in overlying tissue attenuation totalling 10 dB (Hill 1994).

Not all therapeutic applications of ultrasound are based primarily on exploiting thermal mechanisms of achieving tissue modification and an interesting exception is extracorporeal lithotripsy, which is reliant on the localised production of impulses of very high pressure amplitude. A good physical description of the fields achieved in this application has been given by Coleman and Saunders (1993). In this situation extreme conditions of non-linear propagation may arise and it is of interest to note here (Dalecki *et al.* 1991) that acoustic absorption may become predominantly determined by the non-linear properties of the medium, with relatively weak dependence on 'classical' small-signal absorption coefficient.

2.10 MAGNITUDES OF ACOUSTIC FIELD VARIABLES

Hitherto, in both this and the previous chapter, discussion has been rather general. In particular, however, expressions have been derived for a number of quantities that can be used to characterise acoustic fields: particle displacement (ξ), particle velocity (u), particle acceleration (a), particle pressure (p) and condensation (s). It has also been shown that, in the linear approximation, these quantities can often, in principle, be used interchangeably. It will be useful at this stage therefore to summarise the quantitative relationships between these different variables. As will become apparent in subsequent chapters, there are a number of practical medical applications of ultrasound in which finite amplitude ('non-linear') propagation phenomena can be of substantial importance. It will nonetheless generally remain the case that the linear approximation relationships represent a reasonable approximation to reality, and at least give a useful feel for the numbers involved.

A useful presentation of such relationships for plane progressive waves was provided in an early publication by Fry and Dunn (1962), which is no longer readily accessible but from which the following has now been adapted. From the definitions of the acoustic wave variables that have been derived in Section 1.3, it follows that, for a harmonic, plane progressive wave of wave frequency $f = \omega/2\pi$, in the linear approximation, the magnitudes of the different variables are interrelated in the manner indicated in Table 2.2.

Table 2.2. Relationships between acoustic wave variables (see text for conditions of applicability)

	ξ (m)	u (m s^{-1})	p (Pa)	s
Particle displacement (ξ)	1			
Particle velocity (u)	$j\omega$	1		
Particle pressure (p)	$j\omega\rho_0 C*$	$\rho_0 C*$	1	
Condensation (s)	$j\omega/C$	$1/C$	$1/\rho_0 C^2$ *	1
Particle acceleration (a)	$-\omega^2$	$j\omega$	$j\omega/\rho_0 C*$	$j\omega C$

Multiply expressions in the table by the appropriate column heading to obtain the equivalent for a variable listed in the first column. For expressions marked *, the value takes a negative sign for waves travelling in the negative direction.

Table 2.3. Numerical examples of the corresponding amplitudes of the acoustic variables of a plane, progressive harmonic wave in water (at 30°C and normal atmospheric pressure)

Acoustic frequency (MHz)	I (W cm^{-2} or W m^{-2} × 10^4)	P (atm, Pa × 10^5)	D (m × 10^{-8})	U (m s^{-1})	S (× 10^{-4})	A (m s^{-2} × 10^6)
1	1	1.71	1.83	0.115	0.762	0.722
1	100	17.1	18.3	1.15	7.62	7.22
10	1	1.71	0.183	0.115	0.762	7.22
10	100	17.1	1.83	1.15	7.62	72.2

Examples illustrating relationships between the corresponding numerical amplitudes of these quantities are given in Table 2.3, which also lists the quantity acoustic intensity (I), as previously defined in equations (1.41) and (1.42). It will be seen from these equations that the numerical value of an intensity will depend on the value assigned to the integration limit in equation (1.41). It is conventional, and generally convenient, to take this to correspond to an integral number of acoustic cycles, in which case we have, in particular for a harmonic wave:

$$I \equiv \tfrac{1}{2}PU = \tfrac{1}{2}P^2/\rho_0 C \tag{2.10}$$

where P, U are the amplitudes of the particle pressure and velocity fluctuations.

The data in this table nicely illustrate, incidentally, the dictum that 'ultrasound is all acceleration and no movement'.

REFERENCES

Arditi, M., Taylor, W.B., Foster, F.S. and Hunt, J.W. (1982). An annular array system for high resolution breast echography. *Ultrasonic Imaging* **4**, 1–31.

Ballato, A. (1995). Piezoelectricity: old effects, new thrusts. *IEEE Trans*. **UFFC-42**, 916–926.

Beaver, W.L., Dameron, D.H. and Macorski, A. (1977). Ultrasonic imaging with an acoustic lens. *IEEE Trans*. **SU-24**, 235–243.

Benkesser, P.J., Frizzell, L.A., Ocheltree, K.B. and Cain, C.A. (1987). A tapered phased array ultrasound transducer for hyperthermia treatment. *IEEE Trans*. **UFFC-34**, 446–453.

Berlincourt, D.A., Curran, D.R. and Jaffe, H. (1964). Piezoelectric and piezomagnetic materials and their function in transducers. In *Physical Acoustics* Vol. 1A, W. P. Mason (ed.). Academic Press, New York, pp. 169–270.

Brittain, R.H. and Weight, J.P. (1987). Fabrication of non-uniformly excited wide-band ultrasonic transducers. *Ultrasonics* **25**, 100–106.

Burckhardt, C.B., Hoffman, H. and Grandchamp, P.A. (1973). The ultrasound axicon: a device for focusing over a large depth. *J. Acoust. Soc. Amer*. **54**, 1628–1630.

Capineri, L., Masotti, L., Rinceri, M. and Rocchi, S. (1993). Ultrasonic transducer as a black box: equivalent circuit synthesis and matching network design. *IEEE Trans*. **UFFC 40**, 694–703.

Chapeau-Blondeau, F., Greenleaf, J.F., Harrison, W.B. and Hanson, M.R.B. (1989). An experimental study of acoustoelectric transducers with non-uniform distribution of the piezoelectric coefficient. *J. Acoust. Soc. Amer*. **86**, 1223–1229.

Clarke, R.L. (1995). Modification of intensity distributions from large aperture ultrasound sources. *Ultrasound in Med. & Biol*. **21**, 253–263.

Coleman, A.J. and Saunders, J.E. (1993). A review of the physical properties and biological effects of the high amplitude acoustic fields used in extracorporeal lithotripsy. *Ultrasonics* **31**, 75–89.

Dalecki, D., Carstensen, E.L., Parker, K.J. and Bacon, D.R. (1991). Absorption of finite amplitude focused ultrasound. *J. Acoust. Soc. Am.* **89**, 2435–2447.

Davidsen, R.E., Jensen, J.A. and Smith, S.W. (1994). Two dimensional random arrays for real time volumetric imaging. *Ultrasonic Imaging* **16**, 143–163.

Diederich, C.J. and Hynynen, K. (1991). The feasibility of using electrically focussed ultrasound arrays to induce deep hyperthermia via body cavities. *IEEE Trans.* **UFFC-38**, 207–219.

Dietz, D.R., Parks, S.I. and Linzer, M. (1979). Expanding aperture annular array. *Ultrasonic Imaging* **1**, 56–75.

Djelouah, H., Baboux, J.C. and Perdrix, M. (1991). Theoretical and experimental study of the field radiated by acoustic focussed transducers. *Ultrasonics* **29**, 188–200.

Duck, F.A. and Starritt, H.C. (1986). The location of peak pressures and peak intensities in finite amplitude beams from a pulsed focussed transducer. *Ultrasound in Med. & Biol.* **12**, 403–409.

Fan, X. and Hynynen, K. (1992). The effect of wave reflection and refraction at soft tissue interfaces during ultrasound hyperthermia treatments. *J. Acoust. Soc. Am.* **91**, 1727–1736.

Fan, X. and Hynynen, K. (1996). A study of various parameters of spherically curved phased arrays for noninvasive ultrasound surgery. *Phys. Med. Biol.* **41**, 591–608.

Fishell, E.K., Foster, F.S., Connor, T., Khodai, M., Harasciewicz, K. and Hunt, J.W. (1990). Clinical performance of a cone/annular array ultrasound breast scanner. *Ultrasound in Med. & Biol.* **16**, 361–374.

Foster, F.S., Arditi, M., Patterson, M.S., Lee-Chahal, D. and Hunt, J.W. (1983). Breast imaging with a conical transducer/annular array hybrid scanner. *Ultrasound in Med. & Biol.* **9**, 151–164.

Foster, F.S., Larson, J.D., Mason, M.K., Shoup, T.S., Nelson, G. and Yoshida, H. (1989a). Development of a 12-element annular array transducer for realtime ultrasound imaging. *Ultrasound in Med. & Biol.* **15**, 649–659.

Foster, F.S., Larson, J.D., Pittaro, R.J., Carl, P.D., Greenstein, A.P. and Lum, P.K. (1989b). A digital annular array prototype scanner for realtime ultrasound imaging. *Ultrasound in Med. & Biol.* **15**, 661–672.

Foster, F.S., Ryan, L.K. and Turnbull, D.H. (1991). Characterization of lead zirconate titanate ceramic for use in miniature high-frequency (20–80 MHz) transducers. *IEEE Trans.* **UFFC-38**, 446–453.

Freedman, A. (1970). Sound field of plane or gently curved pulsed radiators. *J. Acoust. Soc. Am.* **48**, 221–227.

Fry, W.J. and Dunn, F. (1962). Ultrasound: analysis and experimental methods in biological research. In *Physical Techniques in Biological Research*, Vol. 4, W. L. Nastuk (ed.). Academic Press, New York, pp. 261–394.

Goldberg, R.L. and Smith, S.W. (1994). Multilayer piezoelectric ceramics for two-dimensional array transducers. *IEEE Trans.* **UFFC-41**, 761–771.

Gururaja, T.R., Schulze, W.A., Cross, L.E., Newnham, R.E., Auld, B.A. and Wang, Y.J. (1985). Piezoelectric composite materials for ultrasonic transducer applications. Part 1: resonant modes of vibration of PZT rod–polymer composites. Part 2: evaluation of ultrasonic medical applications. *IEEE Trans.* **SU-32**, 481–498, 499–513.

Hill, C.R. (1994). Optimum acoustic frequency for focused ultrasound surgery. *Ultrasound in Med. & Biol.* **20**, 271–277.

Hill, C.R., Rivens, I., Vaughan, M.G. and ter Haar, G.R. (1994). Lesion development in focussed ultrasound surgery: a general model. *Ultrasound in Med. & Biol.* **20**, 259–269.

Hinkelman, L.M., Liu, D-L., Metlay, L.A. and Waag, R.C. (1994). Measurements of pulse arrival time and energy level variations produced by propagation through abdominal wall. *J. Acoust. Soc. Am.* **95**, 530–541.

Hinkelman, L.M., Liu, D-L., Waag, R.C., Zhu, Q. and Steinberg, B.D. (1995). Measurement and correction of pulse distortion produced by the human breast. *J. Acoust. Soc. Am.* **97**, 1958–1969.

Hunt, J.W., Arditi, M. and Foster, F.S. (1983). Ultrasound transducers for pulse–echo medical imaging. *IEEE Trans.* **BME-30**, 453–481.

Hynynen, K., Watmough, D.J. and Mallard, J.R. (1981). Design of ultrasonic transducers for local hyperthermia. *Ultrasound in Med. & Biol.* **7**, 397–402.

Inoue,T., Ohta, M. and Takahashi, S. (1987). Design of ultrasonic transducers with multiple acoustic matching layers for medical application. *IEEE Trans.* **UFFC-34**, 8–16.

Ito, Y., Kushida, K., Sugawara, K. and Takeuchi, H. (1995). A 100 MHz ultrasonic transducer array using ZnO thin films. *IEEE Trans.* **UFFC 42**, 316–324.

Jaffe, B., Cook, W.R. and Jaffe, H. (1971). *Piezoelectric Ceramics*. Academic Press, New York.

Jones, H.W. and Kwan, H.W. (1985). Ultrasonic lenses for imaging. *Ultrasonics* **23**, 63–70.

Kimura, K., Hashimoto, N. and Ohigashi, H. (1985). Performance of a linear array transducer of vinyledene fluoride trifluoroethylene polymer. *IEEE Trans.* **SU-32**, 566–573.

Kojima, T.A. (1987). A review of piezoelectric materials for ultrasonic transducers. In *Ultrasonics International '87 Conference Proceedings*. Butterworth-Heinemann, London, pp. 888–895.

Krautkramer, J. and Krautkramer, H. (1975). *Ultrasonic Testing of Materials*. Springer, New York.

Lancee, C.T., Souquet, J., Ohigashi, H. and Bom, N. (1985). Transducers in medical ultrasound. Part 1: ferro-electric versus polymer piezoelectric materials. *Ultrasonics* **23**, 138–142.

Lele, P.P. and Parker, K.J. (1982). Temperature distribution in tissues during local hyperthermia by stationary or steered beams of unfocused or focused ultrasound. *Brit. J. Cancer* **45** (Suppl. 5), 108–121.

Lewin, P.A. and Schafer, M.E. (1988). Wide-band piezoelectric polymer acoustic sources. *IEEE Trans.* **UFFC-35**, 175–184.

Li, P-C. and O'Donnell, M. (1994). Efficient two-dimensional blocked element compensation. *Ultrasonic Imaging* **16**, 164–175.

Lockwood, G.R. and Foster, F.S. (1994). Modelling and optimization of high-frequency ultrasound transducers. *IEEE Trans.* **UFFC-41**, 225–230.

Lockwood, J.C. and Willette, J.G. (1973). High speed method for computing the exact solution for the pressure variations in the near field of a baffled piston. *J. Acoust. Soc. Am.* **53**, 735–741.

Lu, J.Y. and Greenleaf, J.F. (1990). Ultrasonic nondiffracting transducer for medical imaging. *IEEE Trans.* **UFFC-37**, 438–447.

Lu, J. and Greenleaf, J.F. (1994). A study of two-dimensional array transducers for limited diffraction beams. *IEEE Trans.* **UFFC-41**, 724–739.

Lu, J-Y., Zou, H. and Greenleaf, J.F. (1994). Biomedical ultrasound beam forming. *Ultrasound in Med. & Biol.* **20**, 403–428.

Lucas, B.G. and Muir, T.G. (1982). The field of a focusing source. *J. Acoust. Soc. Am.*, **72**, 1289–1296.

Lucas, B.G. and Muir, T.G. (1983). Field of a finite amplitude focusing source. *J. Acoust. Soc. Am.* **74**, 1522–1528.

Manes, G., Tortoli, P., Andreuccetti, F., Avitabile, G. and Atzeni, C. (1988). Synchronous dynamic focussing for ultrasound imaging. *IEEE Trans.* **UFFC-35**, 14–21.

Mason, W.P. (1950). *Piezoelectric Crystals and their Application to Ultrasonics*. van Nostrand, New York.

Melton, H.E. and Thurstone, F.L. (1978). Annular array design and logarithmic processing for ultrasonic imaging. *Ultrasound in Med. & Biol.* **4**, 1–12.

Mesdag, P.R., de Vries, D. and Berkhout, A.J. (1982). An approach to tissue characterization based on wave theory using a new velocity analysis technique. In *Acoustical Imaging*, Vol. 12, E. A. Ash and C. R. Hill (eds). Plenum Press, New York, pp. 479–491.

Miller, E.B. and Thurstone, F.L. (1977). Linear ultrasonic array design for echosonography. *J. Acoust. Soc. Am.* **61**, 1481–1491.

Moros, E.G. and Hynynen, K. (1992). A comparison of theoretical and experimental ultrasound field distributions in canine muscle tissue *in vivo*. *Ultrasound in Med. & Biol.* **18**, 81–95.

Moshfeghi, M. (1987). Side-lobe suppression for ultrasonic imaging arrays. *Ultrasonics* **25**, 322–327.

Moshfeghi, M. and Waag, R.C. (1988). *In vivo* and *in vitro* ultrasound beam distortion measurements of a large aperture and a conventional aperture focused transducer. *Ultrasound in Med. & Biol.* **14**, 415–428.

Na, J.K. and Breazeale, M.A. (1994). Ultrasonic nonlinear properties of lead zirconate titanate ceramics. *J. Acoust. Soc. Am.* **95**, 3213–3221.

Ocheltree, K.B. and Frizzell, L.A. (1989). Sound field calculation for rectangular sources. *IEEE Trans.* **UFFC-36**, 242–248.

O'Donnell, M., Busse, L.J. and Miller, J.G. (1981). Piezoelectric transducers. In *Methods of Experimental Physics*, Vol. 19, *Ultrasonics*, P. D. Edmonds (ed.), Academic Press, New York, pp. 29–65.

Ohigashi, H. (1976). Electromechanical properties of polarized polyvinyledine fluoride films as studied by the piezoelectric resonance method. *J. Appl. Phys.* **47**, 949–955.

Oloffson, S. (1963). An ultrasonic optical mirror system. *Acustica* **33**, 361–367.

O'Neil, H.T. (1949). Theory of focusing radiators. *J. Acoust. Soc. Am.* **21**, 516–526.

Patterson, M.S. and Foster, F.S. (1982). Acoustic fields of conical radiators. *IEEE Trans.* **SU-29**, 83–92.

Patterson, M.S. and Foster, F.S. (1983). The improvement and quantitative assessment of B-mode images produced by an annular array/cone hybrid. *Ultrasonic Imaging* **5**, 195–213.

Patterson, M.S., Foster, F.S. and Lee, D. (1982). Sidelobe and speckle reduction for an eight sector conical scanner. *IEEE Trans.* **SU-29**, 169.

Penttinen, A. and Luakkala, M. (1976). The impulse response and pressure nearfield of a curved ultrasonic radiator. *J. Phys. D: Appl. Phys.* **9**, 1547–1557.

Reilly, C.R. and Parker, K.J. (1989). Finite-amplitude effects on ultrasound beam patterns in attenuating media. *J. Acoust. Soc. Am.* **86**, 2339–2348.

Richter, K.P., Millner, R., Holzer, F., Leitgab, N. and Wach, P. (1987). Design, construction and experimental investigation of ultrasonic pulse transducers with different bandwidths. *Ultrasonics* **25**, 229–236.

Rosenberg, L.D. (1962). La génération et l'étude des vibrations ultra-sonores de très grande intensité. *Acustica* **12**, 40–49.

Seyed-Bolorforosh, M.S. (1995). Novel integrated impedance matching layer. *IEEE Trans.* **UFFC-42**, 809–811.

Silk, M.G. (1984). *Ultrasonic Transducers for Nondestructive Testing*. Adam Hilger, Bristol.

Smith, S.W., Pavy, H.G. and von Ramm, O.T. (1991). High-speed volumetric imaging system. Part 1: transducer design and beam steering. Part 2: parallel processing and image display. *IEEE Trans.* **UFFC-38**, 100–108, 109–115.

Smith, S.W., Trahey, G.E. and von Ramm, O.T. (1986). Phased array ultrasound imaging through planar tissue layers. *Ultrasound in Med. & Biol.* **12**, 229–243.

Smith, S.W., Trahey, G.E. and von Ramm, O.T. (1992). Two-dimensional arrays for medical ultrasound. *Ultrasonic Imaging* **14**, 213–223.

Song, T.K. and Park, S.B. (1989). Optimum focusing in an ultrasonic annular array system using a nonspherical lens. *Ultrasonic Imaging* **11**, 197–214.

Stepanishen, P.R. (1971). Transient radiation from pistons in an infinite planar baffle. *J. Acoust. Soc. Am.* **49**, 1629–1638.

Stepanishen, P.R. (1981). Pulsed transmit–receive response of ultrasonic piezoelectric transducers. *J. Acoust. Soc. Am.* **69**, 1815–1827.

Swartz, R.G. and Plummer, J.D. (1980). On the generation of high frequency acoustic energy with polyvinyledine fluoride. *IEEE Trans.* **SU-27**, 295–303.

Swindell, W. (1985). A theoretical study of non-linear effects with focused ultrasound in tissues: an 'acoustic Bragg peak'. *Ultrasound in Med. & Biol.* **11**, 121–130.

Thijssen, J.M., Verhoef, W.A. and Cloostermans, M.J. (1985). Optimisation of ultrasonic transducers. *Ultrasonics* **23**, 41–46.

Turnbull, D.H. and Foster, F.S. (1991). Beam steering with pulsed two-dimensional arrays. *IEEE Trans.* **UFFC-38**, 320–333.

Umemura, S. and Cain, C.A. (1992). Acoustical evaluation of a prototype sector-vortex phased-array applicator. *IEEE Trans.* **UFFC-39**, 32–38.

van Kervel, S.J.H. and Thijssen, J.M. (1983). A calculation scheme for the optimum design of ultrasonic transducers. *Ultrasonics* **21**, 134–140.

Vogel, J., Bom, N., Ridder, J. and Lancee, C. (1979). Transducer design considerations in dynamic focusing. *Ultrasound in Med. & Biol.* **5**, 187–193.

Weight, J.P. (1984). New transducers for high resolution ultrasonic testing. *NDT Int. (GB)* **17**, 3–8.

Weight, J.P. and Hayman, A.J. (1978). Observations of the propagation of very short ultrasonic pulses and their reflection by small targets. *J. Acoust. Soc. Am.* **63**, 396–404 (also **66**, 945–951).

Weyns, A. (1980a, b). Radiation field calculations of pulsed transducers: (a) Part 1: planar circular, square and annular transducers. (b) Part 2: spherical disk- and ring-shaped transducers. *Ultrasonics* **18**, 183–188, 219–223.

Yamaguchi, K., Yagumi, H. and Fujii, T. (1986). New method of time-domain analysis of the performance of multilayered ultrasonic transducers. *IEEE Trans.* **UFFC-33**, 669–678.

Yoon, Y.T. and Benkesser, P.J. (1992). Ultrasonic phased arrays with variable geometric focussing for hyperthermia applications. *IEEE Trans.* **UFFC-39**, 273–278.

Zhang, Q. and Lewin, P.A. (1993). Wideband and efficient polymer transducers using multiple active piezoelectric films. *Proc. IEEE 1993 Ultrasonics Symposium*, pp. 757–760.

3

Detection and Measurement of Acoustic Fields

C. R. HILL

Institute of Cancer Research, Royal Marsden Hospital, UK

3.1 INTRODUCTION

Almost all the practical applications of ultrasound in medicine entail, at some stage, a process of detection or measurement. The need for this can be seen to arise in three broad areas: the derivation of 'diagnostic' information from patients; the measurement of acoustic propagation behaviour in tissues and other materials; and measurement of the ultrasonic fields to which living cells and tissues (including those of patients) may be exposed, where the interest is to relate possible biological change to physical measures of exposure. These various applications will differ in the particular requirements that they place on a measuring technique, for example in resolution of details of a field in space and time, or in traceability of some primary standard of measurement. In addition, aspects of practical convenience will differ for the various applications; for example in relation to portability, ruggedness and the need for direct conversion of an acoustic to an electrical signal.

The two preceding chapters have set out the nature of ultrasonic fields: typically they are space- and time-variant, often with a substantial frequency bandwidth, and may exhibit a wide range of practically interesting amplitude. Such fields may be characterised quantitatively by a set of field vectors – particle displacement, velocity, acceleration and pressure, velocity potential and intensity – which, under certain simplifying conditions only, may be interrelated to an approximate degree and can then be used interchangeably. Thus, ideally, we should like to be able to measure several, and preferably all, of these with high spatial and temporal resolution and with good sensitivity; in fact we are limited to what is practically possible bearing in mind, among other factors, cost and achievable signal-to-noise ratio.

Ultrasound is, by definition, not directly perceptible by the human senses; nor, in particular, is there any convenient ultrasonic equivalent to photographic or X-ray film. It is therefore necessary to exploit some physical phenomenon, or chain of phenomena, that will allow its perception in an appropriate, and generally quantitative way. Here there will be evident practical convenience in considering processes that lead fairly directly to generation of an electrical signal.

A considerable number of usable phenomena exist, and the principal ones of these are listed in Table 3.1. These phenomena will be discussed in some detail below, but it can be

Physical Principles of Medical Ultrasonics, Second Edition. Edited by C. R. Hill, J. C. Bamber and G. R. ter Haar.
© 2004 John Wiley & Sons, Ltd: ISBN 0 471 97002 6

Table 3.1. Physical phenomena of value in detection and measurement of acoustic fields

Effect	Quantity detected	Approximate resolution limits	
		In space (m)	In time (s)
Piezoelectric	p	10^{-3}	10^{-9}
Displacement (capacitance)	ξ	10^{-3}	10^{-7}
Displacement (opt. interference)	ξ	10^{-4}	10^{-7}
Radiation force	I	10^{-3}	1
Calorimetric	I	10^{-4}	10^{-3}
Optical diffraction	p	10^{-4}	10^{-9}
Acousto-electric	I	10^{-3}	10^{-7}

said immediately that the piezoelectric effect is of major importance, particularly in application to diagnostic ultrasound, because of its characteristic of direct, simple and efficient conversion between acoustical and electrical energy. All the effects listed are potentially quantitative, in the sense that they can be implemented in such a way that the measured quantity has an established relationship, using known physical constants, with the acoustic field quantity of interest. Thus, choice of method for a particular purpose becomes a matter of convenience and appropriateness in terms of the particular field quantity that it is required to measure or detect.

The list given in Table 3.1 is not exhaustive and some other examples are briefly referred to below, and described more fully in the literature. The first comprehensive review of the subject resulted from an international workshop held in the USA (Reid & Sikov 1973); more recent and extensive coverage is given in a special issue of *IEEE Transactions* (IEEE 1988; Harris *et al.* 1988) and in a review by Preston (1986).

3.2   PIEZOELECTRIC DEVICES

The piezoelectric effect was described in Chapter 2, in connection with its application, in inverse mode, for generation of acoustic fields. It is also of major importance in its application to acoustic detection. Piezoelectric detectors have been constructed in a wide variety of forms but, most commonly, for medical applications at least, they have the form of thin, parallel-sided plates or films, either plane or appropriately shaped.

For diagnostic use, such detectors, which in practice may also be the radiators or 'projectors' of pulse–echo systems, are usually plates cut to operate in fundamental thickness mode. A modern diagnostic transducer will often be sectioned into a number of elements arranged in a one- or two-dimensional array, but will normally be used with a sufficient number of such elements connected coherently to form an effective aperture equivalent to at least 30 acoustic wavelengths in the propagation medium: the minimum requirement for achieving satisfactory directivity. Diagnostic transducers are normally mounted (e.g. by epoxy resin casting) onto an acoustically matched and attenuating backing block, in order to damp resonances that would otherwise be set up by an incoming acoustic signal, with consequent loss of range resolution. It is common practice also to coat the outer surface of the transducer with one or more $\lambda/4$ acoustic matching layers (Section 1.7.3), a procedure analogous to 'blooming' of optical surfaces. This procedure, however, somewhat counteracts the effect of matched backing, in that it is essentially frequency sensitive and imposes a bandwidth limitation.

It cannot be assumed that a transducer constructed in this manner will have a uniform sensitivity over its aperture: the measured sensitivity even of single-element transducers commonly shows considerable variability, with possible fall-off near the perimeter and anomalies associated with unsuspected flaws in the adhesion of matching and backing layers. Such departures from 'ideal' behaviour will affect the spatial directivity pattern of the detector. Further discussion of the behaviour of piezoelectric detectors in diagnostic-type applications is taken up in Chapter 9.

The property of phase coherence over an extended aperture, which is vital for high spatial resolution diagnostic applications, can prove to be a major drawback when attempts are made to use a transducer in applications that require the quantitative detection of received energy in a manner that is independent of its direction of arrival. This problem can arise where a phase-sensitive receiving transducer is used for quantitative measurement of propagation properties (e.g. attenuation coefficient) of a material such as human tissue, in which inhomogeneities in refractive index can significantly distort the arriving wave front. In such a situation, components of the wave front arriving at different points on the transducer face may tend to cancel at its electrical output, in a manner that is inappropriate for the exact measurement of total intercepted acoustic power (Busse & Miller 1981b). This provides an illustration of the somewhat differing requirements that can be placed on detectors intended for use in 'imaging' and 'metrology' applications respectively, whilst at the same time signalling a need for caution in the quantitative interpretation of imaging data.

Design criteria for detectors intended to be applied for dosimetry and measurement of material properties will generally differ from those intended for diagnostic use, particularly in relaxation of an extreme requirement for sensitivity: in diagnostic application there is always an underlying requirement to maximise the information derived from a given exposure to a patient. Thus, for narrow-band and multiple spot-frequency measurements on materials and solutions, quartz is a good detector in spite of its relatively low coupling coefficient, whilst for measurements directed at 'exposimetry' (see Section 3.8), where small physical size and uniform frequency response are generally important, it is convenient to use miniature ceramic or PVDF detectors ('hydrophones') in essentially non-resonant conditions.

3.2.1 HYDROPHONES

The development and characterisation of hydrophones for medical applications have been subjects of interest for some considerable time (Hill 1970; Reid & Sikov 1973) and have now reached the point of formal international agreement on recommended methods (IEC 1987, 1991a, b).

The measurement of highly inhomogeneous fields calls, ideally, for a device with linear dimensions much less than an acoustic wavelength in the propagation medium (e.g. 0.1 mm for 15 MHz in water). There are, broadly, two approaches to designs that will satisfy this criterion: 'needle' and 'stretched membrane' hydrophones, each of which has an important role, and each of which employs piezoelectric polymer (e.g. PVDF) elements. In the implementation of high spatial resolution designs, of either type, there will be an inevitable trade-off between miniaturisation and a combination of sensitivity and bandwidth. Devices can now be made

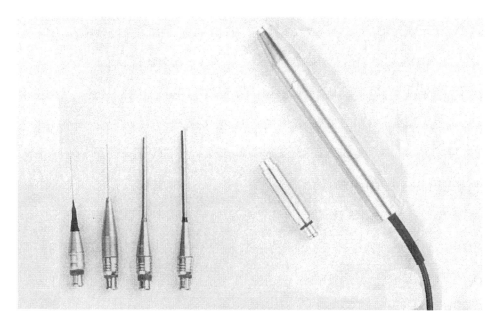

Figure 3.1. A set of needle hydrophones. Each of the four needle probes can be screw-connected to the preamplifier base unit. *Source*: Illustration by courtesy of Precision Acoustics Ltd, Dorchester, Dorset, UK

using polymer thicknesses down to 9 μm, for high bandwidth, and aperture dimensions down to 75 μm, for high spatial resolution (Lum *et al.* 1996), thus requiring an associated preamplifier to compensate for the low sensitivity and high electrical impedance of the device. The preamplifier will also have a role in flattening the overall frequency response.

The sensitive area of a hydrophone can be scanned mechanically over an acoustic field of interest and the device thus forms a very practical, precise and stable measuring system that has found widespread acceptance and use. Knowledge of the directivity of such devices is important and a useful introduction to this topic has been given by Shombert *et al.* (1982).

Needle hydrophones, a set of which is illustrated in Figure 3.1, are constructed by mounting, and electrically connecting, a circular disk of piezo-polymer across the tip of a hypodermic needle. They are widely employed for field plotting and for semi-quantitative field measurement.

In a membrane device (Figure 3.2) the polymer film is stretched over a circular former, and the acoustically sensitive region is defined by an area of overlap between the two conducting electrodes, vacuum deposited on opposing sides of the film (Shotton *et al.* 1980). This arrangement can be extended by forming a linear array of detecting elements, thus simplifying and speeding the use of the device for field plotting. Such a hydrophone, whether single- or multi-element, will have good and stable spatial and frequency response, and is commonly used as a secondary standard device, following calibration against a primary standard, as described below.

When using hydrophones for making any but purely qualitative observations it will be important to have knowledge of their properties and limitations. As mentioned above, they are not point detectors and, unless (as suggested below) measures are taken to account for this fact, their finite size may lead to appreciable errors in measurements of both beam shape and amplitude. In practice, their acoustically effective size can differ substantially from their apparent physical size and Smith (1989), for example, estimates that a hydrophone whose aperture diameter is half the 6 dB width of a beam to be measured may introduce errors of 10–20% in peak pressure (20–35% in intensity). Related errors may arise when using such a finite-aperture hydrophone for determining the characteristics of a beam that is subject to non-linear distortion (Zeqiri & Bond 1992). It is clearly desirable that a hydrophone itself should have a response that is near-linear with respect to acoustic pressure and, although most hydrophones seem to perform quite well in this respect over a substantial amplitude range, their electrical output impedance tends to be very high and serious anomalies can arise due to cable loading if a preamplifier is not used in close electrical proximity (Shombert & Harris 1986; Lewin *et al.* 1987). The frequency response of a membrane hydrophone, when properly connected with a preamplifier, can be constant within ±0.5 dB up to a frequency approaching its thickness-mode resonance, whilst a ceramic device may exhibit fluctuations of several dB (Robinson 1991). Directional response, in both cases, will of course be diffraction dependent and will be determined by the relationship between aperture dimension and wavelength.

An important practical point to bear in mind, particularly when using membrane hydrophones, is that they tend to be very fragile and, in particular, prone to damage by cavitation erosion. It is therefore wise, where possible, to use measurement procedures that avoid exposing the hydrophone to high pressure amplitudes, unless in combination with pulse lengths of no more than a few tens of microseconds.

Another good reason for arranging to use hydrophones in short-pulse, rather than CW fields is to minimise the impact of both acoustic and electromagnetic pickup; the former generally arises from multiple reflections within a sound tank and the latter because even a well-designed hydrophone will often act as a quite effective RF receiving antenna.

A further important practical consideration is to ensure that, in use, a hydrophone is properly 'wetted'. As noted in Chapter 1, even an extremely thin film of trapped air can act as a powerful acoustic reflector.

Calibration of such a hydrophone is achieved by placing it in a series of 'known' acoustic fields, chosen to cover the frequency range of interest, such known fields being themselves referred to a measurement expressible in fundamental quantities (e.g. mass, length, time). Whilst a number of options have been employed for this purpose (Preston *et al.* 1988), two in particular have developed to the point of being acceptable as international standards (IEC 1987, 1991a). The first of these is based on the reciprocity principle, as outlined in the following section, and the second entails recording the output of the hydrophone whilst it is scanned over a defined planar aperture that encompasses a beam whose acoustic power is known by other means, e.g. from a radiation force measurement, as described in Section 3.4.

3.2.2 HYDROPHONE CALIBRATION BY RECIPROCITY METHODS

The theorem of reciprocity in acoustics was originally stated by Rayleigh and has been discussed in detail by McLean (1940) and Foldy and Primakoff (1945, 1947). Its systematic application to the calibration of hydrophones has been described by Ludwig and Brendel (1988) and, for present purposes, it can be stated in the following terms.

If a transducer operated as a projector is driven with a current j, the free-field sound pressure amplitude at a point d metres from the acoustic centre of the projector, and on its acoustic axis within the far-field or spherical-wave region, is given by:

(a)

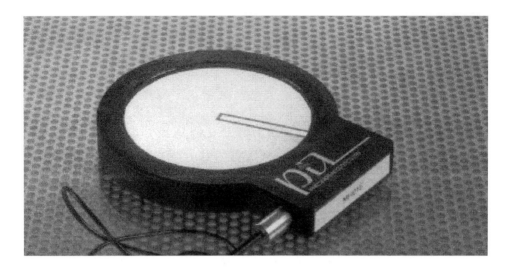

(b)

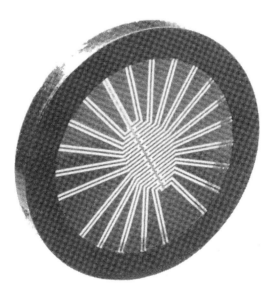

Figure 3.2. (a) A single-element stretched membrane hydrophone. The pair of overlapping, vacuum-deposited conducting electrodes can be seen leading to the preamplifier housing. Multi-element array instruments are of similar construction and will generally employ a common electrode, on one side of the poled polymer film, which is arranged to have an array of sensitive regions of overlap with the tips of a set of

(c)

Single element bilaminar hydrophone

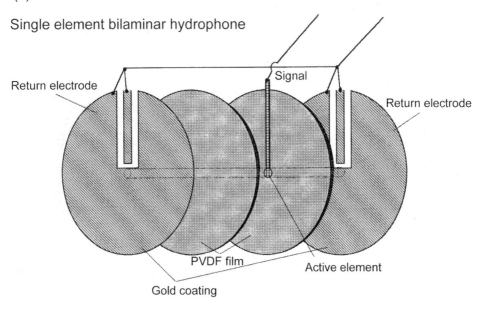

Return electrode

Signal

Return electrode

PVDF film

Active element

Gold coating

(d)

Multi-element bilaminar hydrophone

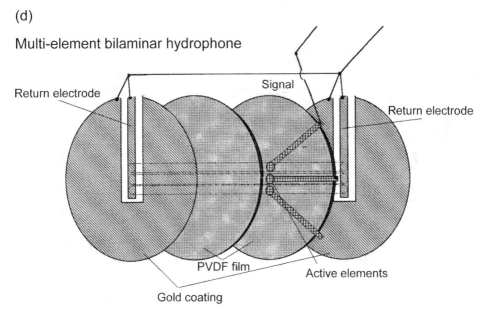

Return electrode

Signal

Return electrode

PVDF film

Active elements

Gold coating

opposing signal electrodes. (b) A 21-element, linear array hydrophone constructed on similar principles. (c, d) Expanded views indicating the principle of construction of single- and multi-element bilaminar hydrophones, respectively. *Source*: (a) Illustration by courtesy of Precision Acoustics Ltd, Dorchester, Dorset, UK. (b–d) By courtesy of R. C. Preston and the UK National Physical Laboratory

$$P = jS/d \tag{3.1}$$

where S is termed the transmitting current response.

For particular transducers of interest, S may be constant over a range of values of P and j, and the transmitting response of the device is then 'linear'.

Similarly, if a transducer operated as a hydrophone is placed with its acoustic centre at a point where the free-field sound pressure amplitude is P, and if its acoustic axis is aligned normal to the wave front at that point, the open circuit voltage across the transducer terminals is given by:

$$e = MP \tag{3.2}$$

where M is termed the hydrophone free-field voltage sensitivity, and corresponding linearity considerations apply.

For reciprocal transducers, the ratio:

$$M/S = J \tag{3.3}$$

where J is a constant termed the spherical-wave reciprocity parameter, which has the value (in SI units):

$$J = 2/\rho f \tag{3.4}$$

where ρ is the density of the propagation medium and f is the frequency at which the measurement is made. Corresponding reciprocity parameters can be defined for plane and cylindrical waves.

That these relationships can be used, at least in principle, to calibrate a hydrophone in terms of fundamental quantities (voltage, current, length) can be seen from the following example. Suppose we have three transducers, designated 1, 2, 3, of which one at least (say no. 3) is reciprocal, and that these are set up in pairs, under free-field conditions, and the transfer impedance of each pair is measured as indicated below:

Projector	Hydrophone	Input current	Output voltage
1	2	j_1	e_{12}
1	3	j_1	e_{13}
3	2	j_3	e_{32}

Then, from the definitions, the measurements give:

$$e_{12} = M_2 P_1 = M_2 j_1 S_1/d \tag{3.5}$$

$$e_{13} = M_3 P_1 = M_3 j_1 S_1/d \tag{3.6}$$

$$e_{32} = M_2 P_3 = M_2 j_3 S_3/d \tag{3.7}$$

From equations (3.5) and (3.6):

$$e_{12}/e_{13} = M_2/M_3 \tag{3.8}$$

Also $M_3/S_3 = J$ (by definition), and thus:

$$M_2 = JS_3 e_{12}/e_{13} \tag{3.9}$$

And thus, from equations (3.4), (3.7) and (3.9):

$$M_2 = (2de_{32}e_{12}/\rho f e_{13} j_3)^{0.5} \tag{3.10}$$

which is the absolute calibration that we require.

Another approach to such a calibration procedure, that of 'self-reciprocity', which involves the use of only one transducer, is outlined in the IEC recommendation previously referred to (IEC 1987), in which detailed accounts of experimental procedures and necessary correction factors are also given.

A requirement of the above approach is that it should be possible to find a suitable transducer that is indeed reciprocal. This is a matter that has been of major concern in underwater acoustics and has been extensively discussed, particularly by Bobber (1970), who states that most transducers that are linear, passive and reversible under appropriate conditions will also be found to be reciprocal (except, perhaps, in the region of a sharp resonance). In practice, it is possible to eliminate any reasonable doubt concerning non-reciprocal behaviour by repeated operation of the above three-transducer calibration, using a number of different transducer combinations, and checking for consistency of the results.

Some additional and complementary methods of hydrophone calibration are outlined in subsequent sections of this chapter.

3.2.3 APPROACHES TO MAKING HYDROPHONE MEASUREMENTS AT A POINT

As noted above, a limitation of most currently available hydrophones arises from their finite size: they do not in fact measure acoustic pressure at a point, but a value integrated over an aperture of finite dimension. A suggested solution to this problem is mathematically to deconvolve the aperture function from the observed response of a finite-aperture device (Miller & Hill 1986).

A small-aperture device, which appears to have the added advantage of sufficient ruggedness to enable it to be used in shock-wave conditions, such as exist in lithotriptor fields, has been suggested by Staudenraus and Eisenmenger (1993). This entails measuring changes in optical reflectivity, resulting from local pressure excursions, that occur at the water/glass interface at the tip of an optical fibre. Such a device, of active diameter 0.1 mm, can operate satisfactorily up to 20 MHz, with wide bandwidth.

3.3 DISPLACEMENT DETECTORS

Particle displacement is another measure of the acoustic field which, under linear plane wave conditions, is simply related to the acoustic pressure, with which it can then be used interchangeably (*cf.* Section 1.3 and Table 2.2). Correspondingly, it can be used as a means of calibrating a pressure-sensitive hydrophone.

An early device to use this approach was the capacitance microphone (Filipczynski 1969), which can be so arranged that an acoustic field is incident normally to one face of an air-gap capacitor, with the resulting deflection then being measurable in terms of known quantities (length, charge). However, the actual capacitance values involved become extremely small if measurement to high spatial resolution is attempted, and the uncertainties become correspondingly large.

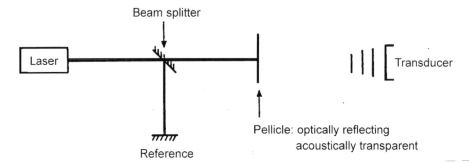

Figure 3.3. Principle of an optical interferometric technique for measuring the acoustic displacement of a thin membrane placed in a transducer field. *Source*: From Zeqiri (1991), reproduced by permission of Springer-Verlag

A more readily quantifiable approach to measurement of particle displacement is that of optical interferometry. This is normally implemented in the manner indicated in Figure 3.3, where the beam of interest is arranged to be reflected near-normally at the 'liquid' surface of a very thin, stretched membrane (or 'pellicle'), forming the boundary between an air space and the propagation liquid. The 'air' side of the membrane is made to be optically reflecting and is raster-scanned, again at near-normal incidence, by a narrow laser beam, which forms one arm of an optical interferometer. Remembering (*cf*. Table 2.3) that an acoustical displacement in water of about one optical wavelength will occur in a field intensity of $10\,\mathrm{mW\,cm^{-2}}$ at $2\,\mathrm{MHz}$, it will be seen that such a device has the potential for rapid mapping, with high spatial and temporal resolution, of most commonly occurring beam profiles. Its practical implementation has proved to be difficult, particularly in respect of isolation from environmental vibration, but an early successful design was described by Mezrich *et al.* (1975) and a more recent arrangement, developed specifically for absolute characterisation of fields used for hydrophone calibration, has been described by Bacon (1988). The principles underlying the method are not entirely straightforward, however and, in particular, the interactions between acoustic and optical wave propagation complicates the precise measurement of details of motion of the pellicle (Bacon *et al.* 1993).

A rather different type of displacement detector has been developed for characterising the very intense fields produced by extracorporeal shock wave lithotriptors (Chapter 13), in which conventional pressure hydrophones can readily be destroyed by the shock wave and associated cavitational action. This consists (Pye *et al.* 1991) of a small stainless steel ball, one pole of which is placed at the field point to be measured whilst the opposite pole is connected mechanically, by a steel rod, to an electromechanical transducer. Displacement of the propagation medium is transferred, through the ball and the rod, to the transducer and, following calibration against a standard hydrophone, the device constitutes a rugged 'field' instrument for routine measurements.

3.4 RADIATION FORCE MEASUREMENTS

A well-known physical phenomenon, discussed in Section 1.8.1, is that of the radiation force experienced by a body that absorbs or deflects a radiant energy beam. Since such a force can be measured very accurately and can also, as will be shown, be related to acoustic parameters, it provides a relatively simple means of evaluating an acoustic field in terms of basic acoustic quantities.

Adequate theoretical description of the radiation force phenomenon has proved to be complicated and has been the subject of controversy (Rooney & Nyborg 1972; Livett *et al.* 1981). This complexity has led many to restrict consideration to linear, plane-wave approximations, but there is reason to believe that their applicability should extend into the transducer's near-field. The method has now been accepted as an international standard for measurement of ultrasonic power in liquids (IEC 1992b, 1993).

The theoretical basis for the radiation force phenomenon has been discussed in Chapter 1, where an expression was derived [equation (1.141)] for the radiation pressure experienced at some point on an ideally absorbing (non-reflective) wall placed normally to the propagation direction of a harmonic plane wave. Generalisation of this expression to a wall of any kind gives:

$$R_P = kI/C \tag{3.11}$$

where k is a constant dependent on the collision geometry, such that $k = 1$ for total absorption of the beam, $k = 2$ for total normal reflection, and $0 < k < 2$ for partial absorption and/or non-normal reflection.

For the practical situation of a beam of intensity varying over its cross-section (but still assuming plane-wave conditions), the total force exerted on a target of finite size placed in the beam is evidently:

$$F = \int_s \langle kI/C \rangle \mathrm{d}s \tag{3.12}$$

where $\langle \rangle$ indicates a time average.

This relationship enables evaluation of an acoustic field parameter (intensity) in terms of fundamental quantities and can thus, in principle, be exploited for absolute acoustic measurement. Such measurements can be considered to fall into two broad categories: (1) measurements of total beam power, where the intercepting 'target' will be designed to extend over all or most of the effective beam cross-section, and (2) measurements of local intensity, where the target should be small in relation to local variations of beam intensity. Measurements with targets of intermediate size are sometimes made but, even if the geometry is sufficiently simple and it is well known that appropriate allowance can be made for a theoretically predictable pattern of variation (e.g. Figure 2.5), considerable uncertainties may arise. Radiation force measurements can also be divided into those where the objective is direct assessment of power or intensity and, secondly, measurements carried out as part of a procedure for calibration of a secondary device, such as a hydrophone.

3.4.1 LARGE-TARGET METHODS

A considerable variety of designs of large-target, total-power measurement devices has been described, mostly using reflecting rather than absorbing targets (to avoid thermal anomalies consequent on heating), and differing principally in their designed sensitivity range and in their method of force measurement. Included here are: devices based on standard analytical balances, as illustrated in Figure 3.4a (Hill 1970; Rooney 1973); electromagnetically compensated null-deflection devices (Farmery & Whittingham 1978); strain gauge instruments (Chivers *et al.* 1989); and compensated Cartesian divers, as shown in Figure 3.4b (Shotton

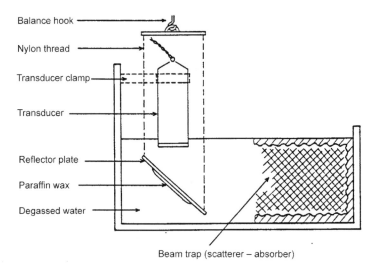

Balance hook

Nylon thread

Transducer clamp

Transducer

Reflector plate

Paraffin wax

Degassed water

Beam trap (scatterer – absorber)

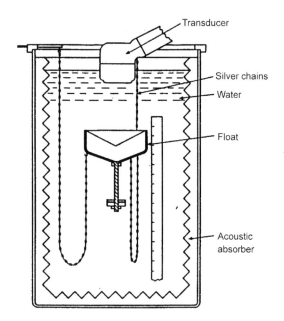

Transducer

Silver chains

Water

Float

Acoustic absorber

Figure 3.4. Two examples of a radiation force balance. (a) Ultrasonic radiometer based on a chemical microbalance and capable of a precision of 0.3 mW. The beam is totally reflected at 45° (above the critical angle for a water/aluminium interface) and surface tension anomalies are minimised by suspending the reflector plate by three fine-nylon filaments. Compensation for temperature dependence of apparent weight of the plate in water is achieved by fusing onto it an appropriate mass of paraffin wax. *Source*: From Hill (1970), reproduced by permission of the Institute of Physics. (b) Cartesian diver radiometer. The buoyancy of the float is balanced, at a particular vertical position, by the sum of the acoustic force and the effective weight of chain supported by the float. Sensitivity of up to 30 mm/W is achievable. *Source*: From Shotton (1980), reproduced by permission of Elsevier

1980; Davidson 1991; Chivers *et al.* 1993). From the point of view of their acoustical behaviour (i.e. excluding any electrical and mechanical uncertainties resulting from their design, and if operation in strongly non-linear propagation conditions is avoided) such devices should be capable of measurement accuracy within about 5%, where this residual uncertainty arises mainly from possible coupling of acoustic energy into the target and anomalous re-radiation.

A radiation force balance can be used as a means of calibrating a hydrophone. The procedure here is, first, to determine the total power crossing a surface of constant phase in the field of a harmonic acoustic source. A hydrophone can then be scanned over the entire aperture previously intercepted by the radiation force balance target, whilst values are measured for e, the open circuit voltage across the hydrophone terminals, given, from equation (3.2), as:

$$e = Mp \tag{3.13}$$

where M is the required free-field hydrophone sensitivity (or 'receiving response') in volts per Pascal.

If it is assumed that there is locally a plane-wave field in the vicinity of the hydrophone aperture (and this can generally be achieved by appropriate design of the calibration field, and checked experimentally), then:

$$I_z = pu_z \tag{3.14}$$

The relationship between p and u_z (Table 2.2) is:

$$u_z = p/\rho_0 c \tag{3.15}$$

Thus, local values for I_z are given by:

$$I_z = p^2/\rho_0 c \tag{3.16}$$

One thus obtains, from equations (3.13) and (3.16):

$$\langle I_z \rangle = \langle e^2 \rangle / \rho_0 c M^2 \tag{3.17}$$

where $\langle \rangle$ indicates the time average.

Integrating the time-average intensity over the constant phase surface would determine the total power, which would also be known by the radiation force measurement method. That is:

$$\langle W \rangle_{\text{RF}} = (1/\rho_0 c M^2) \int_{\text{const.phase}} \langle e^2 \rangle \, dA \tag{3.18}$$

Thus, the receiving response of the hydrophone is:

$$M = \left[(1/\rho_0 c \langle W \rangle_{\text{RF}}) \int_{\text{const.phase}} \langle e^2 \rangle \, dA \right]^{0.5} \tag{3.19}$$

A potential limitation on the accuracy of this approach arises from uncertainty as to edge effects in the target of the force balance. This problem can be minimised, however, if the target size is chosen such that its edges coincide with a null in the intensity field distribution (*cf.* Figure 2.5). Using such precautions, the method has been accepted, in parallel with the reciprocity approach, as the basis for an international standard on the measurement of medical ultrasonic fields (IEC 1993).

3.4.2 SMALL-TARGET METHODS

If a radiation force technique is to be used directly for measurement of local values of intensity, it will be important, first, that the dimensions of the target are reasonably small relative to the local spatial variations of the field and, second, that the wave–target interactions are calculable. The best hope of satisfying the latter requirement is to use a spherical target (commonly a steel ball-bearing). Calculations for this case are available (Hasegawa & Yosioka 1969), and results are generally presented in terms of the dimensionless quantity $Y_p = F_r/\pi a^2 E$: the radiation force, F_r, acting on the sphere, per unit cross-section (where a is the sphere radius) and per unit mean energy density, E.

A convenient implementation of this principle is to suspend the sphere, using two equal-length filaments (e.g. fine nylon thread), to form a pendulum suspended in the propagation liquid. In this case the horizontal force necessary to deflect the sphere by a distance, d, in the horizontal direction can be determined and equated to the radiation force, F_r, as:

$$F_r = mgd/(L^2 - d^2)^{0.5} \tag{3.20}$$

where L is the perpendicular distance from the axis between the filament suspension points to the centre of the sphere (with $L \gg d$), m is the mass of the sphere plus the mass of that fraction of the suspension structure involved, both corrected for buoyancy, and g is the gravitational acceleration.

Thus, F_r can be determined experimentally and is related to the acoustic intensity, I, at the ultrasonic field point of interest as:

$$I = F_r c/\pi a^2 Y_p \tag{3.21}$$

In making such a measurement it will be important that the suspending fibres are sufficiently thin to be essentially unperturbing and that their attachment does not appreciably modify the profile of the sphere or its natural modes of vibration.

Some typical calculated values of Y_p are shown in Figure 3.5, from which it will be seen, first, that the interaction has a complex frequency dependence and, second, that its application with reasonable accuracy will require very good knowledge of the physical properties of the

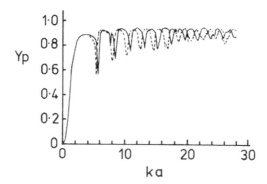

Figure 3.5. Values of Y_p (see text) calculated for spheres made of two grades of steel with slightly differing physical properties: shear wave sound velocity $3252\,\mathrm{m\,s^{-1}}$ (solid line) and $3089\,\mathrm{m\,s^{-1}}$ (dotted line); longitudinal velocity $5949\,\mathrm{m\,s^{-1}}$ in each case. *Source*: From Stockdale and Hill (1976), reproduced by permission of Elsevier

material of the sphere. Such calculations, however, ignore the effects of acoustic attenuation in the material, and it is to be expected that use of a sphere material exhibiting high acoustic attenuation will lead to a damping of the frequency dependence and a less variable behaviour (Anson & Chivers 1980), although the consequences of target heating may be of significance in this case.

3.5 CALORIMETRY

Perhaps the most widely used approach to assessing the energy associated with various physical phenomena is to arrange for complete conversion of such energy to heat, and thus measurable temperature rise. So far as beams of ultrasonic energy are concerned, there are here, as with radiation force measurements, broadly two types of approach which may be adopted: (a) to measure the total power associated with a beam, as defined by a particular aperture, and (b) to measure a local value of intensity at a point within the beam profile, as evidenced by local rate of rise of temperature in a medium of known absorption coefficient.

As in the case of radiation force measurements, a calorimetric method of measuring total beam power has the attraction that, in principle, it can be carried out with direct reference to fundamental physical quantities. If, however, it is to be used as a means of calibrating a secondary device, such as a hydrophone, such calibration will again be subject to uncertainties, first, as to the exact distribution of energy in the low-intensity region of the beam profile and, second, as to edge effects arising at the beam entrance window of the calorimeter.

An application of ultrasonic calorimetry where these problems do not arise is in the measurement of the total acoustic power output of a transducer under conditions where the complete beam can be directed into the calorimeter. This approach was used in early work on calibration of power transducers used for treating Menière's disease (Wells *et al.* 1978). Whilst this particular application does not call for very high sensitivity, calorimetric methods can be developed to be highly sensitive, and a good indication of what is possible is the parallel work that has been carried out with ionising radiation dosimetry (Laughlin & Genna 1966). A moderately sensitive device for use at medical ultrasonic frequencies has been described by Torr and Watmough (1977), but such approaches to total power measurement have generally proved less satisfactory than those based on radiation force, and so seem to have fallen out of favour.

Measurements of local values of intensity by calorimetric methods entail a rather different approach, and one that is additionally of interest in the assessment of the patterns of temperature rise that occur in tissues exposed to both therapeutic and investigative sources of ultrasound (Chapters 13 and 14). Here there is usually a need to achieve good spatial resolution, and fine-wire thermocouple junctions are commonly used, with small thermistors providing an alternative that will give greater temperature sensitivity at the cost of decreased spatial and temporal resolution. Thermocouple dosimetry has been well described by Fry and Fry (1954), who have used it for measuring the spatial profiles and absolute intensities of energetic and highly focused beams. Their technique is to construct a thermocouple junction from wires that have been thinned to approximately 0.01 mm diameter and to embed this in a liquid sound-absorbing medium (e.g. castor oil or a suitable silicone oil) whose absorption coefficient at the operating temperature and frequency is well known, whilst care is also taken that the medium and its container (which may have very thin plastic film windows) are well matched acoustically to the external medium. The sound source is then excited to give a single, square-wave acoustic pulse of about 1 s duration, and the resulting time-course of the

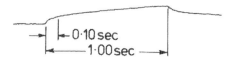

Figure 3.6. Thermoelectric emf recorded from a fine-wire thermocouple embedded in an absorbing medium and exposed to a 1-s burst of ultrasound

thermoelectric potential is recorded. This will generally have the form indicated in Figure 3.6, where the initial rapid rise corresponds to the period of equilibration in the viscous interaction between wire and fluid. The ensuing phase of the temperature sequence is caused by absorption of sound in the body of the fluid medium and its initial, approximately linear slope is a direct measure of local absorption coefficient.

For inhomogeneous, and in particular strongly focused fields, the method is open to a number of complicating influences, including those of heat diffusion, thermal conductivity in the lead wires, and non-linear acoustic behaviour (Hynynen *et al.* 1983; Dickinson 1985). It is worth noting, however that, in a form where the thermocouple or other detector is inserted directly into an 'unknown' medium, the method measures true absorption coefficient and thus provides information complementary to measured data on attenuation coefficient (see Chapter 4 and Drewniak *et al.* 1990).

3.6 OPTICAL DIFFRACTION METHODS

The transient pressure changes in a medium associated with propagation of an acoustic disturbance lead to corresponding changes in the optical refractive index: the Raman–Nath effect (see, e.g., Klein & Cook 1967; Riley & Klein 1967). This phenomenon can be exploited for acoustic metrology using an arrangement such as that illustrated in Figure 3.7. A parallel light beam traverses an acoustic propagation medium, in a direction normal to the axis of the acoustic beam of interest, and is subsequently brought to a focus by means of a lens or mirror. In this situation the sound beam acts as a phase grating, and a proportion of the energy of the

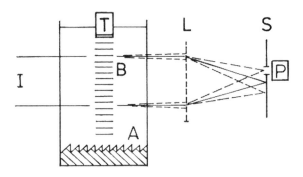

Figure 3.7. Arrangement for measuring optical diffraction due to density variations within an ultrasonic beam. First-order optical diffraction is indicated by dashed lines. I: illuminating source of parallel light; T: ultrasonic source transducer; B: ultrasonic beam in water; A: acoustic absorber; L: converging lens; S: slit; P: photodiode

zeroth order (primary) beam is diffracted into higher orders. The intensity of light in each of such diffraction orders is a function (which can be evaluated under practical conditions typical of most medical ultrasonic beams) of the peak acoustically induced change in optical refractive index and of the length of optical propagation path through the sound beam. Fuller details of this relationship, and references to the literature, are given by O'Brien (1978).

Achievement of quantitative measurements using this principle entails considerable complexity, particularly as pressure amplitude is not uniform across the beam profile. However, Reibold (1977) has reported a comparison of optical and radiation force methods over the frequency range 1–9 MHz and found good agreement between the two except where deviations arise from *a priori* assumptions about the form of the sound field.

In addition to any such quantitative use, the phenomenon provides the basis for a very useful, qualitative means for visualising the shape of an acoustic field, including the potential to observe in real time the form and propagation behaviour of pulse-wave packets. Returning to Figure 3.7, if an optical slit is placed so as to select only light that falls into one particular diffraction order (e.g. the first), and an additional optical stage is provided to form an image of the object plane containing the acoustic beam, such an image will present as a dark field with positive modulation corresponding to optical-path integrals of local values of excursions of pressure amplitude. An example of such a so-called Schlieren (literally 'streak') representation is shown in Figure 3.8.

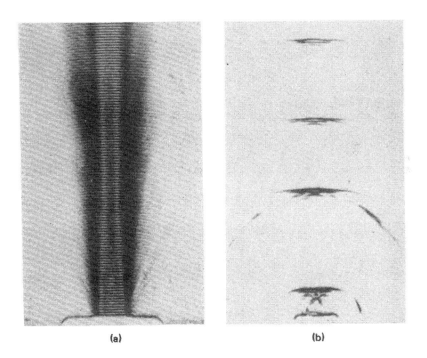

(a)   (b)

Figure 3.8. 'Schlieren' images of acoustic disturbances shown propagating vertically upwards. (a) Continuous wave field from a plane transducer similar to those used for therapy. (b) Pulsed field, from a diagnostic linear array, photographed at four successive time points. Note the separation of the pulsed wave packet into 'plane' and 'edge-wave' components (*cf.* Section 2.4). *Source*: By courtesy of R. C. Preston and the UK National Physical Laboratory

3.7 MISCELLANEOUS METHODS AND TECHNIQUES

There are a considerable number of other physical phenomena that make possible the observation of acoustic fields and measurement of their parameters. It is only possible here to make brief reference to some of these.

A so-called acousto-electric effect can arise as a result of coupling of the energy of an acoustic travelling wave to the system of photo-excited charge carriers within a photosensitive semiconductor crystal such as cadmium sulphide (Weinreich *et al.* 1959). The effect is a consequence of the finite time-lag that exists between the wave and the response of the charge carriers, which are dragged along with the wave, similarly to electrons in a linear accelerator, and gives rise to a unidirectional potential gradient. In the sense that the phenomenon entails a direct transformation of acoustical into electrical energy, it has some analogy to the piezoelectric effect, but it differs in not being phase sensitive. This property has been exploited in the construction of detectors for attenuation coefficient measurement where, as discussed above and in Chapter 4, erratic and unpredictable phase variations over a phase-sensitive detector surface can give rise to anomalous data (Busse & Miller 1981a, b).

One of the major disadvantages suffered by light and X-rays is the absence of any ultrasonic equivalent of the photographic process. Various attempts have been made to find a substitute but none has found any widespread application. It has been shown, for example, that the process of chemical development of a uniformly exposed photographic film is accelerated by ultrasonically induced microstreaming, thus making possible a rather crude recording of intensity variations within an acoustic beam. Another device, the so-called Pohlmann cell, makes use of the tendency of small elongated particles (e.g. microscopic metal flakes) in liquid suspension to take up preferential alignments in a standing wave field, thus leading to local alterations in optical reflectivity of the suspension in a manner that follows local acoustic pressure amplitude.

It may sometimes be desirable to be able to carry out an acoustic field measurement by non-invasive means, for example when the location of interest is within a living body. An approach to achieving this that has been investigated by Gavrilov *et al.* (1988), with promising results, is to make use of a strongly focused ultrasonic receiver.

3.8 MEASUREMENT OF BIOLOGICALLY EFFECTIVE EXPOSURE AND DOSE

An important area of application of acoustical field measurements is that concerned with the changes that ultrasound may induce in cells and tissues, and with related practical questions of safety in diagnostic use and of effectiveness in therapeutic use. Biological and applied aspects of this subject are dealt with in detail in Chapters 12 to 14, but it will be useful here to consider the situation in relation to physical measurements.

It will be clear from reading these later chapters that ultrasound, when it has any observable effect at all, may produce changes in cells and tissues by means of a number of quite distinct mechanisms, each with a characteristic dependence on particular conditions of exposure. It will also be seen that some of these mechanisms are not understood, and that their patterns of relationships between exposure conditions and effect are documented only very sparsely, if at all. As a consequence, it is not at present possible to construct a meaningful and universal system of 'ultrasonic dosimetry'. There is an important, but not always appreciated contrast here with ionising radiation dosimetry, where the quantity 'absorbed energy per unit mass' is generally found to be a quantitatively good predictor of both therapeutic effectiveness and expected damage. Except under certain rather special conditions there is no equivalent quantity for prediction of ultrasonic effects.

Here we need, therefore, to consider briefly the relevance in ultrasound of the terms 'dose' and 'exposure'. Although there seems to be no universal pattern, the ionising radiation analogy suggests that 'exposure' will generally connote an energy or intensity that is incident on a target, whilst 'dose' implies a quantity of energy converted within the target to a biologically effective form, of which heat and ionisation are simply two examples. On this basis it will be seen that the majority of acoustic measurements record exposure rather than dose and that, in spite of a certain inelegance, it is conducive to clarity of thought to refer not to ultrasonic 'dosimetry' but rather to 'exposimetry' (a term originally coined by the present author and subsequently taken into common usage: Hill 1975; IEEE 1988).

In the absence of a satisfactory single dosimetric quantity for ultrasound, the only meaningful way to report experimental exposures in a manner that allows comparison with related experiments, and predictions of practically important consequences, is by inclusion of a complete temporal and spatial description of the acoustic field employed. In most cases the best way to carry out such measurements will be by means of the piezoelectric hydrophones described above, in Section 3.2.

Much current practice, however (apparently deriving from the tradition that a simple radiation force balance is a convenient measuring device), is generally based on the quantity 'intensity' or, perhaps better, 'exposure intensity': the power per unit aperture area entering the region of interest, in $W\,cm^{-2}$. This quantity is now usually qualified as to whether it expresses peak or average intensity, both spatially (within a specified aperture) or temporally (within a specified exposure time). Thus we may have:

SATA intensity: (spatial average, temporal average)
SATP intensity: (spatial average, temporal peak)
SPTP intensity: (spatial peak, temporal peak)
SPTA intensity: (spatial peak, temporal average)

A useful account of procedures for measuring these and related quantities has been given by Harris (1985). It is also becoming apparent that pulse duration and repetition frequencies are important quantities in determining biological effect, and that they therefore also need to be documented, as should be ultrasonic frequency (and its spectral distribution in the case of broadband, i.e. short-pulse, exposures).

There are, nevertheless, certain situations where there is a practical need to express the emission from equipment, or the exposure of a tissue, in terms of a single number. An approach to this that has been adopted in the relevant publication of the World Health Organisation (WHO 1989), and in modified form by the International Electrotechnical Commission (IEC 1992a), is to recommend the use of the following quantities:

> For emissions and exposures due to pulse–echo diagnostic devices: the spatial peak pressure amplitude (in Pascal);

> For therapeutic, surgical, and Doppler diagnostic (continuous wave and pulsed) devices: the 'central beam power' (in watts), which is here defined as 0.541 of the product of the spatial peak, temporal average derived intensity ($w\,cm^{-2}$) and the 6 dB beam cross-sectional area (cm^2). The factor 0.541 follows arithmetically from the assumption of an axially symmetric beam with Gaussian profile and linear, harmonic propagation.

The logic behind the above approach will be substantiated in Chapters 12 and 14 and is based on consideration of biophysical mechanisms of action that are most likely to be effective in a given situation. Pulse–echo exposures seem very unlikely to give rise to appreciable heating and, if they do lead to any observable change, this seems most likely to be through mechanical stress, of which the amplitude of pressure excursions is a reasonable measure. By contrast, the various sources of exposure included in the second of the above groups are all considered to have potential for inducing change by thermal, in preference to mechanical, mechanisms; thus, power, where it is concentrated at the centre of a beam, is likely to be the determining quantity.

In this connection it is important to bear in mind that, from the point of view of actual exposure of a target tissue, it is the *in situ* values of the various field quantities that will be effective, and that these may differ substantially, as a result of attenuation, from the corresponding 'free-field' values that will generally have been measured in a non-attenuating medium such as water (Bacon 1989; Preston *et al.* 1991). Under near-linear conditions of propagation, adjustment between the two values merely entails a simple attenuation correction. However, in applications such as that of focused ultrasound surgery (Chapter 13), quite substantial propagation non-linearity may arise, leading both to anomalous values of attenuation coefficient and to attenuation-dependent changes in beam shape. Thus, in practice, unacceptable uncertainty may arise as to the relationship between the *in situ* and free-field values of field parameters. For this reason, and to try to achieve unambiguous and standardised reporting of exposure conditions, it has seemed appropriate to use the 'linear-equivalent spatial average intensity' (I_{sal}) for this application. This quantity is defined as the ratio of two unambiguously measurable quantities: the full acoustic beam power incident on the target aperture (e.g. as measured by a large-target force balance and with an appropriate diffraction correction for aperture – see Section 3.4.1); and the area of the beam, taken out to the half-pressure-maximum ($-6\,dB$) contour and measured with a hydrophone under small-signal, i.e. 'linear', conditions (Hill *et al.* 1994).

Special considerations may need to be given to acoustic measurements related to some of the other particular medical applications of ultrasound. Its use in physiotherapy, for example, is very extensive and, of course, designed to induce some kind of 'effect', so that it has been important here to develop appropriate, standard measurement methods (see e.g. Hekkenberg *et al.* 1994). Similarly, although in much less widespread application hitherto, there has been need to quantitate the effectiveness of ultrasonic and other sources of tissue heating in the practice of hyperthermic tumour therapy (see e.g. Ocheltree & Frizzell 1987). Finally, the increasingly widespread, but initially rather unquantitative, use of focused ultrasonic beams in so-called extracorporeal shock wave lithotripsy (ESWL) has led to a need for measurement devices sufficiently rugged and reliable to work in the very extreme shock-wave conditions generated by this technique. Lewin *et al.* (1988) have reported an arrangement for this that uses a PVDF sensor and reference has been made above to two other techniques, based respectively on an electromagnetic probe (Pye *et al.* 1991) and the use of fibre optics (Staudenraus & Eisenmenger 1993).

Hitherto, a large fraction of the applied work in ultrasonic exposimetry has been directed at diagnostic exposures. Thus, there are now available good data not only on the ranges of patient exposure due to various classes of current equipment but also on how these have changed over the years (Duck & Martin 1991).

REFERENCES

Anson, L.W. and Chivers, R.C. (1980). The use of absorbing polymeric materials for suspended sphere radiometers. *Acoust. Lett.* **4**, 74–80.

Bacon, D.R. (1988). Primary calibration of ultrasonic hydrophones using optical interferometry. *IEEE Trans.* **UFFC-35**, 152–161.

Bacon, D.R. (1989). Prediction of *in situ* exposure to ultrasound: an improved method. *Ultrasound in Med. & Biol.* **15**, 355–361.

Bacon, D.R., Chivers, R.C. and Som, J.N. (1993). The acousto-optic interaction in the interferometric measurement of ultrasonic transducer surface motion. *Ultrasonics* **31**, 321–325.

Bobber, R.J. (1970). *Underwater Acoustic Measurements*. Naval Research Laboratory Publication, Washington, D.C.

Busse, L.J. and Miller, J.G. (1981a). Response characteristics of a finite aperture, phase insensitive ultrasonic receiver based on the acousto-electric effect. *J. Acoust. Soc. Am.* **70**, 1370–1376.

Busse, L.J. and Miller, J.G. (1981b). Detection of spatially non-uniform ultrasonic radiation with phase sensitive (piezoelectric) and phase-insensitive (acousto-electric) receivers. *J. Acoust. Soc. Am.* **70**, 1377–1386.

Chivers, R.C., Som, J.N., Anson, L.W. and Ogulu, A. (1989). Design considerations for strain-gauge radiation force detectors. *Ultrasonics* **27**, 302–307.

Chivers, R.C., Zell, K., Peake, J.C.F. and Fielding, S.L. (1993). A tethered float radiometer. *Acustica* **79**, 170–174.

Davidson, F. (1991). Ultrasonic power balances. In *Output Measurements for Medical Ultrasound*, R. C. Preston (ed.). Springer, London, pp. 75–90.

Dickinson, R.J. (1985). Thermal conduction errors of manganin–constantan thermocouple arrays. *Phys. Med. Biol.* **30**, 445–453.

Drewniak, J.L., Frizzell, L.A. and Dunn, F. (1990). Errors resulting from finite beamwidth and sample dimensions in the determination of the ultrasonic absorption coefficient. *J. Acoust. Soc. Am.* **88**, 967–977.

Duck, F.A. and Martin, K. (1991). Trends in diagnostic ultrasound exposure. *Phys. Med. Biol.* **36**, 1423–1432.

Farmery, M.J. and Whittingham, T.A. (1978). A portable radiation force balance for use with diagnostic ultrasonic equipment. *Ultrasound in Med. & Biol.* **4**, 273–279.

Filipczynski, L.S. (1969). Absolute measurement of particle displacement, or intensity of ultrasonic pulses in liquids and solids. *Acustica* **3**, 137.

Foldy, L.L. and Primakoff, D. (1945, 1947). A general theory of passive linear electroacoustic transducers, and electroacoustic reciprocity theorem. *J. Acoust. Soc. Am.* **17**, 109 and **19**, 50.

Fry, W.S. and Fry, R.B. (1954). Determination of absolute sound levels and acoustic absorption coefficients by thermocouple probes: theory and experiment. *J. Acoust. Soc. Am.* **26**, 294–310, 311–317.

Gavrilov, L.R., Dmitriev, V.N. and Solontsova, L.V. (1988). Use of focused ultrasonic receivers for remote measurements in biological tissues. *J. Acoust. Soc. Am.* **83**, 1167–1179.

Harris, G.R. (1985). A discussion of procedures for ultrasonic intensity and power calculations from miniature hydrophone measurements. *Ultrasound in Med. & Biol.* **11**, 803–817.

Harris, G.R., Lewin, P.A. and Preston, R.C. (1988). Introduction to special issue on ultrasonic exposimetry. *IEEE Trans.* **UFFC-35**, 85–86.

Hasegawa, T. and Yosioka, K. (1969). Acoustic radiation force on a solid elastic sphere. *J. Acoust. Soc. Am.* **46**, 1139–1143.

Hekkenberg, R.T., Reibold, R. and Zeqiri, B. (1994). Development of standard measurement methods for essential properties of ultrasonic therapy equipment. *Ultrasound in Med. & Biol.* **20**, 83–98.

Hill, C.R. (1970). Calibration of ultrasonic beams for biomedical applications. *Phys. Med. Biol.* **15**, 241–248.

Hill, C.R. (1975). A proposed facility for ultrasound exposimetry and calibration. *Ultrasound in Med. & Biol.* **1**, 476.

Hill, C.R., Rivens, I., Vaughan, M.G. and ter Haar, G.R. (1994). Lesion development in focused ultrasound surgery. *Ultrasound in Med. & Biol.* **20**, 259–269.

Hynynen, K., Martin, C.J., Watmough, D.J. and Mallard, J.R. (1983). Errors in temperature measurement by thermocouple probes during ultrasound induced hyperthermia. *Brit. J. Radiol.* **56**, 969–970.

IEC (1987). Characteristics and calibration of hydrophones for operation in the frequency range 0.5 MHz– 15 MHz. IEC standard no. 866. International Electrotechnical Commission, Geneva.

IEC (1991a). The absolute calibration of hydrophones using the planar scanning technique in the frequency range 0.5 MHz–15 MHz. IEC standard no. 1101. International Electrotechnical Commission, Geneva.

IEC (1991b). Measurement and characterisation of ultrasonic fields using hydrophones in the frequency range 0.5 MHz–15 MHz. IEC standard no. 1102. International Electrotechnical Commission, Geneva.

IEC (1992a). Requirements for the declaration of the acoustic output of medical diagnostic equipment. IEC standard no. 1157. International Electrotechnical Commission, Geneva.

IEC (1992b). Ultrasonic power measurements in liquids in the frequency range 0.5 MHz–25 MHz. IEC standard no. 1161. International Electrotechnical Commission, Geneva.

IEC (1993). Measurement and characterization of ultrasonic fields generated by medical ultrasonic equipment using hydrophones in the frequency range 0.5 to 15 MHz. IEC standard no. 1220. International Electrotechnical Commission, Geneva.

IEEE (1988). Special issue on ultrasonic exposimetry. *IEEE Trans.* **UFFC-35**, 85–269.

Klein, W.R. and Cook, B.D. (1967). Unified approach to ultrasonic light diffraction. *IEEE Trans.* **SU-14**, 123–134.

Laughlin, J.S. and Genna, S. (1966). Calorimetry. In *Radiation Dosimetry*, Vol. 2, F. H. Attix and W. C. Roesch (eds). Academic Press, New York, pp. 389–441.

Lewin, P.A., Schafer, M.E. and Chivers, R.C. (1987). Factors affecting the choice of preamplification for ultrasonic hydrophone probes. *Ultrasound in Med. & Biol.* **13**, 141–148.

Lewin, P.A., Schafer, M.E. and Gilmore, J.M. (1988). Ultrasonic probes for shock wave measurements. *IEEE 1988 Ultrasonics Symposium*, pp. 955–958.

Livett, A.J., Emery, E.W. and Leeman, S. (1981). Acoustic radiation pressure. *J. Sound Vib.* **76**, 1–11.

Ludwig, G. and Brendel, K. (1988). Calibration of hydrophones based on reciprocity and time-delay spectrometry. *IEEE Trans.* **UFFC-35**, 168–174.

Lum, P., Greenstein, M., Grossman, C. and Szabo, T.L. (1996). High frequency membrane hydrophone. *IEEE Trans.* **UFFC-43**, 536–544.

McLean, W.R. (1940). Absolute measurement of sound without a primary standard. *J. Acoust. Soc. Am.* **12**, 140.

Mezrich, R.S., Etzoid, K.F. and Vilkomerson, D.H.R. (1975). System for visualising and measuring ultrasonic wave fronts. In *Acoustical Holography*, Vol. 6, N. Booth (ed.). Plenum Press, New York, pp. 165–191.

Miller, E.B. and Hill, C.R. (1986). Detection and measurement of acoustic fields. In *Physical Principles of Medical Ultrasonics* (1st edn), C. R. Hill (ed.). Ellis Horwood, Chichester, pp. 93–117.

O'Brien, W.D. (1978). Ultrasonic dosimetry. In *Ultrasound: Its Application in Medicine and Biology*, Part 1., F. J. Fry (ed.). Elsevier, Amsterdam, pp. 343–391.

Ocheltree, K.B. and Frizzell, L.A. (1987). Determination of power deposition patterns for localized hyperthermia: a steady-state analysis. *Int. J. Hyperthermia* **3**, 269–279.

Preston, R.C. (1986). Measurement and characterization of the acoustic output of medical ultrasonic equipment. *Med. Biol. Eng. Comput.* **24**, 113–120 (part 1), 225–234 (part 2).

Preston, R.C., Bacon, D.R., Corbett, S.C., Harris, G.R., Lewin, P.A., McGregor, J.A., O'Brien, W.D. and Szabo, T.L. (1988). Interlaboratory comparison of hydrophone calibrations. *IEEE Trans.* **UFFC-35**, 206–213.

Preston, R.C., Shaw, A. and Zeqiri, B. (1991). Prediction of *in situ* exposure to ultrasound. *Ultrasound in Med. & Biol.* **17**, 317–332 (An acoustical attenuation method), 333–339 (A proposed standard experimental method).

Pye, S.D., Parr, N.J., Munro, E.G., Anderson, T. and McDicken, W.N. (1991). Robust electromagnetic probe for the monitoring of lithotriptor output. *Ultrasound in Med. & Biol.* **17**, 931–939.

Reibold, R. (1977). Application of holographic interferometry for the investigation of ultrasonic fields. *Acustica* **38**, 253–257.

Reid, J.M. and Sikov, M.R. (eds) (1973). *Interaction of Ultrasound and Biological Tissues* (Section 4, Ultrasound Dosimetry, pp. 153–201, various authors). DHEW Publication (FDA) 73-8008, US Govt. Printing Office, Washington, D.C.

Riley, W.A. and Klein, W.R. (1967). Piezo-optic coefficients of liquids. *J. Acoust. Soc. Am.* **42**, 1258–1261.

Robinson, S.P. (1991). Hydrophones. In *Output Measurements for Medical Ultrasound*, R. C. Preston (ed.). Springer, London, pp. 57–73.

Rooney, J.A. (1973). Determination of acoustic power outputs in the microwatt–milliwatt range. *Ultrasound in Med. & Biol.* **1**, 13–16.

Rooney, J.A. and Nyborg, W.L. (1972). Acoustic radiation pressure in a travelling plane wave. *Am. J. Phys.* **40**, 1825–1830.

Shombert, D.G. and Harris, G.R. (1986). Use of miniature hydrophones to determine peak intensities typical of medical ultrasonic devices. *IEEE Trans*. **UFFC-33**, 287–294.

Shombert, D.G., Smith, S.W. and Harris, G.R. (1982). Angular response of miniature ultrasonic hydrophones. *Med. Phys.* **9**, 484–492.

Shotton, K.C. (1980). A tethered float radiometer for measuring the output power from ultrasonic therapy equipment. *Ultrasound in Med. & Biol.* **6**, 131–133.

Shotton, K.C., Bacon, D.R. and Quilliam, R.M. (1980). A PVDF membrane hydrophone for operation in the range 0.5 MHz to 15 MHz. *Ultrasonics* **18**, 123–126.

Smith, R.A. (1989). Are hydrophones of diameter 0.5 mm small enough to characterize diagnostic ultrasound equipment? *Phys. Med. Biol.* **34**, 1593–1607.

Staudenraus, J. and Eisenmenger, W. (1993). Fibre-optic probe hydrophone for ultrasonic and shock-wave measurements in water. *Ultrasonics* **31**, 267–273.

Stockdale, H.R. and Hill, C.R. (1976). Use of a sphere radiometer to measure ultrasonic beam power. *Ultrasound in Med. & Biol.* **2**, 219–220.

Torr, G.R. and Watmough, D.J. (1977). A constant-flow calorimeter for the measurement of acoustic power at megahertz frequencies. *Phys. Med. Biol* **22**, 444–450.

Weinreich, G., Sanders, T.M. and White, H.G. (1959). Acousto-electric effect in n-type germanium. *Phys. Rev.* **144**, 33–44.

Wells, P.N.T., Bullen, M.A., Follett, D.H., Freundlich, H.F. and Angell-James, J. (1978). The dosimetry of small ultrasonic beams. *Ultrasonics* **1**, 106–110.

WHO (1989). Ultrasound. In *Nonionizing Radiation Protection* (2nd edn), M. J. Suess and D. Benwell (eds). WHO Regional Publication, European Series No. 25. World Health Organisation, Geneva, pp. 245–291.

Zeqiri, B. (1991). Overview of measurement techniques. In *Output Measurements for Medical Ultrasound* R. C. Preston (ed.). Springer, London, pp. 35–56.

Zeqiri, B. and Bond, A.D. (1992). The influence of waveform distortion on hydrophone spatial-averaging corrections: theory and measurement. *J. Acoust. Soc. Am.* **92**, 1809–1821.

4

Attenuation and Absorption

J. C. BAMBER

Institute of Cancer Research, Royal Marsden Hospital, UK

4.1 INTRODUCTION

Sound wave propagation is determined by the inertial, restoring and loss parameters of the medium, as discussed in Chapter 1. Density and compressibility determine sound speed, variations of which result in refraction. Spatial fluctuations in either density or compressibility (which together determine characteristic acoustic impedance), or sound absorption, may give rise to scattering or reflection. In biological tissues refraction, reflection, scattering and absorption all contribute to the total loss (attenuation) of sound energy due to the tissue. In practice bulk variations of speed, impedance, absorption, scattering and attenuation are used to provide information about tissue structure: in particular they all contribute to the complicated process of formation, and therefore to the appearance, of pulse–echo images. Clearly, therefore, knowledge of these parameters and their variation with frequency, amplitude, temperature, age, pathology, etc. is crucial to our ability to understand and make the most efficient use of present and potential ultrasonic diagnostic techniques. Attenuation and absorption coefficients also play a part in determining the sound power reaching, and deposited in, a particular tissue volume. They thus play an important role in determining the nature and magnitude of the biological effects of ultrasound that are discussed in Chapters 12 to 14. Attenuation of wave energy by any of the above mentioned loss mechanisms leads to a modification of equation (1.49) by a constant factor, α, per unit path length. Thus, for a plane wave propagating in the positive x-direction,

$$u(x, t) = U e^{-\alpha x} e^{i\omega(t-x/c)} \tag{4.1}$$

where the equation has been written in terms of scalar particle velocity, u, rather than acoustic pressure. In addition to these loss mechanisms, since practical situations rarely involve perfectly plane waves, there are almost always additional losses (or gains) of acoustic intensity due to the diffraction field of the sound source (see Chapters 1 and 2). A loss of received energy due to this effect, termed the 'diffraction loss', can lead to an error if one is attempting to measure attenuation or scattering due to the tissue. Similarly, diffraction-derived phase changes constitute errors in speed measurements. Steps taken to reduce the effect of these errors upon the measurements are, if implemented by calculation, termed 'diffraction corrections'. If bulk reflection and refraction are regarded as special cases of a general scattering phenomenon, then the theory of acoustic wave propagation in biological media has

Physical Principles of Medical Ultrasonics, Second Edition. Edited by C. R. Hill, J. C. Bamber and G. R. ter Haar.
© 2004 John Wiley & Sons, Ltd: ISBN 0 471 97002 6

thus far developed along two, largely separate, lines: the study of acoustic absorption and dispersion, and the study of acoustic wave scattering. The specific details of scattering theory will be covered in Chapter 6 although, as mentioned later (see Section 4.3.7), it is not always easy to distinguish between a scattering and an absorption event. This chapter deals broadly with attenuation, absorption and dispersion, and methods of measuring attenuation, whilst methods of measuring the speed of sound are covered in Chapter 5.

4.2   TISSUE–ULTRASOUND INTERACTION CROSS-SECTIONS

In many areas of physics dealing with wave–matter interactions, absorption and scattering are described in terms of fundamental interaction cross-sections for the particles of the medium that interact with the wave. Numerical estimation of individual cross-sections in biological tissues is, in general, not possible, and quantities have to be ascribed which relate to the bulk scattering and absorbing properties of the tissues. These quantities are the macroscopic cross-sections, or interaction cross-sections per unit volume, of the tissue concerned. More specifically, there are three such macroscopic cross-sections: the attenuation cross-section per unit volume, the absorption cross-section per unit volume, and the scattering cross-section per unit volume. In order to illustrate tangibly the physical meaning of these quantities, and to demonstrate one way in which they might be related to individual cross-sections, we consider a medium that is composed entirely of two types of inhomogeneity: those which absorb and those which scatter the acoustic energy. There are n_i scattering inhomogeneities per unit volume, each of scattering cross-section σ_{si}, and n_j absorbing inhomogeneities per unit volume, each of absorption cross-section σ_{aj}. For a single inhomogeneity that both scatters and absorbs, its total interaction (or extinction) cross-section would be the sum $\sigma = \sigma_s + \sigma_a$. Such individual cross-sections are defined as the ratio of the total power absorbed or scattered, by a given inhomogeneity, to the incident intensity. They have dimensions of L^2 and are equal to the cross-sectional area of an incident plane wave that contains the same amount of power as was either scattered or absorbed. Thus, for a beam of approximately constant cross-sectional area S, total power W, and uniform intensity, the power scattered by a scattering inhomogeneity would be $\sigma_{si} W/S$ and the power absorbed by an absorbing inhomogeneity would be $\sigma_{aj} W/S$. The powers scattered and absorbed per unit volume will then be given respectively by $\Sigma_i n_{si} \sigma_{si} W/S$ and $\Sigma_j n_{aj} \sigma_{aj} W/S$. The quantities represented by the summations may therefore be defined (in the absence of multiple scattering) as the scattering cross-section per unit volume μ_s, and the absorption cross-section per unit volume μ_a, respectively:

$$\mu_s = \sum_i n_{si} \sigma_{si} \tag{4.2a}$$

$$\mu_a = \sum_j n_{aj} \sigma_{aj} \tag{4.2b}$$

The powers scattered and absorbed per unit path length will be $\mu_s W$ and $\mu_a W$, respectively. Hence, for a thin target of thickness Δx, the total power scattered will be:

$$\Delta W_s = \mu_s W \Delta x \tag{4.2c}$$

and the total power absorbed will be:

$$\Delta W_a = \mu_a W \Delta x \tag{4.2d}$$

By adding ΔW_s and ΔW_a we obtain the total power ΔW that has interacted with the medium:

$$\Delta W = (\mu_s + \mu_a) W \Delta x \qquad (4.2e)$$

The quantity $(\mu_s + \mu_a)$ is the total interaction (or extinction) cross-section per unit volume of the medium and will be denoted by μ.

When considering a target of finite thickness, equation (4.2e) is integrated. Letting $W = W_0$ (the 'incident power') at $x = 0$ gives:

$$W = W_0 e^{-(\mu_s + \mu_a)x} \qquad (4.3)$$

In other words, the power (and hence plane-wave intensity) is an exponentially decreasing function of the propagation path, the coefficient of attenuation being equal to the total cross-section per unit volume μ. Thus the following relationships hold for the bulk properties of the propagation medium:

$$\mu = \mu_s + \mu_a = 2\alpha \qquad (4.4)$$

$$\mu_s = \frac{1}{\Delta x} \frac{W_s}{W_0} = 2\alpha_s \qquad (4.5)$$

$$\mu_a = \frac{1}{\Delta x} \frac{W_a}{W_0} = 2\alpha_a \qquad (4.6)$$

$$\alpha = \alpha_s + \alpha_a \qquad (4.7)$$

where α is the amplitude attenuation coefficient, α_s is the amplitude scattering coefficient (the attenuation coefficient in the absence of absorption), and α_a is the amplitude absorption coefficient (the attenuation coefficient in the absence of scattering). With respect to the quantities μ_s, μ_a and μ, the terms 'macroscopic cross-section', 'cross-section per unit volume' and 'intensity coefficient' may all be used with equal validity. The units used for each μ and α vary with the field of application and purpose of measurement. For purposes of studying fundamental mechanisms of acoustic wave interactions, units of cm^{-1} are most commonly used. Such units are also known as 'nepers per centimetre' since, by taking the natural or 'napierian' logarithm of equation (4.3), for example, we may obtain:

$$\mu = \mu_s + \mu_a = -\frac{1}{x} \log_e \left(\frac{W}{W_0} \right) \qquad (4.8)$$

For many purposes (e.g. in designing instruments for ultrasonic imaging) it is more convenient to express the ratio W/W_0, or the corresponding ratio of signal amplitudes P/P_0, in decibels. Thus,

$$\mu = -\frac{10}{x} \log_{10} \left(\frac{W}{W_0} \right) \qquad (4.9)$$

and

$$\alpha = -\frac{20}{x} \log_{10} \left(\frac{P}{P_0} \right) \qquad (4.10)$$

where μ and α become numerically equal and are expressed in units of dB cm^{-1}. A coefficient expressed in dB cm^{-1} will therefore be given by $10\log_{10}$ ($= 4.343$) times the equivalent intensity coefficient in neper cm^{-1}, or $20\log_{10}$ ($= 8.686$) times the equivalent amplitude coefficient.

A quantity that has found frequent application in discussions of absorption mechanisms is the specific absorption. This is the absorption coefficient divided by the density, or, for materials in solution, the so-called 'excess' absorption coefficient ($\alpha_{solution} - \alpha_{solvent}$) divided by the concentration by weight of solute in the solvent. Tissues may be assigned a specific attenuation coefficient. They are generally considered, for purposes of calculating an excess attenuation, to be a suspension, with the 'solvent' being water. The specific absorption and attenuation coefficients have units of nepers (or decibels) cm^2 per gram and are designed to facilitate comparison between the attenuation or absorption properties of different materials independently of density or concentration. A related quantity, often used to discuss the ultrasonic absorption of solutions, is the molecular absorption cross-section. Also known as the 'excess absorption per molecule', this is defined as the excess absorption coefficient divided by the number of solute molecules in unit volume of solvent (which may be obtained from the product of the molar concentration and Avogadro's number). Note that in the subsequent discussion of absorption mechanisms (Section 4.3.1), an 'excess' absorption will be defined which is not related to that defined above. This same term is used in the literature for two quite separate meanings, which should not be confused.

There remains one final but very important point to be made in this short section on definitions. The attenuation coefficient as defined by equations (4.3) and (4.4) is strictly a theoretically limiting quantity and can never be measured directly. Correspondingly, the quantity $e^{-\mu x}$ will never actually provide the observed proportional reduction of power in a real measurement situation; there will always be some part of μ_s (the forward scattered part) which gives rise to contributions to the received power at distance x. In fact it is possible to conceive of two opposite theoretically limiting geometries for measuring the attenuation coefficient. One of these is a 'perfect' geometry in which the receiving aperture is either infinitesimally small or is an infinite distance away from the measurement point. None of the scattered power would be received, and the measured quantity would indeed be μ. The other geometry is a totally 'imperfect' one in which the receiver is so large that it effectively surrounds the measurement specimen and records all of the scattered power. The measured quantity then becomes the absorption coefficient μ_a. All real attenuation measurement systems must fall short of perfection and, to a degree dependent upon the geometry, underestimate the attenuation coefficient. As will be noted in Section 4.4, however, there are numerous other reasons why the measured attenuation coefficients are more often in error by over-estimation. In any event a 'perfect' measurement for either dosimetric or ultrasonic imaging purposes (and a measured value of an attenuation coefficient) has meaning, in a strict sense, only with reference to the geometry of the particular measurement system used.

4.3 THEORY OF MECHANISMS FOR THE ABSORPTION OF ULTRASONIC LONGITUDINAL WAVES

A number of excellent reviews have been published on the subject of absorption and dispersion of ultrasound in biological media (e.g. Carstensen 1979; Dunn et al. 1969; Dunn & O'Brien 1978; Fry & Dunn 1962; Johnston et al. 1979; Wells 1975; Woodcock 1979). The basic theory, however, although not specifically relating to biological media, has been covered prior to the appearance of these reviews (e.g. Markham et al. 1951; Hertzfeld & Litovitz 1959). Other useful texts are Matheson (1971) and Dunn and O'Brien (1976). The following treatment draws heavily on the above references and contains only the essential features of the subject, although some recent work is also included in an attempt to be as up-to-date as is possible.

4.3.1 HOMOGENEOUS LIQUID-LIKE MEDIA

Absorption of the wave energy results in its degradation to heat. This occurs when the density fluctuations in the medium get out of phase with the sound pressure fluctuations. In 'homogeneous' media (e.g. solutions of macromolecules) the mechanisms by which this is known to occur are relaxation mechanisms. These are not fully understood even in very simple media but arise from the time-lag that is inherent in the perturbation of any physical or chemical equilibrium initiated by the cyclic fluctuations of the wave parameters. At any instant in time the total wave energy may be viewed as being shared amongst a number of different forms of energy: translational energy, molecular vibrational and structural energy, and lattice vibrational and structural states. As time varies, redistribution of the energy occurs, but at finite rates determined by the precise coupling processes relevant to the propagation medium. The coupling processes themselves constitute the absorption mechanisms, the type and number of which may vary enormously from liquid to liquid.

A general form for the equation describing the absorption at a frequency f (wavelength λ) due to a single process of this kind is

$$\frac{\alpha_R}{f^2} = \frac{A}{1 + (f/f_R)^2} \tag{4.11}$$

where $A = 2[(\alpha_R \lambda)_{max}/cf_R]$ is a constant (sometimes called the *relaxation amplitude*) defined by the maximum value of the wavelength-absorption or absorption per cycle[1] ($\alpha\lambda$), the speed (c) and the relaxation frequency (f_R). Figure 4.1a helps to visualise the form of this equation.

At low frequencies the wave parameters fluctuate slowly enough for the redistribution of energy nearly to 'keep up', energy is returned to the wave from its other shared forms only slightly out of phase, and the absorption is low. As the frequency increases, energy is returned more out of phase and the absorption increases until, at frequencies much higher than the relaxation frequency, the wave does not have time fully to perturb the equilibrium of the medium and there is little sharing of the wave energy from its purely translational form. The wavelength-absorption reaches a maximum value when $f = f_R$.

In an attempt to describe observed absorption versus frequency curves a number of such processes are considered, summed and added to the so-called 'classical absorption coefficient' (as calculated by Stokes and Kirchoff over a century ago). The result is symbolised by:

$$\frac{\alpha_a}{f^2} = \frac{4\pi^2}{\rho_0 c^3} \left[\frac{4\eta_s}{3} + \frac{(\gamma - 1)\chi}{C_P} \right] + \sum_j \frac{A_j}{1 + (f/f_{Rj})^2} \tag{4.12}$$

where η_s is the coefficient of shear viscosity, γ is the ratio of specific heats, C_P is the heat capacity at constant pressure and χ is the thermal conductivity. The quantity α/f^2 is sometimes referred to as the 'frequency-free' absorption.

The first term in the large brackets expresses contributions to absorption due to the fact that it takes a finite time, dictated by the shear viscosity, for the molecules of the medium to move to different local arrangements relative to one another. The thermal conductivity term, which is negligible except for molten metals, describes the loss of energy when heat attempts to flow

---

1 This quantity has been misnamed, being widely referred to as 'absorption per wavelength'.

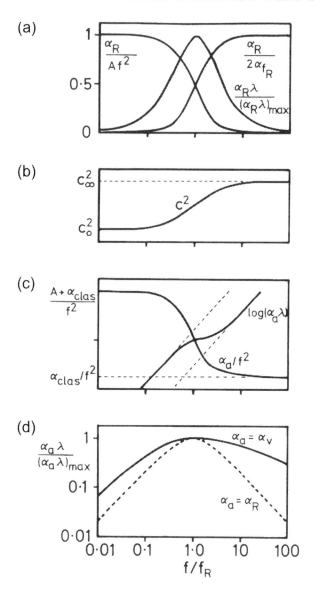

Figure 4.1. Absorption and dispersion representation of a single relaxation process with a time constant $\tau = 1/2\pi f_R$ (a and b), a single relaxation process plus classical processes (c) and a viscous relative motion process compared to a relaxation process (d)

from regions of high acoustic pressure to regions of low pressure. For liquid mixtures there exists, in principle, another absorption term due to the diffusion of molecular species along concentration gradients set up by the sound wave. In reality this contribution is totally negligible and is omitted from equation (4.12). In general these contributions are defined by more precise relaxation expressions which, for frequencies well below the associated relaxation frequencies, reduce to the simple f^2 dependencies of the classical contributions. Consequently, the absorption mechanisms are often, although somewhat incorrectly, referred to separately as 'classical' contributions and 'relaxation' contributions. The inappropriateness of this distinction has been emphasised by Sehgal and Greenleaf (1982) who described the frequency dependencies of ultrasonic absorption in liquids and in tissues (see Section 4.5) in terms of a model based purely on the phase differences which arise between the acoustic pressure and temperature fluctuations when any kind of relaxation process occurs. A closed-form expression for absorption, combining the viscothermal and viscoelastic theories of relaxation processes, has been derived by Jongen *et al.* (1986), who have found it to provide a particularly good fit to experimental data.

In equation (4.12) the values of $A_j = 2[(\alpha_R \lambda)_{\mathrm{max}}/cf_{Rj}]$ and f_{Rj} are constant for each process, but follow distribution functions with frequency and temperature. The forms of these functions at a given temperature are adjusted so that the resulting dependence of α_a ($= \alpha_{class} + \alpha_R$) is a best fit to the experimental data. Figure 4.1c demonstrates schematically the form of equation (4.12) for a single value of j. Thus, departure from linearity of the plot of $\log(\alpha_a/f)$ vs $\log f$ is said to strongly indicate the presence of additional relaxation mechanisms.

For the more complex biological media and soft tissues the slope of $\log(\alpha_a/f)$ vs $\log f$ usually varies between 1 and 1.4 in the frequency range 1 to 10 MHz. The form of the distribution function that needs to be employed in order for equation (4.12) to describe the data, which often approximates to some form of logarithmic square window, is said to provide information about the range of activation energies involved with the relaxation processes that are occurring. For biological media it is not known, however, whether a discrete number of processes is involved or whether the distribution of relaxation frequencies is a continuous function of frequency, in which case the summation in equation (4.12) would be replaced by an integration.

The difference between the measured absorption coefficient α_a and the classical absorption coefficient is usually referred to as the 'excess' absorption (not to be confused with the 'excess' absorption coefficient defined in Section 4.2) and is here attributed to the presence of additional relaxation phenomena. These additional loss mechanisms have the effect of endowing the medium with a bulk, or volume viscosity, η_v.[2] The value of η_v was taken to be zero by Stokes in his original derivation (simply because he had no way of measuring it), but it would have come into the classical expression as a simple summation with the shear viscosity term $(\eta_v + 4\eta_s/3)$ inside the large brackets of equation (4.11).

Molecular relaxation processes have generally been classified into two groups, *viz.* thermal and structural. The detailed discussion of these is beyond the intended scope of this summary, although the two classes of mechanism display some interesting differences, particularly with regard to temperature dependence, which will be mentioned later. Structural mechanisms (reviewed by Litovitz & Davis 1965) involve intermolecular rearrangements and a volume change between different equilibrium states. They predominate in associated liquids such as water and the alcohols, which are of polar molecules and tend to exist with a dynamic short-range crystalline structure, and occur in response to the stress (pressure) fluctuations in the wave. The processes associated with shear viscosity are specific examples of a structural relaxation. Thermal relaxation effects (reviewed by Lamb 1965) are observed in weakly associated or non-associated liquids such as benzene or carbon disulphide, in which the temperature fluctuations of the wave perturb an intramolecular (i.e. chemical) equilibrium.

---

2 Although the terms 'bulk viscosity' and 'volume viscosity' are used here synonymously, there are a variety of such terms to be found in the literature, each defined differently. One example of this is the use Matheson (1971) makes of the term volume viscosity to describe that part of the bulk viscosity due to structural relaxation. Others refer to this part as the 'structural viscosity'.

The intramolecular rearrangements of rotational isomerism and the coupling between translational and internal vibrational forms of energy are both thermal processes. Over a relaxation region of the acoustic frequency spectrum the sound speed is also observed to vary. Such velocity dispersion takes the form, again for a single relaxation process, shown in Figure 4.1b. The existence of such dispersion in homogeneous media may be used as a strong indication of the presence of additional relaxation. The incremental increase in speed over the dispersion region and the absorption peak due to the relaxation mechanism are approximately related in the materials of interest by:

$$\frac{\Delta c}{c} \approx \frac{(\alpha_R \lambda)_{\max}}{\pi} \qquad (4.13)$$

In practice, however, the total variation is usually less than 1% of the actual speed and requires accurate measurement if quantitative deductions are to be made. For a distribution of relaxation frequencies the dependence of c on $\log f$ tends to be roughly linear.

4.3.2 VISCOELASTICITY: SEMI-SOLID MEDIA

In Chapter 1, and thus far in the present chapter, the viscous nature of liquids has been emphasised. In the classical case of a perfectly viscous (Newtonian) liquid the applied stress is always proportional to the rate of change in the resulting strain, but is independent of the strain itself, which is not maintained. The correspondingly ideal, perfectly elastic, solid follows Hooke's law in which stress is always proportional to strain and is independent of the rate of strain. All real materials, however, exhibit some combination of these properties, i.e. the stress depends on the strain and the rate of strain (and higher time derivatives of strain) together, and are therefore viscoelastic in behaviour. Note also that real materials do not respond linearly to stress. The implications of this are discussed in Section 4.3 but, for the present, we continue to assume linearity.

A molecular picture of viscoelasticity may, for example, be gained by considering a liquid between two plates; one fixed and one oscillating to provide a sinusoidal shear stress. At low frequencies of oscillation all the driving energy is dissipated in viscous flow of the different layers of liquid over each other. Such flow occurs as a small directional drift superimposed on the random, thermal, molecular motion. If the frequency of the oscillating stress is increased until it is too fast for any molecular diffusion to occur during the period of shear strain, then the liquid will appear to possess shear rigidity; no energy is dissipated in viscous flow, instead it is stored elastically. The change from viscous to elastic behaviour with increasing frequency, intermediate between these extremes, is called the 'viscoelastic relaxation'. In this case the viscoelastic relaxation time is the diffusional jump-time of the liquid molecules.

With an alternating compression of low frequency the volume fluctuations remain in phase with the applied pressure by flow of molecules between positions of high and low density. At high frequencies the liquid structure is not able to respond to the pressure variations sufficiently quickly; volume or structural relaxation has occurred as the frequency was raised, the relaxation time being the time required for the liquid to adjust itself to its new equilibrium volume following a rapid change in the applied pressure.

An ultrasonic longitudinal wave contains both shear and compressional components, and its propagation may, in general, be discussed in terms of both shear and compressional elastic moduli and relaxation times.

The theory of viscoelasticity is essentially phenomenological and seeks to describe the mechanical behaviour of all macroscopically homogeneous solid and liquid media. Molecular or other mechanisms are not explicitly stated but may include the shear and volume relaxation mechanisms referred to in Section 4.3.1. Viscoelastic theory (Christensen 1971) has probably found its greatest application in describing the mechanical behaviour of polymers (Ferry 1961; Matheson 1971), both in solid form and in solution, which often display the transition from liquid to solid-like behaviour in a spectacular manner. The mainstream medical and biological ultrasonic literature makes little mention of viscoelasticity. However, since the earliest measurements of ultrasonic absorption by biological tissues it has been thought that similar theoretical descriptions might also be applied to tissue (e.g. Hueter 1958). The following is a glimpse of some aspects of viscoelastic theory, which should permit the reading of papers on this subject. The derivations provided are not mathematically rigorous and serve only to illustrate the relationships of results quoted to those in the medical ultrasound literature.

We begin by noting that equation (4.1) can be written in the form

$$u(x,\ t) = U \exp \left\{ i\omega \left(t - x \left[\frac{1}{c} + \frac{\alpha}{i\omega} \right] \right) \right\}$$

which can be written back in the form of equation (4.1), $u(x,\ t) = U e^{i\omega(t-x/c)}$, as c is now a complex quantity given by:

$$\frac{1}{c} = \frac{1}{c'} - \frac{i\alpha}{\omega} \qquad (4.14)$$

where c' is the value that the phase speed took when there was no attenuation. In the presence of attenuation, therefore, the phase speed is frequency-dependent (dispersive) and complex.

The one-dimensional wave equation for sound in solids is:

$$\frac{\partial^2 u}{\partial t} = \frac{M}{\rho_0} \frac{\partial^2 u}{\partial x^2} \qquad (4.15)$$

where $M = K + 4/3G$ is the longitudinal elastic modulus, K is the bulk modulus and G is the shear modulus. Similar equations exist, where M is replaced by K or G, for the propagation of pure compressional or pure shear waves. From the form of the wave equation the propagation speed of sound waves in a solid is given by:

$$c^2 = \frac{M}{\rho_0} = \frac{1}{\rho_0} \left(K + \frac{4}{3}G \right) \qquad (4.16)$$

We see, therefore, that M must also be complex and frequency-dependent. This is also true of K and G. Generally this is written as:

$$\begin{aligned} M &= M' + iM'' \\ K &= K' + iK'' \\ G &= G' + iG'' \end{aligned} \qquad (4.17)$$

The real parts are the elastic or storage moduli, each in phase with a sinusoidally varying strain, and the imaginary parts are those loss moduli, 90° out of phase with the strain.

The components of M may be written in terms of α and c' by combining equations (4.16) and (4.14). If the losses are small enough for $(\alpha c'/\omega)^2 \ll 1$, then the results reduce to:

$$M' = \rho_0 c'^2 \qquad (4.18)$$

and

$$M'' = 2\rho_0 c'^3 \alpha/\omega \qquad (4.19)$$

In the literature on viscoelasticity most experimental results are presented in terms of M' and M'', or the other moduli for non-longitudinal deformations. Equations (4.18) and (4.19) provide a useful means of quickly interpreting such data, in terms of the speed and attenuation coefficient which are usually quoted in biomedical ultrasonics; that is, $c' \propto \sqrt{M'}$ and $\alpha\lambda \propto M''/M' = \tan\delta$ (the 'loss tangent').

Using σ and γ to represent generalised stress and strain quantities respectively, the elastic moduli for perfectly elastic solids are defined by $\sigma_v = K\gamma_v$ and $\sigma_s = G\gamma_s$, and the coefficients of viscosity for a Newtonian liquid are defined by $\sigma_v = \eta_v(d\gamma_v/dt)$ and $\sigma_s = \eta_s(d\gamma_s/dt)$, where the subscripts v and s denote volume and shear deformations respectively.

In modelling the macroscopic aspects of viscoelasticity there are many possible ways of combining the elastic and viscous components (often referred to in this context as 'springs' and 'dashpots' respectively). Two such ways, which have often been used, are known commonly as the Maxwell model and the Voigt model. Elements of these models may be simulated using combinations of 'springs' and 'dashpots' as shown in Figure 4.2a and b. Consideration of these models, or their equivalent electric networks[3] leads to the observation that in the Maxwell element the entire applied stress (voltage) is felt equally by the elastic (capacitance) and viscous (resistance) components, but their strains, or rate of change of strain (current), are additive.

For the Voigt element each component experiences the same strain, but they share the stress (potential division). By inspection of the figures we can write, for the Maxwell model,

$$\frac{d\gamma_s}{dt} = \frac{\sigma_s}{\eta_s} + \frac{1}{G_\infty}\frac{d\sigma_s}{dt} \tag{4.20}$$

and for the Voigt model

$$\sigma_s = \eta_s\frac{d\gamma_s}{dt} + G_\infty\gamma_s \tag{4.21}$$

where shear deformations only have been considered. The subscript infinity is used to indicate the value of the elastic modulus under conditions of totally solid-like behaviour, i.e. at a limiting high frequency.

Solutions to equations (4.20) and (4.21) may be found in texts discussing electrical networks. For example, the transient response of the system described by equation (4.21), when an applied stress is suddenly removed, is given by

$$\gamma_s = \gamma_{so}e^{-t/\tau_{sv}} \tag{4.22}$$

where γ_{so} represents the value of the shear strain at the instant that σ_s is set to zero, and $\tau_{sv} = \eta_s/G_\infty$ is the shear response or relaxation time for the Voigt element. The transient response describes the phenomenon of creep.

Under a sinusoidally varying stress the strain is also sinusoidal, and the frequency-dependent complex elastic moduli corresponding to the two models can be obtained by substituting $\tau_s G_\infty$ for η_s and replacing the time derivatives in equations (4.20) and (4.21) by $i\omega$. Thus, for the Maxwell element,

$$G = \frac{\sigma_s}{\gamma_s} = G_\infty\left[\frac{\omega^2\tau_{sm}^2}{1+\omega^2\tau_{sm}^2} + \frac{i\omega\tau_{sm}}{1+\omega^2\tau_{sm}^2}\right] \tag{4.23}$$

---

3 A description of equivalent electrical and mechanical quantities may be found, for example, in Braddick (1965) p. 42.

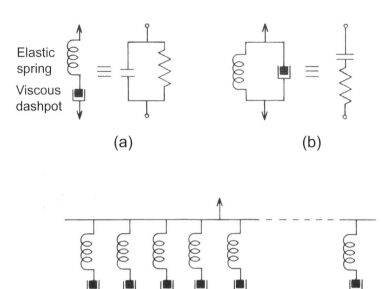

(a)   (b)

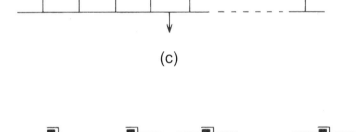

(c)

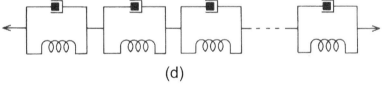

(d)

Figure 4.2. The Maxwell element and its electrical equivalent (a), the Voigt element and its electrical equivalent (b) and their respective generalised models (c and d), which have been used to represent the macroscopic behaviour of viscoelastic materials (adapted from Ferry 1961)

and for the Voigt element

$$G = G_\infty[1 + i\omega^2\tau_{sv}^2]$$ (4.24)

Compressional deformations are dealt with using a model like that of Figure 4.2b, in which the spring represents the zero frequency elasticity (modulus K_0) but the dashpot is replaced by a Maxwell model described by a compressional equivalent of equation (4.20). The combined stress–strain relationship amounts to

$$\sigma_v = K_0\gamma_v + \eta_v\frac{d\gamma_v}{dt} - \frac{\eta_v}{K_\infty}\frac{d\sigma_v}{dt}$$ (4.25)

By defining a bulk relaxation time $\tau_b = \eta_v/K_R$, and assuming the volume to vary sinusoidally, the bulk modulus may be expressed, using equation (4.25), as

$$K = \frac{\sigma_v}{\gamma_v} = K_0 + \frac{K_R \omega^2 \tau_b^2}{1 + \omega^2 \tau_b^2} + \frac{i K_R \omega \tau_b}{1 + \omega^2 \tau_b^2} \tag{4.26}$$

where $K_R = K_\infty - K_0$ is the relaxational part of the bulk modulus.

By combining equation (4.26) with either (4.23) or (4.24), according to (4.16), Maxwell or Voigt expressions for the longitudinal modulus, M, can be obtained. Equations (4.18) and (4.19) can then be used to derive expressions for the propagation speed and attenuation coefficient. This is done in an excellent comparison of the two models provided by Raichel (1971). Usually the two relaxation times τ_s and τ_b are assumed equal.

Both Maxwell and Voigt models yield dispersion relations and relaxation expressions similar to equation (4.11). The essential differences are that greater speed dispersion is predicted by the Maxwell model, which also predicts that the attenuation coefficient should plateau at a maximum high frequency value similar to the curve shown in Figure 4.1a. Attenuation according to the Voigt model, however, has a factor constant with α/f^2 included in the relationship and therefore continues to increase with frequency. An alternative view of this is that α/f^2 for the Maxwell model decreases to zero for infinite frequency, whereas for the Voigt model it decreases to assume a nearly constant high frequency value. This latter behaviour is similar to the curve shown in Figure 4.1c, for a single two-state equilibrium process added to classical processes. The differences as regards speed dispersion can be appreciated by examining equations (4.23), (4.24) and (4.26). When ω approaches infinity, the effective longitudinal modulus, M_∞, can be seen in both models to approach $K_0 + K_R + 4G_\infty/3$. However, if ω is zero, then $M_0 = K_0$ for the Maxwell model, and $K_0 + 4G_\infty/3$ for the Voigt model.

It should be noted that, as is often necessary to describe experimental results, equations (4.24), (4.25) and (4.26) can be generalised to represent distributions of relaxation times (Figure 4.2c and d). Whilst the Maxwell theory has been found adequate for describing sound propagation in liquids, the additional existence of a static shear modulus in the Voigt model seems to provide a better description for tissues. Indeed, Ahuja (1979), using published data on ultrasonic attenuation in tissues, has successfully modelled tissue as a Voigt body using only one relaxation time to describe the data over the medical range of frequencies.

One final point is worthy of note with regard to viscoelasticity. From equation (4.19)

$$\frac{\alpha}{f^2} = \frac{2\pi^2 M''}{\rho_0 c'^3 \omega} \tag{4.27}$$

Expressions for M'', obtained from equations (4.23), (4.24) and (4.26), reduce at low frequencies, for both models, to

$$M'' = \omega \left(K_R \tau_b + \frac{4}{3} G_\infty \tau_s \right)$$

where τ_s is either τ_{sm} or τ_{sv}.

At low frequencies equation (4.27) becomes, therefore,

$$\frac{\alpha}{f^2} = \frac{2\pi^2}{\rho_0 c'^3} \left(K_R \tau_b + \frac{4}{3} G_\infty \tau_s \right) \tag{4.28}$$

which can be expressed as

$$\frac{\alpha}{f^2} = \frac{2\pi^2}{\rho_0 c'^3}\left(\eta_v + \frac{4}{3}\eta_s\right)$$ (4.29)

We have now come full circle, back to the classical expression for absorption in liquids [equation (4.12)].

4.3.3 INHOMOGENEOUS MEDIA, INCLUDING GAS BUBBLES

When the propagation medium is not a homogeneous fluid, mechanisms other than the structural or thermal relaxation of its molecular constituents may contribute to the excess absorption (Morfey 1968). In addition to scattering the sound waves (covered in Chapter 6), inhomogeneities in the inertial or elastic properties of the medium can be responsible for the extraction of the acoustic wave energy by either viscous or thermal processes.[4] Viscous damping results from the relative motion that occurs, between a suspended structure and the embedding medium, when the density of the inhomogeneity is different from that of the medium. If the density of the inhomogeneity is uniform, it will simply attempt to move back and forth along the axis of sound propagation. If the density is not uniform, there will also be a tendency for relative rotational motion to occur. In either case absorption of acoustic wave energy occurs when the velocity amplitude of the relative motion is diminished because of the viscosity of the suspending medium. The process of thermal damping results when, during the cyclic pressure changes of the sound field, alternate compressions and expansions take place and heat is conducted (at a finite rate) between the suspending medium and the inhomogeneity. O'Donnell and Miller (1979) have found, by calculation from estimates of the principal inhomogeneities in specific tissues, that thermal losses appear to be dominated (in the 1 to 10 MHz frequency range) by viscous relative motion losses over a wide range of postulated sizes of inhomogeneity. The ratios of thermal to viscous losses calculated by these authors were of the order of 2% for heart muscle and much less for skin and blood. In applications of the theory of viscous relative motion McQueen (1977) has attempted to explain various experimentally observed phenomena (e.g. the rupture of blood capillaries in rat spinal cord by pulsed ultrasound) of the interaction of ultrasound and soft tissues. Unlike O'Donnell and Miller (1979), who follow a previously used assumption of a suspension of roughly spherical 'particles', McQueen treats the case of a fibrous network permeating a viscous medium; a possibly more realistic starting point for modelling certain tissues.

Another mechanism by which particle suspensions may attenuate ultrasound has been identified by Kol'tsova et al. (1980). If the particles have a high surface activity, then particle ensembles may form which have a mobile structure that responds to the sound pressure fluctuations in a manner that results in ultrasonic absorption of the structural relaxation kind. For particles of silica ($\sim$ 16 nm diameter) in water this contribution to the absorption is about 50 times as great as that from viscous, thermal and scattering losses combined, for the 1 to 10 MHz frequency range. It is not known whether similar processes exist for biologic media.

Since viscous and thermal damping processes involve the cyclic transfer respectively of momentum and heat between the suspended structures and the medium, which takes place at a finite rate, it is perhaps not surprising to find that the equations that describe them may be formulated as relaxation-type expressions. Indeed, Hueter (1958) included these mechanisms as possibly contributing to a viscoelastic model of tissue. The contribution (α_v) to the absorption coefficient by a single mechanism of the viscous relative motion type (see Dunn et al. 1969, p. 235) is given by:

---

4 An alternative interpretation of these phenomena will be provided in Section 4.3.7.

$$\alpha_v = \left(\frac{V_p}{2c}\right)\left(\frac{m_e}{m_p}\right)\frac{(1-\rho_0/\rho_p)^2\omega_0}{\rho_0/\rho_p}\frac{(\omega/\omega_0)^2}{1+(\omega/\omega_0)^2}$$ (4.30)

where $\omega_0 = F/m_p$ and

$$F = 6\pi a\eta_s\left[1+\left(\frac{\rho_0}{2\eta_s}\right)^{0.5}a\omega^{0.5}\right]$$

$$m_p = m_e + m\left[\frac{1}{2}+\frac{9}{4(\rho_0/2\eta_s)^{0.5}a\omega^{0.5}}\right]$$

for spherical particles of radius a, where:

V_p is the volume concentration of the suspended particles
c is the phase speed at frequency $f = \omega/2\pi$
ρ_p and ρ_0 are the densities of the structural elements (particles) and the suspending medium, respectively
m_e is the mass of an element, and
m is the mass of fluid displaced by a particle

Equation (4.30) is applicable in the general case for structural elements of arbitrary shape. The frictional force constant, F, and the effective mass of an element, m_p, are given for the special case where the elements can be approximated as spherical particles. In this case $V_p = 4\pi a^3 n/3$, where n is the number density of particles. A major difference between equation (4.30) and that governing the frequency dependence of absorption due to a simple relaxation process is that, for viscous relative motion, the 'relaxation' frequency ($\omega_0/2\pi$) is itself a function of frequency. As depicted in Figure 4.1d, this results in a relative absorption peak that is much broader than that due to a single molecular relaxation process.

A heterogeneous population of inhomogeneities undoubtedly exists in soft tissues and, as for molecular relaxation processes, the resultant contribution of viscous relative motion losses to the absorption coefficient would be obtained by a summation (or integration) over a range of particle sizes, shapes and densities. An approximately linear dependence of α_v on f in the 1 to 10 MHz range may, however, be predicted (O'Donnell & Miller 1979) by considering only quite a limited range of radii (e.g. 1 to 2 μm for heart muscle myofibrils) for particles all of the same density.

If the inhomogeneities under consideration are gas bubbles, then thermal damping may be more important. Longitudinal wave scattering (known as 'radiation damping' in this context) also becomes important (because of the large difference between the impedance of the gas and that of the liquid, and because bubbles may be of resonant size) and will be treated here as an attenuation mechanism, although scattering in general is dealt with in Chapter 6. For all of the damping mechanisms the dissipation of acoustic power by a bubble is a maximum for the ultrasonic frequency that is equal to the resonant frequency of the bubble, which is given by (Dunn et al. 1969, p. 237):

$$\omega_0 = 2\pi f_0 = \frac{1}{a_0}\left[\frac{3\gamma_g P_0\,g}{\rho_0}\frac{g}{\varepsilon}\right]^{0.5}$$ (4.31)

where:

$$g = 1 + \frac{2T_s}{P_0 a_0}\left(1 - \frac{\varepsilon}{3\gamma_g}\right)$$

$$\varepsilon = 1 + \frac{3(\gamma_g - 1)}{2\xi a_0}\left[1 + \frac{3(\gamma_g - 1)}{2\xi a_0}\right]$$

$$\xi = \left(\frac{\omega_0 \rho_g C_P}{2\chi_g}\right)^{0.5}$$

γ_g is the ratio of specific heats for the gas in the bubble
P_0 and ρ_0 are the static (ambient) fluid pressure and density
T_s is the surface tension
a_0 is the mean bubble radius
ρ_g is the density of the gas
C_P is the specific heat of the gas at constant pressure
χ_g is the thermal conductivity of the gas

Gas bubbles are present in lung and, to a variable extent, in excised tissues, and may arise from cavitation processes. They are also used as echo-enhancing (contrast) agents in medical ultrasound imaging where, to maximise their effectiveness, they should be of resonant frequency. For the medical imaging range of frequencies, a_0 is generally a few μm. For soluble gases such small bubbles dissolve too quickly to be useful and therefore need to be stabilised by coating them with a surfactant or encapsulating them within a thin shell. To account for the additional restoring force due to the shell elasticity, de Jong et al. (1992) added to the fluid pressure, P_0 [for example in equation (4.31)] the term $S_e\pi/3\gamma_g a_0$, where $S_e = 8\pi E\delta a/(1 - v)$, E is the Young's modulus of the shell material, v is its Poisson ratio and δa is the thickness of the shell.

When the population of gas bubbles is of uniform size, their contribution (α_g) to the attenuation coefficient is given by:

$$\alpha_g = \frac{bnc\left(\frac{3\gamma_g P_0}{a_0^2} + \omega^2 \rho_0\right)}{\left[\frac{1}{2\pi a_0}\left(\omega^2 \rho_0 - \frac{3g\gamma_g P_0}{\varepsilon a_0^2}\right)\right]^2 + (2b\omega)^2} \tag{4.32}$$

where b is called the 'total dissipation parameter' and is given by the sum of b_t, b_r and b_v, which are the thermal, radiation and viscous dissipation parameters respectively, and n is the number density of bubbles. When the bubbles are not all of equal size, a summation (or integration) over all radii is necessary (see Section 4.5.2.8). The radiation and viscous dissipation parameters are given by:

$$b_r = \frac{\rho_0 \omega^2}{4\pi c} \tag{4.33}$$

and

$$b_v = \frac{\eta_s}{\pi a_0^3} \tag{4.34}$$

Approximate expressions for the thermal dissipation parameter, b_t are:

$$b_t \approx B_t \frac{\gamma_g - 1}{\gamma_g} \frac{(2\xi a_0)^2}{30} \quad \text{for} \quad \xi a_0 \leqslant 1 \tag{4.35}$$

$$b_t \approx B_t \frac{1 - (1/\xi a_0)}{1 + \left[\dfrac{2\xi a_0}{3(\gamma_g - 1)}\right]} \quad \text{for} \quad \xi a_0 \geqslant 2.5 \tag{4.36}$$

where:

$$B_t = \frac{3\gamma_g P_0 g}{4\pi a_0^3 \omega \varepsilon}$$

de Jong (1997) has calculated the different dissipation parameters as a function of microbubble size, for bubbles of resonant size, and finds that thermal dissipation dominates when $a_0 > 5\,\mu m$ and viscous dissipation dominates when $a_0 < 2.5\,\mu m$. Neglecting surface tension, he notes that the radiation dissipation at resonance is constant with bubble size and its magnitude is small compared with the thermal and viscous dissipation, for bubbles in the size range of interest used as contrast agents. This seems to be qualitatively consistent at least with the data for the ratio of the scattering and attenuation coefficients for contrast agent suspensions, reported later in Section 4.5.2.7. The value of the total dissipation parameter, b, was found to be about 0.15, with little variation about this for resonating bubbles with radius between 2 and $25\,\mu m$.

4.3.4 SOLIDS

Ultrasonic attenuation in solids is generally less than in liquids but may arise from a very large number of possible mechanisms (Mason 1958).

A contribution arises from the thermal conductivity [the Kirchhoff part of equation (4.12)], but this is small except in metals. Particularly at frequencies in the kHz region, a phenomenon known as 'thermoelastic relaxation' may occur. This involves a flow of heat between random local temperature differences that have arisen in adjacent randomly oriented grains, due to the fact that the stress/strain relationships in a crystalline grain are dependent on its orientation. Thermal damping may also arise at dislocations in a crystal lattice. The contribution of these effects to the total attenuation is also small.

A large range of frequency-dependent resonance losses are possible in solids, the specific mechanism being dependent on the properties of the material in question, its shape and its environment. Examples are dislocation loops in crystal lattices, magnetostrictive and piezoelectric effects, and interactions with nuclear and electron spin systems in the presence of an external magnetic field.

Lattice dislocations may also give rise to non-resonant, relaxational-type absorption; and to a hysteresis loss that is independent of frequency but dependent on strain amplitude.

The solid equivalent of structural relaxation involves coupling of the wave energy to a distribution of specific allowable vibrational states (thermal phonons). It is important at gigahertz frequencies and large for solids close to their melting point. Attenuation by direct coupling of the wave energy to charge carriers is an important mechanism in metals at temperatures below about 20 K, and can be varied in semiconductors by doping or altering the optical illumination. In the latter case the momentum transferred from the sound wave to the conduction electrons causes a drift current which is observable as a d.c. electric field in the specimen. This effect, and that of piezoelectricity, are used in the manufacture of detectors of ultrasound (Chapter 3).

In polycrystalline solids, scattering at grain boundaries leads to a non-dissipative loss that can be the major cause of ultrasonic attenuation. At low frequencies, where $\lambda \gg d$ (the mean grain diameter), the attenuation follows the Rayleigh law of being proportional to f^4 and d^3. As the frequency increases, the dependences of the variations of α_s approach f^2 and d^2 over the region where $0.3\lambda < d < \lambda$. After this α_s rises even more slowly and tends towards a constant value with f when $\lambda \ll d$ at which point α_s is inversely proportional to d.

For metals the following law is obeyed in the low MHz frequency range:

$$\alpha = Af + Bf^4 \tag{4.37}$$

The first term represents loss due to plastic hysteresis, A being independent of grain size. In the scattering term B is given by $R_s d^3/c^3$, where c is the sound speed and R_s an elastic anisotropy factor (constant for a given material and kind of wave). Values of B, obtained from a fit of equation (4.37) to experimental data on α vs f, allow metal specimens to be ultrasonically classified according to grain size (Mercier 1975).

Few biological tissues can be regarded as solids, although scattering theory would appear to provide a reasonably quantitative explanation for at least one report of the properties of cancellous bone from human skull (Barger 1979). These measurements of ultrasonic attenuation suggest an f^4 dependence in the region 0.3 MHz to 1.3 MHz and a gradual saturation towards higher frequencies, with an f^2 region between 1.3 MHz and 1.8 MHz.

4.3.5 TEMPERATURE DEPENDENCE

In non-biological media, observed temperature dependences of ultrasonic attenuation vary considerably, depending on the frequency and the mechanisms that are responsible for the attenuation. Very complicated dependences might be expected from biological media on the basis that many mechanisms will be involved, and their relative contributions may also be temperature- and frequency-dependent.

An increase in temperature causes a relaxation time, τ, to shorten according to

$$\tau = \frac{1}{2\pi f_R} = \tau_0 e^{\Delta W/RT} \tag{4.38}$$

where T is absolute temperature, ΔW is the activation energy for the process, R is the gas constant, and τ_0 is a constant. Equation (4.38) is a form of the well-known Arrhenius equation for the rate constant in first-order chemical kinetics (e.g. Moore 1962). Thermal processes tend only to have a single value for ΔW, but the energy required to activate structural changes will depend on local configurations of molecules and will therefore not be a fixed quantity.

Writing $\omega_R = 2\pi f_R$ and $\omega_0 = 1/\tau_0$,

$$\ln \omega_R = \ln \omega_0 - \frac{\Delta W}{RT} \tag{4.39}$$

An 'Arrhenius plot' ($\ln \omega_R$ against the reciprocal of absolute temperature) allows the activation energy for a single relaxation process to be determined from experimental data as the slope, $-\Delta W/R$, of the straight line obtained.

Considering a shift of the $\alpha_R \lambda$ curve in Figure 4.1a, we should expect to find that the temperature coefficient of absorption is negative for observations carried out at frequencies below f_R, and positive for higher frequencies. There is also a change in $(\alpha_R \lambda)_{max}$ with this shift, but generally speaking these dependences are observed. Thermal and structural relaxations display some of their most interesting differences in this regard. Unassociated liquids, which tend to undergo relatively low-frequency chemical relaxations, have a tendency for: $d\alpha/dT$ to be positive, η_v/η_s to be high (10^1 to 10^3), and no correlation to exist between the temperature-dependences of η_v and η_s. Associated liquids, which undergo relatively high-frequency structural and shear relaxations, tend to have: $d\alpha/dT$ negative, η_v/η_s small (1 to 3) and temperature-independent ($d\eta_v/dT$ and $d\eta_s/dT$ both negative). The correlation between η_v and η_s for associated liquids arises because both shear and compressional stresses cause liquid molecules to change their local lattice positions; the same bonds must be broken in both cases, and thus the activation energies are closely related. In some liquids the two types of process coexist, in which case their relative importance within a given frequency and temperature range varies with temperature. For liquids where shear viscosity is the dominant mechanism (i.e. Stokes' formula applies), or in the case of any other dominant high-frequency structural relaxation (i.e. $\alpha \propto f^2$ as in water), α is a negative function of temperature and follows approximately the same temperature dependence as the shear viscosity, *viz.* $\ln \eta_s = B + E/RT$, where B is a constant and E is the activation energy for steady flow.

The speed dispersion (Figure 4.1b) also shifts with temperature and, in combination with decreasing values of c_∞ and c_0, results in dc/dT being negative for very nearly all liquids. The rate of change of c_0 with temperature is between 2 and 4 times that of density, whereas the equivalent factor for c_∞ ranges from 2 to 8. Peculiar exceptions arise in the cases of water, heavy water and aqueous solutions; the speed first increases with temperature to a maximum (at 74°C for pure water) and then decreases (see Figure 5.2). The addition of a solute to water changes the value of the speed maximum and shifts it towards lower temperatures. At low solute concentrations the shape of the curve is parabolic, so that dc/dT has a constant rate of change and may be extrapolated to zero to find the temperature of the maximum if it is out of experimental range. The speed maximum is generally explained on the basis of a two-state model for molecules of aqueous media, involving a loosely packed (ice-like) structure in equilibrium with a more closely packed structure. As the temperature is raised, the overall compressibility (reciprocal of bulk modulus) would increase as for other liquids but for the fact that, initially, the equilibrium shifts in favour of the close-packed structure, which is less compressible than the ice structure. These competing effects result in a minimum in compressibility and hence a maximum in speed.

When a distribution of relaxation times exists, temperature increases would tend, for the above model, to shift the whole curve of $\alpha\lambda$ towards higher frequencies. Where the slope of this curve is slightly positive, a small negative coefficient of absorption ought to be observed. Similarly, a decreasing $\alpha\lambda$ with frequency might lead to a positive temperature coefficient. Although this view is an oversimplification, it will be seen later to permit at least a qualitative interpretation of some experimental data.

The shift in f_R with temperature is often used advantageously in the study of viscoelasticity to effectively enlarge the range of available measurement frequencies beyond the range attainable isothermally. The 'method of reduced variables' (Ferry 1961), as it is known, relies on the ability to superpose a series of isothermal curves of the storage and loss moduli by shifting them on a logarithmic frequency axis. Such time–temperature superposition has been found to apply even when a distribution of relaxation times exists, although this requires all the relaxation times to have approximately the same temperature dependence. If this were true for tissues, and either the shear modulus could be neglected or the shear and volume relaxation times also had roughly the same temperature dependence, the techniques could in principle be applied to extend the measurement range for speed and attenuation data in tissue. In any event, an attempt at superposition often permits the validity of such conditions to be assessed (see Section 4.5.2.6). A significant practical hindrance, however, is the very limited range of temperatures to which tissues may be exposed without irreversible changes taking place.

The above-mentioned expected temperature dependences will be still further complicated if tissue inhomogeneities contribute strongly to the attenuation. We have already seen that, if the predominant mechanism is relative motion of suspended particles, then the attenuation coefficient depends critically on the viscosity of the suspending fluid. O'Donnell *et al.* (1977) have made the suggestion, based upon a series expansion of an equation equivalent to (4.30), that α_v ought to follow a temperature variation which is the square root of that of the viscosity.

The author is unaware of any specific reference to variations with temperature of α_s, the longitudinal wave scattering component of attenuation. It is generally believed that α_s represents a relatively small part of α in many tissues (see Section 4.5.2.2). Exceptions might be those tissues where inhomogeneities consisting of fatty/non-fatty boundaries are prevalent (breast and bone are candidates). Neglecting density variations, α_s becomes proportional to the square of the compressibility fluctuations (see Chapter 6), the compressibility being inversely related to the square of the speed. From the measured variations of speed with temperature in various tissues (Chapter 5) one would not expect $d\alpha_s/dT$ to be negative over the temperature range of interest, and for some tissues it ought to be very strongly positive.

4.3.6 PRESSURE DEPENDENCE

The absorption coefficient and sound speed are functions of ambient pressure as well as of temperature. Although variations of ambient pressure away from atmospheric pressure have in the past not been considered to be applicable to the study of tissues (Dunn *et al.* 1969), such variations have been used deliberately on liquids in attempts to distinguish between possible relaxation processes. In view of the previously mentioned limited temperature range that is applicable, it may well be worth considering deliberate pressure variations for similar purposes in tissues. The author is unaware of anyone yet having attempted to do this although measurement of sound speed as a function of pressure is of course one of the standard methods for measurement of the degree of non-linearity of acoustic propagation in tissues (see Chapter 5).

From the studies on liquids (Litovitz & Carnevale 1958) it appears that, when the ambient pressure is raised, f_R increases for vibrational relaxation, decreases for structural relaxation and remains constant if the mechanism is one of rotational isomerism. When f_R does change with pressure it is typically at a rate of change per atmosphere of between 20% and 50% of its value at normal atmospheric pressure. The values of the absorption coefficient itself and the sound speed are, however, generally decreasing and increasing functions of pressure respectively, making it difficult to distinguish between relaxation models unless the shift in frequency of the relaxation region is actually observed. With the exception of water, the viscosity of liquids generally increases with increasing pressure.

The method of reduced variables, mentioned with regard to temperature variations, has also been applied to pressure variations (Phillippoff 1963).

4.3.7 ABSORPTION, DISPERSION, ATTENUATION AND SCATTERING AS RELATED PHENOMENA

Historically, the subject of the mechanisms of acoustic wave propagation has developed such that the topics of absorption and scattering are usually, as in this book, dealt with separately. Such a distinction between propagation phenomena is, however, in some senses artificial and may become difficult to maintain. As pointed out by O'Donnell *et al.* (1978, 1981), one grey area lies within a general discussion of acoustic loss mechanisms, particularly in relation to speed dispersion. There is no sharp distinction between the various loss mechanisms; a local absorption of energy may be thought of as one limit of a scattering event. Furthermore, phenomenological descriptions exist which define speed dispersion as arising only from the presence of a frequency-dependent attenuation coefficient, which may be due to any of the loss mechanisms described previously (the wave number is derived from a complex speed: $k = \omega/c(\omega) + i\alpha(\omega)$ where $c(\omega)$ is the phase speed). Scattering, in the absence of absorption, may give rise to dispersion. Bergmann (1946), for instance, defines a speed dispersion for a wave propagating in a medium defined only by a variable refractive index:

$$c = \frac{c_0}{n_r}\left(1 + \frac{c_0^2 N_r}{\omega^2 n_r^2}\right)^{-0.5} \tag{4.40}$$

where c is the phase speed, n_r is the index of refraction and N_r is a term which defines the elemental sources of scattered waves [contained within the right-hand side of equation (6.5)]. If there are no refractive index gradients, N_r vanishes and the speed of propagation simply equals c_0/n_r. For the general case, however, the lower the frequency, the more significant will be the reduction in propagation speed due to scattering. By use of the approximate phenomenological relationships:

$$\alpha(\omega) \approx \frac{\pi^2}{2c_1^2}\frac{dc(\omega)}{d\omega} \tag{4.41}$$

and

$$c(\omega) \approx c_1 + \frac{2c_1^2}{\pi}\int_{\omega_1}^{\omega}\frac{\alpha(\omega)}{\omega^2}\,d\omega \tag{4.42}$$

(where ω_1 is some convenient reference frequency and c_1 is the phase speed at this frequency), O'Donnell *et al.* (1978, 1981) have demonstrated that data for sound speed as a function of frequency in a variety of media can be entirely described in terms of the measured frequency dependence of the attenuation coefficient. They conclude, therefore, that it is not valid to use comparisons of attenuation and speed dispersion as the sole means of confirming that the attenuation is due to any particular loss mechanism. Equations (4.41) and (4.42) are approximate relations derived from exact forms under the assumptions that the attenuation and dispersion are sufficiently small and do not change rapidly over the frequency range of interest: assumptions which appear to be valid for many biological media and medical frequencies. The exact forms of these equations are directly analogous to the dispersion relations in electromagnetic wave propagation, which show that the real part of the relative permittivity depends on the variation of the imaginary part over the whole range of frequencies and *vice versa* (Duffin 1968). Equation (4.42) predicts that if the attenuation varies as frequency squared, the incremental increase in speed, $\Delta c = c - c_1$, should vary linearly with frequency (as observed for media exhibiting classical viscous losses only) and, if the attenuation varies linearly with frequency, Δc should vary logarithmically with frequency (which is approximately true for the biological media and soft tissues that have been studied). Discussion of the general causal attenuation–dispersion relationships is considerably extended by Szabo (1995), who compares various theories for a variety of attenuating media.

Another aspect of this poorly defined boundary between scattering and absorption loss phenomena concerns the mechanisms discussed previously under the heading of absorption in inhomogeneous media. The viscous relative motion and thermal damping losses may both be described in terms of scattering phenomena. Morse and Ingard (1968), while evaluating the absorption and scattering cross-sections due to a non-rigid sphere, discuss these effects in terms of scattered shear and thermal waves (of amplitudes sufficient to satisfy the boundary conditions on the temperature and tangential velocity at the surface of the scatterer) that are propagated and then rapidly absorbed in a boundary layer just outside the sphere. The longitudinal scattered wave is only slightly modified from that calculated when these losses are neglected, but the absorption cross-section is entirely dependent on their presence. It appears that the viscous (shear wave) losses occur at density inhomogeneities, while thermal damping arises at fluctuations in the compressibility. The maxima in the $a\lambda$ curves arise at frequencies where the shear and thermal wavelengths are approximately equal to the radius of the particles, if spherical.

4.3.8 NON-LINEAR PROPAGATION

Thus far in our discussion of loss mechanisms a prime assumption has been that the propagation medium is linear in its response to the mechanical stresses imposed by the sound wave. This constitutes an approximation, which is valid only for waves of very small amplitude. We now discuss the conditions for which sound wave propagation in liquids and soft tissues ought to be measurably non-linear, and the effect that this should have on the apparent attenuating properties of the medium.

Some of the references mentioned earlier (Fry & Dunn 1962; Dunn *et al.* 1969) cover aspects of non-linear propagation, and the basics of the subject have been presented in Chapter 1, for non-attenuating media. One of the most comprehensive works on the subject (Beyer 1974) is unfortunately very difficult to obtain. Earlier works (Beyer 1965; Beyer & Letcher 1969), however, still form excellent references. More recently, various workers have turned their attention to studying the non-linearity of propagation under conditions relevant to medical ultrasonics (Carstensen *et al.* 1980; Muir & Carstensen 1980; Goss & Fry 1981; Law *et al.* 1981, 1985; see also both Section 2.9 and Chapter 7 of the present book).

It was shown in Section 1.8 that, for the general case of non-linear propagation, the solution of the wave equation can be obtained using a Taylor series expansion about ambient conditions. Dropping all high-order terms resulted in the first-order, or linear theory [equation (1.17)]. By retaining the quadratic term of the series the second-order, non-linear expression for pressure in terms of condensation, s, was [equation (1.134)] given as

$$p = As + 0.5Bs^2 \text{ (+ higher terms)}$$

where the notation is the same as that used in Chapter 1. Expressed explicitly as a relationship between pressure and density fluctuations (in a lossless medium) this becomes

$$p = c^2 \left[\rho + \frac{B}{2A} \frac{\rho^2}{\rho_0} \right] \qquad (4.43)$$

As a direct consequence of this quadratic relationship between the acoustic pressure and density the wave is predicted to travel with a new phase speed that is a function of the particle velocity (or pressure):

$$c = c_0 \left[1 + \frac{B}{2A} \frac{u}{c_0} \right]^{(2A/B)+1} \tag{4.44}$$

where u is the particle velocity, c_0 now denotes the velocity for linear propagation, $A = \rho_0 c_0^2$ and the ratio B/A is known as the 'parameter of non-linearity' of the medium. This means that the compressions or 'crests' of the wave travel slightly faster than the linear theory would predict, whilst the rarefactions or 'troughs' lag behind with a wave velocity slightly smaller than c_0. Thus each cycle of propagation adds to a cumulative distortion in which the wave, in the region of $u = 0$, becomes progressively steeper until, if unchecked by attenuation, a sawtooth waveform results from a wave that was initially sinusoidal (Figure 4.3a–c).

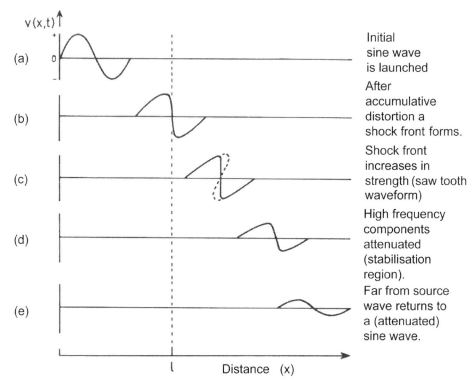

Figure 4.3. The evolution of the shape of a wave that is sinusoidal when launched at distance $x = 0$ and time $t = 0$, in a non-linear, weakly and dispersively attenuating medium. Time, and therefore distance, increase from (a) to (e). Each section shows a single cycle representation of the velocity waveform $u(t)$ at some relative distance from the source (adapted from Beyer 1974)

The change in the shape of a wave that is initially of the form $u(0, t) = U_0 \sin \omega t$ is described by the following solution of the second-order wave equation, due to Fubini (Beyer & Letcher 1969):

$$u = U_0 \sin \left[\omega t - \frac{\omega x}{c_0} + \frac{x}{l} \frac{u}{U_0} \right] \tag{4.45}$$

which can be expressed in terms of a Fourier series expansion:

$$u = 2U_0 \sum_{n=1}^{\infty} \frac{J_n(nx/l)}{(nx/l)} \sin n(\omega t - \omega x/c_0) \qquad (4.46)$$

where l is a constant dependent on the non-linear properties of the medium. Although this solution is valid only for values of $x < l$, equation (4.46) does indicate that, as the wave propagates, there is a decrease in the fundamental component, the energy of which is transferred to the various harmonics.

The point $x = l$ is known as the 'discontinuity distance', given by:

$$l = c_0^2/\omega U_0(1 + B/2A) \qquad (4.47)$$

It is the field position at which, in the absence of attenuation, du/dx becomes negatively infinite. The resulting step in the particle velocity profile is known as the 'shock front'. Beyond $x = l$ more and more of the wave 'piles up' and the shock front increases in strength. Although the above analysis assumes a dissipationless medium, it does shed light, as follows, on some basic relationships of the phenomenon of non-linear propagation.

Firstly, the larger the non-linearity parameter, B/A, the earlier the shock front is formed and the more the wave is distorted at a particular distance from the source. A linear medium is one whose B/A value is equal to zero. As described in Section 5.4, methods for the experimental determination of B/A have either involved observation of the sound speed as a function of temperature and pressure (Madigosky *et al.* 1981; Law *et al.* 1985), or been based on measurement of the development of harmonics (Law *et al.* 1985). Values for B/A for most substances lie in the range 0 to 1 for gases, and 2 to 13 for liquids and solids. Slight increases with increasing temperature or pressure are to be noted. Examples of B/A values are provided in Table 4.1. Few published data yet exist for values corresponding to biological media. Preliminary studies suggest a linear dependence of B/A with concentration of macromolecules and no dependence upon molecular weight (Law *et al.* 1981, 1985). This implies that both

Table 4.1. B/A for some liquids and biologically relevant media (at atmospheric pressure and 20°C unless otherwise indicated)

Propagation medium	B/A	Reference
Distilled water	5.0	Beyer (1974)
Sea water (3.5%)	5.25	Beyer (1974)
Methyl alcohol	9.6	Beyer (1974)
Ethyl alcohol	10.5	Beyer (1974)
Acetone	9.2	Beyer (1974)
Ethylene glycol (30°C)	9.7	Beyer (1974)
Carbon tetrachloride (30°C)	11.54	Bjørnø (1975)
Glycerine	8.8	Bjørnø (1975)
Freon	12.41	Madigoski *et al.* (1981)
RTV 602 silicone rubber (0°C)	13.4	Madigoski *et al.* (1981)
Macromolecules in solution (30°C)	0.053–0.076[a]	Law *et al.* (1981)
Whole blood	6.3	Law *et al.* (1981)
Homogenised liver (23°C and 30°C)	6.8	Law *et al.* (1985), Dunn *et al.* (1982)
Whole liver (23°C and 30°C)	7.8	Law *et al.* (1985), Dunn *et al.* (1982)
Pig fat (30°C)	11.1	Law *et al.* (1985)

[a]The solutes studied were: dextrose, sucrose, dextran, bovine serum albumin and haemoglobin; the values quoted are the range over these solutions for $(B/A_{solution} - B/A_{water})$/concentration (g/100 cm^3). An approximately linear dependence on concentration was observed.

intermolecular and intramolecular solute interactions may not contribute significantly to the value of B/A. Solute–solvent interactions are regarded as a more likely source of non-linearity. Also, the data on whole and homogenised liver suggest that their B/A values are influenced by the presence of large-scale structure in tissue (see also Section 5.4.2).

Secondly, the non-linearities will be observed earlier for sound waves of high frequency than for those of low frequency. This is due to the cumulative build-up of the effects over the distance measured in wavelengths.

Thirdly, the larger the initial amplitude, the shorter the discontinuity distance; as U_0 tends to zero, l tends to infinity and the approximation of linear theory is again reached.

Finally, l will be smaller, and the distortion at a given distance from the source consequently greater, for media of lower sound speed. It has been noted (Beyer 1974; Madigosky *et al.* 1981) that, to a first approximation, B/A for pure non-biological media is a linear function of the reciprocal sound speed. Thus, in general, the non-linear distortion observed varies more widely between media than the documented B/A values alone would suggest. As noted by Law *et al.* (1981), however, B/A increases with increasing speed for water (over the temperature range 0–60°C) and for aqueous solutions of biological macromolecules. Thus, for the biological media studied to date, the speed in fact has a moderating influence on the variation of the amount of non-linear distortion observed.

A not unreasonable estimate for a high temporal-peak source intensity transmitted by pulse–echo imaging equipment used in medical diagnosis is about 20 W cm^{-2}. In water-like media this corresponds to an initial plane wave velocity amplitude, U_0, of approximately 0.5 m s^{-1} (or a pressure amplitude of about 8 atm, or 0.8 MPa). Table 4.2 shows some specific examples of the value of the discontinuity distance, l, calculated assuming this value for U_0. These values give an impression of how rapidly the distortions might build up in the absence of attenuation.

As indicated by Figure 4.3d, e, the effect of frequency-dependent attenuation is to both attenuate the wave and remove the harmonics, the higher harmonics being lost first until, at some distance far from the source, the wave exists as the fundamental only. Amplitude at this time corresponds to propagation according to the infinitesimal theory. For each harmonic there exists a range of propagation distances, known as the 'stabilisation region', during which the rate of energy transference to the harmonic approximately equals its rate of energy loss by attenuation. It is therefore in this region that each harmonic reaches a maximum value and then begins to decay. A variety of methods, all of them approximations and dealing only with continuous waves, have been used to incorporate attenuation in expressions for the variation of the fundamental and harmonic amplitudes with distance (Beyer 1974; Beyer & Letcher 1969). A reasonable impression (at least) of the trends to be observed can be obtained by a method which neglects all energy transference except for that from the fundamental to the second harmonic (Fry & Dunn 1962). The analysis is also strictly applicable only when $x \geq 2l$, but the resulting expression for the intensity of the fundamental,

$$I_1(x) \approx I_0 \frac{4\alpha\, l e^{-2\alpha x}}{(1 + 4\alpha\, l - e^{-2\alpha x})} \tag{4.48}$$

does give I_0 when $x = 0$, and I_1 reduces to $I_0 e^{-2\alpha x}$ when $l \to \infty$.

The ratio of I_{1e} (the intensity of the fundamental that would be expected if propagation was in accordance with the linear theory) to I_1 is then given by:

$$\frac{I_{1e}(x)}{I_1(x)} \approx 1 + \frac{1 - e^{-2\alpha x}}{4\alpha l} \tag{4.49}$$

Table 4.2. Numerical examples of quantities associated with non-linear propagation of ultrasound for a source intensity approximating the peak-pulse intensity to be found in many diagnostic instruments.

	f (Hz)	B/A	c_0 (m s^{-1})	$\rho_0 c_0$ (kg m^{-2} s^{-1})	α (m^{-1})	I_0 (W m^{-2})	U_0 (m s^{-1})	l (m)	$I_1 (2l)$ (W m^{-2})	$I_{le} (2l)/I_1 (2l)$	$(\alpha_{fin} - \alpha)/\alpha$ (%)
Multiply figures in table by:	10^6	1	10^3	10^6	1	10^3	1	10^{-3}	10^3	1	1
Medium:											
Water	1	5	1.5	1.5	0.02	200	0.5	200	99	2.0	4300
	5	5	1.5	1.5	0.5	200	0.5	40	94	2.0	870
	10	5	1.5	1.5	2	200	0.5	20	88	1.9	400
Blood	1	6.3	1.57	1.63	2	200	0.5	190	29	1.5	27
	5	6.3	1.57	1.63	14	200	0.5	40	15	1.4	15
	10	6.3	1.57	1.63	35	200	0.5	20	9	1.3	9
Liver	1	9	1.6	1.67	12	200	0.5	150	0.1	1.1	1
	5	9	1.6	1.67	58	200	0.5	30	0.1	1.1	1
	10	9	1.6	1.67	120	200	0.5	15	0.1	1.1	1
Ethanol	1	10.5	1.12	0.88	0.05	200	0.7	45	99	2.0	7700
	5	10.5	1.12	0.88	1	200	0.7	23	93	2.0	750
	10	10.5	1.12	0.88	5	200	0.7	5	93	2.0	693

In Table 4.2 the specific numerical examples chosen previously are continued in order to illustrate equations (4.48) and (4.49). The last column gives the percentage increase, due to non-linear effects, in the average value of the attenuation coefficient for the path between the source and the position $2l$ from the source, assuming that the fundamental only is observed. This quantity is calculated making use of the relationship:

$$\alpha_{fin} - \alpha = \frac{1}{2x} \ln \left(\frac{I_{1e}(x)}{I_1(x)} \right) \tag{4.50}$$

where α_{fin} is the attenuation coefficient for non-linear propagation. It is thus not surprising that, in certain circumstances, non-linear effects can contribute significant errors to the measurement of attenuation and absorption (Bhadra & Roy 1975; Goss & Fry 1981).

Clearly the magnitudes of the errors introduced into an attenuation measurement by non-linear propagation depend upon a great many variables, including not only the quantities discussed so far (that is, B/A, U_0, f, c_0 and α) but also the distance from the source at which the measurement is made. It can generally be stated that the non-exponential character of the attenuation of finite amplitude waves leads to attenuation coefficients which are close to those for infinitesimal waves at distances both near to and far from the source, and which pass through a maximum in the stabilisation region. The situation is, however, further complicated by the fact that many different measurement methods are employed (see Section 4.4). There are both continuous wave (CW) and pulse methods with the observation being of either peak signal height or spectral energy distribution. The detector may be energy-sensitive and therefore receptive to all harmonics of a CW source, resonant and sensitive to only odd harmonics, have a broad though limited bandwidth, or be narrowband and sensitive to the fundamental only. Each situation requires a different theoretical treatment, some of which have appeared previously (Beyer & Letcher 1969), although perhaps the most general and promising approach is that of numerical analysis using a digital computer (Haran 1981). An example of the application of non-linear propagation behaviour has already been described in Section 2.7.

Further discussion of methods for measuring B/A and experimental data is taken up in Chapter 5. Note that B/A increases rapidly as gas bubbles are introduced into a propagation medium. This is discussed below, but particularly in Section 4.5.2.8.

4.3.9 MICROBUBBLES AND CAVITATION

There are a variety of conditions under which microscopic bubbles may be present in a tissue and substantially alter its propagation behaviour.

One situation where this arises, discussed in Section 4.4.2.5 below, is the tissue autolysis that may take place in *ex vivo* specimens, thus constituting a measurement artefact.

Secondly, deliberate introduction of microbubbles, in the form of 'contrast media', is a common practice (see Chapters 9 and 10), and it is important to know how this intervention modifies propagation behaviour. Theoretical models for this situation have been developed (e.g. de Jong *et al.* 1992) and some experimental measurements are discussed below, in Section 4.5.2.8.

Thirdly, under the oscillatory action of a sound wave, submicroscopic gas bubbles may grow by a process known as 'rectified diffusion': gas diffuses out of solution and into the bubble during the low-pressure rarefaction phase of the passing wave, then back from the bubble and into solution during the high-pressure phase. During the rarefaction phase, however, the surface area of the bubble is greater. This allows more gas to enter the bubble than is able to leave during the compression half-cycle and, over a number of cycles, the bubble grows. Eventually the bubble reaches resonant size for the particular ultrasonic wavelength [according to equation (4.31) this would be about 6 μm diameter for 1 MHz], when its vibration amplitude may be several orders of magnitude larger than that of the incident wave. This is known as 'stable cavitation' and results in a quiet degassing of a liquid containing dissolved gas. It is distinct from another transient or collapse form of cavitation which occurs only at higher pressure amplitudes. Cavitation alters propagation behaviour, producing erroneous results for measurements of attenuation, absorption, speed, scattering and B/A. It is essential when making such measurements that a technique and/or conditions are chosen which ensure that cavitation is not present. The occurrence of cavitation depends on the pressure amplitude of the incident sound field, frequency, temperature, ambient pressure, pulse length, viscosity and the degree to which dissolved gas and submicroscopic gas bubble 'nuclei' are present. The reader is referred to Chapter 12 for a fuller discussion of these details.

4.4 MEASUREMENT OF ATTENUATION AND ABSORPTION COEFFICIENTS IN TISSUE

4.4.1 MEASUREMENT TECHNIQUES

There have been a great many methods devised for making measurements of ultrasonic attenuation in a variety of media, and it is not possible to describe them all here. Relatively few, however, have been suitable for the study of tissues at medical frequencies. Reviews of measurement methods in general for solids, liquids and gases have been given by various authors including Beyer and Letcher (1969), Gooberman (1968), Matheson (1971) and McSkimin (1964). Dunn *et al.* (1969) provide a valuable collection of references in their classification and description of methods of measuring both compressional and shear wave attenuation and speed in terms of the ultrasonic frequency. In another useful reference Goss *et al.* (1979a) provide a comparative description of the various measurement methods of which they have had practical experience.

Since about 1973 a number of fresh approaches to the measurement of attenuation have appeared; in particular, methods for making measurements as a continuous function of frequency, for observing the spatial variation of the attenuation coefficient and for making measurements *in vivo*. All of these are important aspects of the subject in relation to medical ultrasonics, and the following account includes comments on a selection of such newer techniques.

A thorough analysis and presentation of the errors involved in each technique are not possible. Indeed, a number of authors of papers describing measurement techniques do not appear to have properly estimated such errors. Some possible sources of error in attenuation measurements are discussed in Section 4.4.2. It will be necessary to make reference to these when attempting to discuss the relative merits of each measurement method. For many of the methods the apparatus employed may be used also for a measurement of speed of sound and will, therefore, be referred to again in Chapter 5.

4.4.1.1 Absorption in Tissue

With reference to the classification scheme described in Figure 4.4, an initial distinction may be drawn between those methods that yield, for inhomogeneous media, the attenuation coefficient, and those that yield the absorption coefficient as the measured quantity. Of course, an accurate attenuation measurement in a homogeneous medium will yield, numerically, the

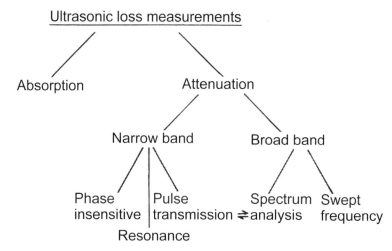

Figure 4.4. The scheme used in the text for classifying the methods used for making ultrasonic loss measurements. Many techniques are related to each other and therefore tend to bridge such partially artificial classifications

absorption coefficient. Very few workers have actually made direct measurements of α_a in tissues (as opposed to indirect estimates from attenuation and scattering measurements). One point to be aware of is that much of the older literature does not distinguish between absorption and attenuation. Fortunately this situation has altered, but careful reading is still sometimes required to avoid confusion.

The method of Fry and Fry (1954a, b), Fry and Dunn (1962), Dunn *et al.* (1969), Goss *et al.* (1979a), which monitors the local rate of rise in temperature using a thermocouple probe, does measure the portion of the ultrasonic energy that is locally absorbed and transformed into thermal energy. Briefly, a probe consisting of a thermocouple junction of small diameter relative to the ultrasonic wavelength is implanted in the sample, which is then exposed to short bursts of plane ultrasonic waves of known frequency. During the first tenth of a second or so of a burst, there is a rapid rise in probe temperature due to absorption by viscous relative motion of the thermocouple wires themselves. This part of the response becomes relatively large at low frequencies and when the absorption is small, and contributes to limiting the lowest frequency of application of the method (about 300 kHz). The subsequent rate of temperature rise, to a duration of about one second, is relatively linear and is due to local sound absorption in the sample. The absorption coefficient is determined from the estimated initial slope of the linear portion (see Figure 3.6). The density, specific heat at constant pressure and acoustic intensity must all be known. An iterative technique is used to estimate α_a, whereby an initial value, calculated using the measured incident intensity, is used as an attenuation coefficient to estimate the true value of I, knowing the propagation distance within the sample to the probe. Successive better estimates of α_a and I are then similarly obtained. Convergence of α_a does not occur if the total attenuation is too large. This, as well as difficulties in producing broad plane sound waves and small thermocouples, imposes the high-frequency limit of the method. Measurements at frequencies up to 7 MHz have been made in tissues. The total uncertainty in the value of $\alpha_a/\rho C_P$ is thought to be of the order of 10–15%.

Apart from being able to measure the absorption coefficient directly, this method also has advantages in that measurements can be made *in situ*, *in vivo* and in small local structures (e.g.

within the mouse spinal cord; Dunn 1962). The presence of gas bubbles in tissue specimens is a severe problem for attenuation measurements but has almost no effect on the thermoelectric measurement of absorption (Frizzell *et al.* 1979).

At high intensities, required to obtain a detectable temperature rise if α_a is very low, care must be taken to exclude the possibility that non-linear effects are contributing to the measurement (see Section 4.3.8). The time resolution of the thermocouple probe is poor, so that simultaneous speed-of-sound measurements are not possible with this apparatus.

Extensions to this method have led to a more complete analysis of the errors involved (Goss *et al.* 1977) and to an automated version of the measurement system (Duback *et al.* 1979).

Also using an embedded thermocouple, Parker (1983) developed an alternative to the rate-of-heating method which he called the 'thermal pulse decay' method. Instead of a long burst of ultrasound, a short (less than 0.1 s) pulse was used. As with the method of Fry and Dunn, viscous heating around the wire occurs simultaneously with true absorption in the tissue. However, after the pulse has passed, the rate of temperature reduction due to conduction of heat away from the region can be analysed to distinguish these contributions. Since viscous heating occurs only in a small volume around the thermocouple, there is an initial rapid drop in thermocouple temperature, which then, within 2 s, becomes a good measure of the decaying temperature in the surrounding tissue. A theoretical fit to the second part of the cooling curve can then be used to determine the total absorbed energy and thus the absorption coefficient. Parker found the results to be 'very close' to those obtained with the rate-of-heating method.

4.4.1.2 Attenuation in Tissue

To assist the present discussion a further classification of measurement techniques will be defined, *viz.* narrowband and broadband.

(a) *Narrowband techniques.* Many early attenuation measurements were made using what can be classed as 'narrowband' techniques. The sense in which this is meant is that the transmitted acoustic signal is *assumed* to contain a sufficient number of cycles of the wave such that the measurement is regarded as being made at a single frequency. The many techniques that exist in this class have been reviewed in the references cited at the beginning of this section. Such techniques previously did not easily permit measurements to be made as a continuous function of frequency but with computer control of experiments, particularly of a function generator driving the transmitting transducer, this is easily possible. Note that although this definition of narrowband can include pulse transmission methods, in some applications described below (e.g. Robinson & Lele 1972; Bhagat *et al.* 1976) the transmitted acoustic signals used had significant bandwidth, so that the frequencies at which the measurements were made were not precisely defined. Furthermore, changes in pulse shape due to dispersive attenuation (Redwood 1963) or phase cancellation (see Section 4.4.2.3) would not have been detected and may have given rise to large errors.

'Pulse transmission' systems form a major class of techniques, within which a distinction has been made (McSkimin 1964; Dunn *et al.* 1969) between so-called 'fixed path' and 'variable path' instruments. The path length referred to is that between the transmitter and the receiver, which may or may not be the same as the sound path through the specimen. Short bursts of sound are transmitted through the sample and received, either with a separate transducer aligned coaxially with the transmitter or with the transmitting transducer after the pulse has been reflected by a plane interface and propagated back through the specimen. The latter configuration has sometimes been referred to as the pulse–echo method, but should not be confused with the *in vivo* pulse–echo attenuation estimating methods mentioned later.

Advantages of using pulses include the ability to eliminate standing waves, multiple echoes in general and heating of the sample due to ultrasonic absorption.

In the *variable path* methods (e.g. Pellam & Galt 1946; Pinkerton 1947; Andreae *et al.* 1958; Kessler *et al.* 1971; Froelich 1977) the rate of change in the logarithm of the amplitude of the received signal with the position of the receiver or reflector provides the value of α, independent of any coefficients of reflection or electromechanical transduction. Variable path methods are capable of yielding absolute values for α, but require corrections for diffraction losses. Such losses introduce errors, which are proportionately worse at low frequencies, and a requirement for relatively large sample volumes (~ 0.5 l). For an accuracy of about $\pm 5\%$ these methods would generally not be used to make measurements at frequencies below about 3 MHz. If only frequencies above 12–15 MHz are used then millilitre sample volumes can be measured by this method without appreciable diffraction errors (Eggers *et al.* 1981). In such a case the main sources of error occur in the calibration of the electronic signal processing, distance measurement, and alignment of transmitting and receiving transducers. Accuracies of around $\pm 0.5\%$ appear to be achievable, however, if the temperature control and homogeneity are good enough. Variable path methods tend not to be suitable for measurements on tissues because of the difficulties of varying the path length in non-fluid media. They have been used to study biologically interesting solutions and liquids at frequencies up to about 200 MHz (e.g. Hawley & Dunn 1969; Sadykhova & El'piner 1970; Lang *et al.* 1978; Goss & Dunn 1980).

In *fixed path* pulse transmission methods, such as the *substitution method* used by Schwan and Carstensen (1952) and the *insertion technique* (Esche 1952; Kremkau *et al.* 1981), diffraction corrections are low (possibly negligible) and alignment tolerances less stringent, but the measurements are relative to the attenuation coefficient of a chosen reference liquid (usually water). The method of Schwan and Carstensen, used to study blood in the frequency range 0.3–20 MHz (Carstensen *et al.* 1953), has the transmitting and receiving transducers mechanically linked so that they move simultaneously, one through the reference liquid and the other through the test liquid. An acoustically transparent window separates the two liquids. In this way only the acoustic path lengths in the two liquids are varied, allowing α to be determined independent of reflection coefficients, etc., with measurement errors that may be as low as $\pm 2\%$. Difficulties still arise for non-fluid tissues, but these can be overcome (Pauly & Schwan 1971) if the process of mincing the tissue is considered not to change significantly its attenuation coefficient. Another problem is that very large sample volumes are required (1–4 l).

The *insertion technique*, on the other hand, is more suited to the study of solid tissues and is far the most widely used method for this purpose. The principle is that of determining the logarithm of the ratio of the received signals when the tissue is present between the transmitter and receiver and when a reference medium only is present. The use of additional reference medium as a buffer between the transducers and the tissue sample, as illustrated in Figure 4.5, minimises the error due to diffraction losses by reducing the relative change in overall acoustic path length when the tissue is inserted. This principle is applied in many of the other measurement systems in the classifications described below, and will be used later as a basis for a general discussion of the errors in attenuation measurement. Disadvantages of the insertion method are that reflections at the specimen faces are included in the measured loss, and accurate cutting of parallel-sided tissue slabs is very difficult. Typical measurement accuracies are in the region of $\pm 10\%$ or worse. This situation may be improved somewhat, and the effect of reflection losses automatically eliminated, if the measurement is repeated for other samples of the same material but of varying thickness, so that α is obtained from the slope of the graph of attenuation vs thickness.

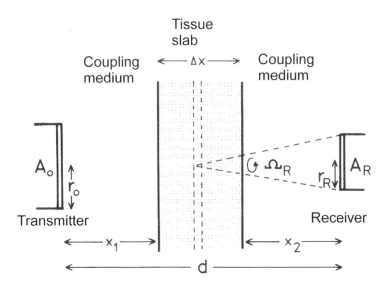

Figure 4.5. A typical experimental configuration for an attenuation measurement by the insertion technique, which is widely used for studying solid tissues. The system may be 'broadband' or 'narrowband'. The receiver may be phase sensitive, power sensitive, or simply a large plane interface that reflects the sound back directly to the transmitter

The narrowband class of techniques also includes various instruments that employ continuous waves and make use of the resulting resonances. These include interferometric and reverberation methods.

Ultrasonic interferometers may be configured with variable path (Dumas *et al.* 1983; Lang *et al.* 1978; see also the reviews cited at the beginning of Section 4.4.1) or variable frequency (Eggers & Funck 1973; review of Goss *et al.* 1979), and the resonant path may be between two transducers or one transducer and a reflector. Wavelength, and hence sound speed, are obtained from the distance, or the frequency difference, between resonance peaks. The variation in the strength of the resonance with distance, or the bandwidth of the resonance, can be used to determine the attenuation coefficient. However, since, in general, diffraction effects and side wall reflections contribute significantly to the measurement, these methods are not absolute and require calibration with a liquid of known properties. Eggers' technique requires only about 10 ml of the test liquid and is able to cover the frequency range 0.2–10 MHz. The method has been used to measure attenuation in collagen suspensions to an estimated accuracy of $\pm 10\%$ over a 0.5–3 MHz frequency range (Goss & Dunn 1980).

Reverberation methods (see the review cited at the beginning of Section 4.4.1) make use of the fact that, if a relatively large, almost lossless, resonant container (e.g. a 5 l thin-walled glass sphere in a vacuum) holding the test liquid is excited into vibration, then the rate of decay of the vibration when the sound source is turned off is primarily determined by the attenuation coefficient of the liquid. Diffraction effects are absent, but wall losses require correction by the use of a reference liquid that has the same acoustic impedance as the test liquid, and absolute values of α are not obtained. The operating frequencies of reverberation methods are generally below 1 MHz.

The use of large area piezoelectric transducers as receivers in the measurement of attenuation in inhomogeneous media introduces artefacts that have become known as 'phase cancellation' errors (see Section 4.4.2.3). In those narrowband techniques that utilise power-sensitive receivers this particular source of error is absent. Normally an insertion technique is employed, using water as the reference. The most commonly used power-sensitive device in attenuation measurements is the radiation pressure balance (Pohlman 1939; Colombati & Petralia 1950; Marcus & Carstensen 1975; Kremkau *et al.* 1981; Pohlhammer *et al.* 1981; Parker 1983). Care must be taken to eliminate errors associated with ultrasonic degassing of the specimen and coupling liquid, acoustic streaming in the coupling liquid and changes in target buoyancy due to ultrasonic heating. Nevertheless, this method is considered to have yielded the most consistent and accurate data for mammalian tissues. Ultrasonic streaming itself may be used to measure α over a wide frequency range, but the method is limited to very large volumes of liquid of which the viscosity must be known (Hall & Lamb 1959; Bhadra & Roy 1975) and accurate results are likely to require correction for diffraction errors (Quan & Watmough 1990). Transient thermoelectric probes (Fry & Fry 1954a, b) may also be used as power-sensitive receivers; they were adopted, for instance, to measure attenuation in lung (Dunn & Fry 1961). Marcus and Carstensen (1975) have pointed out the attractiveness of the cadmium sulphide acoustoelectric receiver, which may be used to measure total power in pulse transmission studies. Miller *et al.* (1976) and Busse and Miller (1981) have followed this up and developed acoustoelectric detectors for their own (phase-insensitive) attenuation measurements on muscle. Although little used as yet, probably the best method of generating a power-sensitive receiver for attenuation measurements is to sum over the powers obtained by sampling the transmitted field at many points, either by scanning with a phase-sensitive receiver of small dimensions relative to the spatial rate of change of phase or by using an array of such receivers.

(b) *Broadband techniques.* Following the introduction of spectral analysis techniques into non-destructive testing, a number of methods were developed utilising a broadband transmitted acoustic signal, plus appropriate signal processing in the receiver, to obtain α as a continuous function of frequency without the necessity of changing transducers (Holasek *et al.* 1973; Papadakis *et al.* 1973; Heyser & Le Croisette 1974; Chivers & Hill 1975; Baboux *et al.* 1976; Lele *et al.* 1976; Lizzi *et al.* 1976; Miller *et al.* 1976; Barger 1979; Foster & Hunt 1979; Kelly Fry *et al.* 1979; and others). In principle this is an attractive prospect and, with the wide availability of digital computers and sophisticated r.f. signal processing equipment, it has become relatively easy to set up an automated system of this kind. Indeed, broadband (spectral) techniques now constitute the most popular class of methods for studying solid tissues. Nevertheless, the experimental difficulties are perhaps easily underestimated, and the theoretical analysis of the errors involved in such a measurement has been incomplete. It is difficult, for instance, to achieve a genuinely wideband system. Baboux *et al.* (1976) have probably done the best in this regard (1.5 to 11 MHz using a single pair of transducers) but devoted some considerable research and development purely to that end (Lakestani *et al.* 1975). Chivers and Hill (1975), using diagnostic transducers at that time, found it necessary to have five transducers to cover the range 1 to 7 MHz. With regard to errors, Papadakis *et al.* (1973) were, for a long time, the only authors to have applied a rigorous analysis of the diffraction corrections involved but this topic underwent a revival of interest in the context of *in vivo* attenuation measurement (see Section 4.4.2.2). The spectral processing applied to the received signal necessitates the use of a phase-sensitive receiver in order to preserve the full r.f. information. Hence it is inevitable that these methods will all suffer from the phase cancellation artefacts already mentioned. However, as will be mentioned later, the spectral approach permits easy recognition of pronounced phase cancellation effects, and spectral averaging and curve fitting also help to lessen the problem. Such features are not available in the pulse transmission methods mentioned previously.

In all of the above broadband systems tissue specimens are examined by an insertion method, using water or saline for coupling purposes. Both two-transducer and reflector configurations are in common use. The sound pulses are converted upon reception to a spectrum of transmitted acoustic frequencies, and the variation of α with frequency is determined from the logarithm of the ratio of the spectra obtained when the tissue is present in the beam and when it is absent. In all but one of the systems used, the transmitted sound pulse contains as few cycles of the wave as possible. Frequency analysis used to be performed using an analogue r.f. spectrum analyser but this is now generally done by first digitising the pulse and then computing the spectrum by means of a discrete Fourier transform algorithm. The digital method is able to preserve the phase information for use in observing speed dispersion although the dynamic range of the measurement, the range of measurable frequencies and the speed of processing will be influenced by the choice of analogue to digital converter and computer. The one exception referred to is the time delay spectrometry (TDS) system of Heyser and Le Croisette (1974), originally devised as a transmission imaging method. In this system, a swept frequency ('chirp') signal is transmitted through a water-bath insertion arrangement. The received signal is both attenuated and delayed by the specimen, so that heterodyning the signal with the transmitted signal results in an audio frequency signal, the amplitude of which is related to the attenuation, and the frequency of which depends on the time delay (i.e. speed).

(c) *Spatial mapping of attenuation.* The measurement methods as discussed thus far in this section provide information at discrete positions and as spatial averages over the sound path. The measurement of the spatial distribution of ultrasonic properties within a specimen is often desirable as, for example, when it is required to compare regions of normal tissue with regions affected by pathological change. Some of the methods may be adapted to achieve this by the use of a suitable scanning arrangement (see, for example, Bamber & Bush 1991; Bush *et al.* 1993). Other systems used have inherently acquired the results in the form of an image. The method of Calderon *et al.* (1976) provided attenuation images of inserted specimens by using a scanned-laser interferometer to measure the displacement amplitude of a fine membrane that had been excited to vibrate by a short (1.5–3 MHz bandwidth) transmitted acoustic pulse. No clear account was given of the errors of the attenuation measurement by this method, which may be considerable.

Images of the attenuation coefficient in the plane of the sound beam may be possible by computerised reconstruction from one-dimensional ultrasonic projections; although artefacts due to refraction and phase cancellation are so severe that speed of sound would appear to be the only parameter which may be imaged in this way with reasonable accuracy (Carson *et al.* 1981; Greenleaf & Bahn 1981; Klepper & Brandenburger 1981).

Foster *et al.* (1984) constructed what they called an ultrasound macroscope. Using a single, strongly focused source/receiver and a plane reflector placed at the focal plane, an insertion technique was applied to produce quantitative images of the distribution of attenuation and sound speed in specimens of excised breast at a frequency of 13 MHz. Similar methods were used by Moran *et al.* (1995) to measure the ultrasonic propagation properties in different structures within human skin after sectioning and, but at much lower frequencies, by Roux *et al.* (1996) to map attenuation and sound speed in bone, resulting in improved reproducibility of ultrasound measurements compared with systems that average using a single line of site. The ultrasonic microscopes mentioned below may well provide the means to spatially map the attenuation coefficient on a much finer scale and at a higher frequency; Daft *et al.* (1989), for example, have reported measurements up to 500 MHz.

(d) *Microscopic measurements.* At a frequency of 100 MHz, measurements of α have also been made on thin (0.3–2.5 mm) tissue specimens using a scanning laser acoustic microscope (Kessler 1973). By using multiple specimens of varying thickness the errors in making average attenuation measurements at 100 MHz with this instrument have been reduced to the level where an accuracy of about ±5% is achieved (Tervola *et al.* 1985a, b). Further discussion of acoustic microscopy is taken up in Chapter 11.

4.4.1.3 *In Vivo* Measurement

As mentioned above, accurate *in vivo* absorption studies are possible with the transient thermoelectric technique. Measurement of the attenuation coefficient of live tissue is also possible, although only under special circumstances is it possible to make accurate measurements. An example of such circumstances is provided by the *in vivo* measurement of the average value of α in breast (Foster & Hunt 1979), where it is possible to place transducers in contact with opposite sides of the organ to measure the average attenuation along the transmission path. For similarly accessible anatomical regions the transmission reconstruction methods (Greenleaf & Bahn 1981) might eventually provide a means of quantitative *in vivo* measurement of local values of α.

All other *in vivo* methods presently available yield what is essentially a statistical estimate of α, and rely on one or more assumptions about the nature of propagation and scattering of the sound waves in the tissue concerned. If these properties of the tissue are approximately constant and uniformly distributed, and the region of interest is large enough (e.g. as in diffuse liver disease), then quite good estimates of the average pulse attenuation coefficients may be obtained from an exponential regression of echo amplitude data (Mountford & Wells 1972a, b).

This approach was subsequently studied more thoroughly by Parker and Waag (1983) who extended it to make measurements as a function of frequency, correcting for the non-linear responses of the signal processing of the ultrasonic scanner from which the raw data were obtained.

Spectrum analysis of sectioned echo trains may be used to estimate the slope of the frequency dependence of α if this is assumed to be constant with frequency, the transmitted sound pulse has a Gaussian shape and the tissue volume in question is macroscopically uniform in its scattering behaviour (Kuc & Schwartz 1979). The frequency dependence of the attenuation coefficient causes a downward shift in the centre frequency of the sound pulse as it propagates, which, if these assumptions are valid, is a linear function of path length. Considerable development of this basic idea has taken place over the years. This has led to extensions of the theory to accommodate non-Gaussian pulses and non-linear frequency dependence of α (Ophir & Jaeger 1982; Narayana & Ophir 1983a; Shaffer *et al.* 1984), a simpler method for determining the spectral shift (Flax *et al.* 1983), compensating for the effects of the diffraction field of the transducer (see Section 4.4.2.2) and clinically implementing the methods on commercial equipment. Bevan and Sherar (2001) have extended the spectral shift method to produce cross-sectional images of the estimated values for the frequency slope of the attenuation coefficient, and have applied it to the problem of localising a region of thermal coagulation in bovine liver. Preliminary reports of *in vivo* clinical data were given by Maklad *et al.* (1984) and Knipp *et al* (1997). Leeman *et al.* (1984) reviewed most of the proposed *in vivo* attenuation estimation techniques, which appear to have changed relatively little since that time. Jones and Leeman (1984) summarised values for ultrasonic attenuation *in vivo*, and variations with 187 pathological conditions.

Spatial averaging of echo spectra, over directions perpendicular to or in line with the sound beam, was used by Lizzi *et al.* (1976) to estimate α as a function of frequency (*cf.* Chapter 9). This method is strongly related to the relative attenuation imaging method known as reflex transmission imaging (RTI), described by Green and Arditi (1985). Green's RTI method relied on employing a strongly focused transducer operating in backscatter mode, acting as a confocal source and receiver. This transducer was scanned in two dimensions, in a constant depth (C-scan) pattern (see Section 9.2.2), and the image obtained by integrating the magnitude of echoes from tissue occupying a range of depths beyond the focus. Such an image signal is strongly related to the attenuation coefficient of the tissue located at constant depth in the focal plane, and effectively employs the tissue beyond the focus as a reference echo-producing structure that is assumed to be spatially homogeneous. The broad region of the beam beyond the focus provides a degree of averaging of any spatial inhomogeneities of backscattering coefficient. Averaging over depth provides additional benefit in this regard, as well as worthwhile speckle reduction (see Chapter 9). The breadth of the beam anterior to the focus helps to average out small-scale attenuation fluctuations present between the transducer and the focal plane. RTI has been employed at high frequencies (20–25 MHz) to make high-resolution attenuation images of skin tumours in a plane that allows direct visual comparison with photographs of the skin surface (Guittet *et al.* 2000), and at low frequencies (3–5 MHz) to visualise regions of tissue that have been thermally ablated using focused ultrasound surgery (Malcolm 1997; Baker 2003). As yet, however, RTI has not been adapted to provide quantitative values of the attenuation coefficient. The effect on the attenuation coefficient of heat coagulation of soft tissue is discussed below in Section 4.5.2.6.

Finally, suggestions also exist in the literature for the *in vivo* separation and measurement of the spatial distributions of the attenuation coefficient and backscattering cross-section per unit volume. These include backscatter reconstruction (Duck & Hill 1979; see also Chapter 11), which neglects diffractive scattering and assumes directional isotropy of the backscattering and other propagation properties, and the use of multiple frequencies (Hill 1975; Levi & Keuwez 1979). The latter method is essentially a reconstruction approach that assumes constant simple functions for the frequency dependences of attenuation and scattering. For automated attenuation compensation in medical pulse–echo imaging it appears to be useful to assume a simple monotonic relationship between attenuation and scattering (Hughes & Duck 1997).

4.4.2 PROBLEMS, ARTEFACTS AND ERRORS

Errors in attenuation measurements may arise from a large number of sources, many of which are difficult to estimate reliably. Hence, particularly in view of the wide variety of measurement techniques just discussed, it should be clear that it will not be possible to deal with all possible sources of measurement error. The widely used insertion technique (Figure 4.5) will therefore be employed as a basis for the following discussion, and some emphasis will be placed on the spectrum analysis method since this has probably suffered a greater neglect of error assessment than have the other methods. First, the equation commonly used for such a measurement configuration will be derived. Following this, the relative importance of the various sources of error in the measurement will be discussed. This discussion will initially focus on primary sources of error, which would arise even if the specimens to be measured were totally homogeneous, then move on to the complications that arise with real (inhomogeneous) tissues and variations in the conditions of specimen preparation and measurement.

4.4.2.1 The Measurement Equation

Considering the situation illustrated in Figure 4.5, the power arriving at the receiver when there is no tissue in the sound path is

$$W_R' = W_T \frac{S_r}{4\pi d^2} G \exp(-d\mu_w) \tag{4.51}$$

where W_T is the acoustic power at the surface of the transmitter, S_r is the area of the receiver, μ_w is the intensity attenuation coefficient of the coupling medium, and d is the geometrical separation of transmitter and receiver. G is a gain factor which, for a small receiver in the far-field of the transmitter, is the amount by which the equivalent isotropically radiated intensity would have to be multiplied to equal the true intensity due to a directional radiator ($= 4\pi S_0/\lambda^2$ for a large radiator of active area S_0). When the receiver is not in the far-field of the transmitter, G may be regarded as also including the modifications due to diffraction effects.

The power received when a slab of tissue is interposed is:

$$W_R = W_T \frac{S_r}{4\pi d^2} GT_{wt}^2 \exp(-[x_1 + x_2]\mu_w - \Delta x\mu) + W_{fs} \tag{4.52}$$

where T_{wt} is the energy transmission coefficient for the boundary between the coupling medium and the tissue, μ is the required attenuation coefficient, Δx is the tissue thickness, x_1 and x_2 are indicated in Figure 4.5 and W_{fs} is the power scattered by the tissue that reaches the receiver (forward scattered power). Equation (4.52) neglects multiple scattering and assumes that both tissue and coupling medium have the same sound speed. By integrating the forward scattering from elemental depth increments, an approximate analysis (Bamber 1979), assuming first-order scattering only and thin specimens lying in a uniform part of the sound beam not close to the receiver, yields

$$W_R = W_T \frac{S_r}{4\pi d^2} GT_{wt}^2 (1 + 4\Delta x\Omega_R\mu_{d(0)}) \exp(-[x_1 + x_2]\mu_w - \Delta x\mu) \tag{4.53}$$

where Ω_R is the solid angle subtended at the receiver by a point at the centre of the specimen, and $\mu_{d(0)}$ is the value of the differential scattering cross-section per unit volume for the forward direction.

No measurements of $\mu_{d(0)}$ are available for any tissues. Estimates of this quantity obtained by extrapolation of differential scattering cross-section measurements at other angles (Campbell & Waag 1984; Nassiri & Hill 1986a, b) vary over several orders of magnitude for different tissues and ultrasonic frequencies. Coupled with the almost limitless number of possible variations of measurement geometry, this means that it is not yet possible to calculate the likely contribution of forward scattering to the measurement of attenuation. It can be shown however, that, in some circumstances, forward scattering might make a significant contribution to the received power. For example the data of Nassiri and Hill (1986a) suggest that $\mu_{d(0)}$ for liver tissue at 6 MHz may be about 10^{-1} cm^{-1} steradian^{-1}. Taking a high but possible value of $\pi/8$ as an estimate for the geometrical factor $\Delta x\Omega_R$, the term in brackets in equation (4.53) comes to approximately $(1 + 2 \times 10^{-1})$; i.e. the error in neglecting the forward scattering contribution to the received power (in this hypothetical case) would be around 20%.

Nevertheless, if we neglect the scattering term, dividing equation (4.51) by (4.52) and taking logs we can obtain

$$\mu = \mu_w + \frac{1}{\Delta x}(\ln W_R' - \ln W_R + 2\ln T_{wt}) \tag{4.54}$$

If a similar analysis is applied to the system where the receiver is replaced by a reflector, then

$$\mu = \mu_w + \frac{1}{2\Delta x}(\ln W_R' - \ln W_R + 4\ln T_{wt}) \tag{4.55}$$

Very often T_{wt} and μ_w are neglected and the variation of the ratio of $W_R : W'_R$ with frequency is assumed to be given by the square of the ratio of the voltage signals measured, $V(f)$ and $V'(f)$, i.e.

$$\alpha(f) = \frac{20}{\Delta x}(\log_{10} V'(f) - \log_{10} V(f)), \quad \text{in units of dB cm}^{-1} \tag{4.56}$$

$20 \log_{10} V'(f)$ and $20 \log_{10} V(f)$ are the logarithmically displayed spectra with and without the specimen, respectively.

4.4.2.2 Errors in Measuring Homogeneous Specimens

4.4.2.2.1 Primary Errors

Neglecting, for the moment, the inhomogeneous nature of tissues, primary errors may be defined as arising from uncertainties in measuring the quantities on the right-hand side of equation (4.56). Although solids and liquids may be more or less easily confined to a known uniform thickness, this is generally not easy to do for soft tissues to an accuracy of much better than about $\pm 10\%$. By contrast, if care is taken in designing the apparatus, the inaccuracies associated with measuring the signals V' and V may be kept very small. It is important here to use wideband calibrated attenuators in order to keep the received signal within the linear region of the receiver amplifier characteristic for both reference and tissue measurements. The uncertainty of defining V' and V is then limited by the calibration of the attenuator and amplifiers (as a function of frequency) and the digitisation accuracy (number of bits) if computer processing is used. Note that when very small total attenuations are being measured as a function of frequency, even relatively minor non-linearities in the receiver gain characteristic may become significant. It is conceivable (but not proven) that these may be the cause of irregularities (lack of smoothness), present but not explained, in virtually all data published from measurements using short-pulse spectral analysis methods. In this regard it is also desirable to use transducers with as flat a response as possible, to avoid working on different parts of the receiver gain characteristic at different frequencies. The effect of this becomes most obvious at the extremes of the bandwidth of a given transducer (especially the high frequency extreme where attenuation is greatest), where the signal drops off rapidly and sits either on the low amplitude 'toe' of the gain characteristic or falls below the noise level of the system. Both cause the apparent measured attenuation to 'level out' at a system-dependent frequency. To assist interpretation of results it is advisable, before making attenuation measurements, to carry out a preliminary measurement of this 'maximum measurable attenuation'. Switching off the transmitter conveniently mimics an infinitely attenuating specimen, although care needs to be taken to ensure that this does not also remove interference contributions to the noise level (see below).

It is important to exclude unwanted acoustic and electrical interference from the measurement. The former may require anechoic lining of the inside of the water tank, careful positioning of the specimen and receiver to avoid coincidence of unwanted reverberations with the desired signal and time-gating of the signal to separate it, prior to amplitude measurement, from non-coincident interference. Reflection systems with analogue spectral processing may require the use of r.f. gated amplifiers, which also require calibration. These possess only a limited ability to suppress unwanted signals such as the large-amplitude excitation signal, and thus may also limit the attenuation that can be measured. Direct measurement from a log spectral display (e.g. with a real-time spectrum analyser) may offer practical convenience but may also limit the precision with which spectral amplitude can be measured (in the region of ± 0.3 dB for analogue analysers).

Also implicit in equation (4.56) is the specification of the frequency of measurement. For studies as a continuous function of frequency, an uncertainty in defining the frequency will be transferred to an error in the measurement of V' or V, which will depend on the slope of the frequency dependence of the received signal. Thus, it is desirable that the system has as flat a response as possible over the frequency range of interest. Data length for digital systems, pulse or gate lengths, and filter characteristics for analogue systems, in addition to any frequency scale or digitisation rate calibration, will all influence the frequency-resolving capability of a system. Voltage spikes, associated with switch-on and switch-off of analogue gates, will interfere with the received pulse, and will cause a corresponding modulation of the frequency spectrum, which will be sensitive to changes in the time relationship of the pulse and gate. The equivalent of this for digital systems is of course the selection of a limited section of the digitised signal surrounding the transmitted sound pulse, which corresponds to multiplying by a rectangular window and causes spectral modulation if the signal does not reach zero, or is not forced to reach zero by an appropriate weighting function, at the edges of the window.

4.4.2.2.2 Errors Due to Invalid Assumptions

A second class of errors may be defined as those due to the fact that some of the assumptions made in arriving at equation (4.56) are not valid. Here we consider: (1) the basic assumptions of linearity of ultrasonic propagation and electroacoustic transduction; (2) the neglect of factors such as reflection at tissue boundaries, the attenuation coefficient of the displaced coupling medium and forward scattering; and (3) problems arising from the assumption that the tissue and coupling medium have the same sound speed.

(1) *Non-linearity*. The effects of non-linear sound propagation on attenuation measurements were discussed in Section 4.3.8, from which it is clear that prediction of such effects is made difficult because of the highly system-specific nature of their dependence on many variables. Since broadband spectral analysis measurement systems make use of short pulses, which contain peaks of high pressure-amplitude, they would seem to be more likely than some of the other methods to suffer from artefacts due to non-linear propagation. Akiyama *et al.* (1983) have studied this possibility, using a computer simulation that repetitively applies a low-pass filter and a rule similar to equation (4.44) to compute the changes in shape of a short pulse as it propagates through an insertion measurement system like that illustrated in Figure 4.5. It appears that, as the peak pressure amplitude is raised, it is within the high and low peripheral regions of the transducer bandwidth where distorted measurements are first observed (as artefactually low values of the attenuation coefficient at these frequencies) but no explanation or thorough discussion of this result was provided.

Although non-linear propagation effects might be minimised by careful positioning of the specimen (away from the stabilisation region), the best course of action clearly is to ensure linear conditions. Linearity of propagation and of transduction may both be checked simply by observing the effect on the measurement of varying the input voltage amplitude to the transmitting transducer. Particular care should be taken of non-linear effects when measuring attenuation in media that are known to possess a high value of the non-linearity parameter B/A, especially those that contain gas bubbles, which may include suspensions of contrast agent microbubbles, inadequately degassed tissue specimens, cavitating or boiling media, or inflated lung. Indeed it may become part of the experiment in such cases to characterise the pressure dependence of the apparent attenuation coefficient, if this is needed for other purposes such as an attenuation correction in the simultaneous measurement of a scattering coefficient. In such a situation short-pulse spectral analysis methods may be undesirable because the acoustic wave pressure launched by the source will vary with frequency, due to the frequency transfer characteristic of the transducer. Austin (2003) has, however, found that this can very effectively be compensated for in a pseudo-CW measurement system, where a function generator and power amplifier were used to excite the transmitting transducer with a long (e.g. 20 cycle) sine wave burst. Using a broadband receiver and by varying the frequency over many bursts whilst keeping the excitation voltage amplitude constant, the frequency transfer characteristic of the transducer was measured, inverted and subsequently used for inverse excitation of the transducer so as to generate, over a limited but useful bandwidth, sine wave bursts with a pressure amplitude that was independent of frequency. This system may have been the first to be designed explicitly to improve the accuracy of measurements of attenuation and scattering coefficients in non-linear media. As an additional benefit, this method is very effective in broadening the bandwidth over which a single transducer can be made to provide useful attenuation measurements.

(2) *Reflection at tissue boundaries.* Quoted values (*cf.* Chapter 1) for the impedance mismatch between water and soft tissue result in a value of $T_{wt} \approx 0.997$, which, if neglected, would result in an over-estimation of the attenuation by only 0.05 dB, even for the reflection system [equation (4.55)]. Specimen holders commonly employ acoustic windows made from polyethylene, Mylar™, Saran™ and similar substances. The attenuation due to a single layer of polyethylene of thickness 25 μm, for example, has been measured over the frequency range 2–10 MHz (Bamber 1979) to be equal to about 0.005 dB MHz$^{-1.2}$. For the reflection system this loss typically would only amount to about 1–2% of the measured attenuation. Losses due to reflection at interfaces are therefore often neglected for soft tissue studies. If, however, the attenuation coefficient of the medium to be measured is low (e.g. as in testis and biological fluids such as blood), or the reflection loss is high (e.g. as for bone or some 'tissue simulating' phantom materials, or due to an 'imperfectly wetted' interface – see Section 1.8.3), then a straight line fitted to the attenuation measured as a function of specimen thickness for different samples of the same material will yield the reflection loss as a constant offset.

Displaced coupling medium. The value of μ_w, if the coupling medium is water, is equivalent only to about 0.002 dB cm^{-1} at 1 MHz. This rises with f^2, and so will become more important at high frequencies, but even at 8 MHz the correction required is still only 0.14 dB cm^{-1}. For accurate measurements on weekly attenuating media at high frequencies, values of μ_w for degassed distilled water, as a function of temperature and frequency, may be obtained from Pinkerton (1947).

Forward scattering. Failure to correct for the energy received as a result of forward scattering by liver tissue was earlier in this section related to an underestimation in α by an unknown amount. This artefact is likely to be most evident where strongly scattering media are concerned (e.g. lung, bone and perhaps breast). Thus for media in which α_s contributes strongly to α, one would expect different measurement systems to give different results for α, depending on such factors as specimen thickness, distance of specimen to receiver and area of the receiver. Perhaps of particular interest here are the materials used in phantoms and chosen to mimic tissue values of attenuation and speed. Some of these consist of a base material such as gelatine, for which α_a is very low, to which scatterers such as powdered graphite are added until the required value of α is obtained.

(3) *Sound speed of tissue.* The difference in sound speeds, between tissue and coupling medium, leads to at least three more potential sources of error: bulk refraction of the sound beam due to misalignment or non-parallelism of the specimen, diffraction losses and phase cancellation due to acoustic path length variations across the beam (Truell & Oates 1963).

Generally speaking, refraction errors will be reduced by the use of focused transducers, thin specimens, large-area receivers and a short tissue-to-receiver distance. The reflection system tends to be less prone to refraction errors than the two-transducer system. One estimate, for a study of soft tissues in a reflection arrangement where parallelism and alignment were both controlled to within $\pm 3°$, put the error due to bulk refraction at 1% or less of the measured attenuation (Bamber 1979).

In some of the variable-path measurement systems, failure to apply corrections for losses associated with the diffraction field of the transmitter can lead to errors as high as 30%. Figure 4.6a is plotted from the theoretical data of Seki *et al.* (1956) and shows the calculated total diffraction loss as a function of distance from the face of the transmitter. The received intensity has been derived from the square of the average pressure over an on-axis receiver of identical shape and area to the transmitter, at distances (Z) expressed in units of r^2/λ, where r is the transducer radius.

Buffered insertion techniques are designed to minimise the change in acoustic path length that occurs between the reference and attenuated measurements. In fixed frequency systems the error resulting from the remaining path length change may be further reduced by placing the receiver at a position of one of the diffraction peaks or troughs, such that any small shift in Z results in only a very small change in the diffraction loss. For coaxially aligned focused transducers, this amounts to placing the receiver so that its focal point is coincident with that of the transmitter (Penttinen & Luukkala 1977). Variable frequency systems that are not strongly focused do not permit such optimum positioning of the receiver and, although the associated errors may still be small when measuring soft tissues, it is instructive to note the form that they take. Remember, however, that the errors may be substantial for media other than soft tissues. Figure 4.6b shows examples of the frequency dependence of the additional signal loss (or gain) due to the differences in the diffraction loss for the received signal with and without the specimen in the sound path (see Figure 4.5) for two kinds of specimen, one having a speed of sound 1600 m s^{-1} (in the upper range for a tissue like liver) and the other having a speed of sound 1350 m s^{-1} (a very low value for fatty tissue). For both situations the speed of sound in the coupling medium was assumed to be 1485 m s^{-1}, the specimen thickness was 3 cm, the transducers were 7.5 mm radius, and the receiver was positioned at the nominal last axial maximum ($Z = 1$) of the transmitter. Several general points are worth noting. Firstly, there is a trend for the diffraction errors to be more severe at lower frequencies. Secondly, the oscillatory nature of this systematic error means that the small corrections encountered will be further reduced by fitting the attenuation data to some smooth function of frequency, leaving in this case a constant negligible offset of about 0.03 dB. This is an advantage of continuously variable frequency systems over narrowband insertion methods. Thirdly, specimens with a sound speed higher than that of the coupling medium will, on average, produce a diffraction loss, whereas those with a sound speed below that of the coupling fluid will result in an average diffraction gain. For focused transducers positioned confocally, however, both types of specimen will produce a diffraction loss. Papadakis (1973) and Brendel and Ludwig (1975) have demonstrated that the troughs and peaks in the diffraction loss curve become progressively less pronounced as the bandwidth is increased. The loss is also decreased and smoothed if the transmitting transducer is 'shaded' (apodised), i.e. the amplitude of vibration decreases monotonically along its radius from the centre to the circumference (Papadakis 1970; see also Chapter 2).

Improved methods for diffraction error correction have been described by Ophir and Mehta (1988), Xu and Kaufman (1993) and Zeqiri (1996), among others. Experimental versions of the diffraction loss curve (Figure 4.6a), but which apply specifically to the measurement system being used, may be obtained by recording the signal $V(f)$, without the specimen present, as one varies the path length between the transmitting transducer and either the receiver or the

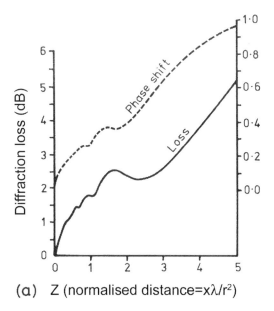

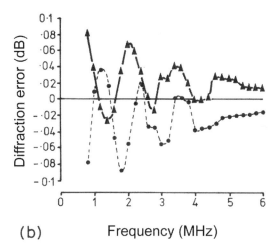

Figure 4.6. (a) Diffraction loss and phase shift from a circular piston of radius r (Seki *et al.* 1956; Papadakis 1966). (b) Diffraction error (i.e. additional apparent attenuation), obtained from (a), for a variable frequency, fixed path, insertion measurement system of the kind illustrated in Figure 4.5. Key: ▲—▲ is for a specimen with a sound speed of 1600 m s^{-1}, ●- - -● is for a specimen with a sound speed of 1350 m s^{-1}. Sound speed in the coupling liquid was set at 1485 m s^{-1}, the specimen thickness at 3 cm, the transducer radii at 7.5 mm, and the total distance, d, at the value of the last axial maximum of the transmitter

plane reflector. Interpolated values from this curve may then be used to apply a 'computed diffraction correction' to the recorded attenuation values, if the change in acoustic path length is also recorded when the specimen is inserted (as described in Chapter 5 for sound speed measurement). Alternatively, after insertion of the specimen, either the transmitter, the receiver or the plane reflector may be physically moved along the acoustic axis so as to correct for the time-shift observed when the specimen is inserted, i.e. to return the acoustic path length to its original value. This technique provides an 'experimental diffraction correction' and has come to be known as 'axial beam translation' (Ophir & Mehta 1988).

A confocally and coaxially arranged pair of matched focused transmitting and receiving transducers represents one of the best geometries for use with the buffered insertion technique, helping to reduce diffraction and other errors. Here the diffraction loss curve is relatively smooth and exhibits a peak at the transducer separation that places the foci at the same point. On the other hand, an example of poor geometry with regard to diffraction errors would be a large plane transmitter and a point receiver such as a hydrophone, in which case the diffraction loss curve becomes the strongly wavelength-dependent on-axis intensity distribution of the transmitter, as seen in Chapter 1.

The *in vivo* methods for measuring α, mentioned in Section 4.4.1.3, will also contain an error due to diffraction loss or gain. The situation is exceedingly complicated, however, and exact corrections may not be possible. The complications are largely due to the facts that the four-dimensional (i.e. frequency-dependent) diffraction field must be considered, the nature of the reflectors over which this field must be integrated is both unknown and spatially variable, and the frequency-dependent attenuation in intervening tissue alters the correction to be applied at any given point in the field. Various approaches to these problems have been published (Cloostermans & Thijssen 1983; Fink *et al.* 1983; Fink & Cardoso 1984; Insana *et al.* 1983; Kuc & Regula 1984; O'Donnell 1983; Zhou *et al.* 1992), although it would seem that a complete solution is intractable without additional independent information on the scattering structure of the tissue. It is possible, however (see for example Zagzebski *et al.* 1993; Mercer 1997), to employ distributed scattering phantoms such as sponges or gels containing suspensions of scatterers, and using a varying water path between the pulse–echo transducer and a scattering volume at a fixed shallow depth within the phantom, to arrive at a reasonable approximation to the calibration that is necessary for an *in vivo* numerical diffraction correction. For *in vivo* use, however, an experimental diffraction correction achieved by the axial beam translation technique described above, if it can be applied, may be more effective than the computational approach. Scanning through a water bath or other suitable stand-off medium may be a necessary inconvenience to achieve this, although for direct skin contact scanning electronic adjustment of the diffraction field produced by an array transducer should in principle be possible.

Phase cancellation, which may be produced in homogeneous specimens if the path length varies across the beam, is dealt with below. Related to this, and also arising from the coherent nature of the ultrasonic irradiation, is the speckle phenomenon (discussed in detail in Chapter 9). The consequence of this for measurement uncertainty, and approaches to mitigating its effects, are discussed by Parker (1986).

The temperature and static pressure experienced by the specimen are further potential variables and sources of error, well recognised in the field of physical acoustics in general but rarely considered when measuring biological media. The author is not aware of any studies of the pressure dependence of α for biological tissues. For liquids, an increase in pressure generally decreases α and for water this variation is about 25% per atmosphere at 30°C and about 64% at 0°C (Matheson 1971). If similar figures apply to tissues, then the pressure variations between experiments, corresponding to the few centimetres of water or saline under which the specimens of tissue are usually suspended (i.e. +8 cm of head of water at 0°C), would not be expected to give rise to variations in α of more than about ±0.5%. This is unlikely to be true for specimens containing gas, and lung in particular requires special consideration (Dunn & Fry 1961). The temperature dependence of α in soft tissues has been investigated as an experimental variable affecting the precision and accuracy of attenuation measurements (Bamber & Hill 1979). The greatest variations observed (for fat at room temperature) correspond to a value of $\alpha^{-1}d\alpha/dT$ of about -5% per °C. Whilst it is very important to state the temperature of measurement for comparison purposes, errors due to slightly inaccurate knowledge of the temperature are likely to be small at 20°C (e.g. $< \pm1\%$ for ±0.2°C) and close to zero at 37°C.

Finally, it should be noted that when the quantity being measured is the *absorption* coefficient, by observation of the temperature rise consequent on irradiation by a narrow focused beam of ultrasound, the effect of heat conduction to surrounding unheated regions may be very substantial. This problem has been analysed and discussed by Parker (1985).

4.4.2.3 Inhomogeneity Effects

The acoustical inhomogeneity of most tissues will give rise to additional errors due to refraction and diffraction by the specimen, and to phase cancellation if the receiver is phase sensitive. The refractive and diffractive nature of an inhomogeneous propagation medium may give rise to local perturbation in the ultrasonic beam parameters, relative to values that would be observed at a given reception point in the reference beam if attenuation were the only modifying factor (Mountford & Halliwell 1973; Foster & Hunt 1979). It would appear that no-one has yet attempted to evaluate the possible errors due to this source, but it is likely that they will only be of any importance for very small area receivers.

Phase cancellation at the receiver may be a consequence of propagation through inhomogeneities either in path length or sound speed, as indicated in Figure 4.7. An apparent attenuation coefficient due solely to the phase cancellation, $\alpha_{phase}(f)$ that occurs at a particular frequency may be defined. For the two situations illustrated in Figure 4.7 this contribution to α may be calculated (Bamber 1979) as:

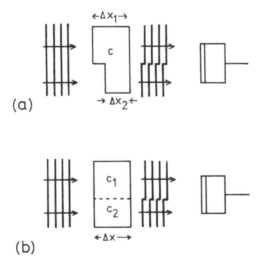

Figure 4.7. A schematic representation of the distortion of an initially plane wave after propagation through a slab of acoustically inhomogeneous material. Two simple, one-dimensional, inhomogeneities are illustrated: (a) a step in specimen thickness $\Delta x(z)$, where $\Delta x(y)$ remains constant, and (b) a step in speed of sound $c_t(z)$, where $c_t(y)$ remains constant

$$\alpha_{phase}(f) = -\frac{10}{\Delta x}\log_{10}\left[g^2 + (1 - g^2) + 2g(1 - g)\cos\left(\frac{f}{2\pi}\Phi\right)\right] \tag{4.57}$$

where g is the proportion of the area of the receiver covered by one phase of the wave (i.e. $g = 0.5$ if the receiver is split exactly in half by the discontinuity in the wave). The quantity Φ is given, for path length fluctuations, by

$$\Phi = \left(\frac{\Delta x_1 - \Delta x_2}{c_w}\right) - \left(\frac{\Delta x_1 - \Delta x_2}{c}\right) \tag{4.58}$$

and, for sound speed fluctuations, by

$$\Phi = \Delta x\left(\frac{1}{c_1} - \frac{1}{c_2}\right) \tag{4.59}$$

where c_w is the speed in the coupling medium. Examples of α_{phase}, for various values of g and variations in speed and path length, are provided in Figure 4.8. It can be seen that even quite small variations in path length or speed may give rise to appreciable measurement errors, particularly at high frequencies.

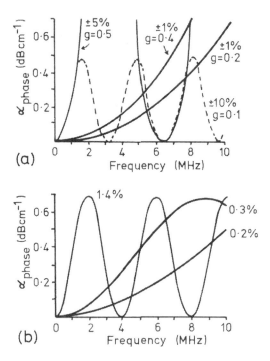

Figure 4.8. Examples of the variation with frequency of the calculated attenuation due to phase cancellation at a circular phase-sensitive receiver. (a) and (b) show respectively the results for the path length fluctuation and velocity fluctuation illustrated in Figure 4.7. For (a) the nominal specimen thickness was 4 cm. The step fluctuations are expressed as percentages of this thickness on each of the curves. The values of g indicate the fraction of the area of the detector covered by one uniform portion of the wave. In (b) the specimen thickness was 2.8 cm and $g = 0.1$. The percentages shown indicate the relative difference in speeds of sound for the two regions of the specimen

Miller *et al.* (1976) have studied in some detail the problem of phase cancellation for transmission measurements on dog heart muscle; observing, on some occasions, over-estimates of α of more than 100%. Marcus and Carstensen (1975) noted, however, that whilst large phase shifts over waves transmitted through muscle were observed, there were no measurable phase differences across waves transmitted through liver. Correspondingly, differences in the value of α measured by these authors using both piezoelectric and radiation force receivers were not observable for liver but ranged up to 380% for muscle tissue. It is clear that the severity of the phase cancellation problem will vary considerably from tissue to tissue, and possibly from specimen to specimen. There are few data as yet regarding acoustic speed inhomogeneity in various tissues and organs. Specific regions within a specimen responsible for gross phase cancellation can, however, easily be recognised with a broadband measurement system, as shown in Figure 4.9, and hence avoided. Processing, in the form of averaging and fitting a smooth curve to the attenuation data, also helps to reduce this problem at specific frequencies, but must inevitably contribute to some general over-estimation of the attenuation coefficient and its frequency dependence. Parallel problems that arise in scattering measurements are referred to in Chapter 6.

Apart from the use of power-sensitive receivers, and broadband techniques as described above, phase-cancellation effects can be minimised by the use of a thin evenly cut specimen, a narrow beam in the vicinity of the specimen (provided by focused transducers), a receiver of small area, and a large distance separating the specimen and the receiver. The last three requirements comprise the condition that the receiver be placed in the 'far-field' (Fraunhoffer region) of the region of phase distortion, and that the phase distorting region be in the far-field of the receiver.

It will be noticed that the solutions to many of the above problems compete with each other. Any measurement system must be the result of a number of compromises.

4.4.2.4 Tests on Standard Materials

In view of the large number of possible sources of error in measuring an attenuation coefficient, and the difficulty of estimating many of them, it is advisable to check any new measurement system by performing measurements on standard materials that have known characteristics that are widely agreed upon. For highly accurate, absolute measuring systems, pure water is usually chosen (data of Pinkerton 1947). For systems designed to make relative measurements on tissues, a phantom incorporating beam distortion and the appropriate amount of scattering is not yet available. Castor oil forms a suitable homogeneous test material, chosen by many for this purpose because there is good agreement on its ultrasonic attenuation properties, and its ultrasonic speed and attenuation are of similar magnitudes to those of many soft tissues. Reviewed by Dunn and Breyer (1962), the data on castor oil reduce to:

$$\alpha_{30C} = 0.5 f^{1.66} \tag{4.60}$$

where α has units of dB cm^{-1}, f is in MHz and covers the range 0.5–500 MHz. Variations with temperature over the range 0–40°C (Dunn *et al.* 1969) may be expressed in Arrhenius form as:

$$\ln \alpha_{1\,\text{MHz}} = 4215 \left(\frac{1}{T} \right) - 4.59 \times 10^{-7} \tag{4.61}$$

where T is in K; or in a more practically useful form as

$$\alpha_{1\,\text{MHz}} = 2.25 \, e^{-0.0493\,T} \tag{4.62}$$

where T is in °C.

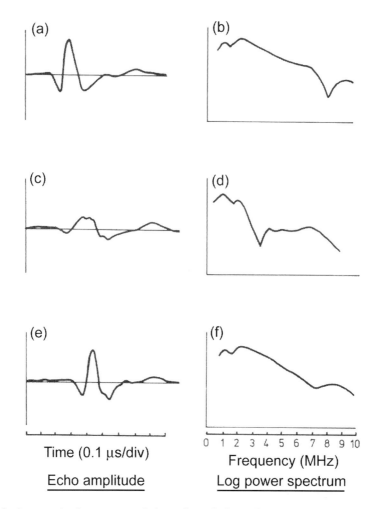

Time (0.1 µs/div)

Echo amplitude

Frequency (MHz)

Log power spectrum

Figure 4.9. An example of a pronounced phase discontinuity, and the consequent phase cancellation, observed during an attenuation measurement on fresh human liver (path length = 4.8 cm). Pulses (a) and (e) were observed on either side of, and pulse (c) was observed directly over, the region in question. The difference in pulse arrival times for conditions (a) and (e) caused the interference and cancellation at about 3.5 MHz observed in the pulse spectrum shown in (d)

The lower attenuation presented by cotton seed oil forms a much more demanding test of system accuracy ($\alpha = 0.035 f^2$ dB cm^{-1} at 26°C; Dunn & Breyer 1962), but this oil is not so readily available as is castor oil.

An alternative approach is to develop a standard material whose properties may be accurately predicted from theory. Hall et al. (1997) chose this method and used suspended polystyrene microspheres for confirming the calibration of broadband attenuation coefficient and backscattering coefficient measurement systems.

4.4.2.5 Influence of Measurement Conditions

As we have seen earlier, accurate measurement of ultrasonic attenuation coefficients generally necessitates work on excised tissue specimens, there being very few situations where *in vivo* measurement is possible. A similar situation also exists for those who wish to measure the speed or scattering of ultrasound. Major problems occur, however, in handling the specimens in ways that facilitate measurement yet yield results characteristic of *in vivo* tissues, and in being able to confirm the measured data at a later time, with perhaps other instrumentation and other specimens. As presented in Table 4.3, this problem area may be divided into two main groups of questions, which will now be reviewed.

There are few studies that can be called upon to provide answers to these questions, and our knowledge in this area is still very far from complete. If no particular precautions are taken either to prepare tissue specimens for measurement, or to select the specimens or measurement positions in any way, or to control the measurement conditions, then very wide variations in α can be observed between and within specimens (Bamber 1981). This is particularly true of both liver and fat, where the variations may be as large as several hundred per cent at a particular frequency. Any or all of the factors quoted in group A of Table 4.3 may contribute to the wide variation of published data for a particular organ (Goss *et al.* 1978).

(a) *Ageing of specimens.* For specimens of a number of organs stored at room temperature (Bamber *et al.* 1977) it has been found that, provided that all evolving gases are removed, ultrasonic attenuation is relatively insensitive to the autolytic processes occurring up to at least 5 days after excision. Time variations attributable to autolysis (i.e. a decrease in α, but not more than -15% in 30 h), were small in comparison to the wide variations between measurements referred to above. Both Frizzell *et al.* (1979) and Bamber *et al.* (1977), however,

Table 4.3. Major groups of questions arising with regard to the handling of tissue specimens for ultrasonic propagation property measurements

Groups of questions	Some potentially relevant factors
A. To what precision and accuracy may the *in vitro* propagation properties themselves be defined, and what are the determining factors? Are the properties stable, and, if not, can they be adequately preserved?	Time after death Temperature of storage Medium of storage Histochemical fixation Freezing Gas inclusion and production Uncertainty of measurement temperature and pressure Selection of specimens (e.g. age at death) Spatial variations within specimens
B. What is the relationship between the acoustic propagation properties measured *in vitro* to those that would be obtained *in vivo*, and how is it determined?	Blood flow and other tissue movement Blood pressure Blood vs other suspending fluids (pH and concentration of solutes) Level of hydration Surrounding tissues and organs Tissue tension (e.g. skin) Temperature difference Factors specific to the death of particular cells and tissues

noted the effects of gas produced by decaying tissue. The effects that are seen when gas is not removed may provide explanations for observed increases in α with time after the excision for beef spleen (Crosby & Mackay 1978) and dog myocardium (O'Donnell *et al.* 1977). In the latter study an average increase of 20% in the first 4 h after death was noted for specimens stored at 35°C, but no significant variations occurred for tissues maintained at 19.5°C. Ageing of human brain stored at 4°C between measurements was reported to cause α to decrease by up to 21% between the first and second measurements (1 day after excision) and to remain unchanged for 4 days thereafter (Kremkau *et al.* 1981), whereas only 8% reduction in 2 days was observed for bovine brain kept at 20°C (Bamber *et al.* 1977).

The speed of sound has been observed to decrease only slightly (about 1% over 5–6 days) with ageing of specimens of human brain (Kremkau *et al.* 1981) and bovine myocardium (Shung & Reid 1978). Backscattering cross-section, on the other hand, may decrease substantially with time after death for tissues kept at 20°C (Bamber *et al.* 1977), but this parameter exhibited no significant changes over 6 days for bovine myocardium kept at 4°C (Shung & Reid 1978).

(b) *Gas bubbles*. A contribution of gas bubbles to the attenuation coefficient of liver has been calculated for various frequencies from equation (4.32) (Bamber & Nassiri 1985). With such a mechanism for attenuation, gassy specimens should display excess attenuation, and almost no frequency dependence of α, at low frequencies. Published data tend to demonstrate features that are consistent with such predictions and that appear not to be dependent on the measurement method. Methods of partial evacuation and manual palpation that are often described in the literature are either unsuccessful or only partially successful in rendering specimens gas free. Refrigeration is an improvement (Frizzell 1976; Frizzell *et al.* 1979; Bamber & Nassiri 1985) since the low temperature increases the solubility of gases in water, and time is available after reheating for measurements to be made before the gas comes out of solution again. Similar logic underlies another method found to be successful by Frizzell (Frizzell 1976; Frizzell *et al.* 1979) and Parker (1983), which involved placing the tissues in an environment of increased pressure. Frizzell used a pressure of 33 bar (3×10^6 Pa) for 90 min; Parker used 27 bar for 30 min and enclosed his samples in a sealed polythene container to prevent additional pressurised gas from dissolving into solution.

Somewhat interestingly the problem of gas production may not be quite so severe for some other tissues as it is for liver (Bamber *et al.* 1977). Nevertheless, the introduction of gas bubbles into the preparation of fresh tissues remains a potential problem.

(c) *Storage and measurement conditions*. The medium in which a tissue sample is stored and measured appears to be important; Frizzell (Frizzell 1976; Frizzell *et al.* 1979) found that samples of liver prepared and measured in water consistently had lower attenuation coefficients than those prepared in physiological saline (6–12% difference). Different levels of swelling of cells and tissue spaces due to osmosis may have been involved here, although the possibility that the saline specimens were more gassy does not appear to have been excluded.

As noted above (see also Pauly & Schwan 1971), the absorption coefficient is influenced by pH, and this factor will be relevant in the present context.

(d) *Freezing*. It is important to know whether tissues may be preserved for measurement by freezing them. Crosby and Mackay (1978) found a substantial increase in soft tissue attenuation coefficient during the freezing process itself, and Miles and Cutting (1974) have shown that a close correlation exists between the sound speed and the percentage of unfrozen water in beef. Freese and Makow (1968) found that attenuation and backscatter from beef and fish tissues differ markedly as between fresh tissue and tissue which has been frozen and then thawed. Increases in both parameters, after thawing, were attributed to small cavities formed by ice crystals and dissolved air which comes out of solution during the freezing process. This is entirely consistent with the observations on liver by Frizzell *et al.* (1979), who also show that proper degassing of the thawed specimens brings the attenuation coefficients down to values nearly equal to the absorption coefficients measured using the transient thermoelectric method, which in turn are approximately equal to the values measured for fresh specimens. In a single specimen of breast tissue, however, the freeze–thaw process was noted to cause a small (4%) decrease in the attenuation coefficient, with no effect on the speed of sound (Foster *et al.* 1984).

(e) *Fixation.* Chemical fixation has been used for many years to preserve tissue specimens for histological and anatomical studies. Various fixatives exist, but the most common, formalin, has also been used by many researchers to preserve specimens for acoustic measurement. The effects of fixation on propagation properties have rarely been the subject of specific investigations. Most of the known facts are summarised by Bamber *et al.* (1979), who studied the action of various fixatives. Large differences between the effects of different fixatives were noticed. Formalin does appear to preserve the acoustic propagation properties of a number of tissues, with perhaps an acceptable level of consistency, although in general the following changes due to fixation were observed: (1) an average increase in the attenuation coefficient of about 10% at 1 MHz and 50% at 7 MHz; (2) an average decrease in speed of about 1.5%; and (3) an average decrease in the backscattering coefficient of about 15% at 1 MHz and 45% at 4 MHz. The results for attenuation and speed are consistent with later findings in human brain (Kremkau *et al.* 1981). Measurements over formalin-fixed specimens tend to have less spatial variation than those for fresh tissues; the increased rigidity due to fixation permits greater precision in cutting the specimens to a uniform thickness. Within the range 5–40°C, the temperature dependence of α has also been measured to be broadly similar for fixed and fresh tissues (Bamber & Hill 1979). A possibly important difference of effect, however, has been noted when acoustically anisotropic tissue is fixed in formalin. A 30% increase in α was observed, due to fixation, when bovine skeletal muscle was measured perpendicular to the line of the muscle fibres, but no measurable change was observed along the fibres (Nassiri *et al.* 1979).

(f) *Temperature and pressure.* The possible influences of temperature and pressure on the precision and accuracy of attenuation measurements were discussed in Section 4.4.2.2. Generally, small temperature fluctuations are not a problem, but major differences in the measurement temperature may account for some of the variations in published data for certain tissues, particularly fat (see Bamber & Hill 1979).

(g) *Inherent biological variability.* Little work has been done specifically to evaluate the statistical variability of the ultrasonic propagation properties of otherwise 'normal' organs and tissues, which may be taken from subjects of varying species, sex, race, age at death, and so on. For example, collagen content in heart and liver (von Ehrenberg *et al.* 1954), and water content in brain (Altman & Dittmer 1972) are known to vary with age. The latter phenomenon would appear to be responsible for the observation that attenuation in human infant brain is about one-third that for adult brain (Kremkau *et al.* 1981). Speed in breast is known to decrease with age (see Section 5.3.3). Further variations may be expected for samples extracted from different locations and/or orientations within certain organs. There appears, however, to be little species difference for the absorption coefficient, at least as revealed by measurements of liver and tendon (Goss *et al.* 1979b).

(h) *Changes in death.* Although much work remains to be done in the areas mentioned above, our knowledge at present of the second of the major questions, regarding the relationship between the live and dead states, is almost non-existent. The list of parameters presented in group B of Table 4.3 is therefore speculative and awaits amendment in the light of future experience. For some purposes cessation of blood flow may render the tissue of interest unusable (Lomonaco *et al.* 1975), though both von Gierke (Dunn 1965) and Robinson and Lele (1972) found no significant change in either speed of sound or attenuation coefficient between the living and dead states. It has been suggested by Heimburger *et al.* (1976) that differences in the vasculature of grey and white matter accentuate the impedance mismatch and so make the grey–white borders more visible to pulse–echo imaging of live brain than of excised brains, although the latter were formalin fixed. The pulsation of the living brain was also considered by these authors to be important in determining its echo properties. The temperature dependence of the ultrasonic parameters (Bamber & Hill 1979; Gammell *et al.* 1979; Kremkau *et al.* 1981) may be expected to account for a large proportion of observed differences, if *in vitro* measurements are not made at body temperature. However, at 0.97 MHz, a 7 to 25% increase in the attenuation coefficient of dog brain, after sudden death, has been observed by Yosioka *et al.* (1968), which apparently could not be accounted for simply on the basis of a temperature change. Miles and Fursey (1974), on the other hand, found the speed of sound through the limbs of living animals, consisting almost entirely of skin, fat and muscle, to lie between those determined at body temperature on excised fat and muscle. Furthermore, absorption coefficients determined by the transient thermoelectric method for mouse liver *in vivo* and immediately after death show no statistically significant differences (Frizzell *et al.* 1979). McNeely and Noordergraff (1981) have measured an average decrease in the attenuation coefficient of cat muscle kept at 38°C, during the period from living to about 4 h after death. The total change during this time, however, was about −24% (1.75 MHz) as compared to an initial variation over measurements between five cats of about ±53%. There was some evidence that after the 4-h period the attenuation was beginning to increase again.

4.5 PUBLISHED DATA ON ATTENUATION AND ABSORPTION COEFFICIENTS

Excellent discussions of this subject already exist (Carstensen 1979; Dunn *et al.* 1969; Dunn & O'Brien 1976; Johnston *et al.* 1979; Wells 1975), and a number of tables of published data on ultrasonic properties of tissues have been compiled, notably those due to Duck (1990), but see also publications by Chivers and Parry (1978), Goldman and Hueter (1956), Goss *et al.* (1978, 1980). This material will not be reproduced here in detail, although it does form the basis for the whole of this section. The attempt here is to place emphasis on those areas that were missed or glossed over in the original reviews, and those for which data have since become available. An important example of data in the latter class has just been discussed in Section 4.4.2.5. Figure 4.10 should be referred to whilst reading this section.

---

figure. The examples provided were chosen for illustrative purposes only and, as such, serve to indicate the general trends with frequency and the relationships between tissues. Key to references for these data: lung (Dunn 1974); skull bone (Hueter 1952); tendon (Dussik & Fritch, obtained from Goss *et al.* 1978); skin (Dussik & Fritch, obtained from Goss *et al.* 1978; note: more recent data on skin are reviewed by Moran *et al.* 1995); breast mean value (as reviewed by Bamber 1983); skeletal muscle parallel to the fibres (Colombati & Petralia, Dussik *et al.*, Buschmann *et al.*, Hueter, obtained from Chivers & Parry 1978); fixed cardiac muscle at 100 MHz (Yuhas & Kessler 1979); adult brain (Bamber 1981; Kremkau *et al.* 1981); liver at 1–10 MHz (Pauly & Schwan 1971); liver at 100 MHz (Tervola *et al.* 1985b; see also Pohlhammer *et al.* 1981); kidney at 100 and 220 MHz (Kessler 1973); spleen (Bamber 1981); testis (Bamber 1981); infant brain (Kremkau *et al.* 1981); whole blood (Carstensen & Schwan 1959); breast cyst liquid (Lang *et al.* 1978; note: 9.4% protein solution from analysis); blood plasma (Carstensen & Schwan 1959); 10% haemoglobin solution at 25°C (as reviewed by Kremkau & Carstensen 1972 and by Wells 1977); range of values for amino acids in solution (as reviewed by Kremkau & Carstensen 1972); water (Pinkerton 1947).

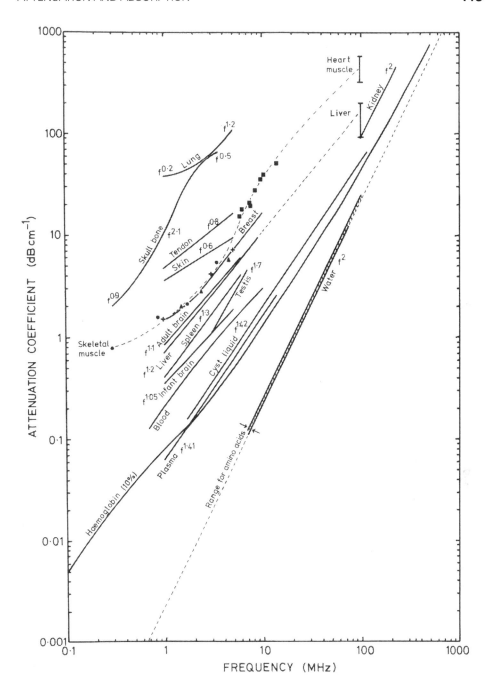

Figure 4.10. Attenuation coefficients of various tissues and biologically relevant liquids as a function of frequency. For most soft tissues the variability in the reported results is such that the data do not permit one tissue type to be separated from another. The data for bone also cover a wide range, not indicated in the

4.5.1 BIOLOGICALLY RELEVANT 'SIMPLE' MEDIA

Hueter (1958) appears to have been the first to point out that a positive relationship exists between the attenuation coefficient and the structural 'complexity' of biological media. The 'simple' media referred to above are water and biological molecules in aqueous solution or suspension. Because of a suspected predominant involvement of molecular relaxation mechanisms in determining ultrasonic attenuation in tissues, the ultrasonic study of aqueous solutions of macromolecules has been quite intensive. Pauly and Schwan (1971), in particular, have convincingly demonstrated, by attenuation measurements on liver and on a homogenate of subcellular components of liver, that most of the attenuation is due to absorption at the macromolecular level. Further discussion of molecular mechanisms is taken up in Chapter 7.

Some of the properties of water were discussed in Section 4.3.5, where mention was made of the two-state model for structural relaxation by water molecules, proposed by Hall (Hall 1948; Dunn *et al.* 1969). A time constant of about 10^{-12} s appears to characterise the process of reorganisation from one state to another. As a result, the absorption measured at about 1 MHz is proportional to f^2, but α/f^2 ($= 15.7 \times 10^{-17}$ s^2 cm^{-1} at 37°C) is greater than that predicated by purely classical mechanisms.

4.5.1.1 Intramolecular Absorption

At medical frequencies and below, the absorption of ultrasound by the water present within tissues represents a negligible contribution to the total attenuation. Whole biopolymers represent the first significant contribution as one progresses up the scale of biological complexity. Monomers such as amino acids in aqueous solution, although interesting because they may (at appropriate pH) display an absorption behaviour that can be described by a single relaxation frequency, barely modify the magnitude and frequency dependence of the absorption in water, even when they are present in the same number, type and concentration to be found in the complete polymers. Proteins, nucleic acids and polysaccharides all appear to display this (what has been termed) 'whole much greater than the sum of the parts' behaviour.

The detailed situation is more complex than this, however. The specific absorption coefficient of any particular biopolymer increases with molecular weight only over a restricted molecular weight range, which is at least as small as, if not smaller than, a factor of 100 in molecular weight (Kremkau & Cowgill 1984). On either side of this range the specific absorption coefficient is not correlated with molecular weight (i.e. within groups such as amino acids or proteins). The properties of molecules responsible for absorption differences within these groups have not been fully identified. However, in the important case of proteins, Kremkau and Cowgill (1985) have found evidence that the alpha-helix structure plays an important role, at least in linear proteins, but with the suggestion that the tertiary structure of globular proteins reduces absorption because of inhibited solvent interactions. Molecular conformation thus appears to determine some of the properties, though to an uncertain extent. Gelatin, which is a denatured form of collagen and assumes a simple random coil structure in aqueous solution, has a much smaller specific absorption than that of globular proteins possessing tertiary and quarternary structures. Intact collagen and DNA (deoxyribonucleic acid) in aqueous suspension or solution possess even higher specific absorptions. Both of these molecules have very high levels of structure (a triple helix and a double helix, respectively). Yet the specific absorption of molecules of the polysaccharides dextran and ficoll of the same molecular weight is approximately equal, even though dextran is long chain and ficoll is globular. The classical viscous contributions to absorption for these molecular configurations are quite different. Shear viscosity of solutions of macomolecules in general has no correlation with ultrasonic absorption.

The frequency dependence of ultrasonic absorption is similar for all biopolymers that possess higher-order structuring; a fact which has led authors to suggest that a common absorption mechanism, different from that in gelatin, for example, might be responsible. The form of this frequency dependence (nearly linear) suggests a distribution of relaxation times, but the specific mechanisms are unknown. It is widely considered that, at normal physiological levels of pH, the most important contributions probably arise from ultrasonically-induced perturbations of the hydration layers of macromolecules. Redistribution of this region of highly-structured water surrounding each molecule results in energy absorption by a structural relaxation process. It is possible that the ultrasonic absorption is determined by those aspects of molecular conformation that influence the number of water molecules involved in the free-bound equilibrium. Such mechanisms are often termed solute–solvent interactions. Strom-Jensen and Dunn (1984) observed small negative temperature coefficients of absorption that are consistent with a hypothesis of structural relaxation.

Although lipids, in one form or another, constitute the second most prevalent component of the dry weight of many soft tissues (the first being proteins), their acoustic propagation properties have received relatively little attention. The studies available concern themselves with those lipids and structures associated with the cell membranes, utilising suspensions of phospholipids such as lecithin in the form of bilayers within liposomal structures. Under these conditions the absorption phenomena may be described by either single (Gamble & Schimmel 1978) or multiple (Hammes & Roberts 1970) relaxation processes, with relaxation frequencies in the region of 1.6 to 16 MHz. Probable mechanisms concern conformal changes associated with the crystalline–liquid crystalline phase transition. This transition takes place at a temperature of about 41.3°C, at which point the relaxation amplitude is maximal and the speed of sound reaches a local minimum having just exhibited a very large negative temperature coefficient (Mitaku 1981; Maynard et al. 1985). It seems that no additional relaxation processes of significant amplitude occur at frequencies higher than 150 MHz.

For acoustic waves of finite ('non-linear') amplitude, absorption in simple biomolecular materials can become – consistent with the theoretical model discussed in Section 4.3.8 above – largely determined by source amplitude, and only weakly dependent on the small-signal absorption coefficient (Dalecki et al. 1991).

4.5.1.2 Intermolecular Absorption

At low concentrations of macromolecules in solution there is often, though not always, a region of nearly linear dependence of absorption on concentration (i.e. the specific absorption is approximately constant). This is the region where the intramolecular absorption mechanisms discussed above predominate. If solutions are not dilute, then the specific absorption increases with concentration; a phenomenon believed to be due to an increased tendency for some as yet unspecified interaction to occur between the macromolecules themselves. It has been suggested that, at concentrations pertinent to the molecules present in intact tissues, intermolecular absorption mechanisms (also called solute–solute interactions) might form the major macromolecular contribution to the absorption properties of tissues.

There is other evidence in support of the idea that macromolecular interaction is important. Kremkau and Carstensen (Kremkau & Carstensen 1972; Kremkau et al. 1973) have summarised the evidence available at that time, some of which concerns the treatment of macromolecular solutions with chemicals that are known to increase the level of molecular interaction. One class of such chemicals is the histological fixatives, which promote cross-linkages between adjacent protein molecules, and so stiffen and preserve tissues. The acoustical effects of formalin fixation of whole tissues, discussed in Section 4.4.2.5, may be regarded as providing additional support for the suggestions made by Kremkau and Carstensen. The cross-linking of proteins appears to increase the absorption but (anomalously) decrease the speed of sound. Skeletal muscle tissue is an interesting case of relevance, since contraction of the muscle fibres is associated with an increase in the attenuation coefficient (Bhagat *et al.* 1976; Glueck *et al.* 1985) and, in some circumstances, a small decrease in the speed of sound (Section 5.3.1). Although the specific mechanism is not understood there would appear to be similarities between the actin–myosin cross-bridge formation of muscle contraction and the action of polymerising fixatives (Bamber 1979).

As usual, there is evidence to confuse the situation. For example, denaturation and dehydration of the proteins within tissues, due to the action of ethyl alcohol (Bamber *et al.* 1979) and heat or changes in pH (Pauly & Schwan 1971; Lele & Senapati 1977), cause the attenuation and absorption to increase. The effect of heating tissue to high temperatures is discussed further below, in Section 4.5.2.6.

4.5.2 TISSUES

4.5.2.1 Importance of Measurement Method

Considerable variation exists in published data on ultrasonic absorption and attenuation coefficients of solid tissues, even for what are supposedly the same organs from the same species of animal. This has hampered attempts to pool data in order to enable relevant theories to be tested or accurately to guide ultrasonic instrument design. Caution in interpreting the findings is necessary whenever one attempts to do this.

Much of the variation is almost certainly associated with differences in measurement conditions, as discussed in Section 4.4.2.5. An additional, and important, contribution to this variation arises from the existence and use of a great variety of measurement methods (Section 4.4.1). Probably the most important distinction is between the so-called phase-sensitive and phase-insensitive methods, when used to measure the same tissue specimens. Pohlhammer *et al.* (1981) have shown that, using different phase-insensitive methods, self-consistent results for the attenuation coefficients of bovine liver can be obtained over a wide frequency range (1–100 MHz). Nevertheless, the published data from soft tissues in general do not permit the required biological variation to be easily distinguished from variation due to systematic errors. To examine the dependence of an acoustical parameter on other tissue properties, or on state variables (such as temperature), it is desirable therefore (though often not possible) to confine one's attention to data from one laboratory where that particular dependence has been specifically investigated.

4.5.2.2 Contribution of Scattering to Attenuation

An assessment of the contribution that scattering makes to the total attenuation in a given tissue would appear to be the first sensible step towards an understanding of the ultrasonic scattering and absorption mechanisms present within that tissue. Surprisingly, for the majority of tissues, the ratio μ_s/μ is either unknown or has been the subject of dispute. Much of the disagreement has almost certainly been due to the problems of comparing published data from different laboratories and to the difficulty of making direct measurements of the quantity μ_s

(see Chapter 6). We should also remember that there is in fact only a tenuous definition of a measured attenuation coefficient, the quantity being a variable one depending on the measurement geometry (see Sections 4.2 and 4.4.2.1).

There are several tissues over which there is little, or no, dispute regarding the value of μ_s/μ. Firstly, a number of uniform media within the body (in the absence of pathology) appear not to scatter the sound at all, at least at frequencies in the normal range of medical use. Examples are amniotic fluid, aqueous humour, vitreous humour, the lens of the eye (internal) and cyst liquids. Secondly, there is no dispute that it is the presence of air/tissue interfaces in the inflated lung that is responsible for the very high ultrasonic attenuation in this organ. The equations for attenuation due to gas bubbles (Section 4.3.3) were used by Dunn and Fry (1961) to model the level and frequency dependence of attenuation in lung, although a predicted minimum in the region of 4–7 MHz was not later observed experimentally (Dunn 1974). Instead, attenuation in lung increases progressively with frequency over the 1–6 MHz range. In any event, it has been observed that the measured attenuation coefficient in lung increases strongly with level of inflation (Dunn 1986).

Thirdly, there is agreement that the presence of intact cells in the blood is responsible for only a small component of the attenuation, and that most of this is due to viscous relative motion losses (see next section). We shall note below the directly measured absolute values for μ_s/μ in blood. Interesting variations in the value of μ_s occur with changes in haematocrit – a maximum occurs at about 26% red cell concentration, i.e. less concentrated than normal blood (Shung *et al.* 1976).

Possible approaches to estimating the individual contributions of absorption and scattering may be classified into direct and indirect methods. Direct methods of measuring the absorption coefficient were described in Section 4.4.1.1. Measurement of the scattering coefficient without reference to the absorption and attenuation coefficients is difficult and has been attempted for only a few tissues. In measuring an absolute scattering cross-section per unit volume, severe problems arise in accurately estimating the correction factors required to yield results independent of the instrumentation that is used both for obtaining an absolute value for the differential scattering cross-section per unit volume at a given scattering angle (backscattering is often used for this purpose), and for obtaining an accurate average angular distribution of scattering (strongly influenced by sample geometry and the variation with angle of the overlap of receiver and transmitter directivities). Nevertheless, the results from direct scattering measurements probably represent the most accurate estimates of the μ_s/μ ratio that are currently available. Campbell and Waag (1984) find that μ_s/μ in the frequency range 3–7 MHz is about 2% for calf liver; Nassiri and Hill (1986) find (approximately) 19%, 17% and 0.3% for human liver, muscle and blood in the range 4–7 MHz respectively. Such data are very important as a double check on values obtained from direct measurements of μ_a and μ. Parker (1983) has made direct measurements of both μ_a and μ in samples of beef liver, and comments that, at 1.1 and 3.3 MHz, the values are statistically indistinguishable (by comparison with the variance of the two data sets), although at 5.6 MHz a significant difference (equivalent to a value of $\mu_s/\mu = 18\%$) was observed.

There are numerous possible indirect approaches to this problem, but they generally offer little more than circumstantial evidence. Probably the most convincing of these was the classic study by Pauly and Schwan (1971) of the reduction in attenuation in whole beef liver produced by homogenising the tissue. It may be inferred from their results (Hill *et al.* 1978) that μ_s/μ in liver is about 30% (over 1–10 MHz). Even this study, however, assumed that the homogenising process, whilst removing all scattering structures (down to the subcelluar level), did not affect the absorption coefficient. This is unlikely, since contributions to absorption may arise from viscous relative motion losses at tissue inhomogeneities.

Nevertheless, the value of 30% is useful since it represents an upper bound on possible values for μ_s/μ in liver against which to judge other estimates.

Comparisons of published measurements of μ_a and μ have been attempted. Note, however, that even when phase-insensitive attenuation data are chosen for the μ estimate there are dangers such as the fact that attenuation measurements are strongly influenced by the presence of gas bubbles (and other measurement artefacts) whereas absorption measurements are not. Results of μ_s/μ in the frequency range 0.5–10 MHz fall in the range 23–61% for liver (Goss *et al.* 1979b; Pohlhammer *et al.* 1981). Lower values than this could easily have been obtained by appropriate choice of data from the literature.

Other indirect estimates have included modelling the frequency dependence of attenuation in liver according to equation (4.37) used for solids in Section 4.3.4 (Narayana & Ophir 1983b) and the matching of changes which take place in the levels of absorption, backscattering and attenuation when tissues decay or are fixed histochemically (Bamber 1979). Ophir's analysis assumes that μ_s is proportional to f^4 and provides an estimate of the value of the coefficient B in equation (4.37) that is required to produce the frequency dependence of μ in liver demonstrated by published data. Resulting values for μ_s/μ come to about 1% in normal liver and 8–13% in fatty liver, over a 1–5 MHz frequency range. Bamber's analysis assumes that during tissue decay, neither the absorption coefficient nor the angular distribution of scattering vary significantly. For fixation in formalin, changes in the absorption coefficient (Lele & Senapati 1977) were included. Resulting values for μ_s/μ, again for liver, varied between 9% and 16% at 4 MHz.

Unsurprisingly, introduction of a particulate contrast medium into a tissue such as liver increases the scattering contribution to attenuation, although in a quantitative manner that suggests an inhomogeneous biodistribtion of the particles (Tuthill *et al.* 1991). The value of μ_s/μ for microbubble contrast agents is discussed below, in Section 4.5.2.8.

Attenuation coefficients of ultrasound in bone may be between 2 and 20 times those in soft tissues, and there is disagreement regarding the frequency dependence. More than one investigator (Barger 1979; Hueter 1952) has noted that the frequency dependence of attenuation in bone follows a similar relationship to that expected when the attenuation is dominated by scattering from grain-like structures (see Section 4.3.4). One author, however, felt that viscous relative motion losses (next section) could account for the behaviour observed by Hueter (Fry 1952).

4.5.2.3 Contribution of Structural Inhomogeneities to Absorption

Section 4.3.3 described possible mechanisms, other than longitudinal wave scattering, by which small structural inhomogeneities could contribute to the absorption of sound energy. Here the evidence for the relative importance of such mechanisms in intact tissues is briefly discussed.

About 19% of the attenuation of ultrasound in blood (at normal haematocrit and over a frequency range 0.7–4 MHz) cannot be accounted for by absorption by the blood proteins, and has to be regarded as being due to the presence of intact cells (Carstensen & Schwan 1959). Rough estimates of the absorption due to viscous (and thermal) interaction between the cells and the surrounding fluid appear to account for something in the region of 10% (O'Donnell & Miller 1979) whilst, of the remainder, only somewhat less than 1% can be attributed to longitudinal wave scattering.

Using muscle myofibrils and collagen fibrils as structures for heart muscle and skin respectively, O'Donnell and Miller have also attempted to estimate the inhomogeneity losses for these organs. Their approximate results were about 60% of published values of attenuation in both cases, and demonstrate that, for many soft tissues, the attenuation due to this mechanism is not to be neglected.

Skeletal muscle is an interesting case in that the attenuation is greater, by about 160% at 0.3 MHz rising to 200% at 8 MHz, for waves propagating parallel to the muscle fibres, than for those propagating across the fibres (Goldman & Hueter 1956; Nassiri *et al.* 1979). Similar observations have been made in tendon (Miles 1996) and in myocardium (Mottley & Miller 1990). The mechanism of this anisotropy is unknown, but it is interesting to note that the calculations of Ahuja and Hendee (1978) demonstrate that viscous relative motion losses for suspensions of asymmetrical particles are greater for particles moving 'end-on' to the sound field than for those 'broadside' to the field (see Section 5.3.1 for details of the anisotropy of speed of sound in muscle).

4.5.2.4 Frequency Dependence

The frequency dependence of attenuation in some tissues and other biological media was discussed above, demonstrating that the value of m in a representation of the form

$$\mu = bf^m \tag{4.63}$$

can assist the discussion of the likely relative contributions of different attenuation mechanisms. As may be seen from Figure 4.10, most soft tissues and body liquids exhibit a value of m close to unity. For some tissues that have been studied over a wide enough frequency range, this value applies up to frequencies beginning to approach those for which the absorption by water may start to become important. If the measurement frequencies are extended still further, we should expect to see the value of m begin to increase towards 2 for these tissues.

The approximately constant absorption per cycle ($\alpha\lambda$) for soft tissues over this frequency range has received explanations from different authors, using all of the theories of absorption described in Sections 4.3.1–4.3.3. The present state of the published data, however, does not permit any of these to be examined to the desired level of detail.

Examination of individual examples of published data from soft tissues often demonstrates that equation (4.63) is not always the best fit to attenuation values as a function of frequency, which often show tendencies towards a lower value of m (sometimes zero) at the lower frequencies and higher values of m at the higher frequencies. Although such a frequency dependence is characteristic of measurement artefact due to the presence of gas bubbles, there are some examples which suggest that the effect is a real property of the tissue concerned. Note that for muscle, even the pooled data exhibit this effect (Figure 4.10), resulting in $\alpha\lambda$ possessing a minimum value at about 3 MHz. This is suggestive that there may exist a low frequency relaxation region (in addition to others) at around 40 kHz (Hueter 1958). Truong *et al.* (Truong 1972; Truong *et al.* 1978) have demonstrated that most of the relaxing elements of muscle structure do have characteristic frequencies in the region of 31 kHz.

4.5.2.5 Temperature Dependence

Section 4.3.5 outlined, for the known absorption and scattering mechanisms, the expected consequences of temperature variation. Data on tissues, with which to compare these predictions, are very scarce.

Most of the information available at the time regarding soft tissues was summarised by Bamber and Hill (1979), although additional data largely supporting their statements have since been published (e.g. Gammell *et al.* 1979; Bamber 1983). At temperatures (T) between 6 and 40°C, and frequencies above about 2 MHz, the attenuation coefficient is a monotonically decreasing function of temperature, with the slope ($d\mu/dT$) a decreasing function of frequency and temperature. A more complex behaviour is apparent at lower frequencies, with absorption, and possibly attenuation, sometimes increasing with temperature. Similar observations exist for egg white, where absorption below about 4 MHz exhibits a small positive temperature coefficient and, above this frequency, shows a negative temperature coefficient of absorption (Javanaud *et al.* 1984). Fat exhibits the largest negative value for $d\mu/dT$ (at 3 MHz, nearly 300% increase from body to room temperature, compared to about 20% for other tissues). For individual lines of beam propagation at particular frequencies in the complex fat/non-fat structure of the breast, $d\mu/dT$ is completely unpredictable, sometimes being positive even at high frequencies. The average properties of the breast, however, bear a sensible relationship to the data on other tissues.

Above the temperature range 40–50°C, $d\mu/dT$ for fresh tissues becomes positive, even at high frequencies, possibly because of heat denaturation of macromolecules. This is discussed further in Section 4.5.2.6 below.

No single absorption or scattering mechanism has yet been used to explain the observed temperature dependences of attenuation in soft tissues. Different mechanisms must be presumed to predominate under different conditions of temperature and frequency. Above 3 MHz the temperature dependence for non-fatty tissues is reminiscent of that for absorption in blood plasma (Carstensen *et al.* 1953). A model assuming a general shift of relaxation frequencies with temperature provides qualitative agreement with this trend, since above 3 MHz the slope of $\log(\alpha\lambda)$ vs f is indeed slightly positive (see Section 4.3.5). Intriguingly, as was noted in Section 4.5.2.4, below this frequency some tissues exhibit a slight negative slope of $\log(\alpha\lambda)$ vs f. This would be consistent with the positive temperature coefficients of absorption mentioned above.

For frequencies above 3 MHz and temperatures above 20°C the attenuation for most soft tissues decreases with temperature in proportion to the square root of viscosity; a result used by O'Donnell *et al.* (1977) to infer that viscous relative motion losses could be responsible. Fat, and other tissues at temperatures less than 20°C, display a negative $d\mu/dT$ much steeper than the square root of viscosity (Bamber 1979). Combined data on absorption and attenuation in *in vivo*, fresh *in vitro* and fixed tissues of the central nervous system of mouse, cat and man are presented in Figure 4.11. It is undesirable to have to compare in one graph data on different quantities, from different species, obtained under different conditions, but the scarcity of data leaves no alternative.

The behaviour demonstrated in Figure 4.11 is peculiar in that, although the centre of a possible low-frequency relaxation region seems to increase with temperature, the average relaxation amplitude would appear to be a negative function of temperature and, as pointed out by Carstensen (1979), the shape of the relaxation curve changes with temperature. None of these observations is understood at present.

The temperature dependence of attenuation in bone was observed as positive in the frequency range 1.4–4.5 MHz (Kishimoto 1958). This has been said possibly to be associated with a slight negative slope for $\log(\alpha\lambda)$ vs f in bone (Carstensen 1979), but could just as easily have been used as evidence for scattering mechanisms of attenuation (Barger 1979).

4.5.2.6 Heat-Induced Tissue Coagulation

When soft tissues are heated beyond 40–50°C, i.e. temperatures above which both macromolecules are known to denature (and cell death is known to occur), marked increases

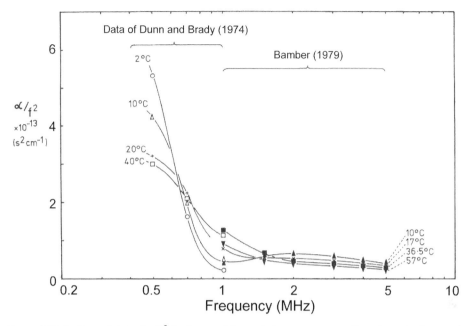

Figure 4.11. Isothermal plots of α/f^2 for tissues of the central nervous system. Data shown for frequencies below 1 MHz are for absorption in mouse spinal cord (Dunn & Brady 1974) and those above 1 MHz are for attenuation in fixed bovine brain (Bamber & Hill 1979). Data of Robinson and Lele (1972), for attenuation in cat brain at 4.2 MHz in the temperature range of approximately 30°C to 50°C, and of Kremkau *et al.* (1981) for human brain, confirm the trends shown but are not plotted, so as to maintain the clarity of the figure

in the attenuation coefficient are seen to occur as the temperature is further increased (Robinson & Lele 1972; Bamber & Hill 1979). These changes in the ultrasonic attenuation coefficient depart substantially from the trends seen at temperatures below 40–50°C, described above. For example, when heating from just above 50°C to about 80°C, the attenuation coefficient at 4.2 MHz in cat brain *in vivo* was observed by Robinson and Lele (1972) to increase about five-fold, compared with a decrease of just a few per cent when the temperature was raised from 30°C to 50°C. The increase was found to reverse to some extent on cooling but showed hysteresis, with the final attenuation coefficient of the tissue after it had returned to body temperature remaining about 50% higher than the value that existed prior to heating. These authors also observed that the attenuation coefficient depends on the time for which the tissue is held at temperatures above 50°C; the attenuation coefficient appears to have increased nearly four-fold between 20 min and 120 min at a constant 55°C.

The temperature dependence of ultrasonic propagation properties has long been of interest for non-invasive measurement and imaging of temperature for assisting clinical procedures such as hyperthermia (e.g. Cetas & Connor 1978). This application seems to have met with relatively little success, possibly due both to the difficulty in making accurate measurements and to the biological variability in the temperature coefficients of interest. The situation looks more promising, however, for applications where absolute temperatures are not required, e.g. for visualising the position and shape of the heated region in thermal ablation systems when they are run at relatively low (pre-ablative) temperatures (e.g. Miller *et al.* 2002, 2003).

For temperatures above those that produce irreversible damage to tissue, imaging the altered ultrasonic propagation properties (post-ablation) may help to confirm the volume of tissue that has successfully been treated. Bush *et al.* (1993) measured the ultrasonic propagation properties of freshly excised porcine liver treated using a focused ultrasound ablation system. They showed that, so long as all gas is removed from the tissue specimens (including gas generated as a result of cavitation or boiling), exposing the tissue to a spatially averaged intensity of about 200 W cm^{-2} at 1.7 MHz for 1–2 min produced on average a doubling of the attenuation coefficient and a small (0.5%) but consistent increase in sound speed, but no useful change in the backscattering coefficient. Similar results were later obtained Malcolm (1997).

There is considerable scope for further study in this area. For example, the author is not aware that use has been made of the sign of the temperature coefficient of attenuation, which as mentioned above, reverses above the temperature region of interest. Monitoring the sign of the rate of change of the attenuation coefficient with time (and hence temperature) during continuous heating might provide a means to measure when tissue coagulation (and cell death) have occurred. Additional confirmation might be provided during the cooling period after heating has ceased, from both the sign of the time dependence of the attenuation coefficient and the reversibility of the phenomenon relative to the heating period. Once again, however, it is apparent that the incomplete state of knowledge from published data on ultrasonic attenuation in biological tissues does not permit a fully informed judgment to be made of the feasibility of such suggestions.

4.5.2.7 Role of Specific Tissue Components

For tissues in general (although excluding some, such as fat, lung and bone) approximate empirical relationships have been shown to exist between the ultrasonic propagation properties and the concentrations of particular structural components (Dunn 1976; Goss *et al.* 1980a; O'Brien 1977; Pohlhammer & O'Brien 1981). There is a tendency, on moving from liquids (such as blood) through to tendon and cartilage, for an increase in the structural protein (collagen) content, which correlates with increasing ultrasonic attenuation and speed of sound. Within parenchymal tissues, for which the collagen content is relatively small, the attenuation and speed appear to be governed by the overall globular protein content, or to be inversely related to the water content (see also Bamber *et al.* 1981). Collagen has, for some time, been regarded as likely to be an acoustically important tissue component, particularly where scattering is concerned (Fields & Dunn 1973), primarily because its low frequency (static) elastic modulus is apparently more than 1000 times greater than that found in measurements of large volumes of intact soft tissues. Measured specific absorption and speed per unit concentration of collagen in aqueous solution have since been determined to be respectively about four and two times those for globular proteins (Goss & Dunn 1980). Increased collagen content has also been found to be associated with pathologically significant high levels of ultrasonic attenuation, for example in some primary breast cancers (Kobayashi 1979), in the aortic wall (Bridal *et al.* 1997) and in infarcted myocardium at the period in time of scar formation (Miller *et al.* 1976). In another study of breast tumours, attenuation coefficients were found to be relatively high for fibrous and parenchymal tissues, low for fat, and with intermediate values in regions of infiltrating duct carcinoma (D'Astous & Foster 1986).

A detailed study of local values of absorption coefficient in ovarian tissues from six different species found values at 1 MHz ranging from 0.017 cm^{-1} for the follicle to 0.050 cm^{-1} for the corpus luteum, largely reflecting macromolecular content, and with little species variation (Carnes & Dunn 1988).

Glycogen is a protein that is known to have a high specific absorption coefficient, and *in vivo* studies have shown, correspondingly, a significant increase – of the order of 10% – in the attenuation coefficient of human liver, as between fasting and well-fed individuals, where the latter have stored glycogen that may constitute up to 10% of liver wet-weight (Tuthill *et al.* 1989).

For some tissues, the fat content is also important, largely because of its very low values for sound speed (see Chapter 5). Increasing fat content in the liver can reduce sound speed, even though the water content may be low, and tends to further increase the attenuation and scattering coefficients (Bamber & Hill 1981; Bamber *et al.* 1981; Freese & Lyons 1977; Narayana & Ophir 1983b; Tervola *et al.* 1985b; Wilson *et al.* 1984). Tissues which possess a high proportion of fat, with a large number of fat/non-fat interfaces, such as breast (Kossoff *et al.* 1973; Bamber 1983), will tend to possess, relative to other soft tissues, a low average speed of sound and high attenuation and scattering coefficients.

4.5.2.8 Microbubble Contrast Agents – 'Aerosomes'

As already mentioned in Section 4.3.9, there is widespread use of ultrasonic contrast agents consisting of encapsulated gas microbubbles, sometimes referred to as aerosomes, and there is a substantial and growing literature on their acoustical characteristics. Aspects of their physical behaviour have been reviewed, for example, by de Jong *et al.* (1991), de Jong (1997), Forsberg (1997), Chang and Shung (1999). Their predominant, useful physical attribute is their strong scattering behaviour, but this influences, and is influenced by, attenuation. A theoretical model for this situation has been developed by de Jong *et al.* (1992) and shown to correlate well with experimental measurements. Some aspects of the relevant theory were discussed in Section 4.3.3.

For concentrations, C, of microbubbles at least to 21×10^6 microbubbles per ml, the attenuation coefficient for microbubble suspensions has been observed to increase linearly with C (e.g. Bleeker *et al.* 1990; Marsh *et al.* 1999). The frequency dependence, however, exhibits a peak in the region of 2–3 MHz (see Figure 4.12, *cf.* Figure 4.10). A single microbubble exhibits an extremely strong resonant behaviour (e.g. μ_s drops by a factor of more than 100 with only a few per cent departure from the resonant frequency). This leads to the often-used assumption that for a distribution of microbubble sizes in suspension the attenuation at any given frequency will be largely due to only the bubbles whose size makes them resonant at that frequency. Hence data such as those shown in Figure 4.12 have been interpreted, via equation (4.31), as relative number density distributions of bubble radii, $n(a)$. The results appear to agree reasonably well with measurements of the size distribution made with optical particle sizing methods (Schlief *et al.* 1994).

A suspension of microbubbles is a situation where equations (4.2a) and (4.2b) may in principle be applied directly to relate the acoustic interaction cross-sections of individual bubbles to the interaction coefficients of the volume suspension, where each bubble both absorbs and scatters sound, so that both n_{ia} and n_{is} in these equations become the number density distributions of bubble radii, $n(a)$. The property μ_s/μ, but known in this context as the scattering-to-attenuation ratio or STAR, has been proposed as an equipment-independent measure of one aspect of the relative potential usefulness of various microbubble contrast agents (Bouakaz *et al.* 1998). Because n_{ia} and n_{is} are both equal to $n(a)$, and so long as a suspension of bubbles does not become so concentrated that either multiple scattering or bubble–bubble interaction occur,

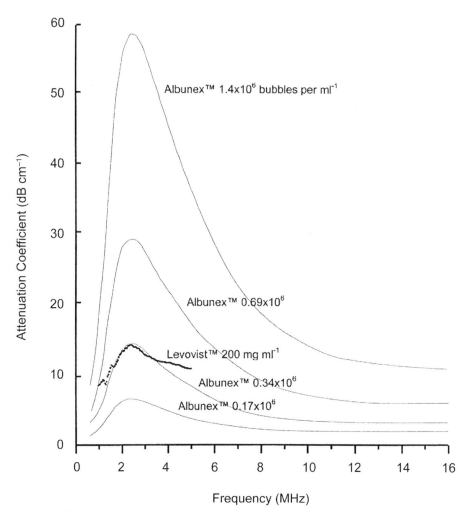

Figure 4.12. Attenuation coefficient as a function of frequency for volume suspensions of two commercially available microbubble contrast agents. The data were re-drawn with permission, for Levovist™ from Schlief *et al.* (1994) (as cited by Forsberg *et al.* 1997) and for Albunex™ from Marsh *et al.* (1999). Similar results may be found for Albunex™ in Chang and Shung (1999), and for MRX-115™ in Unger *et al.* (1997). The peak at around 2–3 MHz is usually taken to indicate that the most predominant size of microbubble in these suspensions is in the region of 3 μm diameter. This correlates well with measurements made with independent particle-sizing devices

$$\frac{\mu_s}{\mu} = \frac{1}{1 + \sum_a n(a)\sigma_s(a) / \sum_a n(a)\sigma_a(a)} \tag{4.64}$$

and μ_s/μ should therefore be independent of concentration. Marsh *et al.* (1999) have confirmed this for the contrast agent Albunex™. Values for μ_s/μ were obtained by measuring at 'low' insonifying pressure amplitudes (see comment below, about non-linearity) the attenuation coefficient, μ, and the backscattering coefficient, μ_{bs}, and then computing $4\pi\mu_{bs}/\mu$.

This assumes isotropic (monopolar) scattering (see Chapter 6 and Bamber 1997, 1998). They found the value of μ_s/μ to increase nearly linearly with frequency over the range studied, from about 5% at 1 MHz to about 45% at 16 MHz, suggesting that Albunex^{TM} (stabilised by a relatively stiff shell of albumin) should be more useful at higher frequencies, with decreasing effects from acoustic shadowing. Levovist^{TM} on the other hand (stabilised by a surfactant, palmitic acid) appears to exhibit a maximum value of μ_s/μ at around 1 MHz (Bouakaz *et al.* 1998). Marsh *et al.* warn that μ_s/μ alone is not sufficient to define the comparative efficacy of a contrast agent for enhancing backscattered signal strength; the full concentration dependence of the attenuation and scattering coefficients is required. This is because the acoustic power backscattered from within an attenuating medium is given by

$$W_{bs} = K_1 \mu_{bs}(C) e^{-K_2 \mu(C)} \tag{4.65}$$

where K_1 and K_2 are constants for fixed acoustic range and include factors such as the acoustic power at the source, the solid angle over which the backscattered power is received, diffraction corrections and other losses in the acoustic path (Bamber 1997, 1998). The equation has been modified to include the bubble concentration dependence of both backscattering and attenuation, but assuming a fixed acoustic frequency and pressure amplitude. Thus, even when both μ_{bs} and μ are proportional to C, their contributions to W_{bs} compete; at low concentrations the low attenuation allows W_{bs} to rise as concentration increases but at higher concentrations the strong exponentially decreasing attenuation term causes W_{bs} to decrease rapidly as concentration is further increased. This creates an optimum concentration at which W_{bs} is maximum, the concentration for which varies with the contrast agent, the frequency and the path length through the intervening microbubble suspension.

An interesting, and potentially valuable property of microbubble suspensions is their strongly non-linear acoustic behaviour. For two different commercial contrast agents, Wu and Tong (1998) measured B/A values of 600 and 2000 respectively. It has been shown that useful levels of both sub-harmonic and second harmonic signals are present in scattered radiation (Krishna & Newhouse 1997; Shankar *et al.* 1998), and the phenomenon has been shown experimentally to be capable of substantially improving visualisation of blood flow in small vessels (Ragavendra *et al.* 1997). As a consequence of this strong non-linearity, however, measurements such as those reported above for μ_{bs} and μ produce results that are dependent on the amplitude of the ultrasonic pressure field, requiring special care to be taken in this respect. Microbubbles also require careful and consistent handling. They may be destroyed at high insonating acoustic pressure amplitudes and results are expected to be dependent on ambient temperature and pressure. Sboros *et al.* (2002), in particular, raise important issues regarding the difficulty of relating characteristics measured for volume suspensions of microbubbles, especially at high concentrations, to those of single bubbles. Their experimental results also demonstrated that some agents are more non-linear in their response than others and may in fact consist of two simultaneously existing populations of bubbles, one of encapsulated bubbles with their shells intact and another of free bubbles, where the relative number of bubbles in the two populations is dependent on the incident acoustic pressure.

4.6   CONCLUSION

The subject of attenuation and absorption of ultrasonic longitudinal waves in biological media and tissues is extremely complex and remains poorly understood. At the present time no completely satisfactory explanation exists for the variation of attenuation with any physical or tissue parameter (i.e. frequency, temperature, etc.).

The attenuation coefficient is an elusive quantity to define, and it is difficult to be sure that one has measured it accurately. Different measurement methods result in different values of the attenuation coefficient for the same specimens. Although these differences are due to systematic error, it is not true that the method having the greatest accuracy will give rise to the most appropriate estimate of ultrasonic loss in all situations (diagnostic imaging, for example).

The practical consequences of the phenomena and data described in this chapter (and the next) are too numerous to have been discussed here. Simple examples would be the inability to use ultrasound efficiently to image through and within lung or bone, and the ease with which liquid-filled cavities may be identified. More involved examples would be the ultrasonic beam degradation and resolution impairment imposed by the frequency dependence of the attenuation (Foster & Hunt 1979), and the use of the data to optimise the frequency for imaging a particular organ or to construct ultrasound phantoms suitable for test or training purposes.

The *in vivo* measurement techniques described in Section 4.4.1.3 are beginning to form a basis for quantitative imaging and tissue analytical techniques, to be discussed in Chapter 9.

REFERENCES

Ahuja, A.S. (1979). Tissue as a Voigt body for propagation of ultrasound. *Ultrasonic Imaging* 1, 136–143.

Ahuja, A.S. and Hendee, W.R. (1978). Effects of particle shape and orientation on propagation of sound in suspensions. *J. Acoust. Soc. Am.* **63**, 1074–1080.

Akiyama, I., Nishida, Y., Nakajima, M. and Yuta, S. (1983). On the measurement of frequency dependent attenuation in biological tissue using broadband pulsed ultrasound. *IEEE Ultrasonics Symposium Proc.* **2**, Cat. No. 83CH1947-1, 80–805.

Altman, P.L. and Dittmer, D.S. (1972). *Biology Data Book* (2nd edn), Vol. I. FASEB, Washington, D.C., p. 392.

Andreae, J.H., Bass, R., Heasell, E.L. and Lamb, J. (1958). Pulse techniques for measuring ultrasonic absorption in liquids. *Acustica* **8**, 131.

Austin, J.C. (2003). Prospects for acoustic signature recognition of microbubble contrast agents. Ph.D. thesis, University of London.

Baboux, J.C., Lakestani, F., Fleischmann, P., Perdix, M., Guillaud, C. and Goutte, R. (1976). An ultrasonic spectroscopy device: application to tissue differentiation. In *Proc. 2nd European Congress on Ultrasonics in Medicine*, E. Kazner *et al.* (eds). American Elsevier Publishing, New York, pp. 108–114.

Baker, L.A.S. (2003). Ultrasonic reflex transmission imaging with commercial linear arrays for monitoring minimally invasive ablation therapies. Ph.D. thesis, University of London.

Bamber, J.C. (1979). Ultrasonic characterization of structure and pathology in human soft tissues. Ph.D. thesis, University of London.

Bamber, J.C. (1981). Ultrasonic attenuation in fresh human tissues (letter). *Ultrasonics*, **July**, 187–188.

Bamber, J.C. (1983). Ultrasonic propagation properties of the breast. In *Ultrasonic Examination of the Breast*, J. Jellins and T. Kobayashi (eds). John Wiley, Chichester, pp. 37–44.

Bamber, J.C. (1997). Acoustical characteristics of biological media. In *Encyclopaedia of Acoustics*, M.J. Crocker (ed.), Ch. 141. John Wiley, New York, pp. 1703–1726.

Bamber, J.C. (1998). Ultrasonic properties of tissues. In *Ultrasound in Medicine*, F.A. Duck, A.C. Baker, H.C. Starritt (eds). IoP Publishing, Bristol, pp. 57–88.

Bamber, J.C. and Bush, N.L. (1991). Quantitative imaging of acoustical and histological properties of excised tissues. In *Acoustical Imaging*, H. Lee and G. Wade (eds), Vol. 18. Plenum Press, New York, pp. 17–25.

Bamber, J.C. and Hill, C.R. (1979). Ultrasonic attenuation and propagation speed in mammalian tissue as a function of temperature. *Ultrasound Med. Biol.* **5**, 149–157.

Bamber, J.C. and Hill, C.R. (1981). Acoustic properties of normal and cancerous human liver: dependence on pathological condition. *Ultrasound Med. Biol.* **7**, 121–133.

Bamber, J.C., Hill, C.R., Fry, M.J. and Dunn, F. (1977). Ultrasonic attenuation and backscattering by mammalian organs as a function of time after excision. *Ultrasound Med. Biol.* **3**, 15–20.

Bamber, J.C., Hill, C.R. and King, J.A. (1981). Acoustic properties of normal and cancerous human liver – II. Dependence on tissue structure. *Ultrasound Med. Biol.* **7**, 135–144.

Bamber, J.C., Hill, C.R., King, J.A. and Dunn, F. (1979). Ultrasonic propagation through fixed and unfixed tissues. *Ultrasound Med. Biol.* **5**, 159–165.

Bamber, J.C. and Nassiri, D.K. (1985). Effect of gaseous inclusions of the frequency dependence of ultrasonic attenuation in liver. *Ultrasound Med. Biol.* **11**, 293–298.

Barger, J.E. (1979). Attenuation and dispersion of ultrasound in cancellous bone. In *Ultrasonic Tissue Characterisation 11*, M. Linzer (ed.). National Bureau of Standards, Spec. Publ. 525, US Govt. Printing Office, Washington, D.C., pp. 197–201.

Bergmann, P.G. (1946). The wave equation in a medium with a variable index of refraction. *J. Acoust. Soc. Am.* **17**, 329–333.

Bevan, D.P. and Sherar, M.D. (2001). B-scan ultrasound imaging of thermal coagulation in bovine liver: frequency shift attenuation mapping. *Ultrasound Med. Biol.* **27**, 809–817.

Beyer, R.T. (1965). Nonlinear acoustics. In *Physical Acoustics: Principles and Methods*, W.P. Mason (ed.), Vol. II, Part B, Ch. 10. Academic Press, New York, pp. 231–264.

Beyer, R.T. (1974). *Nonlinear Acoustics*. Naval Ship Systems Command, US Department of the Navy.

Beyer, R.T. and Letcher, S.V. (1969). *Physical Ultrasonics*. Academic Press, New York.

Bhadra, T.C. and Roy, B. (1975). Attenuation of ultrasonic energy in liquids by the streaming method. In *Ultrasonics International Conference Proc.*, IPC Science and Technology Press, Guildford, pp. 253–256.

Bhagat, P., Hajjar, W. and Kadaba, M. (1976). Measurement of the acoustic properties of a nerve–muscle preparation as a function of physiological state. *Ultrasonics*, **Nov.** 283–285.

Bjørnø, L. (1975). Non-linear ultrasound – a review. *Ultrasonics International Conference Proc.*, IPC Science and Technology Press, Guildford, pp. 110–115.

Bleeker, H., Shung, K. and Barnhart, J. (1990). On the application of ultrasonic contrast agents for blood flowmetry and assessment of cardiac perfusion. *J. Ultrasound Med.* **9**, 461–471.

Bouakaz, A., de Jong, N. and Cachard, C. (1988). Standard properties of ultrasound contrast agents. *Ultrasound Med. Biol.* **24**, 469–472.

Braddick, H.J.J. (1965). *Vibrations, Waves, and Diffraction*. McGraw-Hill, London.

Brendel, K. and Ludwig, G. (1975). Measurement of ultrasonic diffraction loss for circular transducers. *Acustica* **32**, 110.

Bridal, S.L., Fornes, P., Bruneval, P. and Berger, G. (1997). Correlation of ultrasonic attenuation (30 to 50 MHz) and constituents of atherosclerotic plaque. *Ultrasound Med. Biol.* **23**, 691–703.

Bush, N.L., Rivens, I., ter Haar, G.R. and Bamber, J.C. (1993). Acoustic properties of lesions generated with an ultrasound therapy system. *Ultrasound Med. Biol.* **19**, 789–801.

Busse, L.J. and Miller, J.G. (1981). Detection of spatially nonuniform ultrasonic radiation with phase sensitive (piezoelectric) and phase insensitive (acoustoelectric) receivers. *J. Acoust. Soc. Am.* **70**, 1377–1386.

Calderon, C., Vilkomerson, D., Mezrich, R., Etzold, K.F., Kingsley, B. and Haskin, M. (1976). Differences in the attenuation of ultrasound by normal, benign, and malignant breast tissue. *J. Clinical Ultrasound* 249–254.

Campbell, J.A. and Waag, R.C. (1984). Measurements of calf liver ultrasonic differential and total scattering cross-sections. *J. Acoust. Soc. Am.* **75**, 603–611.

Carnes, K.I. and Dunn, F. (1988). Absorption of ultrasound by mammalian ovaries. *J. Acoust. Soc. Am.* **84**, 834–837.

Carson, P.L., Meyer, C.R. and Scherzinger, A.L. (1981). Breast imaging in coronal planes with simultaneous pulse echo and transmission ultrasound. *Science*, **214**, 1141–1143.

Carstensen, E.L. (1979). Absorption of sound in tissue. In *Ultrasonic Tissue Characterization II*, M. Linzer (ed.). National Bureau of Standards, Spec. Publ. 525. US Govt. Printing Office, Washington, D.C., pp. 29–40.

Carstensen, E.L., Law, W.K., McKay, N.D. and Muir, T.G. (1980). Demonstration of nonlinear acoustical effects at biomedical frequencies and intensities. *Ultrasound Med. Biol.* **6**, 359–368.

Carstensen, E.L., Li, K. and Schwan, H.P. (1953). Determination of the acoustic properties of blood and its components. *J. Acoust. Soc. Am.* **25**, 28–289.

Carstensen, E.L. and Schwan, H.P. (1959). Absorption of sound arising from the presence of intact cells in blood. *J. Acoust. Soc. Am.* **31**, 185–189.

Cetas, T.C. and Connor, W.G. (1978). Thermometry considerations in localized hyperthermia. *Med. Phys.* **5**, 79–91.

Chang, P.P. and Shung, K.K. (1999). Interaction of ultrasound and contrast agents. In *Trends in Contrast Media*, H.S. Thomsen, R.N. Muller and R.F. Mattrey (eds), Ch. 26. Springer-Verlag, Berlin, pp. 311–320.

Chivers, R.C. and Hill, C.R. (1975). Ultrasonic attenuation in human tissue. *Ultrasound Med. Biol.* **2**, 25–29.

Chivers, R.C. and Parry, R.J. (1978). Ultrasonic velocity and attenuation in mammalian tissues. *J. Acoust. Soc. Am.* **63**, 940–953.

Christensen, R.M. (1971). *Theory of Viscoelasticity*. Academic Press, New York.

Cloostermans, M.J.T.M. and Thijssen, J.M. (1983). A beam corrected estimation of the frequency dependent attenuation of biological tissues from backscattered ultrasound. *Ultrasonic Imaging* **S**, 136–147.

Colombati, S. and Petralia, S. (1950). Assorbimento di ultrasuoni in tessunti animali. *La Ricerca Scientifica Anno* **20** (1–2), 71–78.

Crosby, B.C. and Mackay, R.S. (1978). Some effects of time post-mortem on ultrasonic transmission through tissue under different modes of handling. *IEEE Trans. Biomed. Eng.* **BME-25**, 91–92.

Daft, C.M., Briggs, G.A. and O'Brien, W.D. (1989). Frequency dependence of acoustic attenuation measured by acoustic microscopy. *J. Acoust. Soc. Am.* **85**, 2194–2201.

Dalecki, D., Carstensen, E.L., Parker, K.J. and Bacon, D.R. (1991). Absorption of finite amplitude focused ultrasound. *J. Acoust. Soc. Am.* **89**, 2435–2447.

D'Astous, F.T. and Foster, F.S. (1986). Frequency dependence of ultrasound attenuation and backscatter in breast tissue. *Ultrasound Med. Biol.* **12**, 795–808.

de Jong, N. (1997). Physics of microbubble scattering. In *Advances in Echo Imaging Using Contrast Enhancement* (2nd edn), N.C. Nanda, R. Schlief, B.B. Goldberg (eds), Ch. 3. Kluwer Academic, Dordrecht, pp. 39–62.

de Jong, N., Hoff, L., Skotland, T. and Bom, N. (1992). Absorption and scatter of gas-filled microspheres: theoretical considerations and some measurements. *Ultrasonics* **30**, 95–103.

de Jong, N., Ten Cate, F.J., Lancee, C.T., Roelandt, J.R. and Bom, N. (1991). *Ultrasonics* **29**, 324–340.

Duback, D.W., Frizzell, L.A. and O'Brien Jr. W.D. (1979). An automated system for measurement of absorption coefficients using the transient thermoelectric technique. *IEEE Ultrasonics Symposium Proc.*, Cat. No. 79CH 1482-9SU, 388–391.

Duck, F.A. (1990). *Physical Properties of Tissue*. Academic Press, London.

Duck, F.A. and Hill, C.R. (1979). Mapping true ultrasonic backscatter and attenuation distributions in tissue: a digital reconstruction approach. In *Ultrasonic Tissue Characterization 11*, M. Linzer (ed.), National Bureau of Standards Spec. Publ. 525. US Govt. Printing Office, Washington, D.C. pp. 247–251.

Duffin, W.J. (1968). *Advanced Electricity and Magnetism*. McGraw-Hill, London, pp. 172–174.

Dumas, G.A., Thiry, P.S. and Drouin, G. (1983). Interferometric measurement method of ultrasonic attenuation in small liquid samples. *IEEE Trans. Son. Ultrasan.* **30**, 59–68.

Dunn, F. (1962). Temperature and amplitude dependence of acoustic absorption in tissue. *J. Acoust. Soc. Am.* **34**(10), 1545–1547.

Dunn, F. (1965). Ultrasonic absorption by biological materials. In *Ultrasonic Energy: Biological Investigations, and Medical Applications*, E. Kelly (ed.). University of Illinois Press, Urbana, pp. 51–65.

Dunn, F. (1974). Attenuation and speed of sound in lung. *J. Acoust. Soc. Am.* **56**, 1638–1639.

Dunn, F. (1976). Ultrasonic attenuation, absorption and velocity in tissues and organs. In *Ultrasonic Tissue Characterization*, M. Linzer (ed.), National Bureau of Standards Spec. Publ. 453. US Govt. Printing Office, Washington, D.C., pp. 21–28.

Dunn, F. (1986). Attenuation and speed of ultrasound in lung: dependence upon frequency and inflation. *J. Acoust. Soc. Am.* **80**, 1248–1250.

Dunn, F. and Brady, J.K. (1974). Temperature and frequency dependence of ultrasonic absorption in tissue. In *Proc. 8th Intl. Congress on Acoustics*. Goldcrest Press, Trowbridge, Vol. I, p. 366c.

Dunn, F. and Breyer, J.E. (1962). Generation and detection of ultra-highfrequency sound in liquids. *J. Acoust. Soc. Am.* No. **34**(6), 775–778.

Dunn, F., Edmonds, P.D. and Fry, W.J. (1969). Absorption and dispersion of ultrasound in biological media. In *Biological Engineering*, H.P. Schwan (ed.), McGraw-Hill, New York, pp. 205–332.

Dunn, F. and Fry, W.J. (1961). Ultrasonic absorption and reflection by lung tissue. *Phys. Med. Biol.* **5**, 401–410.

Dunn, F., Law, W.K. and Frizzell, L.A. (1982). Nonlinear ultrasonic propagation in biological media. *Br. J. Cancer* **45**(suppl. V), 55–58.

Dunn, F. and O'Brien, W.D. (eds) (1976). Ultrasonic biophysics. *Benchmarkpapers in Acoustics* Vol. 7. Hutchinson and Ross ISBN: 0879332069.

Dunn, F. and O'Brien, W.D. (1978). Absorption and dispersion. In *Ultrasound: Its Application in Medicine and Biology*, W.J. Fry (ed.). Elsevier, Amsterdam, Ch. 3, p. 393.

Eggers, F. and Funck, T. (1973). Ultrasonic measurements with milliliter liquid samples in the 0.5–100 MHz range. *Rev. Sci. Instrum.* **44**, 969–977.

Eggers, F., Funck, T. and Richmann, K.H. (1981). Ultrasonic absorption measurements with a millilitre short-path pulse cell. *J. Phys. E.: Sci. Instrum.* **14**, 113–116.

Ehrenberg, von R., Winnecken, H.G. and Biebricher, H. (1954). Der Altemsgang des Bindegewebes in menschlichen Organen. *Zeitschrift für Naturforschung* **9b**, 492–495.

Esche, R. (1952). Untersuchungen zur Ultraschallabsorption in tierischen Geweben und Kunststoffen. *Akustische Beihefte* **1**, 71–74.

Ferry, J.D. (1961). *Viscoelasticproperties of Polymers*. John Wiley, New York.

Fields, S. and Dunn, F. (1973). Correlation of echographic visualizability of tissue with biological composition and physical state. *J. Acoust. Soc. Am.* **54**, 809–812.

Fink, M.A. and Cardoso, J.F. (1984). Diffraction effects in pulse echo measurement. *IEEE Trans. Son. Ultrason.* **SU-31**, 313–329.

Fink, M., Hottier, F. and Cardoso, J.F. (1983). Ultrasonic signal processing for *in vivo* attenuation measurement: short time Fourier analysis. *Ultrasonic Imaging* **5**, 117–135.

Flax, S.W., Pelc, N.J., Glover, G.H., Gutmann, F.D. and McLachlan, M. (1983). Spectral characterization and attenuation measurements in ultrasound. *Ultrasonic Imaging* **5**, 95–116.

Forsberg, F. (1997). Physics of ultrasound contrast agents. In *Ultrasound Contrast Agents*, B.B. Goldberg (ed.), Ch. 2. Martin Dunitz, London, pp. 9–20.

Forsberg, F., Wu, Y., Makin, I.R., Wang, W. and Wheatley, M.A. (1997). Quantitative acoustic characterization of a new surfactant-based ultrasound contrast agent. *Ultrasound Med Biol.* **23**, 1201–1208.

Foster, F.S. and Hunt, J.W. (1979). Transmission of ultrasound beams through human tissue – focussing and attenuation studies. *Ultrasound Med. Biol.* **5**, 257–268.

Foster, F.S., Straban, M. and Austin, G. (1984). The ultrasound macroscope: initial studies of breast tissue. *Ultrasonic Imaging* **6**, 243–261.

Freese, M. and Lyons, E.A. (1977). Ultrasonic backscatter from human liver tissue: its dependence on frequency and protein/lipid composition. *J. Clin. Ultrasound* **5**, 307–312.

Freese, M. and Makow, D. (1968). Ultrasonic backscatter in fresh and thawed animal tissue. *J. Fish. Res. Bd., Canada* **25**, 605–607.

Frizzell, L.A. (1976). Ultrasonic heating of tissues. Ph.D. thesis, University of Rochester, NY.

Frizzell, L.A., Carstensen, E.L. and Davis, D. (1979). Ultrasonic absorption in liver tissue. *J. Acoust. Soc. Am.* **65**, 1309–1312.

Froelich, B. (1977). A simple apparatus for automatic pulse echo tracking. *J. Phys. E. Scient. Inst.* **10**, 210–211.

Fry, W.J. (1952). Mechanism of acoustic absorption in tissue. *J. Acoust. Soc. Am.* **24**, 412–415.

Fry, W.J. and Dunn, F. (1962). Ultrasound analysis and experimental methods in biological research. In *Physical Techniques in Biological Research*, Ch. 4. Academic Press, New York, pp. 261–394.

Fry, W.J. and Fry, R.B. (1954a). Determination of absolute sound levels and acoustic absorption coefficients by thermocouple probes – theory. *J. Acoust. Soc. Am.* **26**, 294–310.

Fry, W.J. and Fry, R.B. (1954b). Determination of absolute sound levels and acoustic absorption coefficients by thermoelectric probes – experiment. *J. Acoust. Soc. Am.* **26**, 311–317.

Gamble, R.C. and Schimmel, P.R. (1978). Nano-second relaxation processes of phospholipid bilayers in the transition zone. *Proc. Natl. Acad. Sci. USA* **75**, 3011–3014.

Gammell, P.M., Le Croisette, D.H. and Heyser, R.C. (1979). Temperature and frequency dependence of ultrasonic attenuation in selected tissues. *Ultrasound Med. Biol.* **5**, 269–277.

Glueck, R.M., Mottley, J.G., Sobel, B.E., Miller, J.G. and Perez, J.E. (1985). Changes in ultrasonic attenuation and backscatter of muscle with state of contraction. *Ultrasound Med. Biol.* **11**, 605–610.

Goldman, D.E. and Hueter, T.F. (1956). Tabular data of the velocity and absorption of high frequency sound in mammalian tissues. *J. Acoust. Soc. Am.* **28**, 35–37.

Goobermann, G.L. (1968). *Ultrasonics Theory and Application.* English Universities Press, London, Ch. 8.

Goss, S.A., Cobb, J.W. and Frizzell, L.A. (1977). Effect of beam width and thermocouple size on the measurement of ultrasonic absorption using the thermocouple technique. *IEEE Ultrasonics Symposium Proc.*, Cat. No. 77CH 1264-lSU, 206–211.

Goss, S.A. and Dunn, F. (1980). Ultrasonic propagation properties of collagen. *Phys. Med. Biol.* **25**, 827–837.

Goss, S.A., Frizzell, L.A. and Dunn, F. (1979b). Ultrasonic absorption and attenuation in mammalian tissues. *Ultrasound Med. Biol.* **5**, 181–186.

Goss, S.A., Frizzell, L.A. and Dunn, F. (1980a). Dependence of the ultrasonic properties of biological tissue on constituent proteins. *J. Acoust. Soc. Am.* **67**, 1041–1044.

Goss, S.A. and Fry, F.J. (1981). Nonlinear acoustic behaviour in focussed ultrasonic fields: observations of intensity dependent absorption in biological tissue. *IEEE Trans. Son. Ultrason.* **SU-28**, pp. 21–26.

Goss, S.A., Johnston, R.L. and Dunn, F. (1978). Comprehensive compilation of empirical ultrasonic properties of mammalian tissues. *J. Acoust. Soc. Am.* **64**, 423–457.

Goss, S.A., Johnston, R.L. and Dunn, F. (1980). Compilation of empirical ultrasonic properties of mammalian tissues. II. *J. Acoust. Soc. Am.* **68**, 93–108.

Goss, S.A., Johnston, R.L., Maynard, V., Nider, L., Frizzell, L.A., O'Brien Jr., W.D. and Dunn, F. (1979a). Elements of tissue characterization, Part II. Ultrasonic propagation parameter measurements. In *Ultrasonic Tissue Characterization 11*, M. Linzer (ed.), NBS Spec. Publ. 525. US Govt. Printing Office, Washington, D.C., pp. 43–51.

Green, P.S. and Arditi, M. (1985). Ultrasonic reflex transmission imaging. *Ultrason. Imaging*, **7**, 201–214.

Greenleaf, J.F. and Bahn, R.C. (1981). Clinical imaging with transmission ultrasonic computerized tomography. *IEEE Trans.* **BME-28**(2), 177–185.

Guittet, C.M., Bamber, J.C., Bush, N.L., Bell, D.S. and Mortimer, P.S. (2000). High frequency reflex transmission imaging: feasibility for eventual application to the diagnosis of skin tumours. In *Acoustical Imaging*, Vol. 25, M. Halliwell and P.N.T. Wells (eds). Kluwer Academic/Plenum Publishers, New York, pp. 325–330.

Hall, C.S., Marsh, C.S., Hughes, M.S., *et al.* (1997). Broadband measurements of the attenuation coefficient and backscatter coefficient for suspensions: a potential calibration tool. *J. Acoust. Soc. Am.* **101**, 1162–1171.

Hall, D.N. and Lamb, J. (1959). Measurement of ultrasonic absorption in liquids by the observations of acoustic streaming. *Proc. Phys. Soc.* **73**, 354–364.

Hall, L. (1948). The origin of ultrasonic absorption in water. *Phys. Rev.* **73**, 775.

Hammes, G.G. and Roberts, P.B. (1970). Ultrasonic attenuation measurements in phospholipid dispersions. *Biochim. Biophys. Acta* **203**, 220–227.

Haran, M.E. (1981). Distortion of finite amplitude ultrasound in tissue (Abstract). 101st Meeting of the Acoust. Soc. Amer. *J. Acoust. Soc. Am.* **69**(suppl. 1), S4.

Hawley, S.A. and Dunn, F. (1969). Ultrasonic absorption in aqueous solutions of dextran. *J. Chem. Phys.* **50**, 3523–3526.

Heimburger, R.F., Fry, F.J., Franklin, T.D., Sanghvi, N.T., Gardner, G. and Muller, J. (1976). Two dimensional ultrasound scanning of excised brains – I. Normal anatomy. *Ultrasound Med. Biol.* **2**, 279–285.

Hertzfeld, K.F. and Litovitz, T.A. (1959). *Absorption and Dispersion of Ultrasonic Waves.* Academic Press, New York.

Heyser, R.C. and Le Croisette, D.H. (1974). A new ultrasonic imaging system using time delay spectrometry. *Ultrasound Med. Biol.* **1**, 119–131.

Hill, C.R. (1975). Echoes from human tissues. *Proc. Ultrasonics International.* IPC Science and Technology Press, Guildford, pp. 20–22.

Hill, C.R., Chivers, R.C., Huggins, R.W. and Nicholas, D. (1978). Scattering of ultrasound by human tissues. In *Ultrasound: Its Application in Medicine and Biology*, F.J. Fry (ed.). Elsevier, Amsterdam, Ch. 9.

Holasek, E., Jennings, W.D., Sokollu, A. and Purnell, E.W. (1973). Recognition of tissue patterns by ultrasonic spectroscopy. In *Proc. IEEE Ultrasonics Symposium, Monterey.* IEEE, New York, pp. 73–76.

Hueter, T.F. (1952). Messung der Ultraschallabsorption in Menschlichen Schadelknochen und ihre Abhängigkeit von der Frequenz. *Naturwissenschaften* **39**, 21. (Translation to be found in *Ultrasonic Biophysics*, F. Dunn and W.D. O'Brien Jr. (eds). Dowden, Hutchinson and Ross.)

Hueter, T.F. (1958). *Visco-elastic Losses in Tissue in the Ultrasonic Range.* Wright Air Development Centre, Wright-Patterson AFB, Ohio. Tech. Rept. No. 57-706, ASTIA, Doc. No. AD142171.

Hughes, D.I. and Duck, F.A. (1997). Automatic attenuation compensation for ultrasonic imaging. *Ultrasound Med. Biol.* **23**, 651–664.

Insana, M.I., Zagzebski, J. and Madsen, E. (1983). Improvements in the spectral difference method for measuring ultrasonic attenuation. *Ultrasonic Imaging* **5**, 331–345.

Javanaud, C., Rahalkar, R.R. and Richmond, P. (1984). Measurement of speed and attenuation of ultrasound in egg white and egg yolk. *J. Acoust. Soc. Am.* **76**, 670–675.

Johnston, R.L., Goss, S.A., Maynard, V., Brady, J.K., Frizzell, L.A., O'Brien, W.D. and Dunn, F. (1979). Elements of tissue characterization, Part I. Ultrasonic propagation properties. In *Ultrasonic Tissue Characterization 11*, M. Linzer (ed.). National Bureau of Standards, Spec. Publ. 525. US Govt. Printing Office, Washington, D.C., pp. 19–27.

Jones, J.P. and Leeman, S. (1984). Ultrasonic tissue characterization: a review. *Acta Electronica* **26**, 3–31.

Jongen, H.A., Thijssen, J.M., van den Aarssen, M. and Verhoef, W.A. (1986). A general model for the absorption of ultrasound by biological tissues, and experimental verification. *J. Acoust. Soc. Am.* **79**, 535–540.

Kelly Fry, E., Sanghairi, N.T., Fry, F.J. and Gallager, H.S. (1979). Frequency dependent attenuation of malignant breast tumours studied by the fast Fourier transform technique. In *Ultrasonic Tissue Characterization 11*, M. Linzer (ed.). National Bureau of Standards, Spec. Publ. 525. US Govt. Printing Office, Washington, D.C., pp. 85–91.

Kessler, L.W. (1973). VHF ultrasonic attenuation in mammalian tissue. *J. Acoust. Soc. Am.* **53**, 1759–1760.

Kessler, L.W., Hawley, S.A. and Dunn, F. (1971). Semi-automatic determination of ultrasonic velocity and absorption in liquids. *Acustica* **24**, 105–107.

Kishimoto, T. (1958). Ultrasonic absorption in bones. *Acustica* **8**, 179–180.

Klepper, J.R. and Brandenburger, G.H. (1981). Application of phase insensitive detection and frequency-dependent measurements to ultrasonic attenuation tomography. *IEEE Trans. Biomed. Eng.* **BME-28**, 186–201.

Knipp, B.S., Zagzebski, J.A., Wilson, T.A., Dong, F. and Madsen, E.L. (1997). Attenuation and backscatter estimation using video signal analysis applied to B-mode images. *Ultrason. Imaging* **19**, 221–233.

Kobayashi, T. (1979). Diagnostic ultrasound in breast cancer, analysis of retrotumorous echopatterns correlated with sonic attenuation by cancerous connective tissue. *J. Clin. Ultrasound* **7**, 471–479.

Kol'tsova, I.S., Mikhailov, I.G. and Trofimov, G.S. (1980). Structural acoustic relaxation in suspensions of interacting particles. *Sov. Phys. Acoust.* **26**, 319–322.

Kossoff, G., Kelly Fry, E. and Jellins, J. (1973). Average velocity of ultrasound in the human female breast. *J. Acoust. Soc. Am.* **53**, 1730–1736.

Kremkau, F.W., Barnes, R.W. and McGraw, C.P. (1981). Ultrasonic attenuation and propagation speed in normal human brain. *J. Acoust. Soc. Am.* **70**, 29–38.

Kremkau, F.W. and Carstensen, E.L. (1972). Macromolecular interaction in sound absorption. In *Interaction of Ultrasound and Biological Tissues*, Workshop Proc., J.M. Reid and M.R. Sikov (eds), DHEW publication (FDA) 73-8008 BRH/DBE 73-1. US Govt. Printing Office, Washington, D.C., pp. 37–42.

Kremkau, F.W., Carstensen, E.L. and Aldridge, A.G. (1973). Macromolecular interaction in the absorption of ultrasound in fixed erythrocytes. *J. Acoust. Soc. Am.* **53**, 1448–1451.

Kremkau, F.W. and Cowgill, R.W. (1984; 1985). Biomolecular absorption of ultrasound. I. Molecular weight; II. Molecular structure. *J. Acoust. Soc. Am.* **76**, 1330–1335; **77**, 1217–1221.

Krishna, P.D. and Newhouse, V.L. (1997). Second harmonic characteristics of the ultrasound contrast agents albunex and FS069. *Ultrasound Med. Biol.* **23**, 453–459.

Kuc, R. and Regula, D. (1984). Diffraction effects in reflected ultrasound spectral estimates. *IEEE Trans. Biomed. Eng.* **BME-31**, 527–545.

Kuc, R. and Schwartz, M. (1979). Estimating the acoustic attenuation coefficient slope for liver from reflected ultrasound signals. *IEEE Trans. Son. Ultrason.* **SU-26**, 353–362.

Lakestani, F., Baboux, J.C. and Fleischmann, P. (1975). Broadening the bandwidth of piezoelectric transducers by means of transmission lines. *Ultrasonics* **July**, 176–180.

Lamb, J. (1965). Thermal relaxation in liquids. In *Physical Acoustics*, Vol. 2A, W.P. Mason (ed.). Academic Press, New York, pp. 203–280.

Lang, J., Zana, R., Gairard, B., Dale, G. and Gros, Ch.M. (1978). Ultrasound absorption in the human breast cyst liquids. *Ultrasound Med. Biol.* **4**, 125–130.

Law, W.K., Frizzell, L.A. and Dunn, F. (1981). Ultrasonic determination of the nonlinearity parameter B/A for biological media. *J. Acoust. Soc. Am.* **39**, 1210–1212.

Law, W.K., Frizzell, L.A. and Dunn, F. (1985). Determination of the nonlinearity parameter B/A of biological media. *Ultrasound Med. Biol.* **11**, 307–318.

Leeman, S., Ferrari, L., Jones, J.P. and Fink, M. (1984). Perspectives on attenuation estimation from pulse-echo signals. *IEEE Trans. Son. Ultrason.* **SU-31**, 354–361.

Lele, P.P., Mansfield, A.B., Murphy, A.I., Namery, J. and Senapati, N. (1976). Tissue characterization by ultrasonic frequency-dependent attenuation and scattering. In *Proc. Seminar on Ultrasonic Tissue Characterization*, M. Linzer (ed.), National Bureau of Standards, Spec. Publ. 453. US Govt. Printing Office, Washington, D.C., pp. 167–196.

Lele, P.P. and Senapati, N. (1977). The frequency spectra of energy backscattered and attenuated by normal and abnormal tissue. In *Recent Advances in Ultrasound in Biomedicine*, Vol. I, D.N. White (ed.). Research Studies Ross, Oregon, pp. 55–85.

Levi, S. and Keuwez, J. (1979). Tissue characterization *in vivo* by differential attenuation measurements. In *Ultrasonic Tissue Characterization 11*, M. Linzer (ed.), National Bureau of Standards, Spec. Publ. 525. US Govt. Printing Office, Washington, D.C., pp. 121–124.

Litovitz, T.A. and Carnevale, E.H. (1958). Effect of pressure on ultrasound relaxation in liquids, II. *J. Acoust. Soc. Am.* **30**, 134–136.

Litovitz, T.A. and Davis, C.M. (1965). Structural and shear relaxation in liquids. *Physical Acoustics*, Vol. 2A, W.P. Mason (ed.). Academic Press, New York, pp. 281–349.

Lizzi, F.L., Kate, L., St. Louis, L. and Coleman, D.J. (1976). Applications of spectral analysis in medical ultrasonography. *Ultrasonics* **March**, 77–80.

Lomonaco, A., Kline, P., Halpern, S. and Leopold, G. (1975). Nuclear medicine and ultrasound: correlation in diagnosis of disease of liver and biliary tract. *Sem. Nucl. Med.* **5**, 307–324.

McNeely, W.D. and Noordergraaf, A. (1981). *In vivo* attenuation measurement in pre- and postmortem muscle using ultrasound. *IEEE Trans. Son. Ultrason.* **SU-28**, 237–241.

McQueen, D. (1977). Applications of a simple theory of acoustic motion of fibrous networks in viscous media. *Ultrasonics* **15**, 175–178.

McSkimin, H.J. (1964). Ultrasonic methods of measuring the mechanical properties of liquids and solids. In *Physical Acoustics: Principles and Methods*, W.P. Mason (ed.), Vol. I, Part A, Ch. 10. Academic Press, New York, pp. 271–334.

Madigosky, W.M., Rosenbaum, I. and Lucas, R. (1981). Sound velocities and B/A in fluorocarbon fluids and in several low density solids. *J. Acoust. Soc. Am.* **69**, 1639–1643.

Maklad, N.F., Ophir, J. and Balsara, V. (1984). Attenuation of ultrasound in normal liver and diffuse liver disease *in vivo. Ultrasonic Imaging* **6**, 117–125.

Malcolm, A.L. (1997). An investigation into ultrasonic methods of imaging the tissue ablation induced during focused ultrasound surgery. Ph.D. thesis, University of London.

Marcus, P.W. and Carstensen, E.L. (1975). Problems with absorption measurements of inhomogeneous solids. *J. Acoust. Soc. Am.* **58**, 1334–1335.

Markham, J.J., Beyer, R.T. and Lindsay, R.D. (1951). Absorption of sound in fluids. *Rev. Mod. Phys.* **23**, 353–411.

Marsh, J.N., Hughes, M.S., Brandenburger, G.H. and Miller, J.G. (1999). Broadband measurement of the scattering-to-attenuation ratio for albunex® at 37°C. *Ultrasound Med. Biol.* **25**, 1321–1324.

Mason, W.P. (1958). *Physical Acoustics and the Properties of Solids.* Van Nostrand, New York.

Matheson, A.J. (1971). *Molecular Acoustics.* John Wiley, London.

Maynard, V.M., Magin, R.L. and Dunn, F. (1985). Ultrasonic absorption and permeability for liposomes near phase transition. *Chem. Phys. Lipids* **37**, 1–12.

Mercer, J. (1997). Ultrasound scatterer size imaging of skin tumours – potential and limitations. Ph.D. thesis, University of London.

Mercier, N. (1975). Ultrasonic classification of metals by grain size. In *Ultrasonics International Conf. Proc.* IPC Science and Technology Press, Guildford, pp. 64–67.

Miles, C.A. (1996). Ultrasonic properties of tendon: velocity, attenuation and backscattering in equine digital flexor tendons. *J. Acoust. Soc. Am.* **99**, 3225–3232.

Miles, C.A. and Cutting, C.L. (1974). Technical note: changes in the velocity of ultrasound in meat during freezing. *J. Fd. Technol.* **9**, 119–122.

Miles, C.A. and Fursey, G.A. (1974). A note on the velocity of ultrasound in living tissue. *Amin. Prod.* **18**, 93–96.

Miller, J.G., Yuhas, D.E., Mimbs, J.W., Dierker, S.B., Busse, L.J., Laterra, J.J., Weiss, A.N. and Sobel, B.E. (1976). Ultrasonic tissue characterization: correlation between biochemical and ultrasonic indices of myocardial injury. *Ultrasonics Symp. Proc. IEEE*, Cat. No. 76-CH1120-5SU, 33–43.

Miller, N.R., Bamber, J.C. and Meaney, P.M. (2002). Fundamental limitations of noninvasive temperature imaging by means of ultrasound echo strain estimation. *Ultrasound Med. Biol.* **28**, 1319–1333.

Miller, N.R., Bamber, J.C. and ter Haar, G.R. (2003). Noninvasive temperature imaging by means of ultrasound echo strain estimation: preliminary *in vitro* results. *Ultrasound Med. Biol.* (in press).

Mitaku, S. (1981). Ultrasonic studies of lipid bilayer phase transition. *Mol. Cryst. Liq. Cryst.* **70**, 21–28.

Moore, W.J. (1962). *Physical Chemistry* (4th edn). Longmans, Green and Co., London, Ch. 8.

Moran, C.M., Bush, N.L. and Bamber, J.C. (1995). Ultrasonic propagation properties of excised human skin. *Ultrasound Med. Biol.* **21**, 1177–1190.

Morfey, C.L. (1968). Sound attenuation by small particles in a fluid. *J. Sound Vib.* **8**, 156–170.

Morse, P.M. and Ingard, K.U. (1968). *Theoretical Acoustics.* McGraw-Hill, New York.

Mottley, J.G. and Miller, J.G. (1990). Anisotropy of the ultrasonic attenuation in soft tissues: measurements *in vitro. J. Acoust. Soc. Am.* **88**, 1203–1210.

Mountford, R.A. and Halliwell, M. (1973). Physical sources of registration errors in pulse–echo ultrasound systems. Part II – beam deformation, deviation and divergence. *Med. Biol. Eng.* **January**, 33–38.

Mountford, R.A. and Wells, P.N.T. (1972a). Ultrasonic liver scanning: the quantitative analysis of the normal A-scan. *Phys. Med. Biol.* **17**, 14–25.

Mountford, R.A. and Wells, P.N.T. (1972b). Ultrasonic liver scanning: the A-scans in the normal and cirrhosis. *Phys. Med. Biol.* **17**, 261–269.

Muir, T.G. and Carstensen, E.L. (1980). Prediction of nonlinear acoustic effects at biomedical frequencies and intensities. *Ultrasound Med. Biol.* **6**, 345–357.

Narayana, P.A. and Ophir, J. (1983a). Spectral shifts of ultrasonic propagation: a study of theoretical and experimental models. *Ultrasonic Imaging* **5**, 22–29.

Narayana, P.A. and Ophir, J. (1983b). On the frequency dependence of attenuation in normal and fatty liver. *IEEE Trans. Son. Ultrason.* **SU-30**, 379–383.

Nassiri, D.K. and Hill, C.R. (1986a). The differential and total bulk acoustic scattering cross sections of some human and animal tissues. *J. Acoust. Soc. Am.* **76**, 2034–2047.

Nassiri, D.K. and Hill, C.R. (1986b). The use of acoustic scattering measurements to estimate structural parameters of human and animal tissues. *J. Acoust. Soc. Am.* **76**, 2048–2054.

Nassiri, D.K., Nicholas, D.N. and Hill, C.R. (1979). Attenuation of ultrasound in skeletal muscle. *Ultrasonics* **17**, 230–232.

O'Brien Jr., W.D. (1977). The relationship between collagen and ultrasonic attenuation and velocity in tissue. *Ultrasonics International Conference Proc.* IPC Business Press, Guildford, pp. 194–205.

O'Donnell, M. (1983). Effects of diffraction on measurements of the frequency dependence of ultrasonic attenuation. *IEEE Trans. Biomed. Eng.* **BME-30**, 320–326.

O'Donnell, M., Jaynes, E.T. and Miller, J.G. (1978). General relationships between ultrasonic attenuation and dispersion. *J. Acoust. Soc. Am.* **63**, 1935–1937.

O'Donnell, M., Jaynes, E.T. and Miller, J.G. (1981). Kramers–Kronig relationships between ultrasonic attenuation and phase velocity. *J. Acoust. Soc. Am.* **69**, 696–701.

O'Donnell, M. and Miller, J.G. (1979). Mechanisms of ultrasonic attenuation on soft tissue. In *Ultrasonic Tissue Characterization 11*, M. Linzer (ed.), NBS Spec. Publ. 525. US Govt. Printing Office, Washington, D.C., pp. 37–40.

O'Donnell, M., Mimbs, J.W., Sobel, B.E. and Miller, J.G. (1977). Ultrasonic attenuation of myocardial tissue: dependence of time after excision and on temperature. *J. Acoust. Soc. Am.* **62**, 1054–1057.

Ophir, J. and Jaeger, P. (1982). Spectral shifts of ultrasonic propagation through media with nonlinearly dispersive attenuation. *Ultrasonic Imaging* **4**, 282–289.

Ophir, J. and Mehta, D. (1988). Elimination of diffraction error in acoustic attenuation estimation via axial beam translation. *Ultrason. Imaging* **10**, 129–152.

Papadakis, E.P. (1966). Ultrasonic diffraction loss and phase change in anisotropic materials. *J. Acoust. Soc. Am.* **40**, 863–876.

Papadakis, E.P. (1970). Effects of input amplitude profile upon diffraction loss and phase change in a pulse–echo system. *J. Acoust. Soc. Am.* **49**, 166–168.

Papadakis, E.P. (1973). Ultrasonic diffraction loss and phase change for broad-band pulses. *J. Acoust. Soc. Am.* **3**, 847–849.

Papadakis, E.P., Fowler, K.A. and Lynnworth, L. (1973). Ultrasonic attenuation by spectrum analysis of pulses in buffer rods: methods and diffraction corrections. *J. Acoust. Soc. Am.* **53**, 1336–1343.

Parker, K.J. (1983). Ultrasonic attenuation and absorption in liver tissue. *Ultrasound Med. Biol.* **9**, 363–369.

Parker, K.J. (1985). Effects of heat conduction and sample size on ultrasonic absorption measurements. *J. Acoust. Soc. Am.* **77**, 719–725.

Parker, K.J. (1986). Attenuation measurement uncertainties caused by speckle statistics. *J. Acoust. Soc. Am.* **80**, 827–834.

Parker, K.J. and Waag, R.C. (1983). Measurement of ultrasonic attenuation within regions selected from B-scan images. *IEEE Trans. Biomed. Eng.* **BME-30**, 431–437.

Pauly, H. and Schwan, H.P. (1971). Mechanism of absorption of ultrasound in liver tissue. *J. Acoust. Soc. Am.* **50**, 692–699.

Pellam, J.R. and Galt, J.K. (1946). Ultrasonic propagation in liquids: I. Application of pulse technique to velocity and absorption measurements at 15 megacycles. *J. Chem. Phys.* **14**, 608–614.

Penttinen, A. and Luukkala, M. (1977). Diffraction losses associated with curved ultrasonic transducers. *J. Phys. D: Appl. Phys.* **10**, 665–669.

Phillippoff, W. (1963). Viscoelasticity of polymer solutions at high pressures and ultrasonic frequencies. *J. Appl. Phys.* **34**, 1507–1511.

Pinkerton, J.M.M. (1947). A pulse method for the measurement of ultrasonic absorption in liquids: results for water. *Nature* **160**, 128–129.

Pohlhammer, J. and O'Brien Jr., W.D. (1981). Dependence of the ultrasonic scatter coefficient on collagen concentration in mammalian tissue. *J. Acoust. Soc. Am.* **69**, 283–285.

Pohlhammer, J.D., Edwards, C.A. and O'Brien Jr., W.D. (1981). Phase insensitive ultrasonic attenuation coefficient determination of fresh bovine liver over an extended frequency range. *Med. Phys.* **8**, 692–694.

Pohlman, R. (1939). Über die Absorption des Ultraschalls im menschlichen Gewebe und ihre Abhängigkeit von der Frequenz. *Physik Z.* **40**, 159–161.

Quan, K.M. and Watmough, D.J. (1990). Determination of ultrasonic absorption coefficient by means of acoustic streaming: the need to consider the effect of diffraction on streaming velocity. *Meas. Sci. Technol.* **1**, 1084–1086.

Ragavendra, N., Chen, H., Powers, J.E., Nilawat, C., Robert, J.M., Carangi, C. and Laifer-Narin, S.L. (1997). Harmonic imaging of porcine intraovarian arteries using sonographic contrast medium: initial findings. *Ultrasound Obstet. Gynecol.* **9**, 266–270.

Raichel, D.R. (1971). Sound propagation in Voigt fluid. *J. Acoust. Soc. Am.* **52**, 395–398.

Redwood, M. (1963). A study of waveforms in the generation and detection of short ultrasonic pulses. *Appl. Mat. Res.* **April**, 76–84.

Robinson, T.C. and Lele, P.P. (1972). An analysis of lesion development in the brain and in plastics by high-intensity focused ultrasound at low megahertz frequencies. *J. Acoust. Soc. Am.* **51**, 1333–1351.

Roux, C., Fournier, B., Laugier, P., Chappard, C., Kolta, S., Dougados, M. and Berger, G. (1996). Broadband ultrasound attenuation imaging: a new imaging method in osteoporosis. *J. Bone & Mineral Research* **11**, 1112–1118.

Sadykhova, S.Kh. and El'piner, I.E. (1970). Absorption of ultrasonic waves in aqueous solutions of biopolymers. *Soviet Physics-Acoustics* **16**, 101–107.

Sboros, V., Ramnarine, K.V., Moran, C.M., Pye, S.D. and McDicken, W.N. (2002). Understanding the limitations of ultrasonic backscatter measurements from microbubble populations. *Phys Med Biol.* **47**, 4287–4299.

Schlief, R., Schurmann, R., Balzer, T., *et al.* (1994). Saccharide-based contrast agents and their application in vascular Doppler ultrasound. *Advan. EchoContrast* **3**, 60–76.

Schwan, H.P. and Carstensen, E.L. (1952). Ultrasonics aids diathermy experiments. *Electronics* **July**, 216.

Sehgal, C.M. and Greenleaf, J.F. (1982). Ultrasonic absorption and dispersion in biological media: a postulated model. *J. Acoust. Soc. Am.* **72**, 1711–1718.

Seki, H., Granato, A. and Truell, R. (1956). Diffraction effects in the ultrasonic field of a piston source and their importance in the accurate measurement of attenuation. *J. Acoust. Soc. Am.* **28**(2), 230–238.

Shaffer, S., Pettibone, D.W., Havlice, J.F. and Nassi, M. (1984). Estimation of the slope of the acoustic attenuation coefficient. *Ultrasonic Imaging* **6**, 126–138.

Shankar, P.M., Dala-Krishna, P. and Newhouse, V.L. (1998). Advantages of subharmonic over second harmonic backscatter for contrast-to-tissue echo enhancement. *Ultrasound Med. Biol.* **24**, 395–399.

Shung, K.K. and Reid, J.M. (1978). Ultrasonic scattering from tissues. In *IEEE Ultrasonics Symposium Proc.*, Cat. No. 77 CH 1264159, 230–233.

Shung, K.K., Sigelmann, R.A. and Reid, J.M. (1976). Scattering of ultrasound by blood. *IEEE Trans. Biomed. Eng.* **23**, 460–467.

Strom-Jensen, P.R. and Dunn, F. (1984). Ultrasonic absorption by solvent–solute interactions and proton transfer in aqueous solutions of peptides and small proteins. *J. Acoust. Soc. Am.* **75**, 960–966.

Szabo, T.L. (1995). Causal theories and data for acoustic attenuation obeying a frequency power law. *J. Acoust. Soc. Amer.* **97**, 14–24.

Tervola, K.M.U., Foster, S.G. and O'Brien Jr., W.D. (1985a). Attenuation coefficient measurement technique at 100 MHz with the scanning laser acoustic microscope. *IEEE Trans. Son. Ultrason.* **SU-32**, 259–265.

Tervola, K.M.U., Grurnmer, M.A., Erdman Jr., J.W. and O'Brien Jr., W.D. (1985b). Ultrasonic attenuation and velocity properties in rat liver as a function of fat concentration. A study at 100 MHz using a scanning laser acoustic microscope. *J. Acoust. Soc. Am.* **77**, 307–313.

Truell, R. and Oates, W. (1963). Effect of lack of parallelism of sample faces on the measurement of ultrasonic attenuation. *J. Acoust. Soc. Am.* **35**, 1382–1386.

Truong, X.T. (1972). Extensional wave propagation characteristics in striated muscle. *J. Acoust. Soc. Am.* **51**, 1352–1356.

Truong, X.T., Jarrett, S.R. and Rippel, D.V. (1978). Longitudinal pulse propagation characteristics in striated muscle. *J. Acoust. Soc. Am.* **64**, 1298–1302.

Tuthill, T.A., Baggs, R.B. and Parker, K.J. (1989). Liver glycogen and water storage: effect on ultrasound attenuation. *Ultrasound Med. Biol.* **15**, 621–627.

Tuthill, T.A., Baggs, R.B., Violante, M.R. and Parker, K.J. (1991). Ultrasound properties of liver with and without particulate contrast agents. *Ultrasound Med. Biol.* **17**, 231–237.

Unger, E., Fritz, T., McCreery, T., Sahn, D., Barrette, T., Yellowhair, D. and New, T. (1997). Liposomes as myocardial perfusion ultrasound contrast agents. In *Ultrasound Contrast Agents*, B.B. Goldberg (ed.), Ch. 6. Martin Dunitz, London, pp. 57–74.

Wells, P.N.T. (1975). Absorption and dispersion of ultrasound in biological tissue. *Ultrasound Med. Biol.* **1**, 369–376.

Wells, P.N.T. (1977). *Biomedical Ultrasonics*. Academic Press, London.

Wilson, L.S., Robinson, B.E. and Doust, D.B. (1984). Frequency domain processing for ultrasonic attenuation measurement in liver. *Ultrasonic Imaging* **6**, 278–292.

Woodcock, J.P. (1979). *Ultrasonics*. Adam Hilger, Bristol.

Wu, J. and Tong, J. (1998). Measurements of the nonlinearity parameter B/A of contrast agents. *Ultrasound Med. Biol.* **24**, 153–159.

Xu, W. and Kaufman, J.J. (1993). Diffraction correction methods for insertion ultrasound attenuation estimation. *IEEE Trans. Biomed. Eng.* **40**, 563–570.

Yosioka, K., Ohmura, A., Hasegawa, T. and Oka, M. (1968). Absorption coefficient of ultrasound in soft tissues and their biological conditions. *Proc. 6th International Congress on Acoustics, Tokyo, Japan.* Paper M1–3, pp. M-S–M-8.

Yuhas, D.E. and Kessler, L.W. (1979). Acoustic microscope analysis of myocardium. In *Ultrasonic Tissue Characterization 11*, M. Linzer (ed.), NBS Spec. Publ. 525. US Govt. Printing Office, Washington, D.C., pp. 73–79.

Zagzebski, J.A., *et al.* (1993). Quantitative backscatter imaging. In *Ultrasonic Scattering in Biological Tissues*, K.K. Shung and G.A. Thieme (eds). CRC Press, Boca Raton, pp. 451–486.

Zeqiri, B. (1996). Validation of a diffraction correction model for through-transmission substitution measurements of ultrasonic absorption and phase velocity. *J. Acoust. Soc. Am.* **99**, 996–1001.

Zhou, K., Zhang, D., Lin, C. and Zhu, S. (1992). Ultrasonic attenuation estimation *in vivo* using the difference ratio correction method. *J. Acoust. Soc. Am.* **92**, 2532–2538.

5

Speed of Sound

J. C. BAMBER

Institute of Cancer Research, Royal Marsden Hospital, UK

5.1 INTRODUCTION

Various aspects of the subject of ultrasonic speed in tissues have been covered in earlier chapters. Specifically, Chapter 4 provided a combined treatment of the biophysical mechanisms of ultrasonic absorption and dispersion, and presented some information on the variation in measured speed of sound in tissues with factors associated with measurement conditions. This chapter confines its attention primarily to two topics: sound speed measurement and published data.

It is worth remembering that there is, strictly speaking, no simple definition of sound speed. Previous chapters have described both group and phase speeds, and it is known that, for waves of finite amplitude, the sound speed is amplitude dependent. Nevertheless, the simplistic viewpoint that has commonly been adopted throughout the field of medical ultrasonics is that there is a single value of sound speed that can be measured for any given medium. The initial sections of this chapter also adopt this viewpoint; the implications of finite amplitude behaviour are taken up in Section 5.4.

5.2 MEASUREMENT OF THE SPEED OF ULTRASOUND IN TISSUES

The speed of sound is a quantity that is easy to measure at moderate levels of precision (say 1%) but difficult if good absolute accuracy and/or higher precision are required. In the case of biological tissues, for example, the precision of the methods used by many workers is rarely good enough to observe velocity dispersion over the frequency range of medical interest. Incidentally, the term *speed of sound* is used here where other authors refer to *sound velocity*. This implies no difference of quantity and use of the former term is maintained simply for consistency. Since, however, the quantity under discussion is a scalar property of the propagation medium, it may well be preferable to reserve the term velocity for use as a vector quantity to describe the speed and direction of travel of the sound energy or the particles of the medium.

Physical Principles of Medical Ultrasonics, Second Edition. Edited by C. R. Hill, J. C. Bamber and G. R. ter Haar.
© 2004 John Wiley & Sons, Ltd: ISBN 0 471 97002 6

5.2.1 MEASUREMENT TECHNIQUES

As was mentioned in Chapter 4, in many cases of sound speed measurement the apparatus used is identical to that used for an associated attenuation measurement. Excellent summaries of the various basic methods of measuring the speed of sound are provided in reviews mentioned previously for attenuation measurement methods (Beyer & Letcher 1969; Dunn *et al.* 1969; Goss *et al.* 1979; McSkimin 1964; Matheson 1971). Many of the comments made in Section 4.4.1.2, with regard to factors such as the range of ultrasonic frequency over which the techniques may be used, or their applicability to measurements on tissues, also apply here. It is intended that the following description should be read in conjunction with Section 4.4.1.2.

5.2.1.1 Absolute Methods

Absolute measurement methods permit direct measurement of sound speed in the medium of interest, without reference to the speed of sound in some previously characterised medium. Pulsed and continuous wave methods exist, as well as the use of the fixed-path and variable-path techniques, as described in Chapter 4.

The most common methods are variants of a general pulse transit-time, or time-of-flight (TOF), measurement, initially developed as a variable-path technique for liquids (Pellam & Galt 1946). The speed of sound is obtained from the difference in round-trip transit times as the path length between the transmitting and receiving transducers, or between the transmitting transducer and a plane reflector, is varied by a measured amount. Alternatively, for a known fixed path length, either a single transit time or the transit times of multiple reflections between the two planes may be observed. The main differences between systems occur in the degree of sophistication applied to determining the TOF and to applying diffraction and other corrections. However, an accuracy of the order of ±0.5% can be obtained by merely measuring the TOF using the time delay of an oscilloscope (Ludwig 1950). Using more sophisticated systems sound speed has been determined typically to within ±0.2%. In the pulse superposition method the pulse repetition rate is adjusted so that successive multiple echoes are superposed (Beyer & Letcher 1969). The round-trip transit time is obtained from the time between pulses. The pulse echo-overlap method (Papadakis 1964) utilises an oscilloscope whose time base is triggered externally. No acoustic superposition takes place but, by varying the trigger rate, successive echoes can be made to overlap. Again, the time between trigger pulses provides the measure of TOF. In an automated version, known as the sing-around system (Greenspan & Tschiegg 1957), separate transmitting and receiving transducers are used, and the received pulse is shaped to be fed back as a trigger for the transmitting transducer. The repetition period is thus self-adjusting to provide the acoustic transit time directly. Van Venrooij (1971) used this technique to make measurements of sound speed *in vitro* on various biological fluids and on brain tumours. For homogeneous media a 0.1% uncertainty was claimed.

A highly accurate and convenient instrument for sound speed determination in the 1 to 100 MHz range is the continuous wave ultrasonic interferometer (see Section 4.4.1.2). Accuracies better than ±0.1% are relatively easily attained. Some of the most accurate measurements of sound speed in pure water have been made using a variable path interferometer (Del Grosso & Mader 1972). Such a method has even been applied to solid soft tissues, keeping the compressional distortion of the tissue to within 25% during the measurement (Goldman & Richards 1954).

5.2.1.2 Relative Methods

The absolute measurement techniques discussed above are generally (though not always) unsuitable for studying solid tissues, where it is difficult either to measure the path length accurately or to vary it. Relative methods are made possible because reliable published data of absolute speed of sound values are available for a number of substances, which may be used as reference media in the measurement scheme. The most common of these reference media is pure water, but saline of known sodium chloride concentration is also used. The accuracy of a relative measurement method will ultimately be limited to the accuracy of the measurement made on the reference medium. For water this is about ±0.03%, but this is not a problem for materials of interest in medical ultrasonics and, as discussed in Section 5.2.2, both accuracy and precision are usually limited much more severely by other considerations (see later).

A simple means of obtaining a speed of sound measurement relative to some reference medium, and one very often used for measurements on tissues, is a variation on the pulse TOF technique discussed above. Various geometrical configurations involving either one or two transducers are possible (e.g. Kossoff *et al.* 1973; Nasoni *et al.* 1979; Zimmerman & Smith 1983). An example is one that uses the specimen and transducer arrangement of the insertion attenuation measurement scheme shown in Figure 4.5. All that is required is an oscilloscope with a fast delayed timebase capable of measuring the time shift, Δt, in the position of received sound pulse with and without the tissue specimen in place. A timebase sweep of 0.1μs cm^{-1} would be sufficiently fast for most purposes. Then, with a knowledge of the speed of sound in the tank water (or other reference medium), c_w, the average speed of sound over the total tissue path traversed by the sound beam, Δx, may be calculated from:

$$\frac{1}{c_t} = \frac{1}{c_w} - \frac{\Delta t}{\Delta x} \tag{5.1}$$

This kind of approach, although often using a focused transducer and sometimes with the specimen placed against a plane reflector, has been used by various authors to obtain macroscopic images of the distribution of speed of sound (plus attenuation and backscattering coefficients) in slices of excised soft tissue and bone (Foster *et al.* 1984; Bush *et al.* 1993; Laugier *et al.* 1997). *In vitro* speed of sound images of tissue slices have also been produced using time-delay spectrometry (Heyser & Le Croisette 1974; see Section 4.4.1.2).

In Section 4.4.1.2 reference was made to the Schwan and Carstensen narrowband method of measuring attenuation in fluids, which minimises diffraction effects by maintaining a fixed path between transmitter and receiver; as the path length in the test liquid is varied it is compensated for by an equivalent path of reference liquid. The same technique provides a highly accurate method of measuring phase speed (as good as the accuracy with which the speed of the reference liquid is known) and phase dispersion in liquids; the received signal is mixed with an electronic reference copy of the transmitted signal in order to detect their difference in phase as the relative path length is varied (Carstensen 1954).

A further example of a relative method for sound speed measurement, that allows phase speed to be determined from a pulse TOF measurement and is applicable for appreciably inhomogeneous media, is described below, at the end of Section 5.2.2.2. Droin *et al.* (1997) employed such an approach to characterise dispersion of sound speed in trabecular bone and, by scanning, produce images of the amount of dispersion.

5.2.1.3 Microscopic Measurements

Various reasons exist for wishing to make measurements of the speed of sound at the microscopic level. For instance the specimens of interest may be available only in small quantities, or one may wish to obtain measurements of the microscopic spatial distribution of speed (and density) so as to aid understanding of the macroscopic ultrasound scattering behaviour of the specimen (see Chapter 6).

The scanning laser acoustic microscope ('SLAM' – see Chapter 11) has been used to measure the spatial distribution of the speed of sound in tissue specimens of thicknesses 300–900 μm over a 3 mm by 2 mm field of view at an ultrasonic frequency of 100 MHz (Embree *et al*. 1985). For homogeneous media the method has a precision of the order of ±0.3% and tends to over-estimate the absolute value, but not by more than 2%. The SLAM produces acoustic transmission (attenuation-related) images of a specimen by using a scanning laser system to monitor the microscopic spatial distribution of the normal displacement amplitude of the lower surface of a mirror-like glass coverslip placed over the specimen. Displacements of the coverslip are produced by a sound wave that has passed obliquely through the specimen from below.

In another mode of use, an interference image is produced by electronically mixing the laser detector output with a 100 MHz reference signal. The image then consists of light and dark fringes which, for a uniform medium, are straight and equally spaced. Slices of tissue are placed in a background of saline of known concentration and, from the direction and magnitude of the shift in the position of any of the fringes, relative to its position in the saline, the speed of sound at a given point in the tissue may be computed relative to the speed of sound in the saline.

Grant and Bernardin (1981) have adapted the interferometric mode of using the SLAM, for measurements of sound speed in very small volumes of liquids (e.g. 0.05 ml), by attaching a spacer to one end of the coverslip to produce a wedge-shaped interferometer cell. The method was used to measure speed of sound as a function of protein concentration in solutions of bovine serum albumin, to a precision of better than ±0.2%, although no figures for accuracy were given.

The more standard scanning acoustic microscope ('SAM' – see Chapter 11), which uses a mechanically scanned focused ultrasound receiver, has also been used in an interference mode for speed of sound measurements (Chubachi 1981). The preparation of specimens of accurately known and uniform thickness may, however, be a considerable problem. In the SLAM technique this is dealt with by using the weight of the coverslip to make the tissue conform to a thickness defined by a spacing washer surrounding the specimen. To avoid such problems with the SAM, Sinclair *et al*. (1982) devised a technique which allows the instrument to be used to measure, at a given point on the specimen, the critical angle (i.e. the angle of incidence at which total internal reflection occurs) for transmission from a low speed of sound reference medium to the tissue. Snell's law then gives the sound speed in the tissue, which is said to be relatively independent of specimen thickness. Further details of both the SLAM and SAM methods of acoustic microscopy are presented in Chapter 11.

5.2.1.4 *In Vivo* Measurement

Until comparatively recently the primary medical ultrasonic interest in the speed of sound in tissues was to provide a figure for time-range calibration of echographic imaging devices. It is now recognised that sound speed is possibly a very useful tissue-specific characteristic in its own right, and many methods have been devised to measure speed, or even to image its spatial distribution, in the body.

Some through-transmission measurements, providing speed estimates that are averages over all tissues in the path of the sound beam, have been made on various parts of the body where this is possible. Kossoff *et al.* (1973) have used the relative TOF method described above to make measurements of average speed of sound in the female breast. Extensions of this approach, by scanning the sound beam to obtain multiple TOF projections, make it possible to reconstruct tomographic images of the speed of sound in coronal planes through the breast (Greenleaf & Bahn 1981; Carson *et al.* 1981; Glover & Sharp 1977; Koch *et al.* 1983). Images so produced appear to provide information complementary to the echographic imaging process. The sing-around method has also been used *in vivo* to study the dependence of sound speed on contractility in the human biceps muscle (Mol & Breddels 1982). Liver is another organ where knowledge of the speed of sound would provide additional information valuable for diagnosis (see Section 5.3.4) but direct through-transmission measurements have been thought to be impossible (see next paragraph). For some subjects, however, it has been shown that a sub-costal B-scan may be used to visualise and measure the relative TOF to a target placed in a rear inter-costal space (Bamber *et al.* 1987). In this method the operator may use the echo image also to confirm whether the path of sound transmission is occupied mainly by liver tissue.

Despite the methods described above, it remains difficult to make the desired direct through-transmission measurements in human liver and other organs. For such situations a variety of ways of average sound speed determination, utilising ultrasonic echoes from the tissue itself, have been explored. The first to appear was the method of Robinson *et al.* (1982), in which a suitable object, such as a blood vessel, is located within the tissue of interest and imaged in two pulse–echo scans obtained from different directions, through a water path. Owing to the difference in sound speed between the water and the tissue, and the difference in the angle of incidence of the sound at the water–tissue boundary for each image, the two images of the chosen object will not appear in exact registration. By measuring the amount of misregistration and the angles of incidence, Snell's law of refraction may be used to compute an average speed of sound in the tissue over the combined path length for the images concerned. The repeatability of the measurement *in vivo* was about 1%. The system has been used to measure the speed of ultrasound in normal and diffusely diseased livers and spleens (Doust *et al.* 1985; Manoharan *et al.* 1985). An adaptation of this method, for use with a conventional real-time linear scanner, has been proposed by Bamber and Abbott (1985). This scheme effectively produces two misregistered images by placing an acoustic biprism, of known geometry and properties, between the linear array probe face and the tissue.

The crossed beam method (Haumschild & Greenleaf 1983; Iinuma *et al.* 1985; Akamatsu *et al.* 1985; Ohtsuki *et al.* 1985) relies on a statistical estimation of pulse transit time over a path including scattering from a region of the tissue defined by overlapping beams from strongly directive transmitting and receiving transducers. Estimations of accuracy after averaging over 100 pulses in a homogeneous phantom are in the region of ±0.5%. Somewhat improved performance, in terms of both measurement accuracy and localisation, may be achievable by using a tracking crossed beam method (Ophir 1986).

Two schemes exist for determining average sound speed by observation of focusing behaviour whilst obtaining wide aperture (high resolution) pulse–echo images of the tissue. In the method of Hayashi *et al.* (1985) a specially adapted real-time scanner provided the user with a manual control of the digital delay lines used for generating the focused sound beam and receiving directivity. After calibration, the average speed of sound in the tissue was obtained from the delay settings required to produce the sharpest image, as judged by visual observation. Again the error, in homogeneous media, was estimated as ±0.5%. The other focusing scheme is complex but probably the most flexible approach of all, perhaps eventually permitting some crude *in vivo* mapping of sound speed from echo data. A 'minimum entropy' criterion was used to automate the judgement of sharpness of images generated by varying the assumed speed of propagation at the reconstruction stage of a synthetic aperture imaging technique (Mesdag *et al.* 1982). Exploitation of the information in the full set of data received across a transducer array is also the basis of the technique developed by Anderson and Trahey (1998).

5.2.2 PROBLEMS, ARTEFACTS AND ERRORS

5.2.2.1 Errors in Measuring Homogeneous Specimens

(a) *Path length estimations.* As for attenuation measurement, when measuring specimens of biological tissues the final precision and accuracy are strongly influenced by the difficulty in defining the path length. In the experimental arrangement relevant to equation (5.1) it is often difficult to define the path length. The advantage of relative methods of this kind is that even an error in the path length of about ±10% would result in a speed error of less than ±1%, if the surrounding medium were water or saline.

(b) *Knowledge of speed in the reference medium.* For relative measurement methods, most of the inherent precision and accuracy of the method comes from the fact that accurate published values are available for the speed of sound in the reference medium. One must be aware of the temperature and purity of the reference medium but, for water, even using a standard laboratory mercury-in-glass thermometer to measure the temperature, the error from this source is unlikely to be greater than ±0.4% at 20°C.

(c) *Definition of pulse-arrival time.* Pulse TOF measurements have been established for some time as a simple, but accurate, means of obtaining ultrasonic speed measurements. Yet the technique suffers from one basic disadvantage: that, to measure the position in time of the sound pulse, some reference point on its shape must be chosen, or some other criterion used to define the time of its arrival. A single reference point will be of less use if the shape of the pulse changes after propagation through the medium under investigation. Homogeneous or inhomogeneous media may alter the shape of a transmitted sound pulse if either the speed of sound or the attenuation coefficient is dispersive. Fortunately, in biological tissues the dispersion of speed alone is not strong enough to cause noticeable pulse distortion. This in turn means that it is difficult to make measurements of speed dispersion using pulse TOF. Ultrasonic attenuation in tissues is, however, strongly frequency-dependent and, as pointed out by Redwood (1963), the preferential removal of the high frequencies from the pulse will lead to a progressive stretching of the pulse as it travels. In practical terms it will be important, therefore, to calibrate the measurement system in a manner that takes into account the possibility of such changes in pulse shape and height.

Figure 5.1b shows what the 10 MHz pulse of initial shape shown in Figure 5.1a would look like after travelling 5 cm in a medium whose attenuation coefficient is linearly dependent on frequency with a value of $1 \, \mathrm{dB} \, \mathrm{cm}^{-1} \, \mathrm{MHz}^{-1}$. This simple example, which was computed using a zero phase-shift frequency-domain filter, shows that, if the centre of the pulse is chosen as a reference point, then the errors due to pulse stretching will be minimised. However, recognition of the centre of the pulse is difficult if the pulse shape changes, and other reference points are often chosen, particularly if the method is to be automated. Greenleaf *et al.* (1975), for instance, used as their TOF reference point the first time that the signal appears to rise out of noise, while Bowen *et al.* (1979) detected the occurrence of the first zero crossing. In the situation illustrated in Figure 5.1 these criteria would have led to under-estimates in the TOF equivalent to about 0.5λ and 0.6λ respectively. The use of earliest time of arrival by Greenleaf

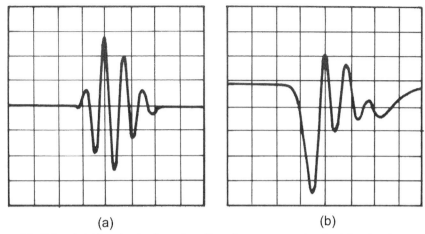

(a)   (b)

Figure 5.1. Pulse stretching due to dispersive attenuation – a computer simulation has been used to demonstrate the effect. The frequency dependence of the attenuation coefficient was modelled using a Fourier domain filter in which $\alpha/f = 1\,\mathrm{dB}\;\mathrm{cm^{-1}\,MHz^{-1}}$. The shape of the reference pulse (centre frequency 10 MHz) is shown in (a), whilst (b) illustrates what the same pulse would look like after travelling 5 cm in the attenuating medium. Both synthesised pulses were displayed on an oscilloscope, with an arbitrary vertical gain setting, using a digital-to-analogue converter

et al. is, however, said to reduce a number of other artefacts that occur in TOF reconstructions. For the experimental arrangement relating to equation (5.1), and for a specimen path length of 4 to 5 cm, the use of earliest time of arrival results in over-estimation of the acoustic speed by about 4%, but this will depend on the precise value of the frequency slope of the attenuation coefficient over the path of interest. This topic will be discussed further in Section 5.2.2.2.

Although often neglected, a further potential cause of pulse shape distortion is non-linear propagation (see Sections 4.3.8 and 5.4). If such distortion is significant, errors may result from the distortion being different when the specimen is present compared to when the propagation path consists of reference medium only. Modelling of this effect in a given measurement set-up is likely to be complex, being dependent on factors such as the nature of the reference medium, the pressure amplitude, frequency spectrum and focusing properties of the source, distance of the specimen from the source, the frequency dependence of attenuation in the specimen and the distance of the receiver from the specimen. It can of course be reduced by decreasing the source pressure amplitude.

(d) *Diffraction corrections.* Diffraction phase corrections, similar in origin to the diffraction corrections applied in attenuation measurements, are made in variable-path speed measuring systems (Papadakis 1966). Calculations of the diffraction phase error may be obtained, for a plane circular transducer, from Seki *et al.* (1956) and are shown in Figure 4.6. Verhoef *et al.* (1985) have performed calculations for focused transducers. In systems using the pulse overlap and the pulse superposition methods the diffraction phase errors can be up to 0.25 of the r.f. period (Papadakis 1972). For insertion techniques the diffraction phase errors are usually neglected.

The effect of diffraction on accuracy of speed of sound measurement by the interferometric method is important for frequencies below about 3 MHz. Subrahmanyam *et al.* (1969) reviewed early work on the subject and, in a study of their own, found the effects to be more than three times as serious as predicted theoretically (the maximum measured excess speed due to diffraction was about 0.5%).

(e) *Transducer effects on TOF and path length estimation.* For single TOF fixed path measurements it is strictly necessary to allow for any quarter-wave impedance matching or insulating layers on the surfaces of the transducers, and for errors in pulse-arrival time arising from internal reflections within the receiving transducer (Kittinger 1977). The application of differential techniques solves this problem and that due to any phase shift which occurs on reflection from the target (Beyer & Letcher 1969).

It is not wise to use large area or strongly focused transducers for speed of sound measurements, since there may be an uncertainty as to which part of the transducer was responsible for first detecting the sound wave, and thus a path length ambiguity may arise.

An indication of the likely quality of current published data, taking into account the impact of the above sources of error, comes from the results of an interlaboratory comparison (Madsen *et al.* 1986) of measurements on tissue-mimicking material, which gave a spread of measured sound speeds of about 0.3%.

5.2.2.2 Inhomogeneity Effects

Phase cancellation effects were mentioned in Chapter 4 as being a potentially serious source of artefact in attenuation measurements. Their effect is likely to be equally serious in TOF measurements, since they may be associated with some of the grossest changes in pulse shape that can be observed. This is also a reason for adopting the earliest time of arrival as the measurement criterion, in preference to an amplitude peak (Ragozzino 1981) or to some zero crossing (Bowen *et al.* 1979; Kremkau *et al.* 1981).

The statistics of electromagnetic and optical pulse arrival times in turbulent, strongly scattering media were studied theoretically by Liu and Yeh (1980), where excess delay times were observed, caused mainly by pulse spreading rather than by pulse wandering. In this case the time centroid of the pulse, defined by the first temporal moment of the signal, underwent relatively small fluctuations as compared to the excess time delay of the pulse caused by the spreading of the pulse. By analogy this suggests that there could be an advantage in defining acoustic pulse arrival time by a similar 'centre of mass' criterion, using a square-law detected version of the r.f. pulse. It is also worth noting that Chenevert *et al.* (1984) obtained considerable improvements in fidelity of reconstruction of speed of sound distributions by adopting an estimator of pulse propagation time which utilises the cross-correlation of received signals with a reference signal of known transit time.

A Fourier domain equivalent of this last approach exists where, in a substitution-type relative measurement, the phase spectrum of the received sound pulse (obtained by digitising the pulse and taking its Fourier transform) is subtracted from the phase spectrum of the pulse propagating through the reference medium. A number of methods exist for utilising such phase difference spectra for computing the phase and group speeds, and there was a suggested method for estimating a correction factor for the phase speed at a given frequency, said to be required when significant dispersion exists (Verhoef *et al.* 1985). The correct phase speed was estimated using a first guess at the dispersion, calculated using the general relationship, and described by equation (4.42), between dispersion and the frequency dependence of attenuation.

5.2.2.3 Tests on Standard Materials

It is advisable to check the precision and accuracy of a measurement system, in the absence of some fundamental standard, by making measurements on materials that have been studied by

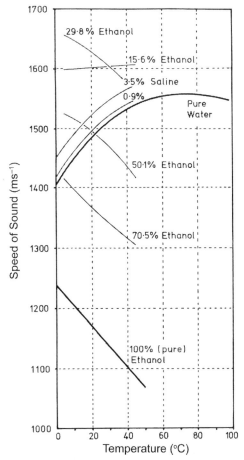

Figure 5.2. Variation of speed of sound with temperature in media which have been used for reference purposes, or to check the accuracy and precision of speed of sound measurement systems. Data obtained from Del Grosso and Mader (1972) for water; Coppens (1981) for saline; Giacomini (1947) for ethanol–water mixtures (% saline refers to g dry salt per 100 cc water; % ethanol refers to concentration by weight of ethyl alcohol in water). For all data the hydrostatic pressure is 1 atm

other people and for which the measured properties are widely agreed upon. The most commonly used substance for the purpose of checking speed of sound measurements is pure water, but saline of known sodium chloride concentration has also been employed. It is important to know the temperature at which the measurement is made; but controlling and varying the temperature can provide a convenient means of testing the system over a range of speeds of sound. Figure 5.2 is a graphical presentation of the data on speed of sound as a function of temperature in pure water, saline and some ethyl alcohol–water mixtures. Del Grosso and Mader (1972) obtained a fifth-order polynomial fit to measured data, which may be used to calculate the speed of sound at normal atmospheric pressure in pure water at a temperature T, over the range 0–100°C, to within 0.015 m s^{-1}. This equation, which was used to plot the curve for water in Figure 5.2, is given by:

$$c_{water} = \sum_{i=0}^{5} k_i T^i \tag{5.2}$$

where the coefficients are:

i	k_i (m s^{-1})
0	$+1402.38754$
1	$+5.03711129$
2	$-5.80852166 \times 10^{-2}$
3	$+3.34198834 \times 10^{-4}$
4	$-1.47800417 \times 10^{-6}$
5	$+3.14643091 \times 10^{-9}$

Most of the data for sound speed in aqueous salt solutions have arisen from an interest in underwater acoustics and sound propagation in the sea. It is common practice to use such data for reference purposes when measuring solutions of NaCl in the laboratory. Millero and Kubinski (1975) provided tabulations of sound speed as a function of salt concentration and temperature at atmospheric pressure, whilst Coppens (1981) presented easy to use empirical equations for computing the sound speed, given the temperature, saline concentration and the depth below the water surface. Assuming atmospheric pressure (zero depth) the equation reduces to (in the form quoted in Kinsler *et al.* 1982):

$$c_{saline} = 1449.05 + 45.7T' - 5.21T'^2 + 0.23T'^3 + (1.333 - 0.126T' + 0.009T'^2)(10S - 35) \tag{5.3}$$

where $T' = T/10$ (T in °C) and S is the salt concentration in g dry salt per 100 ml water.

Mixtures of ethyl alcohol and water form a useful method of generating a wider range of test speeds. As shown in Figure 5.2, pure ethanol has a low sound speed with a negative temperature coefficient. As the amount of water in the mixture increases, the sound speed increases and the temperature coefficient decreases. Eventually the sound speed reaches a maximum (higher than the speed in pure water) and the temperature coefficient reverses. At a concentration of 17% ethanol (by weight) the temperature coefficient is zero, a property which prompted Giacomini (1947) to consider the mixture useful as a standard for propagation speed.

5.2.2.4 Influence of Measurement Conditions

Major difficulties in measuring accurately, and in comparing data on, speeds of sound in biological tissues may occur owing to the wide range of possible conditions of measurement. Factors such as whether the specimen is excised or *in vivo*, time since death, condition or storage and temperature may affect the measured values. The reader is referred to Section 4.4.2.5, where the state of knowledge on the influence of measurement conditions on speed of sound, attenuation and scattering measurements is summarised.

5.3 PUBLISHED DATA FOR SPEED OF SOUND VALUES

5.3.1 GENERAL OBSERVATIONS

A valuable compendium of published values for the speed of sound has been provided by Duck (1990). Typical ranges for these values are shown here in Figure 5.3, where data have been chosen from measurements on a variety of tissues of both man and other mammalian species. For comparison, values for a few non-biological media have also been included in the figure. No particular species variation for the speed of sound in a given tissue type has been noted, although the sparseness of the data, and the lack of control of experimental conditions in such comparisons, may not permit such variation to be apparent, and it has not been the subject of any specific investigation. Much of the range given for any particular tissue could easily have arisen, for example, from variations in measurement temperature, as we shall see in the next section.

Broadly, three classes of tissue are apparent in Figure 5.3: lung, which has a speed of sound commensurate with its high gas content (Dunn 1986); bone, which is a truly hard solid tissue; and all other liquid or soft (liquid-like) tissues of the body. The large differences between the sound speed and density values on either side of soft tissue/bone or soft tissue/lung boundaries give rise to very high levels of scattering from such interfaces. Thus the sound speed in the first two material classes combines with the associated high attenuation coefficients (see Chapter 4) to make it extremely difficult (often impossible) to obtain useful ultrasonic images through lung (or other gas) or bone. Within the last group (of liquid and soft tissues) speed varies over a total range of only about ±10% of the mean value. Designers of echographic systems for imaging a particular part of the body therefore make a normally reasonable assumption of a constant value for the sound speed, in computing the depth coordinate of the displayed signal. Nevertheless, even some time ago it was felt worthwhile attempting some kind of average speed calibration measurement prior to imaging each patient (Jellins & Kossoff 1973). This was primarily because an incorrect value for the assumed speed of sound led to misregistration of compound scans and consequent blurring of the compound image (see Chapter 9). More recent examples of this have arisen in systems that employ a speed of sound map to make refraction corrections to improve image quality in backscatter computed tomography (e.g. Kim *et al.* 1984; Jago & Whittingham 1992). Similarly, in wide-aperture systems that electronically focus the signals received on a number of transducer elements, a blurred image will result if the speed of sound is not known accurately. As mentioned above, in Section 5.2.1.4, the converse use of this phenomenon provides a means of using echo images to determine average sound speed. If the distribution of sound speed is sufficiently inhomogeneous, such as may be the case when a mixture of fat and other tissues is present in the sound path, substantial apparent energy loss due to phase cancellation in the receiver (Chapter 4) and other image artefacts due to wave aberration (Chapter 9) may occur. Such effects are likely to be strongly temperature dependent (see next section).

Other points worthy of note from Figure 5.3 are that most liquids and soft tissues except fat, which has the lowest speed of sound in this class, have a sound speed higher than that for water, and that the highest speed of sound within the class is possessed by muscle tendon.

Muscle itself is an interesting case since it is both anisotropic and contractile. There are different opinions as to whether the speed is higher along or across the fibre direction. Ludwig (1950) found no significant difference between sound speeds measured in these two directions for beef tongue, whereas Goldman and Richards (1954) observed higher speeds for propagation perpendicular to the fibres in dog and rabbit skeletal muscle, and Mol and Breddels (1982) observed the speed to be higher in the direction parallel to the fibres for various types of muscle. Furthermore, contraction caused the speed to increase for human biceps *in vivo* (Mol & Breddels 1982) and either slightly decrease (Bhagat *et al.* 1976) or not change (Mol & Breddels 1982) for frog muscle *in vitro*. The increase *in vivo* was postulated as being due to varying blood content in the muscle.

As a convenient model for studying the consequences, for acoustic propagation, of anisotropy in arrangement of collagen fibres, mammalian tendon has been chosen by some authors. Miles (1996), for example, measured speeds of 1733 and 1650 m s^{-1} along and across

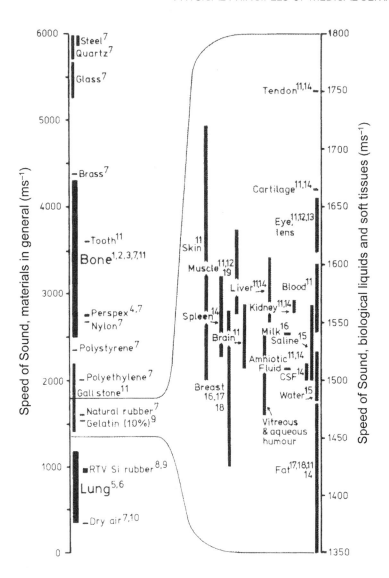

Figure 5.3. Ranges of values for the speed of sound in various biological media. Data for some non-biological media are also provided, some for purposes of comparison and others because they are used in ultrasound research laboratories. The data for soft tissues and biological liquids, which fall within a very narrow range, are presented on the right of the figure, using an expanded scale. Note that tissues were not all from the same species of mammal, the ultrasound frequency may have been in the range I to 10 MHz, and the measurement temperature range was 20–37°C. All data are, however, from either *in vivo* or freshly excised sample preparations. The key to the numbered references is (1) Goldman and Hueter (1956); (2) Barger (1979); (3) Yoon and Katz (1979); (4) Robinson and Lele (1972); (5) Dunn and Fry (1961); (6) Dunn (1974); (7) Kaye and Laby (1966); (8) Edmonds *et al.* (1979); (9) Eggleton and Whitcomb (1979); (10) Kinsler *et al.* (1982); (11) Goss *et al.* (1978); (12) Chivers and Parry (1978); (13) Thijssen *et al.* (1985); (14) Johnston *et al.* (1979); (15) see Figure 5.2 for the data regarding water and saline; (16) Kossoff *et al.* (1973); (17) Bamber (1983a); (18) Greenleaf and Bahn (1981); (19) Mol and Breddels (1982)

the fibres, respectively. Consistent with these data are those of Hoffmeister *et al.* (1994), who express their results in terms of elastic stiffness coefficients and find values of 4.51 and 3.08 GPa for the coefficients C_{33} and C_{11}, again along and across the fibres, respectively.

As has already been noted, speed of sound does not vary strongly with frequency for biological soft tissues, and few systems have been designed to make accurate enough measurements for dispersion to be observed. Figure 5.4 provides examples of measured dispersion in haemoglobin solution and in human brain. Applications of relaxation theory [see equation (4.13)] and general relationships between ultrasonic attenuation and dispersion [equation (4.42)] have been used to show that these results are close to the expected dispersion (Kremkau *et al.* 1981). From average measurements on sheep and cat livers using the SLAM, Frizzell and Gindorf (1981) concluded that there is negligible difference between the sound speed at 100 MHz and that at low MHz frequencies.

The high speed of sound and attenuation (see Section 4.5.2.2) in bone is accompanied by a relatively large degree of dispersion – believed to be predominantly due to scattering (Barger 1979; Yoon & Katz 1979). This makes it particularly important to distinguish between group speed and phase speed when discussing sound propagation in bone. Bone structure may be highly anisotropic; dispersion of longitudinal sound speed varying between about 1% and 12% over the 1 to 3 MHz frequency range (*cf.* 0.2% over the same frequency range for brain in Figure 5.4), depending on the bone type and the direction of sound propagation. Transverse waves may be propagated in bone. The speed of such waves also varies with direction but,

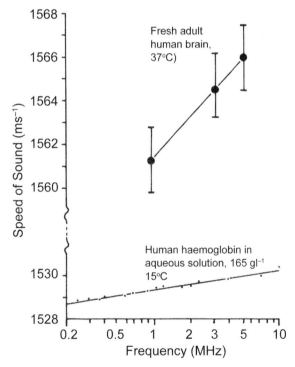

Figure 5.4. Dispersion in the speed of longitudinal sound waves in human haemoglobin solution (Carstensen & Schwan 1959) and in human brain (Kremkau *et al.* 1981). Data for sound speed dispersion in bone are described in the text (Section 5.3.1) but have been omitted from the figure because of the considerable change of scale which would be required to accommodate them

varying between 1700 and 2200 m s^{-1}, it is always lower than the corresponding longitudinal wave speed, and there is relatively little directional variation of shear wave dispersion.

5.3.2 TEMPERATURE DEPENDENCE

The parabolic shapes of the curves of speed vs. temperature for water and dilute aqueous solutions, discussed in Section 4.3.5, are shown in Figure 5.2. Figure 5.5 demonstrates the main features of the temperature dependence of sound speed in soft tissues. It is seen that fat tissue is distinguished not only in having a low sound speed but also in having a negative temperature coefficient (dc/dT), whereas dc/dT is positive for all of the non-fatty tissues that have been measured. This gives rise to unpredictable and variable temperature dependences of sound speed in complex structures such as breast parenchyma (Bamber 1983a). Scattering from fat/non-fat interfaces might be expected to be very strongly temperature dependent, as would the degree of aberration for waves propagating through such media. Practical applications of these observations might occur, since deliberate manipulation of the temperature could lead to reduced image artefacts or improved tissue characterisation based on measurements of speed, attenuation or scattering.

Kremkau *et al.* (1981) observed a minimum in sound speed in human adult brain at 15°C but not in infant brain. They postulated that this might be due to the relatively higher lipid content of adult brain and that, at low temperatures, the dc/dT for the lipid dominates, but at higher temperatures it is the non-fatty tissue component that determines dc/dT. The results for foetal brain (Wladimiroff *et al.* 1975), which has a very high water content, show only the typical non-fatty tissue dependence of sound speed on temperature.

The acoustical characteristics of fat also depend on whether it is in a solid, liquid or melting state. All three phases are believed to be present in the body. Johnson *et al.* (1977) suggested that the data on sound speed in fatty breast tissue demonstrated a solid–liquid phase transition at temperatures in the region of 35°C (see Figure 5.5).

It has also been thought that the temperature dependence of sound speed might be useful in the area of non-intrusive temperature measurement and mapping for purposes of monitoring dose and dose distribution in localised hyperthermia (Johnson *et al.* 1977). Unfortunately, absolute sound speed images have been made successfully *in vivo* only for extremities of the body such as the breast. Difficulties also arise due to the substantial variation of the sound speed at a given temperature from tissue to tissue and from specimen to specimen. There was a suggestion that dc/dT is sufficiently better behaved as to be useful (Bowen *et al.* 1979; Cetas & Connor 1978; Nasoni *et al.* 1979), particularly if one has prior knowledge of regional distributions of particular tissue types and if the differential speed information is combined with differential attenuation data (Haney & O'Brien 1982). If all that is required is an image to show the position of a localised alteration of temperature with time, then such images can be made using echo strain estimation methods to measure the spatial distribution of echo stretching or contraction due to localised heating or cooling (Seip *et al.* 1996; Bamber *et al.* 1997; Miller *et al.* 2002, 2003). Even for this task, however, difficulties may arise due to the small values of, or unpredictable nature of dc/dT, as described above.

The shapes of the curves of c vs. T for non-fatty soft tissues, and the appearance of a maximum in the region of 40–50°C, parallel the behaviour of dilute aqueous salt solutions (Stuehr & Yeager 1965). Fat behaves more like most other, non-aqueous, liquids (see, for example, the data on alcohols in Litovitz & Davis 1965), presumably because of its low water content.

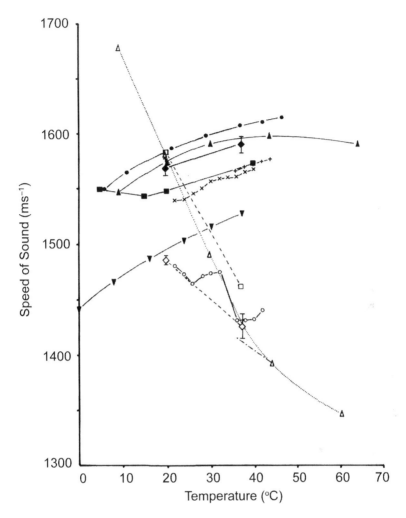

Figure 5.5. Examples of the measured variation with temperature of the speed of ultrasound in mammalian soft tissues. Hollow symbols have been used for fatty tissues; non-fatty tissues are represented by solid symbols. Key to references:

	Fatty tissues		Non-fatty tissues	Reference
△	Bovine peritoneal fat	●	Human liver	Bamber and Hill (1979)
		▲	Bovine liver	Bamber and Hill (1979)
◇	Human breast fat	◆	Human breast carcinoma (error bars show ± one standard error)	Bamber (1983a)
○	Human breast fat	×	Non-fatty human breast parenchyma	Johnson et al. (1977)
—·—·—	Canine stomach fat	+	Canine kidney	Bowen et al. (1979)
☐	Human orbital fat			Buschmann et al. (1970)
		■	Human adult brain (75–79% water)	Kremkau et al. (1981)
		▼	Human foetal brain (90% water)	Wladimiroff et al. (1975)

Although not strictly a temperature dependence, it is appropriate to mention here that heat denaturation or coagulation of tissues has been noted to produce a small but measurable decrease in sound speed (Bush *et al.* 1993).

5.3.3 PRESSURE DEPENDENCE

Speed of sound in general increases with increasing hydrostatic pressure – a fact that leads to the non-linear behaviour of sound propagation (see Sections 4.3.6, 4.3.8 and 5.4). Observations of the changes in sound speed with pressure have been used to measure the non-linearity parameter, B/A (see Section 5.4.2 below), in tissues and solutions of macromolecules, where it was found that among the soft tissues measured, fat has a B/A value which appears to be significantly higher than the values for non-fatty soft tissues (Law *et al.* 1985) – an interesting result in view of the major differences, noted above, regarding the temperature coefficient for sound speed in fatty and non-fatty tissues.

5.3.4 ROLE OF SPECIFIC TISSUE COMPONENTS

Examination of the data for soft tissues (excluding fat) presented in Figure 5.3 reveals, as was discussed in Section 4.5.2.7, that increasing speed of sound from one tissue to another correlates with an increasing protein content, particularly the structural protein collagen, and with a decreasing water content (Dunn 1976; Goss *et al.* 1979; O'Brien 1977). Variations within a particular tissue such as liver, on the other hand, are little influenced by the collagen content and appear to be primarily determined by the water content (Sarvazyan *et al.* 1987; see Section 4.5.2.7). The same was found to apply within brain tissue, where differences in water content provide reasonable explanations for the differences in the speed of sound between adult and infant or foetal brain (Kremkau *et al.* 1981; Wladimiroff *et al.* 1975; see also Figure 5.5). This is not apparently so for arterial tissue, where speed of sound correlates positively with collagen content and negatively with percentage cholesterol, and the collagen content is a major determinant of the speed (Rooney *et al.* 1982).

The very low speed of sound in fat results in it, also, being an acoustically important component of some tissues. In the normal and pathologically abnormal liver a low water content produces an increased speed of sound, unless accompanied by a high fat content, in which case the speed of sound is found to be reduced (Bamber *et al.* 1981; Zimmermann & Smith 1983). The female human breast, which has a high proportion of fat, tends to possess a low average speed of sound, which decreases with the age of the women due to progressive replacement of glandular tissue with fat (Bamber 1983a; Kossoff *et al.* 1973). Lactating breast, with its high milk content and glandular tissue proliferation, has a raised speed of sound (see Figure 5.2). Images of the spatial distribution of ultrasonic properties in thin slices of excised breast tissue (Foster *et al.* 1984) demonstrate very well how the fat distribution is a major determinant of both normal and pathological variations of sound speed and other acoustic characteristics.

For purposes of quantitative imaging and tissue characterisation one ideally requires as many of the ultrasonic propagation properties as can be accurately measured (Bamber 1983b). However, where it has been possible to make measurements of sound speed and/or its distribution (Bamber & Hill 1981; Foster *et al.* 1984; Greenleaf & Bahn 1981; Sehgal *et al.* 1986), this particular tissue characteristic has often been found to be more useful for discriminating between normal and pathological tissues than are the attenuation or backscattering coefficients. This may be due, in part, to the fact that, when the circumstances permit a measurement of sound speed to be made, it is possible to obtain a higher precision and accuracy than are obtainable in the measurement of attenuation or scattering. Preliminary results for pathological variations of human liver suggested that sound speed may indeed be more useful than the attenuation coefficient for assisting diagnosis of diffuse liver disease. Excellent separation of results was found for normal liver, fatty liver and cirrhosis (Hayashi *et al.* 1985). Doust *et al.* (1985), however, obtain quite different results for cirrhotic livers, and suggested that this may be due to differences in the causes of cirrhosis (and therefore type of cirrhosis) in the populations of Australia and Japan, the countries where the two studies were carried out. This suggestion might have been consistent with the findings of Zimmermann and Smith (1983), from measurements on fixed human liver specimens, that cirrhosis affects sound speed in a non-linear fashion: slight and moderate grades of cirrhosis depress the speed of sound relative to that in normal liver, whereas marked cirrhosis is indistinguishable from normal, and extreme cirrhosis produces a slightly elevated sound speed.

Few other tissues have been studied specifically in relation to pathological variations. Brain has possibly received the greatest attention, where most abnormal conditions (except haemorrhage and hydrocephalus) produce an elevated sound speed – although not many abnormalities have been studied by more than one author (Kremkau *et al.* 1979).

5.4   FINITE AMPLITUDE ('NON-LINEAR') PROPAGATION

Hitherto in this chapter we have implicitly assumed a linear stress–strain relationship in the acoustic propagation process. We have seen, however, in previous chapters (Sections 1.8.3 and 4.3.8) that this is only true to a first approximation and that, if higher order terms are taken into account – as they need to be when amplitudes of propagation parameters are no longer vanishingly small – relationships become non-linear and, in particular, particle velocity becomes pressure-dependent [equation (1.134)]. The concept of 'sound speed' thus becomes more complex and, as already discussed, the quantitative measure commonly used to express the influence of any particular propagation medium on this non-linear behaviour is the ratio 'B/A' of the second to first-order coefficients of the propagation equation [equations (1.134) and (4.44)].

5.4.1. MEASUREMENT OF NON-LINEARITY

There are two main methods for determining the parameter B/A.

The finite amplitude method, of which there have been various embodiments (Law *et al.* 1981; Cobb 1983; Cain *et al.* 1986; Zhang & Dunn 1987), is based on the measurement of the second harmonic generated during propagation of a sinusoidal wave [equation (4.46)]. Two transducers are used, as in the variable path attenuation measurement (Section 4.4.1.2). The second harmonic pressure, $p_2(z)$, as a function of propagation distance, z, is (Zhang & Dunn 1987):

$$p_2(z) = \frac{\pi f(2 + B/A)}{2\rho_0 c^3} p_1^2(0) z \, \exp[-\alpha_{a1} + \alpha_{a2}/2)z] DIFF(z) \tag{5.4}$$

where $p_1(0)$ is the acoustic pressure output of the transmitting transducer at the fundamental frequency, α_{a1} and α_{a2} are the absorption coefficients of the measured medium, at the fundamental and second-harmonic frequencies respectively, and $DIFF(z)$ is the diffraction correction (see Section 4.4.2.2). By analogy with the insertion method of attenuation measurement (Section 4.4.1.2), comparison of the second-harmonic pressure determined for a sample with that of a reference medium having a known B/A value and acoustic impedance close to that of the sample (e.g. 10% NaCl solution) circumvents transducer calibrations.

The thermodynamic method, also known as the 'pressure-jump method', requires measurement of the rate of change with ambient pressure of sound speed in the sample $(\partial c_{finite}/\partial p)_s$ when the pressure is decreased rapidly enough (approximately $10\,\text{MPa s}^{-1}$) to approximate an adiabatic depressurisation (Zhang & Dunn 1987; Sehgal *et al.* 1986). Then:

$$B/A = 2\rho_0 c \left[\frac{\partial c_{finite}}{\partial p}\right]_s \qquad (5.5)$$

Not surprisingly, the finite amplitude and thermodynamic methods have many sources of error in common with those for attenuation and sound speed estimation. The total systematic error is of the order of $\pm 8\%$ for the finite amplitude method and about $\pm 5\%$ for the thermodynamic method (although these are likely to worsen with the effect of any sample inhomogeneity: see Law *et al.* 1985). The two measurement methods have been compared by measuring B/A for a 23% bovine serum albumin solution and found to agree within $\pm 3\%$ (Zhang & Dunn 1987). When studying relative non-linear properties of solutions, extremely precise relative sound velocity measurement methods may be used, yielding relative thermodynamic measurements of B/A with a precision better than $\pm 0.3\%$ (Sarvazyan *et al.* 1990). There appears to be no significant difference between *in vivo* and *in vitro* values (Zhang *et al.* 1991).

5.4.2 PUBLISHED DATA FOR NON-LINEARITY PARAMETER

Examples of reported measurements of the non-linearity parameter, B/A, for biological and other relevant media, are presented in Figure 5.6 (see also Table 4.1 and chapter 7). Values for B/A increase slightly with sound speed, and with temperature over the range 0–40°C, for water, for aqueous solutions of macromolecules, and for most tissues (*cf.* Figure 5.3). For fat, however, B/A is greater than for aqueous media, whilst sound speed is lower. By inference from the temperature dependence for fatty liver, this behaviour rather resembles that for pure non-biological media, where B/A is inversely correlated with sound speed (Sehgal *et al.* 1986; Madigoski *et al.* 1981). For solutions of biological compounds, B/A depends on the concentration and on the type of solute but is independent of molecular weight. Solute–solvent interactions are therefore regarded as the most likely source of non-linearity in such media, rather than inter- or intra-molecular interactions, with the solute hydration shell structure playing an important role (Sarvazyan *et al.* 1990). B/A has been shown to result from a linear combination of the contributions due to various chemical components. Measurement of both sound speed and B/A enables chemical composition to be estimated, in terms of the volume fractions of water, fat and residual components such as proteins and carbohydrates (Sehgal *et al.* 1986). Values for whole and homogenised liver suggest that B/A is influenced by the presence of large-scale structure in tissue. According to Zhang and Dunn (1987), of the value of B/A obtained after that due to water had been subtracted, 26% was due to cell–cell adhesive force, 20% due to hepatocyte cellular structure and 15% due to secondary and tertiary protein structure.

Finally, it is of interest to contrast the B/A values for normal tissues as recorded in Figure 5.6, generally in the range 5–10, with those found in microbubble-based contrast media. Here, for example, Wu and Tong (1998) have reported B/A values of 600 and 1000 respectively for suspensions of two commercial contrast agents, reflecting the extremely non-linear behaviour of gas bubbles in an acoustic field.

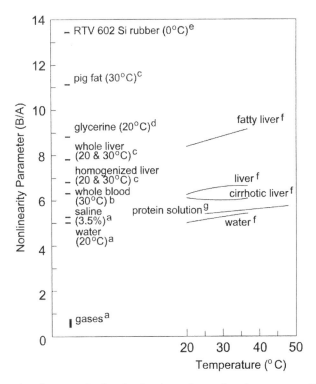

Figure 5.6. Examples of measured values for the ultrasonic non-linearity parameter, B/A, at atmospheric pressure. References are: (a) Beyer (1974); (b) Law *et al.* (1981); (c) Law *et al.* (1985); (d) Bjørnø (1975); (e) Madigoski *et al.* (1981); (f) Sehgal *et al.* (1986); (g) Zhang and Dunn (1987)

5.5 CONCLUSION

The speed of sound is a very important tissue characteristic. It is closer to being a fundamental acoustic propagation characteristic of tissues than either the attenuation or scattering characteristics, in that these are influenced to some extent by variations in sound speed. A great many different methods have been devised for the measurement of sound speed, although many of these are difficult to apply to biological tissues, and *in vivo* measurements on a broad range of tissues are only just beginning to be made. When it is possible to make a measurement of sound speed, it tends to be easier to achieve good accuracy and precision in this measurement than in that of attenuation or scattering.

Efforts to overcome the difficulties of *in vivo* measurement and quantitative imaging of sound speed may well be rewarded by improved diagnostic accuracy. Furthermore, correcting for the sound speed fluctuations that otherwise cause blurring and misregistration may enhance echo images.

Temperature is an important variable to consider when making measurements of sound speed. Conversely, the temperature coefficient of speed may be used in remote monitoring of relative temperature distributions.

Except in the first approximation, 'sound speed' is a complex concept, whose detailed documentation calls for study of the non-linear nature of the response of propagation media to acoustic stress: a phenomenon that, in turn, can be highly informative about the physical nature of such media. Further discussion of this issue is taken up in Chapter 7.

REFERENCES

Akamatsu, K., Miyauchi, S., Nishimura, N., Ohkubo, H. and Ohta, Y. (1985). A simple new method for *in vivo* measurement of ultrasound velocity in liver and its clinical usefulness. In *Proc. 4th Meeting of the World Federation for Ultrasound in Medicine and Biology*, R.W. Gill and M.J. Dadd (eds). Pergamon Press, Sydney, p. 522.

Anderson, M.E. and Trahey, G.E. (1998). Direct estimation of sound speed using pulse–echo ultrasound. *J. Acoust. Soc Am.* **104**, 3099–3106.

Bamber, J.C. (1983a). Ultrasonic propagation properties of the breast. In *Ultrasonic Examination of the Breast*, J. Jellins and T. Kobayashi (eds). John Wiley, Chichester, pp. 37–44.

Bamber, J.C. (1983b). Ultrasonic tissue characterization in cancer diagnosis and management. *RNM Images* Oct, 12–19.

Bamber, J.C. and Abbott, C. (1985). The feasibility of measuring average speed of sound in tissues using a real-time scanner. In *Proc. 4th Meeting of the World Federation for Ultrasound in Medicine and Biology*, R.W. Gill and M.J. Dadd (eds). Pergamon Press, Sydney, p. 517.

Bamber, J.C., Cosgrove, D.O., Page, J. and Bossi, C. (1987). *In vivo* sound speed in normal human liver by whole body transit-time measurements using a real-time scanner. *Eurosn '87, Conference Proceedings*, S. Bondestam, A. Alanen and P. Jouppila (eds). Finish Society for Ultrasound in Medicine and Biology, Helsinki, p. 306.

Bamber, J.C. and Hill, C.R. (1979). Ultrasonic attenuation and propagation speed in mammalian tissues as a function of temperature. *Ultrasound Med. Biol.* **5**, 149–157.

Bamber, J.C. and Hill, C.R. (1981). Acoustic properties of normal and cancerous human liver – I. Dependence on pathological condition. *Ultrasound Med. Biol.* **7**, 121–133.

Bamber, J.C., Hill, C.R. and King, J.A. (1981). Acoustic properties of normal and cancerous human liver – II. Dependence on tissue structure. *Ultrasound Med. Biol.* **7**, 135–144.

Bamber, J.C., Meaney, P., Doyley, M.M., Clarke, R.L. and ter Haar, G.R. (1997). Non-invasive temperature imaging using ultrasound echo strain: preliminary simulations. In *Acoustical Imaging*, Vol. 23, S. Lees and L. Ferrari (eds). Plenum Press, New York, pp. 25–33.

Barger, J.E. (1979). Attenuation and dispersion of ultrasound in cancellous bone. In *Ultrasonic Tissue Characterization 11*, M. Linzer (ed.), NBS Spec. Publ. 525. US Govt. Printing Office, Washington, D.C., pp. 197–201.

Beyer, R.T. (1974). *Nonlinear Acoustics*. Naval Ship Systems Command, US Department of the Navy.

Beyer, R.T. and Letcher, S.V. (1969). *Physical Ultrasonics*. Academic Press, New York.

Bhagat, P., Hajjar, W. and Kadaba, M. (1976). Measurement of the acoustic properties of a nerve–muscle preparation as a function of physiological state. *Ultrasonics* **Nov.**, 283–285.

Bjørnø, L. (1975). Non-linear ultrasound – a review. In *Ultrasonics International Conf. Proc.*, Z. Novak (ed.). IPC Science and Technology Press, Guildford.

Bowen, T., Conner, W.G., Nasoni, R.L., Pifer, A.E. and Sholes, R.R. (1979). Measurement of the temperature dependence of the velocity of ultrasound in tissues. In *Ultrasonic Tissue Characterization 11*, M. Linzer (ed.), NBS Spec. Publ. 525. US Govt. Printing Office, Washington, D.C., pp. 57–61.

Buschmann, W., Voss, M. and Kemmerling, S. (1970). Acoustic properties of normal human orbit tissues. *Opthalmol. Res.* **1**, 354–364.

Bush, N.L., Rivens, I., ter Haar, G.R. and Bamber, J.C. (1993). Acoustic properties of lesions generated with an ultrasound therapy system. *Ultrasound Med. Biol.* **19**, 789–801.

Cain, C.A. *et al.* (1986). On ultrasonic methods for measurement of the nonlinearity parameter B/A in fluid-like media. *J. Acoust. Soc. Am.* **80**, 685–688.

Carson, P.L., Meyer, C.R. and Scherzinger, A.L. (1981). Breast imaging in coronal planes with simultaneous pulse echo and transmission ultrasound. *Science* **214**, 1141–1143.

Carstensen, E.L. (1954). Measurement of dispersion of velocity of sound in liquids. *J. Acoust. Soc. Am.* **26**, 858–861.

Carstensen, E.L. and Schwan, H.P. (1959). Acoustic properties of hemoglobin solutions. *J. Acoust. Soc. Am.* **31**, 305–311.

Cetas, T.C. and Connor, W.G. (1978). Thermometry considerations in localized hyperthermia. *Med. Phys.* **5**, 79–91.

Chenevert, T.L., Schmitt, R.M., Carson, P.L., Bland, P.H., Meyer, C.R., Adler, D.D. and Samuels, B.T. (1984). The potential of ultrasonic CT for breast cancer diagnosis. *J. Ultrasound Med.* **3**(9), 127.

Chivers, R.C. and Parry, R.J. (1978). Ultrasonic velocity and attenuation in mammalian tissues. *J. Acoust. Soc. Am.* **63**, 940–953.

Chubachi, N. (1981). Mechanically scanned acoustic microscope. *Japan J. Appl. Phys.* **21**(suppl. 21-3), 7–10.

Cobb, W.N. (1983). Finite amplitude method for the determination of the acoustic nonlinearity parameter B/A. *J. Acoust. Soc. Am.* **73**, 1525–1531.

Coppens, A.B. (1981). Simple equations for the speed of sound in Neptunian waters. *J. Acoust. Soc. Am.* **69**, 862–863.

Del Grosso, V.A. and Mader, C.W. (1972). Speed of sound in pure water. *J. Acoust. Soc. Am.* **52**, 1442–1446.

Doust, B., Robinson, D.E., Chen, C.F. and Wilson, L.S. (1985). Ultrasonic speed and attenuation determinations in cirrhosis of the liver. In *Proc. 4th Meeting of the World Federation for Ultrasound in Medicine and Biology*, R.W. Gill and M.J. Dadd (eds). Pergamon Press, Sydney, p. 80.

Droin, P., Laugier, P. and Berger, G. (1997). Ultrasonic attenuation and dispersion of cancellous bone in the frequency range 200 kHz–600 kHz. *Acoustical Imaging*, Vol. 23, S. Lees and L. Ferrari (eds). Plenum Press, New York, pp. 157–162.

Duck, F.A. (1990). *Physical Properties of Tissue*. Academic Press, London.

Dunn, F. (1974). Attenuation and speed of ultrasound in lung. *J. Acoust. Soc. Am.* **56**, 1638–1639.

Dunn, F. (1976). Ultrasonic attenuation, absorption and velocity in tissues and organs. In *Ultrasonic Tissue Characterization*, M. Linzer (ed.), NBS Spec. Publ. 453. US Govt. Printing Office, Washington, D.C., pp. 21–28.

Dunn, F. (1986). Attenuation and speed of ultrasound in lung: dependence upon frequency and inflation. *J. Acoust. Soc. Am.* **80**, 1248–1250.

Dunn, F., Edmonds, P.D. and Fry, W.J. (1969). Absorption and dispersion of ultrasound in biological media. In *Biological Engineering*, H.P. Schwan (ed.). McGraw-Hill, New York, pp. 205–332.

Dunn, F. and Fry, W.J. (1961). Ultrasonic absorption and reflection by lung tissue. *Phys. Med. Biol.* **5**, 401–410.

Edmonds, P.D., Reyes, Z., Parkinson, D.B., Filly, R.A. and Busey, H. (1979). A human abdominal tissue phantom. In *Ultrasonic Tissue Characterization 11*, M. Linzer (ed.), NBS Spec. Publ. 525. US Govt. Printing Office, Washington, D.C., pp. 323–326.

Eggleton, R.C. and Whitcomb, J.A. (1979). Tissue simulators for diagnostic ultrasound. In *Ultrasonic Tissue Characterization 11*, M. Linzer (ed.), NBS Spec. Publ. 525. US Govt Printing Office, Washington, D.C., pp. 323–326.

Embree, P.M., Tervola, K.M.U., Foster, S.G. and O'Brien Jr., W.D. (1985). Spatial distribution of the speed of sound in biological materials with the scanning laser acoustic microscope. *IEEE Trans. Son. Ultrason.* **SU-32**, 341–350.

Foster, F.S., Strban, M. and Austin, G. (1984). The ultrasound macroscope: initial studies on breast tissue. *Ultrasonic Imaging* **6**, 243–261.

Frizzell, L.A. and Gindorf, J.D. (1981). Measurement of ultrasonic velocity in several biological tissues. *Ultrasound Med. Biol.* **7**, 385–387.

Giacomini, A. (1947). Ultrasonic velocity in ethanol–water mixtures. *J. Acoust. Soc. Am.* **19**, 701–702.

Glover, G.H. and Sharp, J.C. (1977). Reconstruction of ultrasound propagation speed distributions in soft tissue: time-of-flight tomography. *IEEE Trans. Son. Ultrason.* **24**, 229–234.

Goldman, D.E. and Hueter, T.F. (1956). Tabular data of the velocity and absorption of high-frequency sound in mammalian tissues. *J. Acoust. Soc. Am.* **28**, 35–37.

Goldman, D.E. and Richards, J.R. (1954). Measurement of high frequency sound velocity in mammalian soft tissues. *J. Acoust. Soc. Am.* **26**, 981–983.

Goss, S.A., Johnston, R.L. and Dunn, F. (1978). Comprehensive compilation of empirical ultrasonic properties of mammalian tissues. *J. Acoust. Soc. Am.* **64**, 423–457.

Goss, S.A., Johnston, R.L., Maynard, V., Nider, L., Frizzell, L.A., O'Brien Jr., W.D. and Dunn, F. (1979). Elements of tissue characterization part II; ultrasonic propagation parameter measurements. In *Ultrasonic Tissue Characterization 11*, M. Linzer (ed.), NBS Spec. Publ. 525. US Govt. Printing Office, Washington, D.C., pp. 43–51.

Grant, D.R. and Bernardin, J.E. (1981). Measurement of sound velocity with the scanning laser acoustic microscope. *J. Acoust. Soc. Am.* **69**, 866–868.

Greenleaf, J.F. and Bahn, R.C. (1981). Clinical imaging with transmissive ultrasonic computerized tomography. *IEEE Trans.* **BME-28**, 177–185.

Greenleaf, J.F., Johnson, S.A., Samayoa, W.F. and Duck, F.A. (1975). Two-dimensional acoustic velocity distributions in tissues using an algebraic reconstruction technique. In *Ultrasonics International Conf. Proc.* IPC Science and Technology Press, Guildford, pp. 190–194.

Greenspan, M. and Tschiegg, C.E. (1957). *Rev. Sci. Inst.* **28**, 897.

Haney, M.J. and O'Brien Jr., W.D. (1982). Ultrasonic tomography for differential thermography. In *Acoustical Imaging*, Vol. 12, E.A. Ash and C.R. Hill (eds). Plenum Press, New York, pp. 589–597.

Haumschild, D.J. and Greenleaf, J.F. (1983). A crossed beam method for ultrasonic speed measurement in tissue. *Ultrasonic Imaging*, **5**, 168.

Hayashi, N., Tamaki, N., Yamammoto, K., Senda, M., Yonekura, Y., Torizuka, K., Ogawa, T., Katakura, K. and Umemura, S. (1985). *In vivo* measurement of sound speed in normal and abnormal livers using a high resolution ultrasonic scanner. In *Proc. 4th Meeting of the World Federation for Ultrasound in Medicine and Biology*, R.W. Gill and M.J. Dadd (eds). Pergamon Press, Sydney, p. 520.

Heyser, R.C. and LeCroisette, D.H. (1974). A new ultrasonic imaging system using time delay spectrometry. *Ultrasound Med. Biol.* **1**, 119–131.

Hoffmeister, B.K., Verdonck, E.D., Wickline, S.A. and Miller, J.G. (1994). Effect of collagen on the anisotropy of quasi-longitudinal mode ultrasonic velocity in fibrous soft tissues: a comparison of fixed tendon and fixed myocardium. *J. Acoust. Soc. Am.* **96**, 1957–1964.

Iinuma, K., Sumino, Y., Hirama, M., Okazaki, K., Sato, T. and Sasaki, H. (1985). A proposal of crossed beam method using a linear array probe for *in vivo* measurement of sound velocity of tissue. In *Proc. 4th Meeting of the World Federation for Ultrasound in Medicine and Biology*, R.W. Gill and M.J. Dadd (eds). Pergamon Press, Sydney, p. 515.

Jago, J.R. and Whittingham, T.A. (1992). The use of measured acoustic speed distributions in reflection ultrasound CT. *Physics Med. Biol.* **37**, 2139–2142.

Jellins, J. and Kossoff, G. (1973). Velocity compensation in water-coupled breast echography. *Ultrasonics* **11**, 223–226.

Johnson, S.A., Christensen, D.A., Johnson, C.C., Greenleaf, J.F. and Rajagopalan, B. (1977). Non-intrusive measurement of microwave and ultrasound induced hyperthermia by acoustic temperature tomography. In *IEEE Ultrasonics Symp. Proc.*, Cat. No. 77Chl264-lSU, 977–982.

Johnston, R.L., Goss, S.A., Maynard, V., Brady, J.K., Frizzell, L.A., O'Brien Jr., W.D. and Dunn, F. (1979). Elements of tissue characterization: Part I, ultrasonic propagation properties. In *Ultrasonic Tissue Characterization 11*, M. Linzer (ed.), NBS Spec. Publ. 525. US Govt. Printing Office, Washington, D.C., pp. 19–27.

Kaye, G.W.C. and Laby, T.H. (1966). *Tables of Physical and Chemical Constants and Some Mathematical Functions* (13th edn). Longmans, Green and Co., London.

Kim, J.H., Park, S.B. and Johnson, S.A. (1984). Tomographic imaging of ultrasonic reflectivity with correction for acoustic speed variations. *Ultrasonic Imaging* **6**, 304–312.

Kinsler, L.E., Frey, A., Coppens, A.B. and Saunders, J.V. (1982). *Fundamentals of Acoustics* (3rd edn). John Wiley, New York, p. 397.

Kittinger, E. (1977). Correction for transducer influence on sound velocity measurements by the pulse echo method. *Ultrasonics*, **15**, 30–32.

Koch, R., Whiting, J.F., Price, D.C., McCaffrey, J.F., Kossoff, G. and Reeve, T.S. (1983). Transmission tomography and B-scan imaging of the breast. In *Ultrasonic Examination of the Breast*, J. Jellins and T. Kobayashi (eds). John Wiley, Chichester, pp. 235–239.

Kossoff, G., Kelly Fry, E. and Jellins, J. (1973). Average velocity of ultrasound in the human female breast. *J. Acoust. Soc. Am.* **53**, 1730–1736.

Kremkau, F.W., Barnes, R.W. and McGraw, C.P. (1981). Ultrasonic attenuation and propagation speed in normal human brain. *J. Acoust. Soc. Am.* **70**, 29–38.

Kremkau, F.W., McGraw, C.P. and Barnes, R.W. (1979). Acoustic properties of normal and abnormal human brain. In *Ultrasonic Tissue Characterization 11*, M. Linzer (ed.), NBS Spec. Publ. 525. US Govt. Printing Office, Washington, D.C., pp. 81–84.

Laugier, P., Droin, P., Leva-Jeantet, A.M. and Berger, G. (1997). *In vitro* assessment of the relationship between acoustic properties and bone mass density of the calcaneus by comparison of ultrasound parametric imaging and quantitative computed tomography. *Bone* **20**, 157–165.

Law, W.K., *et al.* (1981). Ultrasonic determination of the non-linearity parameter B/A. *J. Acoust. Soc. Am.*, **39**, 1210–1212.

Law, W.K., Frizzell, L.A. and Dunn, F. (1985). Determination of the nonlinearity parameter B/A of biological media. *Ultrasound Med. Biol.* **11**, 307–318.

Litovitz, T.A. and Davis, C.M. (1965). Structural and shear relaxation in liquids. In *Physical Acoustics*, Vol. 2A, W.P. Mason (ed.). Academic Press, New York, pp. 281–349.

Liu, C.H. and Yeh, K.C. (1980). Statistics of pulse arrival time in turbulent media. *J. Opt. Soc. Am.* **70**, 168–172.

Ludwig, G.D. (1950). The velocity of sound through tissues and the acoustic impedance of tissues. *J. Acoust. Soc. Am.* **22**, 862–866.

McSkimin, H.J. (1964). Ultrasonic methods of measuring the mechanical properties of liquids and solids. In *Physical Acoustics: Principles and Methods*, Vol. 1, Part A, W.P. Mason (ed.). Academic Press, New York, Ch. 10, pp. 271–334.

Madigoski, W.M., *et al.* (1981). Sound velocities and B/A in fluorocarbon fluids and in several low density solids. *J. Acoust. Soc. Am.* **69**, 1639–1643.

Madsen, E.L., Franck, G.R., Carson, P.L., Edmonds, P.D., Herman, B.A., Kremkau, F.W., O'Brien, W.D., Parker, K.J. and Robinson, R.A. (1986). Interlaboratory comparison of ultrasonic attenuation and speed measurements. *J. Ultrasound Med.* **5**, 569–576.

Manoharan, A., Robinson, D.E., Wilson, L.S., Chen, C.F. and Griffiths, K.A. (1985). Ultrasonic characterization of splenic tissue: a clinical study in patients with myelofibrosis. In *Proc. 4th Meeting of the World Federation for Ultrasound in Medicine and Biology*, R.W. Gill and M.J. Dadd (eds). Pergamon Press, Sydney, p. 113.

Matheson, A.J. (1971). *Molecular Acoustics*. Van Nostrand, New York.

Mesdag, P.R., de Vries, D. and Berkhout, A.J. (1982). An approach to tissue characterization based on wave theory using a new velocity analysis technique. In *Acoustical Imaging*, Vol. 12, E.A. Ash and C.R. Hill (eds). Plenum Press, New York, pp. 479–491.

Miles, C.A. (1996). Ultrasonic properties of tendon: velocity, attenuation and backscattering in equine digital flexor tendons. *J. Acoust. Soc. Am.* **99**, 3225–3232.

Miller, N.R., Bamber J.C. and Meaney, P.M. (2002). Fundamental limitations of noninvasive temperature imaging by means of ultrasound echo strain estimation. *Ultrasound Med. Biol.* **28**, 1319–1333.

Miller, N.R., Bamber, J.C. and ter Haar, G.R. (2003). Noninvasive temperature imaging by means of ultrasound echo strain estimation: preliminary in vitro results. *Ultrasound Med. Biol.* (in press).

Millero, F.J. and Kubinski, T. (1975). Speed of sound in seawater as a function of temperature and salinity at 1 atm. *J. Acoust. Soc. Am.* **57**, 312–319.

Mol, C.R. and Breddels, P.A. (1982). Ultrasound velocity in muscle. *J Acoust. Soc. Am.* **71**, 455–461.

Nasoni, R.L., Bowen, T., Conner, W.G. and Sholes, R.R. (1979). *In-vivo* temperature dependence of ultrasound speed in tissue and its applications to noninvasive temperature monitoring. *Ultrasonic Imaging* **1**, 34–43.

O'Brien Jr., W.D. (1977). The relationship between collagen and ultrasonic attenuation and velocity in tissue. In *Ultrasonics International Conference Proc.* IPC Business Press, Guildford, pp. 194–205.

Ohtsuki, S., Soetanto, K. and Okujima, M. (1985). A technique with reference points image for *in vivo* measurement of sound velocity. In *Proc. 4th Meeting of the World Federation for Ultrasound in Medicine and Biology*, R.W. Gill and M.J. Dadd (eds). Pergamon Press, Sydney, p. 521.

Ophir, J. (1986). A beam tracking method for estimation of ultrasound propagation speed in biological tissues. *IEEE Trans. Ultrason. Ferroelectr. Frequency Control* **33**, 359–367.

Papadakis, E.P. (1964). Ultrasonic attenuation and velocity in three transformation products in steel. *J. Appl. Phys.* **35**, 1474–1482.

Papadakis, E.P. (1966). Ultrasonic diffraction loss and phase change in anisotropic materials. *J. Acoust. Soc. Am.* **40**, 863–876.

Papadakis, E.P. (1972). Absolute accuracy of the pulse–echo overlap method and the pulse–superposition method for ultrasonic velocity. *J. Acoust. Soc. Am.* **52**, 843–846.

Pellam, J.R. and Galt, J.K. (1946). Ultrasonic propagation in liquids: I. Application of pulse technique to velocity and absorption measurements at 15 megacycles. *J. Chem. Phys.* **14**, 608–614.

Ragozzino, M. (1981). Analysis of the error in measurement of ultrasound speed in tissue due to waveform deformation by frequency dependent attenuation. *Ultrasonics* **12**, 135–138.

Redwood, M. (1963). A study of waveforms in the generation and detection of short ultrasonic pulses. *Appl. Mat. Res.* **April**, 76–84.

Robinson, D.E., Chen, F. and Wilson, L.S. (1982). Measurement of velocity of propagation from ultrasonic pulse–echo data. *Ultrasound Med. Biol.* **8**, 413–420.

Robinson, T.C. and Lele, P.P. (1972). An analysis of lesion development in the brain and in plastics by high-intensity focused ultrasound at low megahertz frequencies. *J. Acoust. Soc. Am.* **51**, 1333–1351.

Rooney, J.A., Gammell, P.M., Hestenes, J.D., Ghin, H.P. and Blankenhorn, D.H. (1982). Velocity and attenuation of sound in arterial tissues. *J. Acoust. Soc. Am.* **71**, 462–466.

Sarvazyan, A.P., Lyrchikov, A.G. and Gorelov, S.E. (1987). Dependence of ultrasonic velocity in rabbit liver on water content and structure of the tissue. *Ultrasonics* **25**, 244–247.

Sarvazyan, A.P., *et al.* (1990). Acoustic nonlinearity parameter B/A of aqueous solutions of some amino acids and proteins. *J. Acoust. Soc. Am.* **88**, 1555–1561.

Sehgal, C.M., Brown, G.M., Bahn, R.C. and Greenleaf, J.F. (1986). Measurement and use of acoustic nonlinearity and sound speed to estimate composition of excised livers. *Ultrasound Med. Biol.* **12**, 865–874.

Seip, R., VanBaren, P., Cain, C. and Ebbini, E.S. (1996). Noninvasive real-time multipoint temperature control for ultrasound phased array treatments. *IEEE Trans. UFFC* **43**, 1063–1073.

Seki, H., Granato, A. and Truell, R. (1956). Diffraction effects in the ultrasonic field of a piston source and their importance in the accurate measurement of attenuation. *J. Acoust. Soc. Am.* **28**, 230–238.

Sinclair, D.A., Smith, I.R. and Wickramasinghe, H.K. (1982). Recent developments in scanning acoustic microscopy. *The Radio and Electronic Engineer* **52**, 479–493.

Stuehr, J. and Yeager, E. (1965). The propagation of ultrasonic waves in electrolytic solutions. In *Physical Acoustics*, Vol. 2A, W.P. Mason (ed.). Academic Press, New York, pp. 351–462.

Subrahmanyam, S.V., Khan, V.H. and Raghavan, C.V. (1969). Interferometric measurement of ultrasonic velocity in liquids – effect of diffraction. *J. Acoust. Soc. Am.* **46**, 272.

Thijssen, J.M., Mol, H.J.M. and Timmer, M.R. (1985). Acoustic parameters of ocular tissues. *Ultrasound Med. Biol.* **11**, 157–161.

Van Venrooij, G.E.P.M. (1971). Measurement of sound velocity in human tissue. *Ultrasonics* **9**, 240–242.

Verhoef, W.A., Cloostermans, M.J.T.M. and Thijssen, J.M. (1985). Diffraction and dispersion effects on the estimation of ultrasound attenuation and velocity in biological tissues. *IEEE Trans. Biomed. Eng.* **BME-32**, 521–529.

Wladimiroff, J.W., Craft, I.L. and Talbert, D.G. (1975). *In vitro* measurements of sound velocity in human fetal brain tissue. *Ultrasound Med. Biol.* **1**, 377–382.

Wu, J. and Tong, J. (1998). Measurements of the nonlinearity parameter B/A of contrast agents. *Ultrasound Med. Biol.* **24**, 153–159.

Yoon, H.S. and Katz, J.L. (1979). Ultrasonic properties and microtexture of human cortical bone. In *Ultrasonic Tissue Characterization 11*, M. Linzer (ed.), NBS Spec. Publ. 525. US Govt. Printing Office, Washington, D.C., pp. 189–196.

Zhang, J. and Dunn, F. (1987). *In vivo* B/A determination in a mammalian organ. *J. Acoust. Soc. Am.* **81**, 1635–1637.

Zhang, J., Kuhlenschmidt, M.S. and Dunn, F. (1991). Influences of structural factors of biological media on the acoustic nonlinearity parameter B/A. *J. Acoust. Soc. Am.* **89**, 80–91.

Zimmermann, K.P. and Smith, J.C. (1983). Ultrasound velocity in fixed human liver: empirical anova and regression modelling on histologically assessed abnormalities. *Ultrasonic Imaging* **5**, 280–294.

6

Reflection and Scattering

R. J. DICKINSON[1] AND D. K. NASSIRI[2]

[1]Department of Bioengineering, Imperial College, London, UK and
[2]Department of Medical Physics and Bioengineering, St. George's Hospital, London, UK

6.1 INTRODUCTION

6.1.1 THE PHENOMENON OF SCATTERING

Scattering is the fundamental information-coding phenomenon that lies at the heart of investigative ultrasound methods. Systematic interest in the subject dates only from the 1970s (Chivers 1977, 1978; Hill *et al.* 1978) and a very useful overview of developments in the field in the ensuing 20 years has been given by Shung and Thieme (1993). In this chapter we shall outline a theoretical basis for understanding the phenomenon (building on the foundations laid in Chapter 1), describe the principal experimental approaches to scattering measurement, and discuss some of the particular implications of scattering behaviour for clinical imaging.

Scattering occurs when a wave travels through a non-uniform medium, and part of the energy in the wave is redirected and appears separately to the original incident wave, either delayed in time or altered in direction. The simple case, when the non-uniformity is a plane interface perpendicular to the incident wave between two different regions is dealt with in Chapter 1 using the concept of acoustic impedance. In the medical context such surfaces are rare, and the non-uniformities are more commonly varied in shape and size, partly random in position and orientation. A major part of the grey-scale B-scan image is formed by scattered waves from such small-scale structures. In addition to pulse–echo images, Doppler and other techniques rely on the phenomenon of scattering, and some of these are described in Chapters 9 and 10.

This section continues with a brief overview of the current state of scattering theory and its application to medical ultrasound. One particular theoretical approach is then examined in more detail, outlining the basic equations and their solutions. The scattering from tissue is difficult to treat exactly because the acoustic properties of tissue on a scale less than that of the acoustic wavelength are not known, and so a number of simple models for tissue are used, and these are examined. The actual scattering measurements that have been made to date are then discussed, together with the conclusions that may be made about the acoustic properties of tissue.

Most theories of scattering deal with a plane single-frequency wave, whereas the B-scan image is produced by the scattering of a pulse. A section of the chapter is devoted to the theory of scattering of pulses, and its relation to the properties of the B scan image, with a discussion of the effects of tissue motion on the scattered wave.

Physical Principles of Medical Ultrasonics, Second Edition. Edited by C. R. Hill, J. C. Bamber and G. R. ter Haar.
© 2004 John Wiley & Sons, Ltd: ISBN 0 471 97002 6

A number of techniques have evolved in recent years which aim to analyse the scattered waves, in order to obtain more quantitative information about the scattering medium, rather than to display them as an 'image' (*cf.* Chapter 9). One such technique, sometimes referred to as 'impediography', is discussed in detail and illustrates the connection between reflection and scattering. Some other techniques are then discussed, with an indication of possible directions for future research.

6.1.2 OVERVIEW OF SCATTERING THEORY

The theory of scattering by human tissue has been reviewed by Chivers (1977) and Insana and Brown (1993), and a brief account of some of the approaches will be given to put in context some of the detailed theories of later sections. Many of these treatments are included in a comprehensive treatise by Ishimaru (1978), who considers scattering of a number of different forms of radiation.

The case when the wavelength used, λ, is much less than the scale of the inhomogeneities, $\hat{a}$ (where $\hat{a}$ is some average scale parameter, such as the correlation length) can be tackled using two techniques. The first, the ray approximation, applies Fermat's principle to predict the effect of velocity fluctuations of the medium, and obtains an expression for the mean square deviation of the ray after travelling through the medium (Chernow 1960). This approximation is only used when $L < \hat{a}^2/\lambda$, where L is the distance the ray travels, and Chivers (1978) applies the method to ultrasound propagation in tissue. The second technique, described by Uscinski (1977), treats the case where the scattering per inhomogeneity is small (that is, $n\hat{a} < \lambda$, where n is the standard deviation of refractive index) but relaxes the restriction on L, so that the total amount of scattering may be very large. The technique thus incorporates a theory of multiple scattering. He derives and solves differential equations for various statistical moments of the field and thereby can predict the influence of the statistics of the acoustic medium. Thus the expression for the first moment of the field gives the attenuation due to scattering, the second moment gives the spatial auto-correlation function, the frequency auto-correlation function gives the average pulse envelope, and the fourth moment gives the intensity fluctuations.

Where the inhomogeneities are on a scale comparable to or less than the acoustic wavelength, as seems to be the case for human tissue, then a significant part of the interaction will involve diffraction, and it will be on this regime of scattering theory that this chapter will concentrate.

Very few measurements of the small-scale structures of tissue as a function of position are available, although the development of acoustic microscopy (Chapter 11) may change this. However, it may be sufficient to consider tissue as a random medium which can be described by its statistics, and this has led to the development of two theoretical models which are amenable to theoretical analysis and aim to simulate the scattering properties of tissue. These models will be investigated in detail in Section 6.4.

Most theoretical treatments use the Born approximation and hence ignore multiple scattering, the justification being the small measured scattering cross-sections of tissue. One effect of multiple scattering, however, will be beam distortion caused by refractive index fluctuations, and a first step towards a complete treatment of scattering can be made by taking these into account (Farrow *et al.* 1995; Manry & Broschat 1996).

In conclusion, the remainder of this chapter deals with the case when $\hat{a} < \lambda$, which can be treated using two tissue models. This is the regime to consider when examining scattering, and in particular backscattering. The case when $\hat{a} > \lambda$ has been covered by Uscinski; this regime covers the case of beam distortion in tissue, and is not discussed here.

6.1.3 SCATTERING IN OTHER FIELDS

No account of theories of ultrasonic scattering is complete without an acknowledgement of the vast amount of work from other fields. Scattering is a phenomenon common to all waves, including electromagnetic radiation, seismic waves, sonar and nuclear particles. Much of the scattering theory of these modalities is similar, with different terms inserted into the relevant wave equation. Much of the theory relevant to pulse–echo ultrasound was initially developed for radar, and many examples of this are contained in Ishimaru's book. Scattering of acoustic fields has been used in sonar interrogation of fish shoals, examination of the ocean bed and non-destructive testing of metals (Hill *et al.* 1978).

6.2 SCATTERING THEORY

6.2.1 BASIC EQUATIONS

Scattering is the result of a wave propagating through an inhomogeneous medium, and the interaction is governed by an inhomogeneous wave equation. The detailed derivation of this is given in Chapter 1, and the formulation given is based on Section 1.2.4. This considers the medium to have no absorption and small fluctuations in density and compressibility ρ_1 and β_1 about constant values ρ_0 and β_0 inside an inhomogeneous volume V. Outside V, ρ_1 and β_1 are zero, so:

$$\rho(\mathbf{r}) = \rho_0 + \rho_1(\mathbf{r}); \quad \beta(\mathbf{r}) = \beta_0 + \beta_1(\mathbf{r}) \qquad\qquad \text{inside } V \text{ (6.1)}$$

$$\rho(\mathbf{r}) = \rho_0; \quad \beta(\mathbf{r}) = \beta_0 \qquad\qquad \text{outside } V \text{ (6.2)}$$

Also

$$\frac{\partial\rho(\mathbf{r})}{\partial \mathbf{n}} = \frac{\partial\beta(\mathbf{r})}{\partial \mathbf{n}} = 0 \qquad\qquad \text{at the boundary of } V \text{ (6.3)}$$

($\mathbf{n}$ is the normal vector perpendicular to the surface of V).
It is convenient to define the parameters

$$\tilde{\rho}(\mathbf{r}) = \frac{\rho_1(\mathbf{r}) - \rho_0}{\rho_0}; \quad \tilde{\beta}(\mathbf{r}) = \frac{\beta_1(\mathbf{r}) - \beta_0}{\beta_0} \qquad\qquad \text{(6.4/1.20, 1.21)}$$

Then the wave equation becomes (Morse & Ingard 1968)

$$\nabla^2 P(\mathbf{r},\ t) - \frac{1}{c^2}\frac{\partial^2 P(\mathbf{r},\ t)}{\partial t^2} = \frac{1}{c^2}\frac{\partial^2 P(\mathbf{r},\ t)}{\partial t^2}\cdot\tilde{\beta}(t) + div[\tilde{\rho}(\mathbf{r})\cdot grad\cdot P(\mathbf{r},\ t)] \qquad \text{(6.5/1.23)}$$

with $c = (\rho_0\beta_0)^{-1/2}$. It can be solved by the methods of Green's functions (Morse & Feshbach 1953) in which the right-hand side is considered a source term, and the Green's function is the solution of the above equation with the right-hand side equal to a point source radiator.
The solution is:

$$P(\mathbf{r},\ t) = P_i(\mathbf{r},\ t) + \int\limits_{-\infty}^{\infty} dt_0 \int\limits_{V}\left\{\frac{1}{c^2}\frac{\partial^2 P(\mathbf{r}_0,\ t_0)}{\partial t^2}\cdot\tilde{\beta}(t_0) + div[\tilde{\rho}(\mathbf{r}_0)\cdot grad\cdot P(\mathbf{r}_0,\ t_0)]\right\}G(\mathbf{r}_0, \mathbf{r}; t_0, t)d^3\mathbf{r}_0$$

where

$$G(\mathbf{r}_0, \mathbf{r}; t_0, t) = \frac{\delta(t - t_0 - |\mathbf{r}_0 - \mathbf{r}|/c)}{4\pi|\mathbf{r}_0 - \mathbf{r}|} \tag{6.6}$$

A solution of the integral equation for P is only possible for certain simple geometrical objects. The general case is solved by making approximations, the most important being the Born approximation: the integral term in equation (6.6) is approximated by replacing $P(\mathbf{r}, t)$ with $P_i(\mathbf{r}, t)$, which is the incident wave that would travel through V if it was homogeneous (so $\tilde{\rho}$ and $\tilde{\beta}$ are zero), and is usually known. The approximation is only valid if the scattering is weak and both $\tilde{\rho}(\mathbf{r})$ and $\tilde{\beta}(\mathbf{r})$ are small. If this is not true then it is possible to solve equation (6.6) by an iterative technique using successive approximations.

So equation (6.6) becomes

$$P(\mathbf{r}, t) = P_i(\mathbf{r}, t) + P_s(\mathbf{r}, t) \tag{6.7}$$

where $P_s(\mathbf{r}, t)$ is the scattered wave, which by the Born approximation is

$$P_s(\mathbf{r}, t) = \int_{-\infty}^{\infty} dt_0 \int_V \left\{ \frac{1}{c^2} \frac{\partial^2 P_i(\mathbf{r}_0, t_0)}{\partial t^2} \cdot \tilde{\beta}(t_0) + div[\tilde{\rho}(\mathbf{r}_0) \cdot grad \cdot P_i(\mathbf{r}_0, t_0)] \right\} G(\mathbf{r}_0, \mathbf{r}; t_0, t) d^3\mathbf{r}_0 \tag{6.8a}$$

It is instructive to examine the case where the incident wave is a plane wave, of angular frequency ω and amplitude p_0.

$$P_i(\mathbf{r}, t) = p_0 e^{i(\mathbf{k}_i \cdot \mathbf{r} - \omega t)} \tag{6.9}$$

Inserting (6.9) in equation (6.8a) gives

$$P_s(\mathbf{r}, t) = p_0 e^{i\omega t} \int_{V_0} \{k^2 \tilde{\beta}(\mathbf{r}_0) - i \, div \, \tilde{\rho}(\mathbf{r}_0) \cdot \mathbf{k}_i\} \left(\frac{e^{i[\mathbf{k}_i \cdot \mathbf{r}_0 - k|\mathbf{r} - \mathbf{r}_0|]}}{4\pi|\mathbf{r} - \mathbf{r}_0|} \right) d^3\mathbf{r}_0 \tag{6.10}$$

where $k = \omega/c = |\mathbf{k}_i|$.

Expanding the exponent for distances from the scattering region large compared with its extent ($|\mathbf{r}| \gg |\mathbf{r}_0|$), and defining the origin of the coordinate system within V, as in Figure 6.1, gives

$$\mathbf{k}_i \cdot \mathbf{r}_0 - k|\mathbf{r} - \mathbf{r}_0| \approx (\mathbf{k}_i - \mathbf{k}_s) \cdot \mathbf{r}_0 - kr \tag{6.11}$$

where $\mathbf{k}_s$ has magnitude k and is pointed in the direction of $\mathbf{r}$ (Figure 6.1).

Hence:

$$P_s(\mathbf{r}, t) = p_0 \frac{e^{i(kr - \omega t)}}{4\pi r} \int_{V_0} \{k_i^2 \tilde{\beta}(\mathbf{r}_0) - i \, div \, \tilde{\rho}(\mathbf{r}_0) \cdot \mathbf{k}_i\} e^{i(\mathbf{k}_i - \mathbf{k}_s) \cdot \mathbf{r}_0} d^3\mathbf{r}_0 \tag{6.12}$$

6.2.2 ANGULAR DEPENDENCE

Equation (6.12) has the form of a spherical wave emanating from the origin (see Section 1.4.2) but with an anisotropic angular distribution determined by the integral shown.

Defining:

$$\beta(\mathbf{k}) = \int_V \tilde{\beta}(\mathbf{r}) e^{i\mathbf{k} \cdot \mathbf{r}} d^3\mathbf{r} \tag{6.13}$$

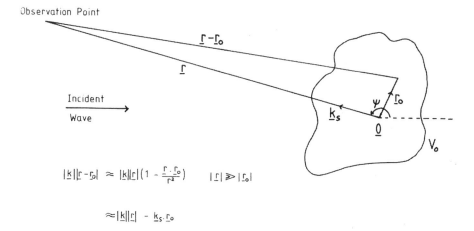

Figure 6.1. Geometry used in Born approximation of Section 6.2.1

$$\rho(\mathbf{k}) = \int_V \tilde{\rho}(\mathbf{r}) e^{i\mathbf{k}\cdot\mathbf{r}} \mathrm{d}^3\mathbf{r} \tag{6.14}$$

$$P_s(\mathbf{r},\, t) = p_0 \frac{e^{i(\omega t - kr)}}{4\pi r} k^2 [\beta(\mathbf{K}) + \rho(\mathbf{K}) \cos \Psi] \tag{6.15}$$

where

$$\mathbf{K} = \mathbf{k}_s - \mathbf{k}_i \qquad \cos \Psi = \frac{\mathbf{k}_i \cdot \mathbf{k}_s}{|\mathbf{k}_i||\mathbf{k}_s|}$$

and Ψ is the angle between the incident and scattered waves.

The scattered wave is a function of the scattered wave vector $\mathbf{K}$ and the scattering angle Ψ. It is convenient to express both the incident and scattered wave vectors in polar coordinates, with the coordinate system defined such that one of the axes coincides with the incident wave. There will be four angles that uniquely define the geometry of the situation. The angles ϕ_s, θ_s are the azimuth and elevation of the scattered wave, and are the scattering angles (Figure 6.2). Ψ is related to ϕ_s, θ_s. For example, if the y axis coincides with $\mathbf{k}_i$:

$$\cos \Psi = (\cos \phi_s \sin \theta_s) \tag{6.16}$$

The angles ϕ_i, θ_i represent the orientation of the scatterer relative to the incident wave, and are the polar coordinates of the incident wave vector $\mathbf{k}_i$ relative to a set of axes embedded in the scatterer.

Thus $\mathbf{K}$ is a function of $|k_i|$ and the angles ϕ_s, θ_s. One scattering measurement will give a single value of $[\beta(\mathbf{K}) + \rho(\mathbf{K}) \cos \Psi]$. The functions $\beta(\mathbf{K})$ and $\rho(\mathbf{K})$ will themselves depend on ϕ_i, θ_i [equations (6.13) and (6.14)].

It is possible to draw some conclusions from this result. First, if the density and compressibility fluctuations are sufficiently small and random, then $|\beta(\mathbf{K})|$ and $|\rho(\mathbf{K})|$ will be constant over a significant range of $\mathbf{K}$; the scattered amplitude will have a k^2 dependence, and hence the intensity (or cross-section, cf. Section 6.2.5) will have a k^4 (or f^4) dependence. This is

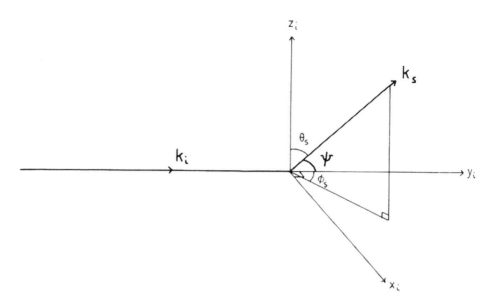

Figure 6.2. Scattering angles used in Section 6.2.1, where ϕ_s and θ_s are the polar coordinates of the scattering vector $\mathbf{k}_s$ relative to $\mathbf{k}_i$. The coordinate system is defined such that $\mathbf{k}_i$ is coincident with the y-axis. There is a similar set of axes, not shown, embedded in the scatterer that define the orientation of the incident wave $\mathbf{k}_i$ relative to the scatterer, giving two angles ϕ_i and θ_i

known as a Rayleigh dependence, and is common to many fields of scattering where the scatterers are much smaller than the wavelength of the incident wave.

The angular dependence is determined by the spatial fluctuations of the compressibility and density. If the compressibility fluctuations are isotropic then they give isotropic scattering. Isotropic density fluctuations give dipole scattering, concentrated in the forward and backward directions. The assumption is often made that density fluctuations can be ignored relative to fluctuations in compressibility. However, if this were the case, then the intensity scattered back to the transducer ($\Psi = \pi$) would be similar to that scattered at right angles ($\Psi = \pi/2$). The experimental findings discussed in Section 6.3.3 indicate that density fluctuations are not in fact negligible.

To obtain the function $[\beta(\mathbf{K}) + \rho(\mathbf{K}) \cos \Psi]$ over a wide range of K values, measurements must be taken at a range of frequencies, to vary $|k_i|$, and angles, to vary (ϕ_s, θ_s). Then $\beta(\mathbf{r})$ and $\rho(\mathbf{r})$ can be reconstructed through Fourier transformation, a process generally known as inverse scattering or diffraction tomography (*cf.* Chapter 11). In many situations it is not possible to obtain all this information, and only a subset of $|k_i|$, ϕ_s, θ_s is available. For a pulse–echo system $\phi_s = 0$ and $\Psi = \pi$, and thus any backscattering measurement will only give information about $\beta(\mathbf{r}) - \rho(\mathbf{r})$. Furthermore, most parts of the body have a limited acoustic access window, limiting the range of scattering angles ϕ_s, θ_s.

Finally, the maximum frequency that may be used is limited by attenuation, which will limit the spatial resolution of $\rho(\mathbf{r})$ and $\beta(\mathbf{r})$. Thus the information about $\rho(\mathbf{r})$ and $\beta(\mathbf{r})$ obtainable from scattering measurements is restricted, and many experiments only measure some averaged parameter such as a scattering cross-section.

6.2.3 SCATTERING OF A PULSE

The scattering so far considered has been concerned with monochromatic incident waves, which give no axial resolution. The most useful instrument in medical ultrasound, the pulse–echo B-scanner, uses a wideband pulse and records the time variation of echoes. This section examines the theory and properties of the backscattered signal obtained with a conventional pulse–echo instrument. For this, we need to derive the tissue impulse response.

If the solution for a monochromatic incident wave is known, then the solution for a broadband pulse of finite width can be obtained by superimposing the correct Fourier components. The approach given here, however, is a direct one, in some respects similar to that taken in Chapter 1 (Section 6.2; see also Gore & Leeman 1977), except that the solution is in the time domain and the effect of the receiving transducer is included.

The scattered wave is given by equation (6.8a), which can be rewritten:

$$P_s(\mathbf{r}, t) = \int_{-\infty}^{\infty} dt_0 \int_V \{\nabla P_i(\mathbf{r}_0, t_0) \cdot \nabla \tilde{\rho}(\mathbf{r}_0) + \nabla^2 P_i(\mathbf{r}_0, t_0)[\tilde{\rho}(\mathbf{r}_0) + \tilde{\beta}(\mathbf{r}_0)]\} G(\mathbf{r}_0, \mathbf{r}; t_0, t) d^3\mathbf{r}_0$$

$$(6.8b)$$

The received signal, or A-scan $V(t)$, is given by the integral of the backscattered pressure over the transducer face $S(r)$. For convenience let the transducer be placed at the origin (Figure 6.3), then:

$$V(t) = \int_S P_s(\mathbf{r}, t) dS \qquad (6.17)$$

The incident pressure wave, P_i, is produced by the same transducer and is given by the following expression [see Chapter 1, equation (1.67); also Stephanishen 1970], known as the Rayleigh's integral

$$P_i(\mathbf{r}, t) = \int_S \frac{a_n(t - |\mathbf{r} - \eta|/c)}{4\pi|\mathbf{r} - \eta|} dS(\eta) \qquad (6.18)$$

where $a_n(t)$ is the acceleration of the piston, assuming a plane piston in an infinite baffle. Inserting these into equation (6.8b) gives:

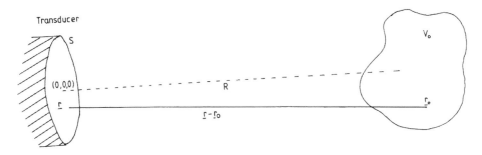

Figure 6.3. Geometry used in the pulse–echo calculations of Section 6.2.3

$$V(t) = \int_{s(r)} dS \int_{-\infty}^{\infty} dt_0 \int_{V_0} \left\{ \nabla\tilde{\rho}(\mathbf{r}_0) \cdot \nabla \int_{S(\eta)} \frac{a_n(t - |\mathbf{r}_0 - \eta|/c)}{4\pi|\mathbf{r}_0 - \eta|} dS(\eta) + [\tilde{\rho}(\mathbf{r}_0) + \tilde{\beta}(\mathbf{r}_0)]\nabla^2 \right.$$

$$\left. \times \int_{S(\eta)} \frac{a_n(t - |\mathbf{r}_0 - \eta|/c)}{4\pi|\mathbf{r}_0 - \eta|} dS(\eta) \right\} G(\mathbf{r}_0, \mathbf{r}; t_0, t) d^3\mathbf{r}_0 \qquad (6.19)$$

This is a sum of two terms, each of which will be considered separately.

Inserting the Green's function into the first term and performing the t_0 integration, we obtain

$$\int_{V_0} \left\{ \nabla\tilde{\rho}(\mathbf{r}_0) \cdot \nabla \int_{S(r)} dS(r) \int_{S(\eta)} \frac{a_n(t - |\mathbf{r}_0 - \eta|/c - |\mathbf{r} - \mathbf{r}_0|/c)}{(4\pi)^2|\mathbf{r}_0 - \eta||\mathbf{r} - \mathbf{r}_0|} dS(\eta) \right\} d^3\mathbf{r}_0 \qquad (6.20)$$

Now the term

$$q(\mathbf{r}, t) = \int_{S(r)} dS(r) \int_{S(\eta)} \frac{a_n(t - |\mathbf{r}_0 - \eta|/c - |\mathbf{r} - \mathbf{r}_0|/c)}{(4\pi)^2|\mathbf{r}_0 - \eta||\mathbf{r} - \mathbf{r}_0|} dS(\eta) \qquad (6.21)$$

is the pulse–echo response from a point reflector at a position $\mathbf{r}_0$, and can also be expressed as

$$q(\mathbf{r}, t) = a(t)*H(\mathbf{r}, t)*H(\mathbf{r}, t) \qquad (6.22)$$

where $*$ represents convolution with t, and $H(\mathbf{r}, t)$ is the impulse response of the transducer [see Chapter 1; equation (1.78)]. In the notation used here

$$H(\mathbf{r}, t) = \int_S \frac{\delta(t - |\mathbf{r} - \eta|/c)}{4\pi|\mathbf{r} - \eta|} dS(\eta) \qquad (6.23)$$

In the far field $q(\mathbf{r}, t)$ can be approximated using the beam profile/axial pulse description (cf. Section 1.6.5)

$$q(\mathbf{r}, t) \approx Q\left(t - \frac{2x}{c}, y, z\right) \qquad (6.24)$$

and expression (6.20) becomes

$$\int_{V_0} \left\{ \nabla\tilde{\rho}(\mathbf{r}_0) \cdot \left[\frac{1}{2}\frac{\partial^2}{\partial x_0^2} + \frac{\partial^2}{\partial y_0^2} + \frac{\partial^2}{\partial z_0^2}\right] Q\left(t - \frac{2x}{c}, y, z\right) \right\} d^3\mathbf{r}_0 \qquad (6.25)$$

or, after integration by parts

$$\int_{V_0} \left\{ Q\left(t - \frac{2x}{c}, y, z\right) \cdot \left[\frac{1}{2}\frac{\partial^2}{\partial x_0^2} + \frac{\partial^2}{\partial y_0^2} + \frac{\partial^2}{\partial z_0^2}\right] \tilde{\rho}(\mathbf{r}_0) \right\} d^3\mathbf{r}_0 \qquad (6.26)$$

A similar treatment of the second part of equation (6.19) gives

$$-\int_{V_0} \left\{ Q\left(t - \frac{2x}{c}, y, z\right) \cdot \left[\frac{1}{4}\frac{\partial^2}{\partial x_0^2} + \frac{\partial^2}{\partial y_0^2} + \frac{\partial^2}{\partial z_0^2}\right] [\tilde{\rho}(\mathbf{r}_0) + \beta(\mathbf{r}_0)] \right\} d^3\mathbf{r}_0 \qquad (6.27)$$

Combining the two terms gives

$$V(t) = \int\limits_{V_0} \left\{ Q\left(t - \frac{2x_0}{c}, y_0, z_0\right) T(x_0, y_0, z_0) \right\} \mathrm{d}^3 \mathbf{r}_0 \tag{6.28}$$

$$T(\mathbf{r}_0) = \frac{1}{4} \frac{\partial^2}{\partial x_0^2} [\tilde{\rho}(\mathbf{r}_0) - \beta(\mathbf{r}_0)] - \left[\frac{\partial^2}{\partial y_0^2} + \frac{\partial^2}{\partial z_0^2}\right] \beta(\mathbf{r}_0) \tag{6.29}$$

The backscattered image, or B-scan, is obtained from the A-scan by scanning the transducer. If a simple linear scanning geometry is considered, the transducer axis will remain parallel to the x-axis, and its position will be $(0, y, z)$. The A-scan will now be given by:

$$V(t, y, z) = \int\limits_{V_0} \left\{ Q\left(t - \frac{2x_0}{c}, y - y_0, z - z_0\right) T(x_0, y_0, z_0) \right\} \mathrm{d}^3 \mathbf{r}_0 \tag{6.30}$$

The A-scan $V(t)$ is converted to an image line $I(x)$ via the transformation $x = ct/2$, giving:

$$I(x, y, z) = \int\limits_{V_0} \left\{ Q\left(\frac{2x}{c} - \frac{2x_0}{c}, y - y_0, z - z_0\right) T(x_0, y_0, z_0) \right\} \mathrm{d}^3 \mathbf{r}_0 \tag{6.31}$$

Finally the actual A-scan displayed is a demodulated version of the raw A-scan, formed by rectifying and smoothing with a low pass filter $F(x)$:

$$I'(x, y, z) = \int |I(x', y, z)| F(x' - x) \mathrm{d}x' \tag{6.32}$$

The result expressed by equations (6.28) and (6.29) is important because it gives an expression for the B-scan in terms of a convolution between the transducer pulse–echo response Q and a tissue impulse response T. This suggests that the results of imaging theory and image enhancement can be applied to B-scans, and the B-scan can be related to the fundamental acoustic properties of the tissue.

The tissue impulse response T involves the second differential of the acoustic properties of the tissue, and unexpectedly contains terms involving variations in compressibility perpendicular to the propagation direction, such as $\partial^2\beta/\partial y^2$. This corresponds to 90° scatter due to a pressure gradient perpendicular to the transducer axis. For a beam of ultrasound there is such a perpendicular pressure gradient associated with the beam width, albeit small compared to the axial pressure gradient. No such term exists for the density term, because density fluctuations give dipole scattering, with no 90° component, whereas compressibility fluctuations cause monopole scattering.

6.2.4 SCATTERING FROM A SINGLE SPHERE

For simple geometrical shapes, it is possible to solve the wave equation to give explicit expressions for the scattering cross-sections. The exact solution for a spherical scatterer is known as Mie theory (Kerker 1969), and together with the theory for a cylindrical scatterer is covered by Morse and Ingard (1968, Chapter 8). Solutions for a limited range of other shapes do exist, but spheres and cylinders can approximate a wide range of scatterers found in biology. The solution of a spherical scatterer using the Born approximation will be outlined here.

Using equations (6.12)–(6.15):

$$f(\theta) = \int k_i^2[\tilde{\beta}(\mathbf{r}_0) + \tilde{\rho}(\mathbf{r}_0)\cos\theta]e^{i\mathbf{K}\cdot\mathbf{r}_0}d^3\mathbf{r}_0 \tag{6.33}$$

where $\mathbf{K} = \mathbf{k}_i - \mathbf{k}_s = 2k\sin\theta/2$. In this case it is convenient to define polar coordinates with the origin at the centre of the sphere and the z-axis pointing in the $\mathbf{K}$ direction:

$$\begin{aligned}
\tilde{\beta}(\mathbf{r}_0) &= \hat{\beta}; & \tilde{\rho}(\mathbf{r}_0) &= \hat{\rho}; & |\mathbf{r}_0| &\leqslant a \\
\tilde{\beta}(\mathbf{r}_0) &= 0; & \tilde{\rho}(\mathbf{r}_0) &= 0; & |\mathbf{r}_0| &> a
\end{aligned} \tag{6.34}$$

$$f = \int_0^a \int_0^{2\pi} \int_0^\pi [\hat{\beta} + \hat{\rho}\cos\theta]e^{i2K(\sin\theta/2\cos\theta)s}s^2\sin\theta\,d\theta\,d\phi\,ds \tag{6.35}$$

$$= 2\pi \int_0^a s^2[\hat{\beta} + \hat{\rho}\cos\theta] \int_{-1}^{+1} e^{is\mu\alpha}d\alpha ds \tag{6.36}$$

$$\mu = 2k_s\sin\theta/2; \qquad \alpha = \cos\theta \tag{6.37}$$

$$= k^2\frac{4\pi}{\mu^3}[\sin\mu a - \mu a\cos\mu a][\hat{\beta} + \hat{\rho}\cos\theta] \tag{6.38}$$

in the small scatterer limit $\mu a \to 0$

$$f \to 4\pi[\hat{\beta} + \hat{\rho}\cos\theta]k^2 V \tag{6.39}$$

and the scattering is isotropic if there are no density fluctuations. V is the volume of the sphere. The scattered power is proportional to $k_i^4 V^2$.

The angular distribution of the scattered power is shown in Figure 6.4 for a range of values of k_i. Here the scattering is not incoherent, as it is proportional to V^2, not V.

6.2.5 COLLECTIONS OF SCATTERERS: DIFFRACTION THEORY

If the scattering volume contains a collection of scatterers, then the waves scattered by each will interfere, and the overall scattering will depend on the configuration of the set of scatterers. In particular if there is some degree of regularity in that configuration, this will have some specific influence on that behaviour. To model this in a first approximation, we can consider N scatterers in a volume, giving (ignoring multiple scattering) a scattering distribution:

$$F(\theta,\ \phi) = f(\theta,\ \phi)\sum_{i=1}^N e^{i\mathbf{k}\cdot\mathbf{r}_i} \tag{6.40}$$

where

$$f(\theta,\ \phi) = k^2 \int [\hat{\beta} + \hat{\rho}\cos\theta]e^{i\mathbf{k}\cdot\mathbf{r}}d^3r \tag{6.41}$$

is the single scatterer response.

If the scatterers are arranged in a three-dimensional lattice, then

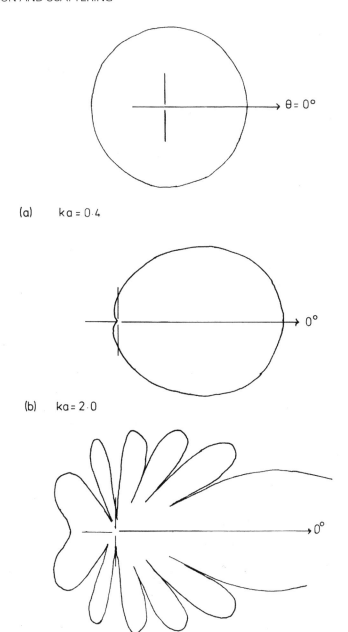

(a)   ka = 0.4

(b)   ka = 2.0

(c)   ka = 10.0   log scale

Figure 6.4. Polar plots of the differential scattering cross-section for a sphere, using the Born approximation, for three different values of *ka*. Note that for *ka* = 10.0 a log scale is used

$$\mathbf{r}_i = l\mathbf{a} + m\mathbf{b} + n\mathbf{c} \tag{6.42}$$

l, m, n are integers, $\mathbf{a}$, $\mathbf{b}$, $\mathbf{c}$ are repeat vectors.

$$F(\theta, \phi) = f(\theta, \phi) \sum_{l=1}^{L} \sum_{m=1}^{M} \sum_{n=1}^{N} e^{i\mathbf{k}(l\mathbf{a} + m\mathbf{b} + n\mathbf{c})} \tag{6.43}$$

F will have maxima when $\mathbf{k} \cdot (l\mathbf{a} + m\mathbf{b} + n\mathbf{c}) = 2\pi.$integer.

The solutions of equation (6.43) are covered in texts on X-ray crystallography (e.g. Gay 1971), as is the inverse problem of inferring $\mathbf{a}$, $\mathbf{b}$ and $\mathbf{c}$ from $F(\theta, \phi)$.

In practice it is difficult to measure $F(\theta, \phi)$, as two transducers are required (Nassiri & Hill 1986a), but it is possible to obtain information from the backscattering cross-section (where $\theta = \pi$ and $\mathbf{K} = 2\mathbf{k}_i$). The dependence of $F(\pi)$ on the orientation of the array has been examined by Nicholas (1979), both theoretically and practically. He uses a narrow band of frequency, and his results will be discussed in Section 6.3.3. The dependence of backscattering on frequency and orientation has been examined theoretically by Koch (1982) for two-dimensional arrays with random perturbations about periodicity.

6.2.6 SCATTERING CROSS-SECTION

In order to be able to relate the above theoretical discussion to experimental observation, it is necessary to develop appropriate definitions for measured scattering parameters.

If a wave of intensity (energy flow per unit area) I is incident on a scatterer, then the total power scattered, S, will be proportional to I. The constant of proportionality is the *total scattering cross-section*, σ_s, which has dimensions of area:

$$\sigma_s = S/I \tag{6.44}$$

It is also possible to define a *differential cross-section* $\sigma_d(\phi_s, \theta_s)$. If $dS(\phi_s, \theta_s)$ is the total power scattered into a solid angle $d\Omega$ in angular direction (ϕ_s, θ_s), then

$$\sigma_d(\phi_s, \theta_s) = \lim_{d\Omega \to 0} \frac{dS(\phi_s, \theta_s)}{I d\Omega} \tag{6.45}$$

One such differential cross-section is the *backscattering cross-section*

$$\sigma_{bs} = \sigma_d(0, \pi) \tag{6.46}$$

The *absorption cross-section* is defined as the total power removed from the incident beam per unit incident flux, and converted to heat at the site of removal:

$$\sigma_a = \text{Power absorbed}/I \tag{6.47}$$

The *attenuation cross-section* is the total power removed from the incident flux by both scattering and absorption:

$$\sigma_t = \sigma_s + \sigma_a \tag{6.48}$$

These definitions of cross-sections apply to any scatterer in a uniform plane wave, and apply equally to single objects and ensembles of scatterers. For certain media, where the scatterers are randomly positioned and the volume contains sufficient scatterers, the power scattered will be proportional to the volume of the media, and the scattering is termed incoherent (Foldy 1945). Then a measure of the scattering of an ensemble can be defined as the scattering cross-section per unit volume, called the scattering coefficient μ_s, with units of m^{-1}. In a similar way a differential scattering coefficient μ_d, backscattering coefficient μ_{bs}, absorption coefficient μ_a, and attenuation coefficient μ_t can be defined. It should be stressed that these coefficients are meaningful only for media that scatter incoherently.

If a wave of intensity $I(x)$ and area A are incident on a slab, of thickness dx, of incoherently scattering material, then the total power removed between x and $x + dx$ is given by:

$$dW = \mu_t I(x) A dx \tag{6.49}$$

This reduction in intensity is $dI = -dW/A$, giving

$$I(x) = I_0 e^{-\mu_t x} \tag{6.50}$$

assuming that energy removed from the incident wave is not returned to it by multiple scattering processes. The scattering cross-section can be calculated from the scattered pressure.

The most convenient geometry for scattering experiments is to measure the pressure in the far-field of the scatterer where the scattered wave can be expressed as a spherical wave, as in equation (6.15):

$$P_s = \frac{f(\theta, \phi) p_0 e^{i(\omega t - kr)}}{4\pi r} \tag{6.51}$$

The intensity of this wave is $P^2/\rho c$ so the rate of energy lost from a volume V is

$$W_{scat} = \int_S \frac{|P_s|^2}{\rho c} dS \tag{6.52}$$

where S is a surface enclosing the volume

$$W_{scat} = \frac{p_0^2}{\rho c} \int |f(\theta, \phi)|^2 \sin \theta \, d\theta \, d\phi \tag{6.53}$$

The scattering coefficient is given by this expression, normalised to the incident intensity, $p_0^2/\rho c$, and scattering volume V:

$$\mu_s = \frac{1}{V} \int |f(\theta, \phi)|^2 \sin \theta \, d\theta \, d\phi \tag{6.54}$$

and

$$\mu_d(\theta, \phi) = \frac{1}{V} |f(\theta, \phi)| \tag{6.55}$$

For the Born approximation as used in Section 6.2.2, the total scattering cross-section is given by (see 6.15)

$$\mu_s = \frac{1}{V} \int \{k_i^2[\beta(\mathbf{k}) + \rho(\mathbf{k}) \cos \psi]\}^2 d\phi \sin \theta \, d\theta \tag{6.56}$$

Each of the scattering cross-sections is so far only defined for a particular orientation of the scattering medium ϕ_i, θ_i. However, because the cross-section is an average scattering parameter, it is appropriate to average the cross-sections over a number of orientations, according to the symmetry of the scatterer. Thus, for an isotropic tissue such as liver, we can average over all angles:

$$\mu_d(\theta_s, \phi_s) = \langle \mu_d(\theta_s, \phi_s, \theta_i, \phi_i) \rangle_{\theta_i, \phi_i} \tag{6.57}$$

For a tissue with cylindrical symmetry, such as muscle, it is appropriate to define two sets of scattering cross-sections, one where the incident wave is parallel to the muscle fibres and one where it is perpendicular to the fibres.

In addition there are some other averaged cross-sections which are amenable to experimental measurement, and these are discussed in the next section.

6.3 SCATTERING MEASUREMENTS

6.3.1 EXPERIMENTAL METHODS

The scattering cross-sections of importance have been defined in Section 6.2.6, and it is one of the aims of scattering experiments to measure these cross-sections independently of the method or equipment. The scattering cross-section, in addition to being a function of the two scattering angles, ϕ_s, θ_s, is also a function of both the orientation of the sample, ϕ_i, θ_i, and the ultrasonic frequency. It is possible to define a number of scattering cross-sections derived from this by averaging over one or more of the angles mentioned, and these cross-sections can then be identified with a particular measurement geometry. A measurement of particular importance is the backscattering cross-section averaged over tissue orientation, and this can be defined as:

$$\langle \mu_d(0, \pi, \theta_i, \phi_i) \rangle_{\theta_i, \phi_i}$$

Scattering measurements are made either with one transducer, for backscattering measurements, or with two for other geometries. A pulse is emitted and the received echo train gated so that the scattering volume is defined by the intersection of the two beams (*cf.* Figure 2.1), and is a complicated function of gate length, pulse length and beam width (Nassiri & Hill 1986a). The emitted pulse may be a tone-burst or a wide-band pulse, in which latter case the received signal must be spectrum analysed to yield the scattered power as a function of frequency. Sigelmann and Reid (1973) discuss the use of tone-burst signals to measure ultrasound backscattering, and also the use of substitution methods, in which signals are compared with those from a known target such as a plane reflector. Indeed, many scattering measurements are still reported in terms of decibels relative to a specified plane reflecting interface. The reference plane reflector should be placed at the same distance from the transducer as the scatterer, and both should be in the far-field of the transducer in order to minimise problems with phase cancellation.

There are two intrinsic sources of error in scattering measurements. The first arises as a trade-off between spatial and frequency resolution. If the gate time is τ, giving a spatial resolution of $c\tau/2$ for $180°$ scattering, then the frequency spectrum will be convolved by sinc $\pi f \tau$, limiting the frequency resolution to $1/\tau$.

The second source of error arises from phase cancellation at the receiving transducer. The cross-section is expressed in terms of the scattered intensity, whereas most piezoelectric transducers are phase-sensitive: any phase fluctuations across the transducer aperture, due to the inhomogeneities in the tissue or other propagation medium, will result in underestimation of the received intensity, and thus of the cross-section. The magnitude of the error can be reduced by performing measurements in the far-field of the transducer, so that the scattered wave is approximately plane over a small aperture. Using a small receiving transducer, such as a hydrophone, will also reduce the error, as will the use of a phase-insensitive transducer

(Busse *et al.* 1997), although this is less feasible for backscattering than for attenuation measurements (Chapter 4).

Further practical problems in scattering come from the requirement to normalise the scattering to the volume, which involves a complex calculation of the three-dimensional size of the interrogating pulse. There is also the need to average over tissue configurations; this requires, first, an estimate of the number of data points that are required to give results which are representative of an individual specimen and, second, an estimate of the number of specimens required for the measurements to be representative of the whole tissue type. The relative contribution of coherent and incoherent scattering varies with the wide range of scattering structures in the tissue, and this has to be considered in making these estimates.

Transmitting transducers are frequently driven by large pulses, in order to improve the signal-to-noise ratio in scattering measurements. Non-linear propagation of the large transmitting wave, and of the reference wave reflected from a strong reflector, can both introduce errors in the scattering measurements. Further sources of error are uncertainty in the extent of attenuation by overlying tissue (Sigelmann & Reid 1973; Madsen 1993) and non-linearity of the receiving electronics.

Most scattering studies are carried out *ex vivo* with the view of extrapolating the results back to *in vivo* conditions. Preliminary studies on the changes in tissue scattering after death have identified significant changes (Patel 1996; Bamber *et al.* 1979). Initial changes are attributed to loss of blood circulation and consequent collapse of blood pressure and loss of tissue structure. Later changes are attributed to bubble formation and tissue degradation. Such changes are highly dependent on the method of tissue preparation, such as whether the tissue has been degassed by application of a vacuum, and on the nature of any histological fixation procedure that has been used. The presence of gas bubbles, which are highly scattering, is a major source of error in tissue measurements, and these must be removed as far as possible.

The rest of this section looks at some features of the scattering cross-section from tissue and the conclusions that may be drawn from them.

6.3.2 FREQUENCY DEPENDENCE OF SCATTERING

In Section 6.4.3 the frequency dependence of scattering is shown to be dependent on the ratio of the wavelength λ to the correlation distance $\hat{a}$ of the medium. For small $\hat{a}/\lambda$ the scattering cross-section has an f^4 dependence; as $\hat{a}/\lambda$ becomes large the total cross-section approaches an f^2 dependence, whereas the backscattering cross-section decreases as $f^2 e^{-k\hat{a}}$. Thus for a single correlation length $\hat{a}$, the backscattering cross-section will not have a simple frequency dependence. Where this is written as $\mu_{bs} \propto f^m$ and plotted on a log–log scale, the gradient m can be expected to decrease with frequency (Figure 6.5a).

A number of workers have measured the frequency dependence of the backscattering cross-section of liver, and all report similar findings, that m increases monotonically with frequency from $m = 0$ at 1 MHz to 3 at 10 MHz (Bamber 1979a,b) (Figure 6.5a). This suggests that a simple model with two or three correlation lengths must be invoked. For example, liver cells of dimensions 20 µm and the liver lobules (1 mm) represent structures of a different $\hat{a}$ which give the requisite frequency dependence, with larger inhomogeneities such as blood vessels giving a better fit at lower frequencies.

This postulate is one of the many that give a reasonable prediction of observed frequency dependence (*cf.* Figure 6.6). Figure 6.5b illustrates the behaviour of a possible model with three correlation lengths, showing that a judicious choice of their values and corresponding r.m.s. amplitudes [$\hat{a}$ and $\langle \beta \rangle^2$ in equation (6.66)] can give a frequency dependence of scattering

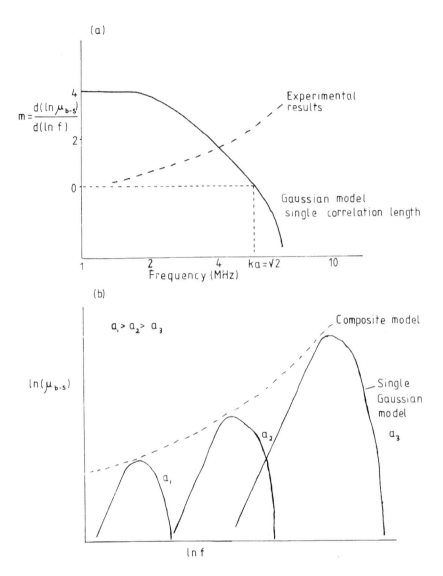

Figure 6.5. Backscattering as a function of frequency for the inhomogeneous continuum model (see Section 6.4.3). (a) Power law dependence of backscattering vs. frequency; observed results and those predicted from tissue with a Gaussian auto-correlation function. (b) Frequency dependence of backscattering for a hypothetical composite model with three levels of structure

that matches the experimental results. A large number of other models could also fit the experimental data. Nicholas (1982) finds that a two-term exponential auto-correlation function fits his experimental data better than the Gaussian, with correlation lengths of similar dimensions, and he also discusses other models.

At higher frequencies, in the range 35–65 MHz, the frequency dependence of scattering from the arterial wall is observed to be between $f^{1.1}$ and $f^{1.4}$ (Lockwood *et al.* 1991). This lower frequency dependence suggests that the ultrasound wavelength is approaching the size of the tissue inhomogeneities.

It is possible to remove the mean trends from the scattering spectrum and examine the residual fluctuations. The periodicities in a spectrum can be examined by a number of techniques including cepstral analysis and correlation analysis (Jones & Kovac 1980). It can be shown that a periodic structure in the spectrum can be related to regular scattering structures, and such periodicities have been observed in spectra from the retina (Lizzi & Coleman 1977; see also Chapter 9) and the liver (Joynt & Sommer 1980). There is evidence, however, that such periodicities in the frequency spectrum are only meaningful for very regular structures (Koch 1982); and a completely random structure will give fluctuations in the scattered spectrum which depend primarily on the bandwidth of the interrogating pulse.

6.3.3 ORIENTATION DEPENDENCE OF SCATTERING

The dependence of backscattering on orientation, $\mu_{bs}(\theta_i, \phi_i)$, has been investigated by Nicholas (1979) who finds for liver a periodicity characteristic of a semi-regular structure with a spacing of the order of 1 mm, and that abnormal liver gives an orientation dependence different from that for normal liver (Waag *et al.* 1976). Nassiri and Hill (1986b) have investigated the angular dependence of scattering in three rather different tissues, liver, skeletal muscle and blood, and have concluded that the scale of structure responsible for scattering in each case is of the order of 55, 74 and 6.0 μm respectively. They also find that the relative magnitude of spatial variation of density in the tissues is comparable to that for compressibility, thus indicating that both variables may need to be taken into account in order to provide a satisfactory understanding of scattering behaviour.

In summary, both the frequency and angular dependence of scattering can provide information on the structure responsible for scattering. Most of the experiments have been performed on liver tissue, and suggest that a range of structures is responsible. The aim of fundamental work on scattering – to completely deduce the tissue structure from the scattered wave, and to localise and characterise the abnormal structures – still remains a long way off. The experimental evidence available concentrates on the frequency range 1–10 MHz, and thus characterises structures on a scale commensurate with the wavelengths in this frequency range, and for a complete scattering description a wider range of frequencies must be employed.

6.3.4 RELATIONSHIP BETWEEN TOTAL SCATTERING CROSS-SECTION AND ATTENUATION

Attenuation consists of two components, energy redirected or scattered, and the energy absorbed and converted to heat (Chapter 4). It is instructive to try to estimate the relative contributions of the two mechanisms, although, as will be seen, very few relevant experimental data are available. In principle it is possible to measure the total attenuation using equation (6.50), and in practice measurements are available to an accuracy of 10%, but the total scattering cross-section and the absorption cross-section are very difficult to measure.

Very few direct measurements of the total cross-section are available. Gramiak *et al.* (1976) and Nassiri and Hill (1986a) have reported on methods of measuring the differential cross-section as a function of angle. The problem in using these results to estimate the total scattering cross-section is that the forward scattering cannot be measured for angles less than 60° in most experimental arrangements, so the result is sensitive to the extrapolation used to estimate the forward scattering. Since some experiments suggest that forward scattering is large, this produces a large error in the total scattering cross-section. The situation is further complicated by the need to correct the measured angular scattering for the changing scattering volume. Nassiri tentatively suggests that, for some tissues, the ratio μ_s/μ_{bs} is in excess of 20, and thus greater than the value of 4π obtained if the scattering is isotropic. There is a further uncertainty due to the spread in measured values of μ_{bs} and μ_a and this puts an upper limit on μ_s/μ_t of $\sim 40\%$ at 1 MHz, but a more accurate estimate is not possible from these data.

The experimental measurement of the backscattering cross-section is much simpler, and it may be possible to relate the scattering coefficient to the attenuation coefficient by observing changes in μ_s and μ_a when the tissue is modified in some way. The significant assumption made is that the absorption and the angular scattering distribution are unchanged by the modification, which is a reasonable assumption if the modification does not affect the spatial distribution of the tissue components, although it may affect the amplitude of density and compressibility variations.

So

$$\mu_{bs} \propto \mu_s, \quad \text{hence:} \quad \delta\mu_{bs}/\delta\mu_t = \mu_s/\mu_t \qquad (6.58)$$

One such change employed by Bamber (1979a) to satisfy such conditions is autolysis, where the backscattering coefficient decreases rapidly with time by up to 95%, whereas the attenuation coefficient decreases by less than 15%, giving $\mu_s/\mu_t < 16\%$. The effects of temperature and fixation have also been investigated (Bamber et al. 1979), but the absorption coefficient is likely to change with these modifications. Pauly and Schwan (1971) have measured the change in attenuation coefficient with homogenisation of liver, which will remove most, but not all, of the scattering structures, again indicating values for μ_s/μ_t in the range 10–20% for liver (Hill et al. 1978). Polkhammer and O'Brien (1981) have measured the total scattering cross-section as the difference between the attenuation and absorption coefficients. This method will be subject to a large error due to the effect of experimental errors on the measured attenuation and absorption coefficients.

In summary, there are a number of methods of estimating the total scattering cross-section; all of them are unsatisfactory, and it is not possible to give an accurate value of μ_s/μ_t with present experimental data.

One tissue where a considerable amount of scattering data is available is blood. The small size of red blood cells relative to the ultrasonic wavelength enables them to be approximated by spheres with the same volume. Ahuja (1972) has derived an expression for their scattering cross-section including the effect of viscosity, and shows the scattering cross-section to be much less than the viscous absorption cross-section. The effect of the haematocrit on scattering is considered by Shung et al. (1976); the scattering cross-section per particle is constant for haematocrits below 8%, and decreases for higher haematocrits, suggesting that multiple scattering may be involved. The cross-section agrees well with the theoretical predictions of Ahuja and Hedee (1977), who also show that at frequencies less than 10 MHz the scattering has a Rayleigh frequency dependence. In a later paper Shung et al. (1977) measure the differential cross-section, and show that the theory of Ahuja (1972) fits the data better than does that of Morse and Ingard (1968), which does not include viscosity.

Measurements at frequencies in the range 35–65 MHz show a frequency dependence of scattering by blood in the range $f^{1.3}$–$f^{1.4}$ (Lockwood et al. 1991). At these frequencies the wavelength (50–25 μm) is approaching the size of the blood cells. The scattering from blood can be observed directly in 30 MHz intravascular ultrasound images and de Kroon et al. (1991) report that scattering level varies during the cardiac cycle, suggesting that there is some degree of higher structure associated with aggregation of groups of blood cells. The agreement between experiment and theory for blood is due to the simple two-phase structure of blood, which enables simple, accurate theoretical models to be used. Other tissues have a much more complex structure, and this sort of analysis has not yet been done.

6.3.5 EFFECT OF DIFFERENT TISSUE CONSTITUENTS

A full characterisation of the size and arrangement of scattering structures may not be required in a clinical situation, where an empirical correlation between scattering cross-sections and tissue components may be sufficient to make a diagnosis. A number of workers have examined the dependence of the scattering properties on different tissue components and on the tissue pathology. For example, Freese and Lyons (1977) find a good correlation between the backscattering and percentage fat content, which is not surprising when the abnormal sound speed in fat is considered (*cf.* Chapter 5). Bamber *et al.* (1981) have found a strong negative correlation with water concentration, which can be considered to dilute the concentration of other tissue components. This is one example of the complex interdependence of the many tissue components in their effect on backscattering, that is also discussed in this chapter. Collagen is often suggested as a major contributor to scattering (e.g. Polkhammer & O'Brien 1981). The effect of different pathologies on scattering coefficients has undergone even less investigation, despite the fact that it is used in B-scan diagnosis. The evidence so far suggests that, at least in the liver, solid tumours scatter less than normal tissue (Bamber & Hill 1981), whereas diffusely diseased tissues scatter more, but there is wide variance on all the values, and more data are required.

In summary, the contributions to our knowledge of the acoustic structure of tissues from measurements of scattering are limited to some indications of the size of the scatterers and to the effect of certain tissue components on the scattering. It does not yet include information on the effect of the spatial arrangement of those components on the scattering properties.

A special case of experimentally observable scattering behaviour arises where tissues have been perfused with microbubble-based contrast media. Here very strong scattering, and associated attenuation, can arise with associated markedly non-linear behaviour. The latter is related to bubble oscillation and resonance, and can lead to strongly frequency-dependent scattering behaviour, with consequent observable shifts in mean frequency of scattered energy relative to that of the interrogating beam (Uhlendorf 1994; Wang *et al.* 1996).

6.3.6 COMPENDIA OF RESULTS

Probably as a result of the experimental problems outlined above, the published data on backscattering coefficients, and on their dependence on factors such as frequency and scattering angle, exhibit considerable differences between the results reported by different authors. Summaries of the available data have been compiled by Duck (1990) and Shung (1993); the latter in some detail.

In Figure 6.6 are plotted some examples of data that have been reported on the absolute values of backscattering coefficients (defined as the power backscattered per unit solid angle, per unit incident intensity and per unit volume of scatterers). These data do illustrate a number of interesting points; the large differences in absolute values as between different tissues, the very close approximation to Rayleigh (fourth power dependence on frequency) behaviour of blood; and the lower, but apparently variable, power dependence of the solid tissues.

Figure 6.7 shows experimental data, with theoretical extrapolations, for dependence on scattering angle. Here blood is seen to be a predominant backscatterer, whilst the solid tissues tend towards forward scattering. As has been discussed in Section 6.2.2, this is a result that can

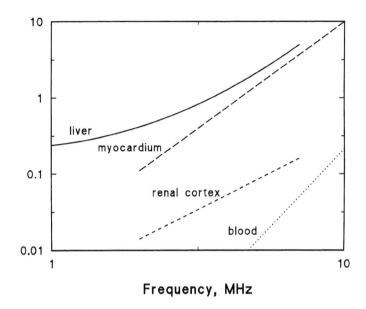

Frequency, MHz

Figure 6.6 Examples of published data on frequency dependence of the backscattering coefficients of various post-mortem mammalian tissues, displayed in units of cm^{-1} $steradian^{-1} \times 10^{-3}$. *Source*: From Shung (1993); reproduced by permission of CRC Press

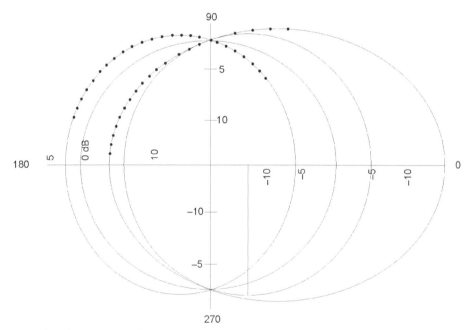

Figure 6.7 Measured data, with corresponding theoretical fits, for the dependence on scattering angle of the scattering coefficient at 6 MHz. Liver, solid line; skeletal muscle, $- - -$; blood, $\cdots$. *Source*: From Nassiri and Hill (1986a), reproduced by permission of the Acoustical Society of America

be understood in terms of the tissue-specific differences in relative contributions of density and compressibility to the scattering behaviour (Nassiri & Hill 1986b).

6.4 MODELS

6.4.1 USE OF MODELS

As we have already seen, tissue is a complex medium whose acoustic properties on a small scale are yet to be measured; to attempt to understand scattering from tissue it is useful to consider certain simple theoretical models. Although some tissues do have a repetitive structure, for example skeletal muscle which consists of a hexagonal array of cylindrical fibrils, no tissue has a perfectly regular structure, and most tissues have a structure somewhere between the two extremes of perfect periodicity and complete randomness. The regular structures can be dealt with using diffraction theory. Two useful models of random structures will be discussed here.

6.4.2 DISCRETE SCATTERING MODEL

This model views the random medium as a number of discrete scatterers embedded at random positions in a homogeneous substrate. The scatterers do not have to be identical, but they must all be small compared to the wavelength. The scattering is given by the superposition of the scattered waves from each individual scatterer. The approach was initiated by Foldy (1945), who introduced the concepts of coherence and incoherence. For any fixed configuration of scatterers, all of the scattering is temporally coherent, but can be divided into coherent and incoherent scattering according to the effect of configurational changes. The coherent part, P_c, is given by the ensemble average of the wave field over different configurations, $\langle P \rangle$, and Foldy shows that it obeys a homogeneous wave equation with the propagation velocity modified by the presence of scatterers, and so will not contribute to the scattered wave. The incoherent part, P_{inc}, is the fluctuating part over different configurations, and is the part that contributes to scattering. Thus (Ishimaru 1978, p. 78)

$$\langle P^2 \rangle = P_c + P_{inc}; \quad \langle P \rangle = P_c \quad \text{and} \quad \langle P^2 \rangle = [\langle P_c \rangle]^2 + \langle [P_{inc}]^2 \rangle \tag{6.59}$$

$$P_{inc}(r, t) = F(\theta, \phi)e^{i(kr-\omega t)} \tag{6.60}$$

$$F(\theta, \phi) = \sum_{n=1}^{N} f_n(\theta, \phi)e^{i\mathbf{k}\cdot\mathbf{r_n}} \tag{6.61}$$

where $|f_n(\theta, \phi)|^2$ and $\mathbf{r_n}$ are the scattering cross-section and position of the nth scatterer. Because each scatterer is small, its scattering can be considered isotropic, hence $fn(\theta, \phi) = k_i^2 a_n$ [from equation (6.39)].

$F(\theta, \phi)$ is a random variable whose ensemble average is zero, and its statistics are discussed in Section 6.2.3 where scattering by a pulse is considered. The ensemble average (or incoherent) intensity is:

$$\langle |F(\theta, \phi)|^2 \rangle = k^4 \left\{ \sum_{n=1}^{N} a_n^2 \right\} \tag{6.62}$$

$$= k^4 N a^2$$

So the scattered intensity is proportional to N, and the scattering has a Rayleigh frequency dependence.

6.4.3 INHOMOGENEOUS CONTINUUM MODEL

In this model the medium is assumed to have small continuous fluctuations of density and compressibility about a constant mean, with a specified auto-correlation function. For such a medium the average incoherent scattering can be calculated. In the following discussion, for the sake of mathematical simplicity, the density is assumed constant, and only compressibility fluctuations are considered. The analysis follows that of Chernow (1960).

From equation (6.15)

$$P_s(\mathbf{r},\,t) = p_0 \frac{e^{i(\omega t - kr)}}{4\pi r} k^2 \beta(\mathbf{K}) \tag{6.63}$$

$P_s(\mathbf{r},\,t)$ and $\beta(\mathbf{K})$ are random functions, so considering their ensemble average

$$\langle |P_s(\mathbf{r})|^2 \rangle = \frac{k^4}{16\pi^2 |r|^2} \langle |\beta(\mathbf{K})|^2 \rangle \tag{6.64}$$

$$\langle |\beta(\mathbf{k})|^2 \rangle = \int_V N_\beta(\mathbf{r}) e^{i\mathbf{k}\cdot\mathbf{r}} d^3\mathbf{r} \tag{6.65}$$

If density fluctuations are included, then equation (6.64) becomes much more complicated, with cross-terms between density and compressibility, and obtaining an analytic solution is more difficult; but in principle the calculation is similar to that given.

N_β is the auto-correlation function of the compressibility fluctuations. Although other functions can be considered, this is often assumed to have a Gaussian form:

$$N_\beta(r) = \langle \beta \rangle^2 e^{-r^2/\hat{a}^2} \tag{6.66}$$

where $\hat{a}$ is the correlation distance.

Inserting (6.66) into equations (6.64) and (6.65) gives

$$\langle |P_s|^2 \rangle = \frac{A_0^2 k^4 \hat{a}^3}{16 r^2 \pi^{1/2}} \langle \beta^2 \rangle \exp\{-\tfrac{1}{4} k^2 \hat{a}^2 \sin^2 \Psi / 2\} \tag{6.67}$$

A number of observations can be made from this equation. For small-scale fluctuations ($k\hat{a} \ll 1$) the scattering is isotropic and proportional to k^4. For large-scale fluctuations the scattering is sharply directed in the forward direction, and most of the power is concentrated within a small solid angle $1/k\hat{a}$.

For no value of $k\hat{a}$ does the backscattered power intensity exceed that forward scattered, so this model is not valid for situations where this is the case, and an alternative model must be used (see Nassiri & Hill 1986a). Including density fluctuations would be one method of making the model more flexible, as would using a more complicated auto-correlation function, not necessarily isotropic. An important practical application of this approach to modelling is in deriving relationships between ultrasound speckle statistics and tissue microstructure (Rao & Zhu 1994). This topic will be considered in more detail in Section 6.5.2.

6.4.4 OTHER MODELS

Neither of the above models can be expected to provide fully satisfactory representations of real situations. In the important case of blood, for example, it appears that an appreciably more accurate description of scattering behaviour can be achieved by the use of a hybrid between the discrete and continuum models (Xu & Emmert 1997). At the same time, for some other tissues, some of the simplifying assumptions incorporated in the above basic models may be inappropriate. Scattering volumes may, for example, contain insufficient scatterers to justify the use of a Gaussian model, with resulting Rayleigh statistics, and indeed the echogenicity of scatterers within the volume may be quite non-uniform (Shankar 1995). Similarly, there is an important group of tissues whose mechanical structure, and thus scattering behaviour, can be strongly anisotropic (Insana & Brown 1993). Finally, a rather different approach to modelling that has been suggested is based on the hypothesis that the structure of some tissues is fractal in nature (Gan 1995).

6.4.5 IMPEDIOGRAPHY

In Chapter 1 the reflection coefficient for a plane wave normally incident on a plane interface is given by equation (1.103):

$$R = \frac{Z_1 - Z_0}{Z_1 + Z_0} \tag{6.68}$$

where Z_1 and Z_0 are the acoustic impedance of the media either side of the discontinuity $(Z = \rho c)$.

If the impedance is a continuous function $Z(x)$ with variations in one dimension only, then it can be treated as a series of small impedance steps. If the incident pulse can be considered as a plane wave, $p(t - x/c)$, and multiple reflections are ignored, then Chapter 1 [equation (1.112)] shows that the backscattered echo train $P_s(t)$ is given by

$$P_s(t) = \int p(t - 2x/c) R(x) \mathrm{d}x \tag{6.69}$$

where

$$R(x) = \frac{1}{2} \frac{\mathrm{d}}{\mathrm{d}x} \ln Z(x) \tag{6.70}$$

This method has been given the name 'impediography' or 'Raylography', and a more detailed treatment incorporating multiple reflections gives:

$$R(x) = \tan h(\tfrac{1}{2} \ln Z(x)) \tag{6.71}$$

The advantage of the impediography approach is that it relates the A-scan to acoustic properties via a convolution integral (Jones 1977) and much work has concentrated on methods of deconvolving equation (6.69) to obtain $R(x)$ (Herment *et al.* 1979). The method is most useful when the object consists of layered structures, such as in the eye, and there are some other *in vivo* applications of impediography (Jones 1977).

Impediography relates the backscattered A-scan to the tissue properties via equation (6.64), which is directly comparable to equation (6.29) in Section 6.2.3, which uses the tissue impulse response. For small fluctuations in density and compressibility, ρ and β, the reflection coefficient becomes:

$$R(x) = \frac{1}{4}\frac{d}{dx}[\hat{\beta}(x) - \hat{\rho}(x)] \tag{6.72}$$

This tissue impulse response is a single differential of the tissue properties, whereas the three-dimensional response [equation (6.29)] is a double differential. This is a direct consequence of the one-dimensional assumptions of the model. The following solution of the one-dimensional wave equation will demonstrate the similarities and differences between the two models.

The solution of the one-dimensional wave equation gives, for the backscattered pressure:

$$P_s(x,\ t) = -\int\int_0^t \left\{ \frac{d\hat{\rho}}{dx_0} \cdot \frac{dP_i(t_0 - x_0/c)}{dt} + [\hat{\rho}(x_0) + \hat{\beta}(x_0)]\frac{1}{c^2}\frac{d^2 P_i}{dt_0^2} \right\} g(x,\ x_0;\ t,\ t_0) dx_0 dt_0$$

$$g = c/2 \quad \text{when} \quad |x - x_0| < c(t - t_0) \tag{6.73}$$
$$= 0 \quad \text{when} \quad |x - x_0| > c(t - t_0)$$

g is the one-dimensional Green's function.
After inserting g and performing the t_0 integration

$$P_s(x,\ t) = -\int \left\{ \frac{d\hat{\rho}}{dx_0}\frac{1}{2}P_i\left(t + \frac{x}{c} - \frac{2x_0}{c}\right) + [\hat{\rho}(x_0) + \hat{\beta}(x_0)] \cdot \frac{1}{2c}\frac{dP_i\left(t + \frac{x}{c} - \frac{2x_0}{c}\right)}{dx_0} \right\} dx_0$$

$$\tag{6.74}$$

After integration of the second term by parts we obtain

$$P_s(x,\ t) = -\int P_i\left(t + \frac{x}{c} - \frac{2x_0}{c}\right)\frac{1}{4}\frac{d}{dx_0}[\hat{\rho}(x_0) - \hat{\beta}(x_0)]dx_0 \tag{6.75}$$

The impulse response obtained here is identical to that obtained by the method of impediography for small variations in ρ and β. Impediography, then, is a scattering model for tissue if it is a one-dimensional medium and is illuminated by a plane wave. If a three-dimensional structure is considered, then the correct treatment is via the tissue impulse response of equation (6.28). To accommodate the three-dimensional nature of ultrasound beams Leeman (1979) has suggested the use of an 'effective impedance' which includes the beam profile and is defined in Chapter 1 equation (1.106). This effective impedance will not be a unique function of the tissue's acoustic properties, but may be a useful parameter in characterising tissue. It should be observed that the impulse response for impediography is a single spatial differential, whereas the tissue impulse response for the three-dimensional case is a second differential. This is a consequence of the difference in solutions between the two wave equations, the one-dimensional Green's function, (6.73) is the integral of the equivalent three-dimensional Green's function (6.6).

An advantage the impediography approach has over the scattering theory of Section 6.2 is that it can deal with multiple scattering via equation (6.71). Impediography can be considered to be a useful bridge between the full-blooded scattering theory of Section 6.2 and simple reflection theory.

6.5   SCATTERING AND THE B-MODE IMAGE

6.5.1 MODELS OF THE B-MODE IMAGE

The expression for the B-scan image, derived in Section 6.2.3, allows its prediction from the tissue impulse response. The inverse solution, however, is difficult and in some cases impossible. One approach to the problem is to insert different tissue impulse responses and compare the resulting computed B-scans with those observed from real tissue (Bamber & Dickinson 1980).

As in Section 6.4, two simple models are common. The first, the discrete scatterer model, has a tissue impulse response $T(\mathbf{r})$ given by

$$T(\mathbf{r}) = \sum_{n=1}^{N} a_n \delta(\mathbf{r} - \mathbf{r}_n) \tag{6.76}$$

The demodulated B-scan of this model is given by

$$I(\mathbf{r}) = \left| \sum_{n=1}^{N} a_n Q(\mathbf{r} - \mathbf{r}_n) \right| \tag{6.77}$$

For a narrowband incident pulse, $Q(\mathbf{r}) \approx A(\mathbf{r})e^{2ik_0 x}$, where A is the pulse envelope and k_0 the centre frequency. At any point in the A-scan the echo amplitude will be a random function determined by the particular arrangement of scatterers within the resolution cell $A(\mathbf{r})$:

$$I(\mathbf{r}) = \left| \sum_{n=1}^{N} a_n(\mathbf{r} - \mathbf{r}_n)e^{2ik_0 x_n} \right| \tag{6.78}$$

This equation is identical to that governing laser speckle, the properties of which are reviewed by Goodman (1976). Laser speckle is formed when a rough surface is interrogated with a laser or other coherent wave such that individual scatterers cannot be resolved, but they interfere to give random fluctuations in intensity, of high contrast. If the same structure is illuminated with incoherent light, the reflections are averaged out to give a mean reflection of low contrast. The same situation arises in ultrasound when individual scatterers cannot be resolved, but because ultrasound is coherent they do interfere to give fluctuations in scattered intensity with position. The first-order statistics of I are given by the Rayleigh probability distribution $\Pi(I)$ (Burckhardt 1978):

$$\Pi(I) = \frac{I}{\langle I \rangle} e^{-I/\langle I \rangle} \tag{6.79}$$

The second-order statistics can be examined by taking the power spectrum of equation (6.78):

$$|I(\mathbf{k})| = N|A(\mathbf{k} - \mathbf{k}_0)|^2 \tag{6.80}$$

The power spectrum, and hence the spatial auto-correlation function, are determined only by the extent of the interrogating pulse, and are independent of the scatterer positions, as long as they are random and sufficiently numerous.

A computer simulation of a B-scan of tissue described by the discrete scatterer model of equation (6.30) is shown in Figure 6.8. It can be seen that the spatial structure bears no obvious relation to the original model. More important, the contrast of the scan is high, even though the structure is not resolved. The histogram of the received amplitude shows the expected Rayleigh distribution, and the ratio of the standard deviation to mean is 2. These properties will be discussed further after considering the inhomogeneous continuum model.

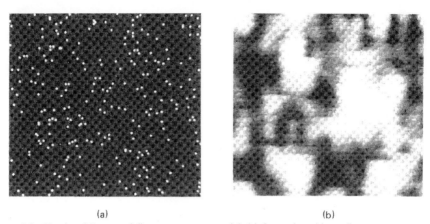

(a)   (b)

Figure 6.8. Simulated B-scan of discrete scatterer model. (a) Scattering object: discrete scatterer model. Mean spacing = 8 pixels. Image area = 128 × 128. (b) Simulated B-scan of (a). Pulse wavelength = 6.0, length = 8.0, beam width = 12.0

In using this model we shall again, for the sake of mathematical simplicity, assume that the density is constant; the compressibility is a random function of position with a specified auto-correlation function, in this case given by a Gaussian function $\exp(-r^2/\hat{a}^2)$. The tissue impulse response is then a second derivative of compressibility, as defined by equation (6.28). Figure 6.9 shows such a random tissue model, with its associated simulated B-scan, which is seen to be similar in appearance to the equivalent scan of the discrete scatterer model. This tissue model can be related to the discrete scatterer model in the following manner.

The tissue impulse response, $T(\mathbf{r})$ is a random variable constrained to have an auto-correlation function $T(\mathbf{r})$. The spatial power spectrum is given by $|T(\mathbf{k})|^2 = F(\tilde{N}_T(\mathbf{r}))$ where F is the Fourier operator, so

$$T(\mathbf{k}) = |F(\tilde{N}_T(\mathbf{r}))|^{1/2} \, e^{i\Phi(\mathbf{k})} \qquad (6.81)$$

where $\Phi(\mathbf{k})$ is a random variable uniformly distributed between 0 and 2π.

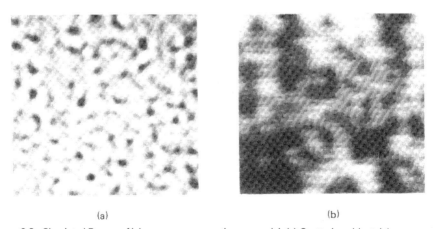

(a)   (b)

Figure 6.9. Simulated B-scan of inhomogeneous continuum model. (a) Scattering object; inhomogeneous continuum model. Gaussian auto-correlation function; correlation length = 6.0. (b) Simulated B-scan of (a); pulse parameters as in Figure 6.5(b)

The properties of the scan of such a model can be determined by considering the power spectrum. Combining (6.81) and (6.31) for a narrowband pulse ($Q(\mathbf{r}) \approx A(\mathbf{r})e^{2ik_0x}$) gives:

$$I(\mathbf{k}) = |T(\mathbf{k})|A(\mathbf{k} - \mathbf{k}_0)e^{i\Phi(\mathbf{k})} \tag{6.82}$$

If the width of the auto-correlation function is small compared to the ultrasonic wavelength and pulse size, then $|I(\mathbf{k})| \approx |A(\mathbf{k} - \mathbf{k}_0)|$, and comparison with equation (6.80) shows that the spatial structure of the two models is identical. The inhomogeneous continuum model thus does have similar properties to the discrete scatterer model for small correlation lengths, and can also model a range of different situations.

6.5.2 PROPERTIES OF THE B-MODE IMAGE

The properties of the B-scan have been investigated for this model by Dickinson (1982) and, for small values of $\hat{a}$, are indeed similar to those of laser speckle. This fact has a number of interesting implications for imaging of tissue. If the tissue has such a random structure, with a small correlation length, then both the first- and second-order statistics will be independent of the tissue structure; the first-order statistics are given by the Rayleigh distribution, and the second-order depend on the incident pulse. Experiments on visual perception suggest that the human visual system is only sensitive to these two statistics (Julesz et al. 1973). Furthermore, even though some of the tissue structure cannot be resolved, the scan will have a high contrast speckle noise, which will obscure any other information in the scan (see Chapter 8). The ratio of the signal (defined as the mean echo level, or mean scattering level) to the noise (defined as the standard deviation of the speckle) will have a constant value of 2 (Burckhardt 1978), and small differences in mean scattering level will be obscured. These properties of the B-scan suggest that the display of echo amplitude is not the best way to present the information contained by ultrasound echoes.

Of course tissue also contains structures of a larger scale, and the B-scan will successfully display these, but for small-scale structures which contribute to the greyscale texture of the B-scan some processing of the echoes will improve the information content of the scan. Abbott and Thurstone (1979) have also examined the properties of speckle with the particular aim of finding methods of speckle reduction by combining uncorrelated scans taken at different positions or frequencies. This subject will be taken up again in Chapter 9, in relation to its practical implications for clinical investigative methods.

Measurements have been made on the properties of echoes from regions of homogeneous tissue and ensembles of small scatterers. Burckhardt (1978) has looked at values of the signal-to-noise ratio of speckle in B-scans, and the effect of logarithmic compression on this. Beecham (1966) has carried out a similar study of the scattered echoes from metal. Smith et al. (1982) have looked at scans of graphite/gelatin phantoms, and have shown that the signal-to-noise ratio is close to the theoretical value of 2. This group also examined the auto-correlation function of the scan, and showed that, in the lateral direction, this function has the predicted shape and dependence on range, whereas in the axial direction the width correlates tolerably well with the pulse length. The effect of frequency on the auto-correlation functions has not been examined, and there is no dependence on scatterer size. A lot more work remains to be done on the relationship between the B-scan texture, the transducer parameters and the tissue structure.

6.5.3 TISSUE MOVEMENT AND ELASTOGRAPHY

The correlation between two A-scans as a function of their separation is a monotonically decreasing function which has been shown to be independent of the tissue structure and depends on the direction of separation and on the transducer pulse and beam shape (Figure 6.10a). If the tissue is moving, then the correlation between two A-scans taken with a stationary transducer at different times will enable the motion in that time interval to be inferred, using Figure 6.10a as a calibration chart. This technique has been used to observe the motion of tissue *in vivo* (Dickinson & Hill 1982), and Figure 6.10b displays the correlation coefficient, R between A-scans separated by 0.1 s, as a function of time, showing the cardiac periodicity of the motion. The form of the motion can be related to the arterial pressure pulse, suggesting arterial pressure fluctuations as the cause of the motion.

Measurement of the de-correlation of ultrasonic A-scans can be combined with an externally applied strain to measure the low frequency elastic shear modulus of soft tissue (Chapter 7): a technique that has been called elastography (Ophir *et al.* 1991). Small, hard inclusions, embedded in a softer medium can be detected using this method (*see Chapter 10 and* Cespedes *et al.* 1993). The technique has been applied to measure the elasticity of arterial wall muscle, with strain applied either by a catheter-based balloon (Shapo *et al.* 1996) or by varying the intra-luminal pressure (Ryan & Foster 1997).

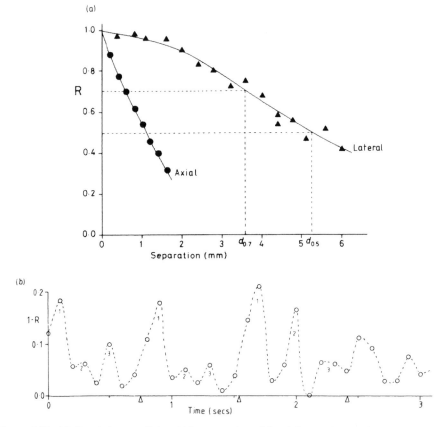

Figure 6.10. (a) Correlation coefficient R between demodulated A-scan from a tissue phantom as a function of their spatial separations, for both axial and lateral motion. Transducer frequency 1.5 MHz; beam width = 3.5 mm. (b) Time dependence of the correlation coefficient R between A-scans separated by 100 ms, relative to the ECG. The parameter $1 - R$ is plotted because this is proportional to the displacement of the tissue between scans. Arrows denote the ECG R-wave

This section has shown how the properties of the B-scan image can be described using tissue models and time-dependent scattering theory. The practical relevance of this theoretical discussion is taken up in Chapters 9 and 10.

6.6 CONCLUDING REMARKS

The information obtained from scattering experiments remains to be completely related via a suitable theory to the acoustic properties of tissue. Although a number of simple theoretical models do exist which give analytical expressions for the scattering cross-section, these models do not fully account for all scattering behaviour. A problem with such models is that, although they give some useful qualitative properties of scattering, it is difficult to make the models fully quantitative because so many parameters are unknown. Thus it is difficult to choose between candidate scattering models on the basis of a single set of scattering measurements.

There are two key areas that will contribute to our understanding of scattering by tissue. The first is acoustic microscopy (Chapter 11), which in principle is capable of making quantitative measurements of acoustic velocity and impedance of *ex vivo* tissue samples, on a scale much less than that corresponding to diagnostic wavelengths. This will enable realistic models of tissue properties to be inserted into scattering parameters identified as relevant in terms of their ability to characterise the microscopic tissue properties. For example, experiments may show that the presence of a particular tissue component, such as fat, correlates with the mean total backscattering cross-section. Acoustic microscopy will give the spatial distribution of that scattering component, and hence the influence of that parameter on the detailed scattering properties.

The second field that will contribute to our understanding of scattering from tissue is reconstruction of acoustic parameters (Chapter 9). This approach attempts to produce quantitative maps of attenuation, sound speed and backscattering coefficient by interrogating from a number of different directions, and using a reconstruction technique analogous to X-ray computed tomography. In addition to producing quantitative parameters, such techniques are inherently capable of greater resolution than conventional B-scanning. The techniques range from those using a ray approximation and an iterative reconstruction algorithm to separate scattering and attenuation (Duck & Hill 1979), to full-scale synthetic aperture techniques, which use phase information across an aperture to reconstruct the scattering cross-sections. The latter can use a reconstructive technique analogous to convolution and back projection in X-ray CT (Norton & Linzer 1979) or use a step-by-step numerical solution of the wave equation, termed wave-field extrapolation, a technique originally developed for seismology (Berkhout *et al.* 1982; Ridder *et al.* 1982). One thing all these techniques share is an attempt to reconstruct the scattering cross-section independently of attenuation, and the particular measurement geometry. Thus they should be able to strengthen the development of our ideas on the structures responsible for scattering. These techniques all make the initial assumption that scattering is isotropic and scattering theory and angular scattering measurements will be useful in determining the fundamental limitations of these techniques, given their assumptions, and in showing what corrections are needed to improve their efficacy.

A more complete understanding and documentation of the scattering properties of tissue will be valuable in defining the fundamental limitations of various techniques of ultrasound diagnosis, including B-scan echography and quantitative methods of tissue characterisation (Chapter 9). There is a trade-off between the speckle noise and resolution, which may be possible to optimise when we have more information on the important scattering parameters.

It can be expected then that, as our understanding of the process of scattering by tissue deepens, our ability to maximise the diagnostic content of ultrasound images will increase, and this is a major reason for continuing our studies of this topic.

REFERENCES

Abbott, J.G. and Thurstone, F.L. (1979). Acoustic speckle: theory and experimental analysis. *Ultrason. Imag.* **1**, 303–324.

Ahuja, A.S. (1972). Effect of particle viscosity on propagation of sound in suspensions and emulsions. *J. Acoust. Soc. Am.* **51**, 182–191.

Ahuja, A.S. and Hedee, W.R. (1977). Effects of red cell shape and orientation on propagation of sound in blood. *Med. Phys.* **4**, 516–520.

Bamber, J.C. (1979a). Theoretical modelling of the acoustic scattering structure of human liver. *Acoust. Lett.* **3**, 114–119.

Bamber, J.C. (1979b). Ultrasonic characterization of structure and pathology in human soft tissue. PhD thesis, University of London.

Bamber, J.C. and Dickinson, R.J. (1980). Ultrasonic B-scanning: a computer simulation. *Phys. Med. Biol.* **25**, 463–479.

Bamber, J.C. and Hill, C.R. (1981). Acoustic properties of normal and cancerous human liver. I: Dependence on pathological condition. *Ultrasound Med. Biol.* **7**, 121–134.

Bamber, J.C., Hill, C.R., Fry, M.J. and Dunn, F. (1977). Ultrasonic attentuation and backscattering by mammalian organs as a function of time after excision. *Ultrasound Med. Biol.* **3**, 15–20.

Bamber, J.C., Hill, C.R. and King, J.A. (1981). Acoustic properties of normal and cancerous human liver. II: Dependence on tissue structure. *Ultrasound Med. Biol.* **7**, 134–144.

Bamber, J.C., Hill, C.R., King, J.A. and Dunn, F. (1979). Ultrasonic propagation through fixed and unfixed tissues. *Ultrasound Med. Biol.* **5**, 159–165.

Beecham, D. (1966). Ultrasonic scatter in metals. Its properties and its application to gain size determination. *Ultrasonics* **4**, 67–76.

Berkhout, A.J., Ridder, J. and van der Wal, L.F. (1982). Acoustic imaging by wavefield extrapolation. I. Theoretical considerations. In *Acoustical Imaging*, Vol. 10, P. Alais and A. Metherell (eds). Plenum Press, New York, pp. 513–540.

Burckhardt, C.B. (1978). Speckle in ultrasound B-mode scans. *IEEE Trans. Son. Ultrason.* **SU-26**, 1–6.

Busse, L.J., Miller, J.G., Yuhas, D.E., Mimbs, J.W., Weiss, A.M. and Sobel, B.E. (1977). Phase cancellation effects: a source of attenuation artefact eliminated by a CdS acousto-electric receiver. In *Ultrasound in Medicine*, Vol. 3, B.D. White (ed.). Plenum Press, New York, pp. 1519–1535.

Cespedes, I., Ophir, J.W., Ponnerkanti, H. and Maklad, N. (1993). Elastography: elasticity imaging using ultrasound with application to muscle and breast *in vivo*. *Ultrason. Imag.* **15**, 73–88.

Chernow, L.A. (1960). *Wave Propagation in a Random Medium*, translated by R.A. Silverman. McGraw-Hill, New York.

Chivers, R.C. (1977). The scattering of ultrasound by human tissues – some theoretical models. *Ultrasound Med. Biol.* **3**, 1–13.

Chivers, R.C. (1978). Phase and amplitude fluctuations in the propagation of acoustic waves in lossless inhomogeneous continua with velocity, density and bulk modulus variations. *Ultrasound Med. Biol.* **4**, 353–361.

de Kroon, M.G.M., Slager, C.J., Gussenhoven, W.J., Serryus, P.W., Roelandt, J.R.T.C. and Bom, N. (1991) Cyclic changes of blood echogenicity in high-frequency ultrasound. *Ultrasound Med. Biol.* **17**, 723–728.

Dickinson, R.J. (1982). A computer model for speckle in ultrasound images: theory and application. In *Acoustical Imaging*, Vol. 10, P. Alais and A.F. Metherell (eds). Plenum Press, New York, pp. 115–130.

Dickinson, R.J. and Hill, C.R. (1982). An ultrasonic technique for measuring soft tissue dynamics. *Ultrasound Med. Biol.* **8**, 263–271.

Duck, F.A. (1990). *Physical Properties of Tissue*. Academic Press, London.

Duck, F.A. and Hill, C.R. (1979). Acoustic attenuation reconstruction from back scattered ultrasound. In *Computer Aided Tomography and Ultrasonics in Medicine*, Ravieri *et al.* (eds). North Holland, Amsterdam, pp. 137–149.

Farrow, C.A., Anson, L.W. and Chivers, R.C. (1995). Multiple scattering of ultrasound in suspensions. *Acustica* **81**, 402–411.

Foldy, L.L. (1945). The multiple scattering of waves. 1. General theory of isotropic scattering by randomly distributed scatterers. *Phys. Rev.* **67**, 107–119.

Freese, M. and Lyons, E.A. (1977). Ultrasonic backscatter from human liver tissue: its dependence on frequency and protein/lipid composition. *J. Clin. Ultrasound* **5**, 307–312.

Gan, W.S. (1995). Acoustical chaotic fractal images for medical imaging. Lecture notes in computer science **945**, 455–462.

Gay, P. (1971). *The Crystalline State*. Oliver & Boyd, Edinburgh.

Goodman, J.W. (1976). Some fundamental properties of speckle. *J. Opt. Soc. Am.* **66**, 1145–1150.

Gore, J.C. & Leeman, S. (1977). Ultrasonic backscattering from human tissue: a realistic model. *Phys. Med. Biol.* **22**, 317–326.

Gramiak, R., Hunter, L.P., Lee, P.P.K., Gerner, R.M., Schenk, E. and Waag, R.C. (1976). Diffraction characterization of tissue using ultrasound. *Proc. Ultrasonics Symp. IEEE* Cat. No. 76, CH1120-SSU, 60–63.

Herment, A., Perronneau, P. and Vayse, M. (1979). A new method of obtaining an acoustic impedance profile for characterization of tissue structures. *Ultrasound Med. Biol.* **5**, 321–332.

Hill, R.C., Chivers, R.C., Huggins, R.W. and Nicholas, D. (1978). Scattering of ultrasound by human tissue. In *Ultrasound: Its Applications in Medicine and Biology*, F.J. Fry (ed.). Elsevier, Amsterdam.

Insana, M.F. and Brown, D.G. (1993). Acoustic scattering theory applied to soft biological tissue. In *Ultrasonic Scattering in Biological Tissues*, K.K. Shung and G.A. Thieme (eds). CRC Press, Boca Raton, pp. 75–123.

Ishimaru, A. (1978). *Wave Propagation and Scattering in Random Media*. Academic Press, New York.

Jones, J.P. (1977). Ultrasonic impediography and applications to tissue characterization. In *Recent Advances in Ultrasound in Biomedicine*, Vol. 1, D.N. White (ed.). Plenum Press, New York, Chapt. 6.

Jones, J.P. and Kovac (1980). A computerized data analysis system for ultrasonic tissue characterization. In *Acoustical Imaging*, Vol. 9, K.Y. Wang (ed.). Plenum Press, New York.

Joynt, C.F. and Sommer, F.G. (1980). A stochastic approach to *in vivo* ultrasonic characterization of human liver tissue in normal and diffusely pathologic states. Abstract in *5th Int. Symposium on Ultrasonic Imaging and Tissue Characterization*. NBS, Gaithersburg.

Julesz, B., Gilbert, E.N., Shepp, L.A. and Frisch, H.L. (1973). Inability of humans to discriminate between visual textures that agree in second-order statistics – revised. *Perception* **2**, 391–405.

Kerker, M. (1969). *The Scattering of Light*. Academic Press, New York.

Koch, I. (1982). Ultrasonic backscattering from non-uniform scatterers. *Ulltrason. Imag.* **4**, 140–162.

Leeman, S. (1979). The impediography equations. In *Acoustical Imaging*, Vol. 8, D.F. Metherell (ed.). Plenum Press, New York.

Lizzi, F.L. and Coleman, D.J. (1977). Ultrasonic spectrum analysis in ophthalmology. In *Recent Advances in Ultrasound in Biomedicine*, D.N. White (ed.). Research Studies, Forest Grove, Chapt. 5.

Lockwood, G.R., Ryan, L.K., Hunt, J.W. and Foster, F.S. (1991). Measurement of the ultrasonic properties of vascular tissues and blood from 35–65 MHz. *Ultrasound Med. Biol.* **17**, 653–666.

Madsen, E.L. (1993). Method of determination of acoustic backscatter and attenuation coefficients independent of depth and instrumentation. In *Ultrasonic Scattering in Biological Tissues*, K.K. Shung and G.A. Thieme (eds). CRC Press, Boca Raton, pp. 205–249.

Manry, C.W. and Broschat, S.L. (1996). FDTD simulations for ultrasound propagation in a 2-D breast model. *Ultrason. Imag.* **18**, 25–34.

Morse, P.M. and Feshback, H. (1953). *Method of Theoretical Physics*. McGraw-Hill, New York.

Morse, P.M. and Ingard, K.N. (1968). *Theoretical Acoustics*. McGraw-Hill, New York.

Nassiri, D.K. and Hill, C.R. (1986a). The differential and total bulk acoustic scattering cross sections of some human and animal tissues. *J. Acoust. Soc. Am.* **79**, 2034–2047.

Nassiri, D.K. and Hill, C.R. (1986b). The use of acoustic scattering measurements to estimate structural parameters of human and animal tissue. *J. Acoust. Soc. Am.* **79**, 2048–2054.

Nicholas, D. (1979). Ultrasonic diffraction analysis in the investigation of liver disease. *Br. J. Radiol.* **52**, 949–961.

Nicholas, D. (1982). Evaluation of backscattering coefficients for excised human tissues: results, interpretation and associated measurements. *Ultrasound Med. Biol.* **8**, 17–28.

Norton, S.J. and Linzer, M. (1979). Ultrasonic reflectivity tomography: reconstruction with circular transducer arrays. *Ultrason. Imag.* **1**, 154–184.

Ophir, J.W., Cespedes, U., Ponnerkanti, H., Yadzi, Y. and Li, X. (1991). Elastography: a quantitative method for imaging the elasticity of biological tissues. *Ultrason. Imag.* **13**, 111–134.

Patel, A.P. (1996). Changes of ultrasound attenuation and backscattering as a function of time after excision after different modes of tissue handling. MSc dissertation, University of Surrey, UK.

Pauly, H. and Schwan, H.P. (1971). Mechanism of absorption of ultrasound in liver tissue. *J. Acoust. Soc. Am.* **50**, 692–699.

Polkhammer, J. and O'Brien, W.P. (1981). Dependence on the ultrasonic scatter coefficient on collagen concentration in mammalian tissues. *J. Acoust. Soc. Am.* **69**, 283–285.

Rao, N. and Zhu, H. (1994). Simulation study of ultrasound speckle statistics with the system point function. *J. Acoust. Soc. Am.* **95**, 1161–1164.

Ridder, J., Berkhout, A.J. and van der Wal, L.F. (1982). Acoustic imaging by wave field extrapolation. II, Practical aspects. In *Acoustical Imaging*, Vol. 10, P. Alais and A. Metherell (eds). Plenum Press, New York, pp. 541–565.

Ryan, L.K. and Foster, F.S. (1997). Ultrasonic measurement of differential displacement and strain in a vascular model. *Ultrason. Imag.* **19**, 1–18.

Shankar, P.M. (1995). A model for ultrasonic scattering from tissues based on the K-distribution. *Phys. Med. Biol.* **40**, 1633–1649.

Shapo, B.M., Crowe, J.R., Skovoroda, A.R., Eberle, M.J., Cohn, N.A. and O'Donnell, M. (1996). Strain imaging of coronary arteries with intraluminal ultrasound: experiments on an inhomogeneous phantom. *Ultrason. Imag.* **18**, 173–192.

Shung, K.K. (1993). *In vitro* experimental results on ultrasonic scattering in biological tissues. In *Ultrasonic Scattering in Biological Tissues*, K.K. Shung and G.A. Thieme (eds). CRC Press, Boca Raton, pp. 291–312.

Shung, K.K., Sigelmann, R.A. and Reid, J.M. (1976). The scattering of ultrasound by blood. *IEEE Trans. Biomed. Eng.* **23**, 460.

Shung, K.K., Sigelmann, R.A. and Reid, J.M. (1977). Angular dependence of scattering of ultrasound from blood. *IEEE Trans. Biomed. Eng.* **24**, 325–331.

Shung, K.K. and Thieme, G.A. (1993). *Ultrasonic Scattering in Biological Tissues*. CRC Press, Boca Raton.

Sigelmann, R.A. and Reid, J.M. (1973). Analysis and measurement of ultrasound backscattering from an ensemble of scatters excited by sinewave bursts. *J. Acoust. Soc. Am.* **53**, 1351–1355.

Smith, S.W., Sandrik, J.M., Wagner, R.F. and Von Ramm (1982). Measurements and analysis of speckle in ultrasound B-scans. In *Acoustical Imaging*, Vol. 10, P. Alais and A.F. Metherell (eds). Plenum Press, New York, pp. 195–212.

Stephanishen, P.R. (1970). Transient radiation from pistons in an infinite planar baffle. *J. Acoust. Soc. Am.* **49**, 1629–1638.

Uhlendorf, V. (1994). Physics of ultrasound contrast imaging: scattering in the linear range. *IEEE Trans. UFFC-41*, 70–79.

Uscinski, B.J. (1977). *The Elements of Wave Propagation in Random Media*. McGraw-Hill, New York.

Waag, R.C., Gramiak, R., Gerner, R.M. and Schenk, E.A. (1976). Tissue macrostructure from ultrasound scattering. *Proc. Conf. on Computerised Tomography in Radiology*, Am. Coll. of Radiology, St. Louis, pp. 175–186.

Wang, S.H., Chang, P.H., Shung, K.K. and Levene, H.B. (1996). Some considerations on the measurements of mean frequency-shift and integrated backscatter following administration of Albunex. *Ultrasound Med. Biol.* **22**, 441–451.

Wright, H. (1973). Impulse response function corresponding to reflection from a region of continuous impedance change. *J. Acoust. Soc. Am.* **53**, 1356–1359.

Xu, S. and Emmert, H. (1997). Models for describing the scattering of ultrasound in blood. *Biomed. Tech.* **42**, 123–131.

7

Physical Chemistry of the Ultrasound–Tissue Interaction

A.P. SARVAZYAN[1] AND C.R. HILL[2]

[1]Artann Laboratories, NJ, USA and [2]Institute of Cancer Research, Royal Marsden Hospital, UK

7.1 INTRODUCTION

In the preceding three chapters we have considered, largely from an empirical and descriptive point of view, phenomena underlying the passive interaction of ultrasound and human tissues, and have arranged the material in three somewhat arbitrary categories: attenuation/absorption, speed of sound and scattering. In this chapter we discuss these phenomena at a rather deeper level: that of the physics and physical chemistry underlying the interactions that ultrasound can have with biologically interesting molecules, which themselves may be behaving either as essentially independent entities or as components of a larger structure. Without understanding phenomena on the molecular level of tissue organisation it is impossible to explore the mechanisms of that interaction and to answer such questions as, why is the absorption of ultrasound in soft tissues so nearly a linear function of frequency?, why is the acoustic non-linearity parameter sensitive to tissue composition? and why does speed of sound in muscle remain so nearly constant during a gross mechanical process such as muscle contraction and relaxation? Furthermore, as we shall demonstrate, seeking answers to such questions is much more than an academic exercise: it can point the way to some new and potentially powerful approaches for applying ultrasound to medical problems.

7.2 ACOUSTIC PROPERTIES REFLECTING DIFFERENT LEVELS OF TISSUE ORGANISATION

Historically, the most extensively studied physicochemical phenomenon related to propagation of sound in tissues is inter- and intramolecular absorption of acoustic waves in biological media. This topic was introduced in Chapter 4. Various molecular mechanisms of absorption of sound in tissues have been discussed and studied, both in experiments with intact and homogenised tissues and also in solutions of biopolymers and their low-molecular-weight derivatives. A methodology for separating contributions to the attenuation of sound that result from molecular and from higher levels of structural organisation of a tissue,

Physical Principles of Medical Ultrasonics, Second Edition. Edited by C. R. Hill, J. C. Bamber and G. R. ter Haar.
© 2004 John Wiley & Sons, Ltd: ISBN 0 471 97002 6

Table 7.1. Sensitivity of acoustic parameters to disintegration of tissue

Parameters insignificantly affected by disintegration	Parameters affected by disintegration
α_a, the absorption coefficient	α_s, the scattering coefficient
K, the bulk modulus	G, the shear modulus
c_l, the speed of longitudinal acoustic waves	c_t, the speed of shear acoustic waves
Z, the acoustic impedance	η, the dynamic shear viscosity
B/A, the acoustic non-linearity parameter	

respectively, was first proposed and utilised in a classical paper of Pauly and Schwan (1971), who measured ultrasonic attenuation coefficients in liver both before and after homogenising the tissue. Using this methodology, one can divide acoustic parameters into two groups: those determined mainly by the molecular composition of tissues and those that are more related to the features of higher structural levels. These two groups are shown in Table 7.1 (Sarvazyan 1989).

Disintegration, i.e. mechanical homogenisation, generally does not lead to substantial, immediate change in the biochemical composition of tissue and has no significant effect on parameters determined by short-range inter- and intramolecular interactions. For example, a parameter such as density, which is mainly determined by the additive contributions of partial volumes of the molecules composing the tissue, is not affected significantly by disintegration.

Another approach to differentiating acoustic parameters of tissues determined mainly by molecular mechanisms from those determined by cellular and higher organisation of tissue is to consider the range of variation of various acoustic parameters of different tissues. Molecular composition of tissues varies much less than their structure: this can be seen clearly by comparing parameters on the left and right sides of Table 7.1. Most soft tissues contain about 80% water and the remaining major molecular components, such as proteins and various organic and inorganic low-molecular-weight components, are basically the same and are often at similar concentrations. In contrast, the range of variability of structural features of tissues, such as geometrical parameters of cells in different tissues and the degrees of heterogeneity and anisotropy, are incomparably greater: the parameters in the right-hand column of Table 7.1 may differ in value between various tissues, and even within one type of tissue, by a few orders of magnitude, whereas those in the left-hand column vary only slightly from tissue to tissue. The bulk modulus and the speed of sound are constant for all the soft tissues within only about 10%. Equally small is the range of variation of characteristic acoustic impedance, which is the product of density and compressibility and, correspondingly, is determined mainly by the molecular content of the tissue. Meanwhile, as discussed in Section 7.5, the shear moduli for different soft tissues vary over four orders of magnitude and, even within one tissue, may change by thousands of per cent during processes such as the development of a tumour or just an ordinary muscle contraction.

Some aspects of the relationship between molecular processes in tissues and their macroscopic acoustic parameters, such as sound absorption, were considered in Chapter 4; other aspects will be discussed in detail later in this chapter. The physical chemistry of ultrasound–tissue interactions includes also those molecular phenomena occurring in acoustic fields that result in observable modifications in the tissue. Some of these phenomena are discussed in Chapter 12, where all the mechanisms of ultrasonic bioeffects are considered comprehensively.

7.3 MOLECULAR ASPECTS OF SOFT TISSUE MECHANICS

From the point of view of mechanics, soft tissue represents an intermediate case between solids and liquids. Similarly to liquids, soft tissues are commonly characterised as 'incompressible' materials, which means that the ratio between shear and bulk moduli is close to zero, i.e. $G \ll K$. Typically, shear moduli of soft tissues are in the range of 10^3–10^7 Pa, whereas bulk moduli are close to that of water and in the narrow range 2–3×10^9 Pa, as indicated in Figure 7.1 (Sarvazyan 1975; Madsen *et al.* 1983). Therefore, when a tissue having an open boundary

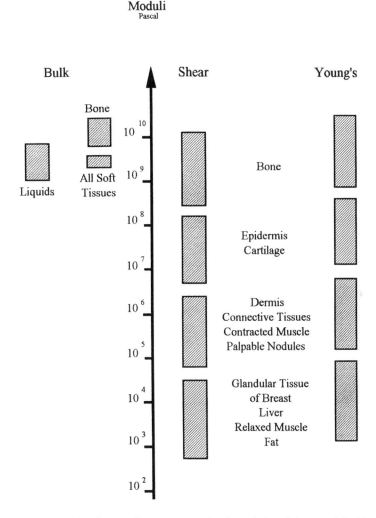

Figure 7.1. Summary of data from the literature concerning the variation of shear modulus, Young's modulus and bulk modulus for various materials and body tissues. Ranges for each of the moduli for a given tissue type are indicated by the shaded regions. *Source*: From Sarvazyan *et al.* (1995), reproduced by permission of Plenum Publishers

is subjected to a stress, it changes its shape, but the volume remains constant within a high degree of precision. Similarly to solids, however, the soft tissues are capable of conserving their shape and of supporting the propagation of both longitudinal and shear waves. This duality of properties of soft tissues is reflected in the terms used to characterise tissues as mechanical objects: they are often called 'semi-solid' or 'liquid-like' media.

Equations relating the mechanical properties of tissues to sound propagation characteristics are presented in Chapter 4. The wave equations describing the propagation of different acoustic waves in solids and liquids differ in the elasticity moduli characterising the stress/strain relationship for each mode of wave motion. The speed of sound of each type of acoustic wave is proportional to the square root of the corresponding modulus:

$$c = (E/\rho)^{1/2}$$

For compressional waves in fluids, E is equal to the bulk modulus K; for shear waves in homogeneous isotropic solids, E is equal to the shear modulus G; and for plane compressional (longitudinal) waves in these solids the modulus is usually denoted as M and called the 'longitudinal modulus'. These moduli are interrelated according to the following equation (Chapter 4):

$$M = K + 4/3G \tag{7.1}$$

It will be helpful at this stage to consider, in terms of a highly simplistic model, the microscopic aspects of elasticity of liquids and solids, and consequently of biological tissues. The stress/strain relationship in a compressed liquid is determined by inter- and intramolecular interactions. The bulk modulus, K, of liquids can be modelled by two springs K_1 and K_2 connected in series, as shown in Figure 7.2a, representing separately intermolecular (K_1) and intramolecular (K_2) forces. Elasticities of springs connected in series are summed as inverse values. In the case of solids and tissues, in addition to short-range inter- and intramolecular interactions, one should consider one more spring related to the shear elasticity modulus representing long-range order and interactions. This is shown schematically in Figure 7.2b, where the lower spring characterises the long-range interactions, added in parallel to the series of springs having the same meaning as in Figure 7.2a.

$$K = (K_1^{-1} + K_2^{-1})^{-1} \tag{7.2}$$

To match the model of Figure 7.2b with equation (7.1) and Figure 7.2a let us assign, to the parallel spring representing long-range interactions, a value of elasticity modulus equal to $4/3G$, and modify Figure 7.2b as shown in Figure 7.2c. This latter figure presents a model of a solid or a tissue with a longitudinal modulus:

$$M = K + 4/3G = (K_1^{-1} + K_2^{-1})^{-1} + 4/3G \tag{7.3}$$

The speed of longitudinal waves in this tissue is equal to:

$$c_1 = (M/\rho)^{1/2} = \{[(K_1^{-1} + K_2^{-1})^{-1} + 4/3G]/\rho\}^{1/2} \tag{7.4}$$

The speed of shear (transversal) waves, c_t, is determined solely by the elasticity modulus G, which characterises structural, supramolecular features of tissue and is equal to:

$$c_t = (G/\rho)^{1/2} \tag{7.5}$$

For most soft tissues, such as muscle, liver, spleen and fat, the parallel spring denoted as $4/3G$ in Figure 7.2c is orders of magnitude 'softer' than the other springs in the model

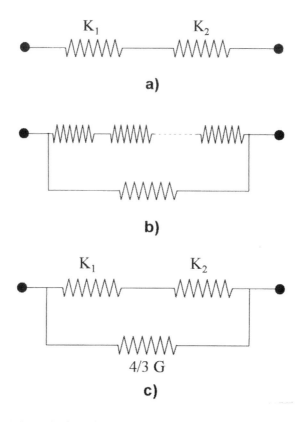

Figure 7.2. Mechanical models of soft tissue (see text)

(Sarvazyan 1975; Madsen *et al.* 1983; Sarvazyan *et al.* 1995). Consequently, as a first approximation, the structural contribution to the tissue bulk elasticity modulus can be neglected and only short-range inter- and intramolecular forces need be taken into account. As far as such bulk properties as compressibility, density and speed of longitudinal waves are concerned, soft tissue may be considered as a structureless aqueous solution having the same molecular composition as that tissue (Sarvazyan *et al.* 1987).

Let us now consider the springs K_1 and K_2 that are connected in series. The value of the elasticity modulus determined by intra-molecular forces (spring K_2) can be estimated by a number of methods, e.g. from the evidence of infrared spectroscopy on oscillation frequences of various molecules, from the shape of interatomic potentials or from the data on the speed of sound in crystals. Nyborg (1975) made an estimate of elasticity from atomic bond stretching and obtained the value of $K_2 = 10^{11}$ Pa, which is about 40 times higher than that for soft tissues or just water. Other estimates yield similar values. It can be concluded therefore that the major influence on the elastic modulus of tissue is the spring K_1 (Figure 7.2a), representing intermolecular interactions, because spring K_2 is over an order of magnitude harder and, as a first approximation, can be neglected. A detailed analysis of the qualitative and quantitative aspects of how intermolecular forces define mechanical and acoustical properties of the tissues is presented in the next section.

In summary, therefore, from the point of view of bulk compressional properties that determine the propagation of ultrasonic waves, soft tissues can be modelled adequately to a first approximation by a structureless fluid: in terms of the model of Figure 7.2, only the spring K_1 matters. The main factor determining compressibility, as well as acoustic impedance and speed of ultrasound in tissues, is intermolecular interactions, specifically the hydration of biological molecules and of their complexes, because water is the major molecular component of soft tissues. Sensitivity of ultrasound propagation parameters to various processes in tissue will depend on whether there are gross changes in the tissue composition. As will be shown later, the situation is very different in the case of the shear properties of tissues.

7.4 RELATIONSHIP BETWEEN ULTRASONIC PARAMETERS AND FUNDAMENTAL THERMODYNAMIC POTENTIALS OF A MEDIUM

The above discussion has been conducted in terms of those features of material behaviour that are measurable by mechanical/acoustic techniques. It will be evident, however (even though the situation has been given surprisingly little attention in the literature), that the acoustically measured data are no more than conveniently obtainable expressions of fundamental material properties that could, in principle, be observed by other means. An illustration of this point, due to Sehgal and Greenleaf (1986), is the close mechanistic relationship, rooted in the hydrogen bond, that exists between sound speed and the NMR chemical shift in tissue-like materials. It is thus of interest here to examine the close relationship that exists between the principal thermodynamic potentials and ultrasonic parameters of media.

In any physics textbook one can find that volume and heat capacity are the first derivatives of the Gibbs free energy G, and enthalpy H, respectively, whereas there is hardly any mention that ultrasound velocity, c, is a simple function of the second derivative of G. For illustrative purposes Table 7.2 lists a series of derivatives for the Gibbs free energy.

A comprehensive physical description of a medium implies establishing relationships between its microscopic molecular and macroscopic thermodynamic properties. To reveal the nature and origin of the acoustic parameters of a medium it is necessary to relate them both to the basic thermodynamic potentials as well as to individual molecular interactions in the medium. The relationship between speed of sound and other thermodynamic parameters, and the derivation of the equation of state (PVT equation) and heat capacity of a medium from sound speed data, have been discussed by a number of authors and reviewed by Tikhonov et al. (1995). In fact, for a well-studied liquid such as water it has been shown that the equation of state derived from sound speeds is more reliable than the presently available directly measured values (Fine & Millero 1973). Obtaining the equation of state is based on the use of the relationship for c^{-2} shown in Table 7.2. After converting adiabatic derivatives into isothermal derivatives, the equation of state can be derived by integration of the pressure dependence of speed of sound.

In physics textbooks, derivation of the principal thermodynamic potentials describing biomolecular structures and interactions (Gibbs free energy ΔG^0, enthalpy ΔH^0 and entropy ΔS^0) is usually described in conjunction with calorimetric measurements, whereas the acoustic

Table 7.2. Derivatives of the Gibbs free energy G

Volume and density (first derivative)	$V = (\partial G/\partial P)_T$ $\qquad$ $\rho = m/V$
Compressibility and sound speed (second derivative)	$\beta_s = \rho^{-1}(\partial \rho/\partial P)_s$ $\qquad$ $c^{-2} = (\partial \rho/\partial P)_s$
Acoustic non-linearity parameter (third derivative)	$B/A = -\beta_s^{-2}(\partial \beta_s \partial P) - 1 = 2\rho c(\partial c/\partial P)_s$

Table 7.3. Calorimetric and acoustic derivations of thermodynamic data

	Calorimetry	Acoustics
Measured	$C_P(T)$	$c(P, T) = (\delta\rho/\delta P)_s^{-0.5} \rightarrow V(P, T)$
Evaluated	$\Delta H^0(T) = \int C_P(T)\mathrm{d}T$	$\Delta G^0(P, T) = \int V\mathrm{d}P$
	$\Delta S^0(T) = \int [C_P(T)/T]\mathrm{d}T$	$\Delta S^0(P, T) = -\int(\delta V/\delta P)_\mathrm{p}\mathrm{d}P$
	$\Delta G^0(T) = \Delta H^0(T) - T\Delta S^0(T)$	$\Delta H^0(P, T) = \int[V - T(\delta V/\delta T)_\mathrm{p}]\mathrm{d}P$

approach is seldom mentioned. Table 7.3 illustrates the complementary nature of the calorimetric and acoustic derivation of thermodynamic data.

To relate macroscopic (thermodynamic) and microscopic (molecular) features of a medium it is necessary to use the language of partial physical parameters, characterising the individual contributions of particular types of molecule into a measurable property, e.g. density, compressibility, or speed of sound. This language comes from the physical chemistry of solutions, where the properties of a solute are studied by measuring a relative change in a physical characteristic, per unit of solute concentration, rather than its absolute value. Data presented here are in the form of such relative concentration values of density, compressibility and sound speed, denoted by square brackets and defined as:

$$[\rho] \equiv (\rho - \rho_0)/\rho_0\kappa$$
$$[\beta_\mathrm{s}] \equiv (\beta_\mathrm{s} - \beta_{\mathrm{s}0})/\beta_{\mathrm{s}0}\kappa$$
$$[c_\mathrm{s}] \equiv (c_\mathrm{s} - c_{\mathrm{s}0})/U_{\mathrm{s}0}\kappa$$

where κ is the concentration of the solute, and parameters related to the solvent are denoted by a subscript '0'. The relationship between these relative increments can be obtained by differentiating the well-known equation

$$c^2 = 1/\rho\beta_\mathrm{s}$$

giving:

$$2[c] = -[\rho] - [\beta_\mathrm{s}]$$

Figures 7.3a and 7.3b, taken from the review paper by Sarvazyan 1991, are plots showing measured values of $[\rho]$, $[\beta_\mathrm{s}]$ and B/A for various classes of molecules in biological tissues (data for four or more particular species per class); Figure 7.3a represents '$[\rho] - [\beta_\mathrm{s}]$ space' and Figure 7.3b '$B/A - [\beta_\mathrm{s}]$ space'.

In interpreting these data it needs to be borne in mind that compressibility, in this context, whether expressed as an absolute or incremental value, will in general reflect contributions from several sources: in particular intrinsic compressibility, related to the core of the solvent molecule; a contribution due to its hydration shell and interaction with other molecules; and a relaxational contribution that may account for some 10% of the total in the case of some large protein molecules (Sarvazyan & Hemmes 1979).

Figure 7.3 demonstrates a rather clear separation, in both presentations, between the different classes of molecule, thus implying significant differences in the corresponding interactions. Closer examination shows that hydration state seems to play an important role in this separation: for example, in Figure 7.3b, electrolytes and (disodium salts of) nucleotides fall in the upper region of the B/A scale while, among the amino acids, there is a progression

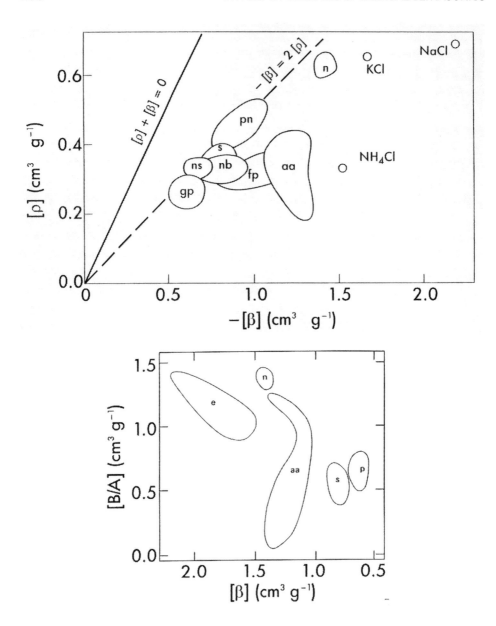

Figure 7.3. Plots showing measured values of $[\rho]$, $[\beta_s]$ and $[B/A]$ for various molecules in aqueous solution, grouped in the following classes: electrolytes (e); amino acids and peptides (aa); proteins (p); globular proteins (gp); nucleosides (ns); nucleic bases (nb); saccharides (s); polynucleotides and DNA (pn); nucleotides (n); fibrillar proteins (fp). Note that parameters displayed here (unlike B/A values in figures 7.4 and 5.6) are partial values, characterising the solute only, and are calculated per unit concentration. *Source:* from Sarvazyan (1991). Reproduced, with permission, from the *Annual Review of Biophysics and Biophysical Chemistry*, Vol. 20, by Annual Reviews Inc

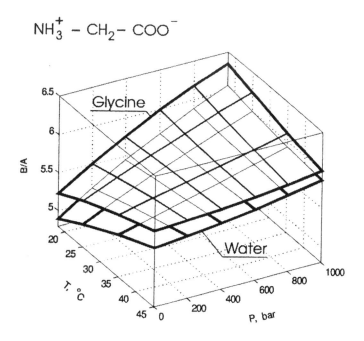

$$NH_3^+ - CH_2 - COO^-$$

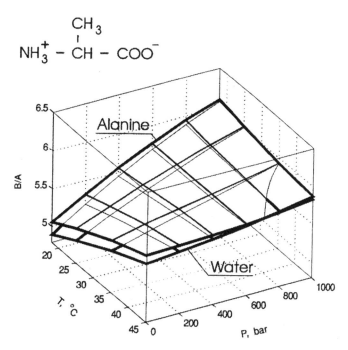

$$NH_3^+ - \underset{\underset{CH_3}{|}}{CH} - COO^-$$

Figure 7.4. Pressure and temperature dependencies of B/A for 5% aqueous solutions of glycine and alanine, illustrating the sensitivity of B/A to apparently small changes in molecular structure

from those with hydrophobic and aromatic residues at low B/A values to others with charged amino and carboxyl groups at the high end. Another strong conclusion that can be drawn from Figure 7.3a relates to the relative contributions of density and compressibility to sound velocity: the solid line corresponds to equal contributions and it can be seen that, for almost all the molecular species examined, the contribution from $[\beta_s]$ to $[U]$ is at least twice that from $[\rho]$.

A final illustration of the remarkable sensitivity of ultrasonic interactions to the thermodynamic behaviour of molecules is presented in Figure 7.4, which plots the pressure and temperature dependence of B/A for two closely related amino acids. Addition of the hydrophobic $-CH_3$ group (in alanine) to a charged zwitterionic molecule of glycine alters the character of the surface of the PT dependence of B/A; indeed, in the region of higher pressures and temperatures, the contribution of the solute to the solution acoustic non-linearity parameter even changes its sign.

7.5 STRUCTURAL CONTRIBUTION TO BULK AND SHEAR ACOUSTIC PROPERTIES OF TISSUES

The foregoing sections presented evidence that, in the first approximation, bulk compressional properties are basically determined by intermolecular forces. Having in mind, however, that current ultrasonic imaging methods are sensitive to changes in acoustic impedance and speed of sound, with resolution of the order of 0.1% or less, it is important to make estimates of the sensitivity of these parameters to structural changes in tissues at the level of the second approximation.

Let us now therefore estimate quantitatively the relative contributions of various types of interactions to the speed of ultrasound in tissue, c_l, using the model of Figure 7.2c. One can separate molecular and structural contributions by estimating the change in c_l caused by disintegration of the tissue, as previously noted. If we homogenise the tissue, thus destroying the structures represented by the lower spring of Figure 7.2c (i.e. long-range interactions) and transforming the tissue into a structureless liquid with bulk modulus K determined by molecular interactions, as shown in equation (7.2), the resulting change in the velocity of ultrasound in tissue will reflect the structural contribution, Δc_{str}, which will be equal to:

$$\Delta c_{str} = c_{tissue} - c_{liquid} = \{[(K_1^{-1} + K_2^{-1})^{-1} + 4/3G]/\rho\}^{1/2} - [(K_1^{-1} + K_2^{-1})^{-1}/\rho]^{1/2} \qquad (7.6)$$

Substituting equations (7.4) and (7.5) into equation (7.6) and taking into account that $K \gg G$, we obtain:

$$\Delta c_{str} = (2/3)(c_t^2/c_l) \qquad (7.7)$$

Literature data on shear elasticity and shear wave velocity in soft tissues are very limited and not very consistent. Because of this and also because of the fact that equation (7.7) has been derived using the simplest mechanical model of tissue, only an order-of-magnitude estimate for c_{str} can be made using this approach. Analysis of available data on the shear velocity in tissues (Madsen *et al.* 1983; Pashovkin & Sarvazyan 1989; Burke *et al.* 1990) shows that, in the ultrasonic range of frequencies, c_t is typically in the range 30–100 m s^{-1}. Consequently, the range for c_{str} estimated from equation (7.7) extends from a fraction of 1 to $\sim$5 m s^{-1}, which is less than 1% of the absolute value of the speed of ultrasound in tissues. In other words, even gross changes in tissue structure will cause less than 1% changes in the speed of sound.

The structural contribution to ultrasound velocity has been studied experimentally and discussed in the literature by several authors (Mol & Breddels 1982; Tamura *et al.* 1982;

Griffiths 1987; Sarvazyan *et al.* 1987; Verdonk *et al.* 1992; Hoffmeister *et al.* 1994), who analysed this problem mainly with respect to the anisotropy of sound velocity in highly structured tissues such as muscle and tendon.

One of the most careful studies of ultrasound velocity in muscle was that of Mol and Breddels (1982). They measured the velocity of ultrasound in various types of muscle as a function of muscle fibre orientation and contraction state. The difference between ultrasound velocity along and across muscle fibres was found to be about 7 m s^{-1}. Change of ultrasound velocity in human biceps muscle *in vivo* during contraction was about 3 m s^{-1}, and the change in ultrasound velocity in isometrically contracting frog muscle was within the 1 m s^{-1} measurement precision. The authors developed a theoretical model to explain their results and derived equations for the difference in the velocities of ultrasound across and along muscle fibres.

The equations that they derived represent, to a certain extent, the same structural contribution to ultrasound as described in equation (7.7). If we rewrite the equations of Mol and Breddels in the same terms as equation (7.7) we obtain:

$$\Delta c_{\mathrm{str}} = (1/3)(c_{\mathrm{t}}^2/c_{\mathrm{l}}) \tag{7.8}$$

Thus, in spite of the great difference between the models used in deriving equations (7.7) and (7.8), they show qualitative agreement. The difference in the factor on the right-hand side of the equations can be explained by the fact that the anisotropy reflected in equation (7.8) represents only a part of the structural contribution to the speed of sound given by equation (7.7).

The finding that c_{l} shows so little dependence on the contraction state of the muscle has been used in neurophysiological studies (Griffiths 1987; Hoffer *et al.* 1989). The transmission time of ultrasound pulses in muscle during contraction depends solely on the muscle length and, consequently, ultrasonic measurements enable physiologists to monitor muscle length in real tissue in the freely walking cat (Hoffer *et al.* 1989).

There are some literature data on significantly higher changes of ultrasound velocity during muscle contraction (Tamura *et al.* 1982) but these results were obtained by low accuracy measurements with an error of about 100 m s^{-1} and the conditions of measurement were not artifact free.

A much greater structural contribution to the speed of sound is seen in highly structured and dense tissues such as tendon (Hoffmeister *et al.* 1994). A high content of collagen, possessing a unidirectional arrangement of fibres and constituting roughly 30% of tendon by wet weight, which is close to that of skin, results in very significant mechanical and acoustic anisotropy. The difference between the velocities of ultrasound along and across collagen fibres reaches 350 m s^{-1} and, clearly, the simplified biomechanical model considered above for other soft tissues is no longer adequate.

7.6 RELEVANCE TO TISSUE CHARACTERISATION

One of the reasons for investigating relationships between acoustic parameters of tissues and their structure and composition is to find possibilities for remotely characterising the conditions of normal and diseased tissues. The main focus in most previous studies of tissue characterisation has been on bulk compressional acoustic parameters. More recently, progress has been made in making use of the great sensitivity of shear acoustic properties of tissues to their physiopathological condition: so-called 'ultrasonic elasticity imaging' (see Chapters 9 and

10). As shown above, bulk properties are determined mostly by the molecular composition of tissue and thus reflect the 'physical chemistry' of tissue, whereas shear properties characterise the mechanical structure, i.e. the 'physics' (mechanics) of tissue organisation. Let us compare these two approaches to tissue characterisation based on 'physical chemistry' and 'physics'.

The data of Figure 7.1 seem to prove the superiority of 'physics' over 'physical chemistry' because the ability of a parameter to differentiate tissues usually depends on the dynamic range of that parameter. The bulk modulus of tissue, as well as the acoustic impedance variations responsible for image contrast in ultrasonic imaging, are 4–5 orders of magnitude less variable than is the shear modulus. But the range of variations of a parameter does not reflect directly its information value; more important is the ratio of that range to the error that is typically involved in its measurement (see Chapter 9 and Hill *et al.* 1990). In the case of bulk elastic properties of soft tissues, the ratio of the variation range (which is about 10%) to the measurement error (of the order of 0.1%) is 100; at the same time, however, the relative error for evaluating the shear elasticity modulus is much greater, typically 20%. Nevertheless, the ratio of variation range to measurement error is over two orders of magnitude greater for shear properties as compared with the bulk: from this point of view, 'physics' is 100 times superior to 'physical chemistry'! The utilisation of this great unexploited potential of shear elasticity in tissue characterisation is attracting considerable research attention, some of which is described here in later chapters. A somewhat more extensive treatment of the subject of the present chapter has been given elsewhere by one of the present authors (Sarvazyan 2001).

REFERENCES

Burke, T.M., Blankenberg, T.A., Sui, A.K.Q., Blankenberg, F.G. and Jensen, H.M. (1990). Preliminary results for shear wave speed of sound and attenuation coefficients from excised specimens of human breast tissue. *Ultrason. Imag.* **12**, 99–118.

Fine, R.A. and Millero, F.J. (1973). Compressibility of water as a function of temperature and pressure. *J. Chem. Phys.* **59**, 5529–5536.

Griffiths, R.G. (1987). Ultrasound transit-time gives direct measurements of muscle fiber length *in vivo*. *J. Neuromusc. Methods* **21**, 159–165.

Hill, C.R., Bamber, J.C. and Cosgrove, D.O. (1990). Performance criteria for quantitative ultrasonology and image parameterization. *Clin. Phys. Physiol. Meas.* **11** (Suppl. A), 57–73.

Hoffer, J.A., Caputi, A.A., Pose, I.E. and Griffiths, R.I. (1989). Roles of muscle activity and load on the relationship beween muscle spindle length and whole muscle length in the freely walking cat. *Progr. Brain Res.* **80**, 75–85.

Hoffmeister, B.K., Verdonk, E.D., Wickline, S.A. and Miller, J.M. (1994). Effect of collagen on the anisotropy of quasi-longitudinal mode ultrasonic velocity in fibrous soft tissues: a comparison of fixed tendon and fixed miocardium. *J. Acoust. Soc. Am.* **96**, 1957–1964.

Madsen, E.L., Sathoff, H.J. and Zagzebski, J.A. (1983). Ultrasonic shear wave properties of soft tissues and tissuelike materials. *J. Acoust. Soc. Am.* **74**, 1346–1355.

Mol, R.C. and Breddels, P.A. (1982). Ultrasound velocity in muscle. *J. Acoust. Soc. Am.* **71**, 455–461.

Nyborg, W.L. (1975). Elasticity from bond stretching. In *Intermediate Biophysical Mechanisms*. Cummings Publishing Company, Menlo Park, CA, p. 201.

Pashovkin, T.N. and Sarvazyan, A.P. (1989). Mechanical characteristics of soft biological tissue. In *Methods of Vibrational Diagnostics of Rheological Properties of Soft Materials and Biological Tissue* V.A. Antonets (ed.). Institute of Applied Physics, Gor'ky, pp. 105–115.

Pauly, H. and Schwan, H.P. (1971). Mechanism of absorption of ultrasound in liver tissue. *J. Acoust. Soc. Am.* **50**, 692–699.

Sarvazyan, A.P. (1975). Low frequency acoustic characteristics of biological tissues. *Mechan. Polym.* **4**, 691–695.

Sarvazyan, A.P. (1989). Acoustical properties of biological tissues and their biochemical composition. In *Proc. 13th Cong. Acoust., Belgrade*, Vol. 4, pp. 171–174.

Sarvazyan, A.P. (1991). Ultrasonic velocimetry of biological compounds. *Ann. Rev. Biophys. Biophys. Chem.* **20**, 321–342.

Sarvazyan, A.P. (2001). Elastic properties of soft tissues. In *Handbook of Elastic Properties of Solids, Liquids and Gases*, Vol. 3, M. Levy, H. Bass and R. Stern (eds). Academic Press, New York, pp. 107–127.

Sarvazyan, A.P. and Hemmes, P. (1979). Relaxational contributions to protein compressibility from ultrasonic data. *Biopolymers* **18**, 3015–3024.

Sarvazyan, A.P. Lyrchikov, A.G. and Gorelov, S.E. (1987). Dependence of ultrasonic velocity in rabbit liver on water content and structure of the tissue. *Ultrasonics* **25**, 244–247.

Sarvazyan, A.P., Skovoroda, A.R., Emelianov, S.Y., Fowlkes, J.B., Pipe, J.G., Adler, R.S., Buxton, R.B. and Carson, P.L. (1995). Biophysical bases of elasticity imaging. In *Acoustical Imaging*, Vol. 21, J.P. Jones (ed.). Plenum Press, New York, pp. 223–240.

Sehgal, C.M. and Greenleaf, J.F. (1986). Correlative study of properties of water in biological systems using ultrasound and magnetic resonance. *Magn. Reson. Med.* **3**, 978–985.

Tamura, Y., Hatta, I., Matsuda, T., Sugi, H. and Tsuchiya, T. (1982). Changes in muscle stiffness during contraction recorded using ultrasonic waves. *Nature* **299**, 631–633.

Tikhonov, D.A., Hatta, I., Matsuda, T., Sugi, H. and Tsuchiya, T. (1995). Ultrasonic approach to obtaining thermodynamic characteristics of solutions. *Ultrasonics* **33**, 301–310.

Verdonck, E.D., Wickline, S.A. and Miller, J.G. (1992). Anisotropy of ultrasonic velocity and elastic properties in normal human myocardium. *J. Acoust. Soc. Am.* **92**, 3039–3050.

8

Ultrasonic Images and the Eye of the Observer

C. R. HILL

Institute of Cancer Research, Royal Marsden Hospital, UK

8.1 INTRODUCTION

This section of the book is concerned with the practical uses of ultrasound for investigating human anatomy and pathology – a topic often referred to, for lack of a better term, as 'diagnostic imaging'. A vitally important contributor to this investigative process, who can all too easily be taken for granted, is the human observer. In fact, the relationship between image and observer is complex, and readily misunderstood, with potentially serious consequences for overall diagnostic performance. It is the purpose of this chapter therefore to examine the role of the observer of 'diagnostic' (or, perhaps better, 'investigative') ultrasonic images and the manner in which observer performance may influence both the design and effectiveness of the overall imaging procedure.

The concept of image making is older than history: the thought that it might be possible to make images of the internal structure of the living human body only became realistic, however, with Röntgen's discovery of X-rays in 1895. Even in the 50 years following that discovery, little beyond empirical development occurred and it is only in the period since about 1950, with the advent of other techniques such as radioisotope imaging, ultrasound, thermography, X-ray CT and NMR/MRI, that the subject has achieved perspective and the beginnings of a unified scientific approach have emerged. An important influence here has been the parallel development, in the field of communications engineering, of a general science of imaging: a development that has occurred in response to the widespread commercial and military interest in the processes of recording, transmitting, displaying and interpreting pictorial information.

This chapter brings together some of the basic concepts that underlie the general process of imaging the human body, and in particular the principles that are available for expressing imaging performance in a quantitative manner and the physical limitations and characteristics of the imaging process. Much of this material is not uniquely relevant to ultrasonic or even medical imaging as opposed to the more general imaging technique, but it seems useful to review it here as an introduction to the detailed treatment given, in subsequent chapters, to the various specific methods of ultrasonic imaging, or 'echography'. For background on how echography fits into the overall framework of medical imaging, an excellent source is the multi-author text edited by Webb (1988).

Physical Principles of Medical Ultrasonics, Second Edition. Edited by C. R. Hill, J. C. Bamber and G. R. ter Haar.
© 2004 John Wiley & Sons, Ltd: ISBN 0 471 97002 6

What follows is necessarily brief and lacking in detail. However, a number of specialised texts deal with particular aspects of the subject. A stimulating introduction (particularly for the physically minded) to methods of image analysis and the essential characteristics of human vision is given in the first part of the book by Pearson (1975), whereas more detailed and comprehensive treatments of visual perception have been provided by Haber and Hershenson (1973) and Cornsweet (1970). Two more engineering-oriented texts that deal, in particular, with the vital factor of signal-to-noise ratio are those of Biberman (1973) and Overington (1976). The specific topic of echographic image formation and perception has been the subject of a special conference publication (Hill & Kratochwil 1981) and, more recently, of a detailed review article (Hill *et al.* 1991). What follows is largely a summary of these publications, which should, in particular, be consulted for more specialised references to the literature.

8.2   QUANTITATIVE MEASURES OF IMAGING AND PERCEPTION

All images are representations, in some particular format, of some aspect of the real world. In the imaging process some quantitative measure of that aspect of the 'real world' (e.g. its optical reflectivity, X-ray absorption coefficient, ultrasonic backscattering coefficient or some complex function of several such quantities) is transposed to a quantitative measure (e.g. luminance) of an image. Thus, for a particular imaging process, it will be important to know the laws that determine the quantitative aspect of that transposition: the grey-scale transformation. Equally important will be statistical measures of that process: its noisiness. Thirdly, one will be concerned with the spatial properties of the process, because points on an object will always, in practice, transform to spatially extended regions of an image, with consequent loss of 'resolution' and, commonly, a degree of spatial distortion. Medical imaging is concerned with living human anatomy, which is itself in a constant state of motion, and human vision is specifically adapted to perception of movement. Thus it will be important to be able to quantify and account for the dynamic nature of the imaging process: a requirement that is particularly relevant to ultrasonic imaging, which lends itself outstandingly to the recording and display of body and tissue movement.

8.2.1 QUANTITATION OF DISPLAYED AMPLITUDE

A practical measure of the displayed amplitude of a particular element of an image is the rate of emission, per unit area of the image, of visible light. This is termed the *luminance* of the image element and is defined in terms of the response of a *standard observer* to light emitted by a black-body radiator at a specified temperature. It is physically equivalent to *brightness*, with the difference that the latter is, by definition, observer dependent (Pearson 1975). Luminance is expressed in units of candela per metre (cd m^{-2}) or milliLamberts (mL: 1 mL = 3.183 cd m^{-2}). Some examples of typical luminance values found in images and the environment are given in Table 8.1.

8.2.2 MEASURES OF SPATIAL CHARACTERISTICS OF IMAGING SYSTEMS

The classical, and apparently most straightforward, approach to expressing the spatial properties of an imaging system – in translating a stimulus in an object space to a signal in the corresponding image space – is to determine the spatial distribution of the image signal that

Table 8.1. Typical environmental and imaging luminance levels

	Luminance (cd m^{-2})
White paper in sunlight:	30 000
Highlights of bright CRT display	1000
Comfortable reading	30
Dark region of low-level CRT display	0.1
White paper in moonlight	0.03

Note: in any one CRT display the ratio of maximum to minimum luminance is seldom more than 100:1, and is typically less.

results from a point object stimulus. Such a distribution is called a *point spread function* (PSF), and a related function, corresponding to an infinitely thin line object, is the *line spread function* (LSF). In dealing with any but the simplest imaging systems, however, the above formulation proves unsatisfactory, particularly as the procedure for computing the combined effect, on the total imaging process, of the set of PSFs contributed by each stage of the process entails a series of mathematical convolutions. Thus it becomes simpler mathematically and computationally, and more intuitively enlightening, to deal with the situation in the spatial frequency domain. The unidirectional Fourier transform of the LSF is the *optical transfer function* (OTF), which is in general a complex quantity whose modulus is termed the *modulation transfer function* (MTF). The MTF for an imaging system, or for any stage of it, is thus the ratio of the amplitudes of the resulting and original set of spatial sine waves, corresponding to the object being imaged, plotted as a function of sine-wave frequency. The MTF for a system made up of a series of stages is now the product of the MTFs of the individual stages.

This approach to analysis of imaging systems has proved to be very powerful, and is dealt with in detail in other texts, such as that by Pearson (1975). It is important to note, however, that its applicability in an exact sense is limited by a number of important conditions that are not fully met in certain medical imaging systems, including those based on ultrasound. Included in these restrictions are that the processes should be *linear* and *space-time invariant* (i.e. the MTF should not vary either with time or over the surface being imaged) and also that they should be *non-negative*. This latter restriction, which implies that an image function should not possess negative values, can be met in imaging systems using coherent radiation (e.g X-rays or radioisotope γ-emissions; see Metz & Doi 1979) but not in those using coherent radiation, which is the case in most ultrasonic systems.

Thus, although frequency domain discussion of the spatial characteristics of ultrasonic imaging systems can be enlightening, and there are recognised methods for overcoming some of the above limitations, care must be taken in attempts at precise analysis.

8.3 IMAGES AND HUMAN VISUAL PERCEPTION

One common factor in almost all forms of imaging is that the image is, at some stage, perceived by the human eye and brain. The properties of the human visual perceptive system are thus central to the subject of imaging and, although the anatomy of the eye, at least in simplified form, is familiar to many, some of the significant facts of visual physiology may not be common currency for many involved in the development and application of medical imaging systems.

The sensitivity and resolution characteristics of vision are closely related to the structure of the retina, in which the sensitive elements include both 'cones' and the relatively more sensitive 'rods'. The central region of the retina, the fovea, which subtends (at the focal plane of the lens) an angle of 1–2°, is lined almost entirely with close-packed cones whereas more peripheral regions contain both rods and cones. Within the fovea the spacing of cones is sufficiently close ($\sim$ 10 μm) to enable grating resolution to be achieved up to about 60 cycles per degree. The behaviour at lower spatial frequencies, for two display luminances, is illustrated in Figure 8.1, in which important features are the peaks in sensitivity (at about 3 and 1 cycles per degree) and the substantial fall-off at lower frequencies.

Some practical implications of this behaviour are that there will be a limit to the degree of fine detail that can be perceived (even if it is present in an image), that very gradual boundaries (e.g. a diffusely infiltrating border of a tumour) may easily be missed unless, perhaps, processing measures are taken to enhance them, and that spatial frequencies roughly in the 1–5 cycles per degree range will be most readily seen. This latter feature may or may not, however, be beneficial, according to whether the structure and magnification of the image are such that the detail in question is anatomical or artefactual (e.g. due to a raster pattern or coherent speckle: see below).

Another important, and related, property of vision is the ability to perceive contrast. Fuller discussion of this topic, in the context of image noise, is taken up in Section 8.3.2, but it may be noted here that contrast perception is very dependent on the sharpness of the contrast boundary. Sharp boundaries, as typified by images of a step-wedge, are relatively well perceived whereas areas contrasting considerably in luminance may not be recognised as such if they are separated by a gradual boundary.

The overall dynamic range of the accommodating human eye is of the order of 80 dB. In imaging practice, however, not all of this may be available. The practical upper limit

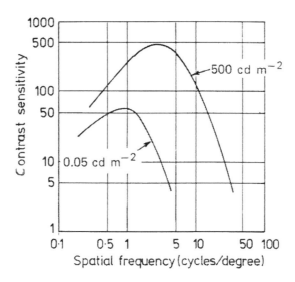

Figure 8.1. Typical contrast sensitivity of the eye for sine-wave gratings. *Source*: From Pearson (1975), reproduced by permission of John Wiley & Sons, Ltd

(corresponding to full brightness on a cathode-ray screen) is about 1000 cd m^{-2} (Table 8.1) whereas below 0.003 cd m^{-2} foveal vision begins to fall off and sensitivity is achieved (by parallel operation of rod sensors over an extended retinal region) increasingly at the expense of spatial resolution.

8.3.1 VISUAL ACUITY AND PERCEPTION OF BRIGHTNESS CONTRAST

The value of about 60 cycles per degree, quoted above for optically achievable grating resolution, represents a limit set by the anatomical structure of the foveal region of the retina and only holds for high levels of illumination and low levels of image noise. Thus, degradation in acuity to below this anatomically determined limit can be seen as arising in two separate ways: from the statistics of the visual averaging process that becomes necessary in the absence of adequate illumination, and from the limitations imposed by image noise. These two factors will be considered here in turn, together with their relevance to the issue of contrast resolution (the ability to discriminate between neighbouring regions of differing image brightness), which is of central importance in several branches of medical imaging.

The definition and measurement of contrast resolution, even in the absence of significant image noise, have been a matter for considerable research. Detailed accounts of the various factors involved are given in specialised texts, e.g. Chapter 5 of Haber and Hershenson (1973). Generally, experiments have been carried out in which observers have been presented with a large screen, illuminated in two different segments at two different brightness levels, and have been tested for their ability to detect a difference in those levels. Contrast resolution threshold, or the 'Weber ratio', $\Delta L/L$, is then determined from the difference in brightness, ΔL, that is just perceivable (reported in 50% of observations) at a given brightness B. The Weber ratio varies considerably with the level of light falling on the retina, in the manner indicated in Figure 8.2.

As these data indicate, the human eye is capable, under ideal conditions (bright illumination and a sharp boundary between two semi-infinite object areas), of discriminating between grey levels separated by as little as 1%. In practical situations, performance is commonly much reduced as a result of four particular factors: the use of sub-optimal illuminance, the absence of sharp boundaries, limited size of the target area for discrimination and the presence of image noise and 'clutter'. The significance of these last two factors will now be considered.

In a classical series of experiments Blackwell (1946) demonstrated the manner in which the ability of a human observer to detect the presence of a circular target against a contrasting background depends on the degree of contrast, the level of illumination and the angular size of the target. For this purpose contrast C is defined as $(B_s - B_0)/B_0$, where B_0 is the brightness of the background, B_s is the brightness of the stimulus (target) and $B_s > B_0$. Alternatively, for $B_s < B_0$, $C = (B_0 - B_s)/B_0$. This dependence is summarised in Figure 8.2. From these data it will be seen in particular that, for a given brightness level, there is an inverse relationship beween the linear size of a target and the degree of contrast necessary for its discrimination. Although this is sometimes stated to be an inverse *linear* relationship, this is clearly an approximation that is valid only over a limited range of target size.

The influence of the noise content of an image on its perception has also been the subject of a great deal of study, particularly in relation to electro-optical imaging and photographic grain noise. In the present context it is convenient to extend the concept of noise to include that of

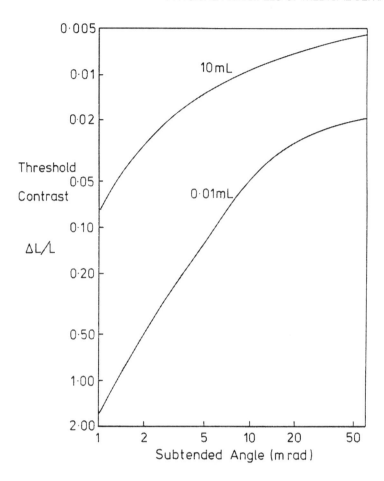

Figure 8.2. Dependence of threshold contrast, $\Delta L/L$ (the 'Weber ratio'), on size of an observed circular disk object for two levels of background luminance, with zero noise and a 6 s viewing time. The effect of added noise and/or of shorter viewing time will generally be to increase the threshold contrast relative to the levels indicated here. *Source*: From Blackwell (1946), reproduced by permission of the Optical Society of America

'clutter': a term that has the more general connotation of an unwanted signal. An important distinction between noise and clutter is that noise, in its restricted sense, is generally incoherent in nature, whereas clutter may exhibit a degree of coherence in relation to the wanted signal.

An important characteristic of image noise, in addition to its magnitude, will be its spatial frequency distribution. Quantitatively, this dependence can be investigated by measuring the amplitude of modulation of a sine-wave bar pattern (raster), as a function of spatial frequency, that is necessary for visual detectability. In the target recognition field this is sometimes referred to as the *noise required modulation* (NRM) or *demand modulation function*.

The application of this concept is illustrated in Figure 8.3, in which NRM is plotted together with the MTF for the corresponding imaging system. Experimentally it is found that the area between these two curves (when plotted on a linear scale), termed the *modulation transfer*

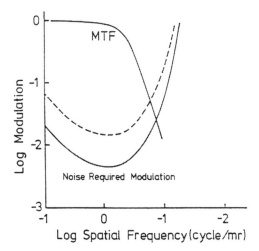

Figure 8.3. Illustrative relationship between the MTF and noise-required modulation in an imaging process. The broken line indicates the effect of an increase in display noise level. The area between the two characteristics is referred to as the modulation transfer function area (MTFA). *Source*: From Biberman (1973), reproduced by permission of Plenum Publishers

function area or **MTFA**, is a good measure of imaging quality for the prediction of operator performance in recognising particular imaged objects (Snyder 1976). It follows from this that noise will have maximum effect in degrading operator performance if it occurs at spatial frequencies for which the MTF has high values: a result whose relevance to particular forms of ultrasonic imaging will become apparent in the following paragraphs.

In experiments in which varying amounts of grain noise are deliberately added to optical images, it is found that an observer, if given the choice, will tend to adjust the viewing magnification in a manner that keeps constant the spatial frequency spectrum of perceived images. This emphasises the importance, in practical system design, of either providing an optimum set magnification or of allowing for operator selection. A rationale for this situation will be outlined in the following section.

8.3.2 NOISE IN ECHOGRAPHY

At this point we need to take a look at the way that one of the particular characteristics of ultrasound images, their noise spectrum, is handled by human visual perception.

As has already been pointed out, ultrasound, unlike the other phenomena used in mainstream medical imaging, is a coherent form of radiation and this has a profound effect on the nature and magnitude of the associated image noise that effectively limits contrast discrimination. As already outlined in Chapter 6 (Section 6.5), and will be discussed again in Chapter 9, the dominant form of noise in an echographic system, which arises directly from the coherent nature of the radiation, is coherent speckle. Its effect is to impose on an image a mottle or speckle with a scale and form that, in itself, is characteristic only of the imaging system. Thus, any small region of interest in the image will contain a small and statistically determined number of speckle centres, with the result that the total signal energy in that region

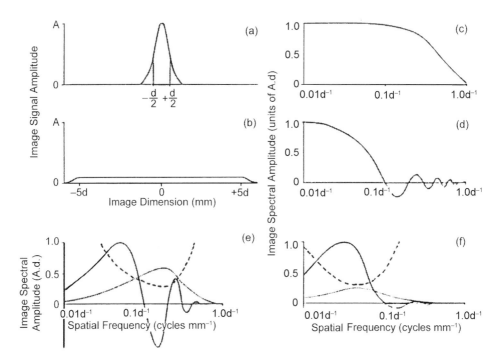

Figure 8.4. Relationship between transfer characteristics and image noise in echographic systems (see text). In this figure, (e) and (f) represent the situation of a normal human subject observing an image characterised by a peak luminance of about 500 cd m^{-2} (*cf.* Figure 7.1) and an LSF full width (i.e. dimension d) of 2 mm, at viewing distances of: (e) 50 cm; (f) 200 cm

will be determined by those statistics. This is analogous to the way in which quantum statistics introduce noise fluctuations into radiographic and radioisotope images.[1]

It follows that the magnitude and spatial frequency shape of speckle noise will be object dependent. An important class of objects in this context is one consisting of large numbers of small (in relation to an acoustic wavelength) and randomly distributed scatterers. In imaging practice this condition of *fully developed speckle noise* can be closely approached when imaging, for example, a volume of blood or an extended volume of parenchymal tissue. In this situation, the autocorrelation function (spatial frequency spectrum) will be almost identical in

---

1 Formal analysis of the behaviour of incoherent, quantum-dependent imaging systems is based on the use of the quantities *Detective Quantum Efficiency* (DQE) and *Noise Equivalent Quanta* (NEQ), which themselves are related to the input and output signal-to-noise ratios (SNR) as:

$$DQE = (SNR_{out})^2/(SNR_{in})^2$$

and

$$NEQ = DQE \times Q$$

where Q is the number of exposure quanta (Wagner 1983). The NEQ can be thought of as the apparent number of quanta that determine the statistics of detector noise. This analysis can be extended to echographic and related coherent imaging systems by recognising that the quantity in such systems analogous to the NEQ is the density of coherent speckle spots in the image (Wagner & Brown 1985).

form to, and thus superimpose on, the imaging system MTF. In an important sense, this result (which minimises values of dynamic range and MTFA and thus of information transfer) is the worst possible, particularly because most soft-tissue echography leads to the generation of speckle noise with broadly similar characteristics.

This point can be illustrated by reference to Figure 8.4. Here, Figure 8.4a illustrates the spread function of the imaging system for a line object, i.e. the LSF, and Figure 8.4b illustrates the spread function that would be produced by the same imaging system for a ribbon-like scattering object having ten times the width, d, of the LSF and the same signal energy as that for the line (i.e. the same areas under the A–d curve). Figure 8.4c is the corresponding MTF of the imaging system and Figure 8.4d is the spatial frequency transform of the extended object (i.e. the Fourier transforms of Figures 8.4a and 8.4b, respectively). The effect of incorporating human vision into the overall description of the imaging system is obtained by multiplication in Fourier space, i.e. as the product of a curve from Figure 8.1 with Figures 8.4c and 8.4d. Representative results are shown in Figures 8.4e and 8.4f for two different viewing distances (i.e. magnification settings) of 50 and 200 cm and assuming (*cf*. Figure 8.1) a reasonably high display luminance.

In Figures 8.4e and 8.4f the resulting (imager plus observer) MTFs are shown dotted and the transformed object functions are depicted by solid lines. The corresponding curves for the NRM, which is inversely proportional to the MTF, are shown dashed and normalised to minima of 0.3. From this it will be seen that the size of the area between the object function and the NRM (the MTFA) is considerably dependent on the viewing distance. Psycho-physically this dependence corresponds to the benefit to be obtained, by optimising viewing distance or magnification, in the perception of objects characterised by spatial frequencies lower than that of the speckle noise.

A quantity related to the MTFA that is also of value as a measure of the available contrast discrimination of a system is the area, expressed as a ratio to the noise spectral area, of the spectrum of the largest image signal that the system can handle without significant distortion. It will be seen that this ratio constitutes a generalised and image-related measure of *system dynamic range* (the limiting value of the SNR for a large signal). In particular, when the two spectra have identical shape, the procedure is equivalent to the more conventional one of taking the ratio in image space of the corresponding r.m.s. signal amplitudes; i.e. in decibel form:

$$SNR = 20 \log_{10}(A_i/A_n)$$

where A_i and A_n are the areas under the spatial frequency spectra (as plotted on linear scales) of the image and noise amplitude, respectively.

Our purpose in discussing the nature and origins of noise in echographic systems has been to shed light on the factors determining contrast resolution: in practical terms, to address questions of the type, 'How small a tumour will I be able to see using this particular scanner?' Evidently, both speckle and electronic noise may contribute to this, and it will be useful here to bear in mind that it is their joint impact on the signal-to-noise ratio that determines the contrast resolution threshold. The result is a dependence on the penetration depth of the approximate form indicated in Figure 8.5. At shallow depth, where receiver electronic noise is not significant, noise is dominated by speckle and the speckle SNR at the receiver input is predicted to be approximately constant with depth. Attenuation of the signal by tissue, which is exponential with depth, causes electronic noise to dominate beyond a certain critical depth and thus reduces the SNR. The actual value of this critical depth will depend on a number of factors, but particularly on the frequency-dependent attenuation coefficient of tissue.

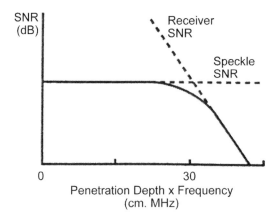

Figure 8.5. Probable form of the dependence on penetration depth of the SNR of an echographic system, for the common situation where signal arises as contrast between different regions of a scattering medium, such as soft tissue

Typically, for abdominal imaging at an acoustic frequency of 3 MHz it may be around 10–12 cm, or about 3 cm for small-part imaging at 10 MHz. The slope of the 'receiver SNR' line will depend on the identity of the penetrated tissue: the example given is typical for liver and similar soft tissues.

8.3.3 THE TIME FACTOR IN VISUAL PERCEPTION

There are at least two separate time-related factors in human visual perception that need to be considered in a discussion of imaging: the response of the visual process itself and the time-course of the pattern- and feature-recognition process that takes place in the higher levels of the brain.

It appears that the human visual process has evolved in a manner that is responsive to specific perception of movement. Quantitatively, this can be measured and expressed (analogously to spatial response) as a temporal frequency function of 'flicker sensitivity' (Pearson 1975). If a small, uniform luminance source is caused to fluctuate sinusoidally in luminance about a mean value L_0, the resulting stimulus will be:

$$L_0 + \Delta L \cos(2\pi f t)$$

where ΔL is the peak amplitude of the fluctuation and f is its frequency. If the value of ΔL that produces a threshold sensation of flicker is determined experimentally as a function of f, a *flicker sensitivity* or *temporal contrast sensitivity* can be derived as the ratio $L_0/\Delta L$.

The typical response of the human eye under representative viewing conditions is illustrated in Figure 8.6. From this it will be seen that, at low brightness levels, the eye behaves as though it were integrating with a time constant of around 0.2 s. By contrast, at higher brightness the system discriminates quite strongly against relatively static aspects of a scene and is maximally sensitive to frequencies around 8 Hz. The criteria for flicker-free viewing will evidently require operation to be on the negative slope of the response curve and relative brightness fluctuation to be below some value set by the flicker frequency. The limitation will be somewhat less stringent at moderate than at high brightness levels.

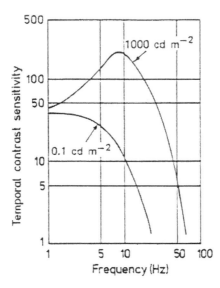

Figure 8.6. Typical flicker sensitivity of the eye for two values of retinal luminance. *Source*: From Pearson (1975), reproduced by permission of John Wiley & Sons, Ltd

8.3.4 MISCELLANEOUS FEATURES OF VISUAL PERCEPTION

Although space does not permit full treatment of visual perception here, it will be useful to bear in mind a number of features of human visual perception that can have a bearing on the performance of an observer of ultrasonic images.

Contrast can arise in either positive (signal brighter than background) or negative forms. There is some evidence that, at least for relatively high contrast and with a suitably trained observer, the eye may be substantially more sensitive to negative contrast, possibly to the extent of halving the angular diameter of an object that is just detectable at a given contrast; this leads potentially to a very significant difference in, for example, tumour detection (Overington 1976; Sanders 1980).

The eye is anisotropic in its sensitivity, being maximally sensitive (particularly for fine detail) to vertical edges and minimally to obliques (Campbell & Kulikowski 1966).

Texture is a complex concept and its quantitative description is made in terms of a number of features at various levels of detail. It seems to be here in particular, for the higher levels of complexity, that 'machine vision' may be able to outperform the human observer (Wagner *et al.* 1991).

Colour differentiation is an important feature of normal human vision, albeit with partial impairment (red/green 'colour blindness') in some 8% of the population. Its exploitation in medical imaging, echography in particular, is generally limited to parametric display, i.e. superimposed display of a second parameter, such as blood flow velocity, simultaneously with the primary imaging parameter, such as backscatter amplitude. Attempts have been made also to transpose from a grey scale to a colour scale display of echo amplitude, but this appears to be of little value in terms of perceptual performance unless, perhaps, means can be found to reduce the impact of speckle noise (Logan-Sinclair *et al.* 1981).

8.3.5 OBSERVERS AND THEIR PERFORMANCE

The concept of operator performance is clearly important in relation to medical imaging because an image here is generally produced to assist in a particular task of detection or recognition of an abnormality. In optical image science it is conventional to define three stages of perception of an object: *detection* (i.e. the object is believed to be present); *recognition* (the class to which the object belongs is discerned, e.g. blood vessel, cyst); and *identification* (the target can be described at a second level of detail, e.g. inferior hepatic vein, cavernous haemangioma). Furthermore, these different degrees of perception have been related empirically to the detectability (using the same imaging conditions and degree of modulation) of bar patterns of given spatial frequency. Thus it is found that detection, recognition and identification occur for approximate target angular widths of $1/v$, $4/v$ and $6.5/v$, respectively, where v is the period of highest detectable spatial frequency (cycles per unit angle). This is, of course, a somewhat simplistic statement and, in practice, performance of such perceptual tasks is influenced by a number of other factors, including the time available for the task and also the *a priori* expectation of finding a particular target in a particular region of a scene. It would be of interest to investigate the practical application of this approach for relating operator performance to imaging system parameters in some particular areas of medical imaging.

The above discussion has been centred around the behaviour and limitations of the human visual faculties. In principle one might expect improved perceptual performance in some respects, for example in contrast-limited resolution by replacing or supplementing human vision by artificial means: extraction of wanted signal from incoherent noise by averaging processes is a well-known example of what is possible here. In this context a distinction is made, in imaging theory, between *real* and *ideal observers*: the latter is assumed to be 'able to use all the information in the noisy image sample, including that in the noise correlations' (Wagner & Brown 1985). It has been estimated that human observers may only be some 60% efficient, as compared with the ideal, whereas the performance of a computational observer may approach 100% (Insana & Hall 1994). In seeking to achieve optimum human investigative performance it is important to know the magnitude of these shortcomings, to understand the reasons for them and to be able to identify the opportunities that may exist for artificial enhancement of performance.

8.4 THE PLACE OF ULTRASOUND IN MEDICAL IMAGING

In the next three chapters we shall describe in some detail particular medical imaging techniques that are based on the use of ultrasound. At this point, therefore, in the light of the above discussion of some aspects of the science of imaging *per se*, we can consider some of the reasons why ultrasound is particularly suited to this purpose.

One of the reasons most commonly put forward in favour of ultrasound methods of imaging in medicine is their relative 'safety'. Some of the evidence on this issue is given in Chapter 14 but at this point we might rephrase the statement in the form that 'for levels of radiation exposure of patients that are associated with a given level of risk, ultrasound will generally be capable of providing a significantly higher image signal-to-noise ratio than will be available from imaging systems based on the use of ionising radiation'. Although such a statement, of course, begs some questions about comparative hazards and risks, it makes the point that, in practice, it is signal-to-noise considerations and their influence on such factors as contrast resolution that ultimately determine the minimum radiation dose levels that are attainable in X-ray and radioisotope imaging. With ultrasound, by contrast, although signal-to-noise ratio is still of fundamental importance, its limitation generally comes from factors other than those connected with radiation safety.

As has been indicated in earlier chapters, the interactions between ultrasound and human tissues are varied and often quite specific: values of parameters such as backscattering and attenuation coefficient, for example, can be distinctly different, as between different but anatomically neighbouring tissue structures. This situation in itself is basic to the potential of ultrasound for providing good degrees of contrast resolution and, for some diagnostic problems, can give it an important advantage over X-ray imaging, where absorption coefficient can be a rather insensitive measure of histopathological change. In ultrasound, as in other branches of medical imaging, there is much interest in methods of so-called 'tissue characterisation' or 'image parameterisation' (see Chapter 9). To some extent the drive here is towards developing more quantitative and objective procedures but, in imaging terms, it can be seen also as a search for imaging parameters that provide clearer differentiation in particular situations and hence the prospect of even better contrast resolution.

Another important consideration that again particularly affects contrast resolution capability is the ability to discriminate against signals from interfering regions of a target (e.g. adjacent or overlying tissue). At least to a useful approximation this ability will be seen to be inherent in the main ultrasonic imaging methods, whereas it is often only attainable at some cost and difficulty (e.g. by computed reconstruction) in X-ray and radioisotope imaging.

Basic requirements on any radiation that is to be used for imaging are that it should propagate in a geometrically predictable manner and without excessive attenuation in the medium of interest, and that it should behave in this way at frequencies for which diffraction-determined directivity is consistent with adequate spatial resolution. In other words, wavelengths must be small in relation to the objects being imaged. It is one of the remarkable features of natural phenomena that these requirements are satisfactorily fulfilled for ultrasound propagating in the soft tissue of the human body. Refractive deflection and deformation of beams do occur but generally not in a manner that significantly affects imaging performance. Equally, attenuation is significant (without it one would have no interactions to use for imaging) but permits penetration in soft tissues to depths of about 300 wavelengths (in the megahertz frequency region) to a sufficient degree to allow imaging with adequate signal-to-noise ratio in either transmission or backscattering modes. In practice, as discussed in detail below, this leads to diffraction-limited resolution of the order of a millimetre.

An additional feature of ultrasound as an imaging mode, which is related both to its facility for engineering implementation and to its apparent freedom from radiation risk, is its potential for generating high-quality, rapid sequential images at a frame-rate above the peak of human flicker sensitivity. In this respect it undoubtedly exceeds any of the other major medical imaging procedures.

8.5   THE SYSTEMATICS OF IMAGE INTERPRETATION

The ultimate justification for trying to form medical images, as indeed for collecting many other forms of medical data, is to optimise the quality of decisions that need to be made about the management of patients. Thus a particular ultrasonic investigative procedure (e.g. making a B-scan of a pregnant abdomen, or measuring the biparietal diameter of a fetal skull) will be used in order to provide answers to particular questions. These may be quite specific (e.g. is the fetus growing at the normal rate?) or somewhat general (e.g. is there any anatomical abnormality in the fetus?), but in any case it is implicitly assumed that there is a correct answer that may be provided by the investigation.

In real life there are very few investigative procedures in medicine that invariably provide the correct answer to questions asked of them. This is partly because all such procedures are inherently noisy. Earlier in this chapter we discussed the physical manifestations of noise in ultrasonic imaging systems, but it needs to be borne in mind also that, where a human interpreter is part of the system, he or she may also constitute a major source of 'noise' in this context, to a degree that is only somewhat diminished as training and experience increase. Thus it becomes useful to discuss systematically the process of decision-making as it relates to the interpretation of medical images and related sets of data.

Several different kinds of decision are involved in the total procedure of image interpretation. The first is that of *detection*: a decision as to whether an abnormality is present. Beyond this, however there is *localisation* (Where is the abnormality?) and *classification* (What sort of abnormality is it?). Of these, the detection process has been discussed most fully and seems to be best understood, although both localisation and classification can be considered usefully as modifications of the detection process.

It is clearly important to be able to assess the quality of investigative decisions that result from a particular imaging (or similar) procedure and a certain formalism has been developed for this purpose, particularly in relation to decisions on detection. This starts from an assumption that a 'true' answer exists to the question of whether an abnormality is present, which is then compared with the actual answer given by the imaging procedure. In this way one can construct the following statistical decision matrix, with associated terminology, covering the four possible situations:

		Is an abnormality truly present?	
		Yes	No
Did the test indicate the presence	Yes	True positive (TP)	False positive (FP)
of an abnormality?	No	False negative (FN)	True negative (TN)

On the basis of this formalism, the following terms and definitions are commonly used to indicate the quality of an investigative procedure.

Sensitivity, or *True Positive Fraction* (TPF)
  $= $ (Number of correct positive assessments)/(Number of truly positive cases)
  $= (NTP)/(NTP + NFN)$

Specificity, or *True Negative Fraction* (TNF)
  $= $ (Number of correct negative assessments)/(Number of truly negative cases)
  $= (NTN)/(NTN + NFP)$

Accuracy
  $= $ (Number of correct assessments)/(Total number of cases)
  $= (NTP + NTN)/(NTP + NTN + NFP + NFN)$

At this point one needs to bear in mind some qualifications as to the objectivity of this kind of analysis. In the first place, particularly if decisions are being made by a human investigator (or even by a programmed machine), one must anticipate the likelihood of bias, deliberate or otherwise. There will always be a certain expectation value for the ratio between normal and abnormal cases, and the assumption of an inappropriate ratio will tend to bias the results. More importantly, however, an investigator may be strongly influenced in decision-making by knowledge of the consequence of a particular decision. Consider, for example, the hypothetical situations of a clinician using an ultrasound scanner, first of all to screen a population of predominantly healthy women for possible signs of breast cancer, and, secondly, to examine a woman with a previously detected breast lump in support of a decision on whether major surgery should be undertaken. In the first case, the statistical expectation of an abnormality will be very low, but the consequence of a high false-positive rate will be the relatively mild one of an excessive number of patients undergoing further examinations. Thus there could be a valid bias towards achieving high sensitivity at the cost of decreased specificity. In the second case the expectation of a serious abnormality will be much higher, but the investigator will need to be able to convey to the referring surgeon the degree of confidence that can be attached to the eventual assessment.

Another important qualification to note is (with Oscar Wilde) that 'truth is rarely pure, and never simple': the assumption implicit in the above, that one can always assume the existence of a 'true' assessment of an abnormality, is unrealistic. The best that one can usually hope for in the way of a definitive diagnosis is a report on histopathology following surgery, biopsy or post-mortem examination. Even this is not always forthcoming and, when it is, may well be open to question.

It is thus clear that a simple measure such as sensitivity, specificity or even accuracy, valuable though it may be when properly interpreted, will not be a truly objective indicator of the quality of the decisions that are available from a particular imaging test procedure. If such an indicator is required, it will be provided rather better by the so-called *receiver operating characteristic* (ROC). This is constructed (Figure 8.7) as a plot of true positive fraction (TPF) against false positive fraction (FPF), the individual points on the curve being obtained by carrying out multiple runs of the test, each with a different degree of bias (or decision threshold) as to the expectation of a positive result. Such a procedure would result in a plot similar to one of those illustrated in the figure. The different curves shown are illustrative of a differing quality in the decision process; the test producing the diagonal straight line would be totally uninformative, whereas lines approaching closest to the FPF = 0 and TPF = 1 axes would be those corresponding to tests exhibiting the best performance (Green & Swets 1966).

The ROC analysis can be used to compare the detectability of different kinds of abnormality and to compare performance (in the sense of facilitating detection decisions) either of imaging systems or of their operators. It can, however, be a very time-consuming procedure and it is useful to note that equally good results can be derived from a considerably faster rating procedure (Chesters 1982; Swets & Pickett 1982; ICRU 1996). In this, the observer is required

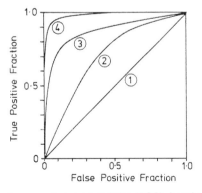

Figure 8.7. Examples of receiver operating characteristics (ROC). Any signal (or test) that generates a ROC curve wholly above and to the left of another is the more powerful

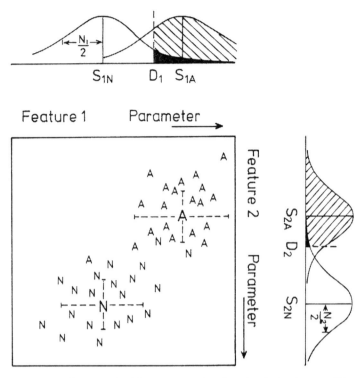

Figure 8.8. Illustration of noise-limited feature separation. The signals for the two different features are characterized by their separations (e.g. $S_{1A} - S_{1N}$) and the widths of their noise spectra (e.g. N_1). Imposing a decision threshold (e.g. D_1) defines the true positive fraction (hatched area) and false positive fraction (solid area). Corresponding distributions in two-dimensional feature space are also shown

to categorise his degree of certainty about his assessment, e.g. almost certainly negative, probably negative, possibly positive, etc.

It is sometimes useful to consider the decision-making procedure in terms of a model in which separation between a normal and an abnormal signal is a noise-limited process (Figure 8.8). In this, the 'signals' may be any of a large number of potentially quantifiable features of an image (e.g. grey level, smoothness of a lesion boundary, etc.) and the noise may originate from the observer, the imaging system and/or variations in the object itself. On this model one can see rather clearly the effect of placing a decision threshold at some particular value on the scale of signal magnitude. This model also illustrates the fact that decisions (whether observer- or machine-implemented) often will be made on the basis of a number of separate features, for each of which there will be a degree of noise-limited signal separation. In this situation the decision will be made (whether in the mind of the observer or in a computer) within the format of a multi-dimensional feature space (shown as two-dimensional in the figure).

REFERENCES

Biberman, L.M. (1973). *Perception of Displayed Information*. Plenum Press, New York.
Blackwell, H.R. (1946). Contrast thresholds of the human eye. *J. Opt. Soc. Am.* **36**, 624–643.

Campbell, F.W. and Kulikowski, J.J. (1966). Orientation selectivity of the human visual system. *J. Physiol.* **187**, 437–445.

Chesters, M.S. (1982). Perception and evaluation of images. In *Scientific Basis of Medical Imaging*, P.N.T. Wells (ed.). Churchill, Edinburgh, pp. 237–280.

Cornsweet, T.N. (1970). *Visual Perception*. Academic Press, New York.

Green, D.M. and Swets, J.A. (1966). *Signal Detection Theory and Psychophysics*. Wiley, New York.

Haber, R.N. and Hershenson, M. (1973). *The Psychology of Visual Perception*. Holt, New York.

Hill, C.R., Bamber, J.C., Crawford, D.C., Lowe, H.J. and Webb, S. (1991). What might echography learn from image science? *Ultrasound Med. Biol.* **17**, 559–575.

Hill, C.R. and Kratochwil, A. (1981). *Medical Ultrasonic Images: Formation, Display, Recording and Perception*. Excerpta Medica, Amsterdam.

ICRU (1996). *Medical Imaging: The Assessment of Image Quality*, ICRU Report No. 54. International Commission on Radiation Units and Measurements, Bethesda, USA.

Insana, M.F. and Hall, T.J. (1994). Visual detection efficiency in ultrasonic imaging: a framework for objective assessment of image quality. *J. Acoust. Soc. Am.* **95**, 2081–2090.

Logan-Sinclair, R., Wong, C.M. and Gibson, D.G. (1981). Clinical application of amplitude processing of echo-cardiographic images. *Br. Heart J.* **45**, 621–627.

Metz, C.E. and Doi, K. (1979). Transfer function analysis of radiographic imaging systems. *Phys. Med. Biol.* **24**, 1079–1106.

Overington, I. (1976). *Vision and Acquisition*. Pentech Press, London.

Pearson, D.E. (1975). *Transmission and Display of Pictorial Information*. Pentech Press, London.

Sanders, R.C. (1980). Comparison between black and white backgrounds for ultrasonic images. *J. Clin. Ultrasound* **8**, 413–415.

Snyder, H.L. (1976). Display image quality and the eye of the beholder. In *Image Analysis and Evaluation*, *Proc. SPSE Conf.*, R. Shaw (ed.), pp. 341–346.

Swets, J.A. and Pickett, R.M. (1982). *Evaluation of Diagnostic Systems: Methods from Signal Detection Theory*. Academic Press, New York.

Wagner, R.F. (1983). Low contrast sensitivity of radiologic, CT, nuclear medicine and ultrasound medical imaging systems. *IEEE Trans.* **MI-2**, 105–121.

Wagner, R.F. and Brown, D.G. (1985). Unified SNR analysis of medical imaging systems. *Phys. Med. Biol.* **30**, 489–518.

Wagner, R.F., Insana, M.F., Brown, D.G., Garra, B.S. and Jennings, R.J. (1991). Texture discrimination: radiologist, machine and man. In *Vision, Coding and Efficiency*, C. Blakemore (ed.). Cambridge University Press, Cambridge.

Webb, S. (1988). *The Physics of Medical Imaging* (2nd edn). Adam Hilger, Bristol.

9

Methodology for Clinical Investigation

C. R. HILL and J. C. BAMBER

Institute of Cancer Research, Royal Marsden Hospital, UK

9.1 INTRODUCTION

The first major international conference on medical ultrasonics, held in 1969 in Vienna, proved to be a turning point in the development of ultrasound for clinical investigation. In the 20 years prior to that date the subject had been explored by a small group of enthusiastic engineers and doctors, supported by a number of specialist manufacturers, but was largely ignored by mainstream clinicians, radiologists and bioengineers (Donald 1974; Wild 1978; Hill 1993). In the years following 1969, however, the subject went through a phenomenal phase of development – not only in its scale but in the scope of its applications and, to a lesser degree, in the understanding of its scientific basis – to the point where ultrasound now accounts for some 20–25% of all imaging-type clinical investigations carried out worldwide and commercially its annual market value has overtaken the X-ray, the previous leader in the field. One particular consequence of this situation, which we shall discuss below, is that the present pattern of use of ultrasound may reflect primarily commercial rather than scientific opportunity.

Over the course of its development hitherto, investigative ultrasound has been based predominantly on the use of the pulse–echo principle: the exploitation of signals received from an interrogated volume following its exposure to a transmitted wave packet. This initially proved to be so practically successful and so comparatively simple to implement (with the ironic consequence that ultrasound tends to be awarded the stigma of 'cheapness'!) that there seemed to be rather little incentive to pursue improvement through better scientific understanding. At the same time, the raw analogue signals that the technique produced accumulated at such a high rate that, at least until the late 1990s, it was impracticable to carry out on the data more than quite simple digital manipulation. Thus, at the time of writing, there are good reasons to believe that there is potential for considerable further developments in the subject. On the one hand there are possibilities, which have hitherto been little explored, for exploiting the underlying physics that we have discussed in earlier chapters. At the same time, there may well be substantial useful information that is not being exploited, even in the signals that are being recorded by present-day techniques.

In this section of the book – the present chapter and the two that follow – we attempt to do two things: to describe in outline the present state of the art; and, to open up discussion on

Physical Principles of Medical Ultrasonics, Second Edition. Edited by C. R. Hill, J. C. Bamber and G. R. ter Haar.
© 2004 John Wiley & Sons, Ltd: ISBN 0 471 97002 6

some ideas and principles that derive from the underlying science that has been set out in previous chapters and that seem to us to have promise for the future.

Any attempt to divide up a subject like this into several 'chapters' must be to some extent arbitrary: there are no very clear boundaries. The scheme that we have adopted is that Chapters 9 and 10 are concerned with approaches that are specifically oriented towards *clinical* investigations (i.e. literally investigations at the bedside: Gk. *klinikos*, a bed). All ultrasonic investigative methods are potentially four-dimensional: here, Chapter 9 discusses general principles and confines descriptions of methods largely to current and prospective pulse–echo practice as applied to the three spatial dimensions; detailed consideration of the time dimension and the study of tissue movement and fluid flow are taken up in Chapter 10. Ultrasound also provides the basis for a variety of other medically and biologically relevant investigative techniques whose application is not, at least primarily, in the clinic; a particularly interesting topic here is what has become known as acoustic microscopy. These are taken up in Chapter 11.

This is not intended to be a 'user handbook'. There are a number of excellent texts that deal with the subject at an essentially practical level (e.g. Bamber & Tristam 1988; Wells 1993; Zagzebski 1996; Dowsett *et al.* 1998; Duck *et al.* 1998; Anglesen 2000) and we have therefore limited our coverage of such material to what seems necessary in order to illustrate underlying principles.

As will be seen, this chapter uses the term 'investigative ultrasound', often in preference to the more commonly used 'diagnostic ultrasound', 'ultrasonic imaging', 'echography', 'sonography', etc. This is deliberate, and is done to press home the point that we are concerned, technically, with much more than just imaging and, clinically, with much more than simply diagnosis.

9.2   IMAGING AND MEASUREMENT: STATE OF THE PULSE–ECHO ART

9.2.1 THE SYSTEM IN OUTLINE

Practical pulse–echo systems can take many forms and it is instructive to consider them – somewhat arbitrarily – to consist of six interrelated parts as indicated in Figure 9.1, operating on an interrogated object or 'target', that itself may need to be accessed through a coupling medium (e.g. a water bath or, more commonly, a thin layer of thixotropic fluid).

The central component in the system is an electro-acoustic transducer, which serves both to propagate an interrogating acoustic pulse towards the 'object' and also to detect the acoustic echoes that subsequently emanate from it. In some early systems the transducer consisted of a single plate of piezoelectric material but now almost invariably comprises a one- or two-dimensional array of cooperating elements. There are certain advantages, particularly in relation to signal-to-noise ratio, in separating the functions of transmit and receive transduction in such arrays. An account of the behaviour of transducers and the nature of their spatial and temporal field patterns has been given in Chapter 2.

To make possible the assembly of echo information into an 'image', it is necessary that the spatial location of a transducer, and/or the orientation of its beam axis, should be known accurately at all times. The scanning process – movement of the beam axis through an interrogated volume – is commonly effected by electronic control of an array transducer, with simultaneous provision of electronic signals that define the beam coordinates. An elegant extension of this scanning process, based on methods of 'speckle tracking' (outlined below), is

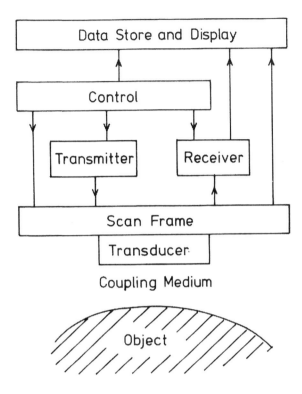

Figure 9.1. Block diagram illustrating the interrelationships of the different main components of pulse–echo diagnostic systems

progressively to build up a scan geometry by reference to landmarks in the previously scanned segments. An example of a scan obtained in this way is shown in Figure 9.10.

The role of the transmitter is to generate a train of electrical pulses (not necessarily identical) of shape and amplitude that will result in acoustic pulse emission from the transducer appropriate to the required interrogation task. Whereas early designs commonly used a fast step function for this purpose, current practice is to so shape the excitation pulse that the transducer output is optimised with respect to the amplitude and frequency spectrum. In particular, different excitation may be required depending on whether the returned echoes are to be used for contributing to B-scan, pulsed Doppler or colour Doppler imaging modes. In some systems special shaping and/or sequencing procedures may be used to exploit opportunities provided by the underlying physics; an example here is *pulse inversion*, where a sequential pair of excitation pulses is used, differing by a 180° phase shift, with the difference between the two echoes characterising propagation or scattering non-linearity in the target tissue (Chapman & Lazenby 1997). In yet other systems, pulse shaping may be to incorporate a code that will allow pulse recognition to overcome the echo position ambiguity referred to below (to increase frame rate or, through signal averaging, signal-to-electronic-noise ratio and penetration depth), or shaping may be specific to elements in a transducer array, for example to permit greater sophistication than a simple single spherical transmit focus. The amplitude of any set of excitation pulses will, in practice, be limited by two factors: the requirement to limit the levels of acoustic energy propagated into the patient (see Chapter 14); and the impact of propagation non-linearity in limiting beam penetration (see Section 9.2.4).

9.2.2 SCANNING

As has been pointed out already, living human anatomy is essentially four-dimensional, with three time-variant spatial dimensions. Ultrasound, with its inherently rapid data acquisition capability, is exceptionally well placed to work in this way. Nevertheless, in order to achieve good spatio-temporal resolution, data will have to be acquired from a great many voxels (volume elements), and a choice is available as to how this can best be achieved for a particular type of application.

It will be useful at this point briefly to consider in more detail this issue of data acquisition rate. The conventional procedure for deriving a pulse–echo image does not make use of coded acoustic pulses or of receiving echoes along multiple lines of sight in parallel. As such, the method employed to distinguish echoes due to one pulse from those due to another, and avoid the echo position ambiguity that would otherwise ensue, is by means of recording a sequential series of image lines, allowing time for all echoes to return along one line before transmitting the next pulse. The time required to obtain a single such line, extending to depth d in the object, is:

$$t_1 = 2d/c \tag{9.1}$$

where c is the speed of sound in the object material. The minimum time to obtain an n-line image is thus:

$$t_i = 2nd/c \tag{9.2}$$

Hence the time to acquire an image of 100 lines (corresponding to rather poor sampling), covering a depth of 10 cm in soft tissues ($c \approx 1500\,\text{ms}^{-1}$), will be approximately 13 ms. Practical considerations will increase this figure somewhat, particularly if, for example, the information to be displayed is not unprocessed echo magnitude and is not available from a single pulse: e.g. when some speckle reduction methods are employed, or when the information is associated with tissue motion or with the degree of propagation non-linearity (see later this chapter and Chapter 10). Nonetheless, it is feasible to obtain good B-scan image quality at frame rates of the order of 10–20 Hz, where human visual sensitivity to brightness modulation is low (see Chapter 8). As was suggested above, there are many schemes for altering the transmit and receive pulse and beam-forming process so as to increase this frame rate but it is an intriguing thought that so-called 'real-time ultrasound' using this simplest of image-forming methods is only made practicable by the apparently fortuitous set of relationships between speed of sound, the scale of human anatomy and the particular physiology of the human eye and brain!

If, as is commonly the case, acquired data are to be presented to a human observer, there will be a choice as to the format in which such presentation will be most appropriate for the investigative task on hand. Some of the earliest scanners simply displayed on an oscilloscope the amplitude of the incoming echo signals, in either r.f. or rectified ('video') form and usually following time-gain compensation (see below) against a time base triggered by the transmit pulse. This so-called 'A-scan' is now rarely, if ever, used apart perhaps from some restricted measurement applications in ophthalmology, where the anatomy lateral to the beam is expected to be reasonably invariant and predictable.

If multiple A-scans are recorded at high repetition rate and over a long time period, very rapid and small movements of tissue structures, which may have been imperceptible on older or lower cost B-scan systems, may be evaluated. This feature has been exploited, particularly for cardiac application, in the M (movement)-scan, in which the time of arrival of the echo from a selected anatomical entity (e.g. a heart valve) is displayed against a slow time base (Figure 9.2). An important feature of this mode of data acquisition is that, even in systems of modest cost, it can be carried out at a repetition rate sufficiently high to follow the very fast movement of heart structures. Techniques such as parallel beam-forming that increase frame rate, and looped digital memory that makes inter-frame motion replay and comparison possible, have made the M-scan almost obsolete but at increased hardware cost.

The principle of the B-scan is well known because it is the basis of virtually all contemporary medical ultrasonic investigation. It can be seen, again, as a development of the A-scan, in which the video echo train is used to brightness-modulate a line in the image plane that is made to correspond instantaneously with the ultrasonic beam axis in the object plane. Thus a 'scan' of this axis across the object plane will build up a corresponding brightness-modulated image.

It is worth bearing in mind at this stage that this procedure, although of great practical value, is in a sense arbitrary and has evolved through considerations of convenience rather

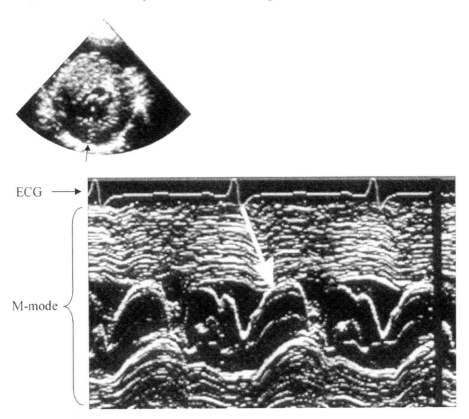

Figure 9.2. An M-mode display (lower picture) showing systolic anterior motion of the mitral valve, where the valve can be seen (white arrow) to be hitting and maintaining contact with the septum. The black arrow in the upper, cross-sectional B-scan indicates the acoustic line of sight to which the M-mode pertains. This example has historical importance although, with modern high frame rate scanners, such a diagnosis might now be made from real-time B-mode imaging alone. *Source*: Images are courtesy of P. Nihoyannopoulos

than from scientifically based strategy. It should become evident from later discussion that there may well be potential imaging parameters that, although at present less easy to implement in practice, could in some applications be more sensitive or reliable indicators of anatomy and pathology than a map of the modulus of echo amplitude, modified to an indeterminate extent by tissue attenuation.

The physical 'scanning' process referred to above – movement of the beam axis within a scanning frame – can be effected in two basic ways: by actual movement of a transducer having a fixed beam axis or by electronically controlled movement of a beam axis relative to an array-type transducer whose position is essentially fixed in space. The former approach has a long and creditable history but arrays are now in virtually universal use.

Array transducers in common use are broadly of two types, so-called 'linear' and 'phased' arrays, the terminology referring to the method by which scanning of the beam is achieved. The principles of these two arrangements are illustrated in Figure 9.3. In a linear array (Figure 9.3a), successive, spatially limited groups of array elements execute successive transmit–receive sequences, with the selected group being progressed, usually by one element width per image line, along the length of the array, thus acquiring a complete image frame by translating the point of origin of the beam from one end of the array to the other. As illustrated in Figure 9.3b, some degree of focusing in the array plane may be achieved by appropriately adjusting

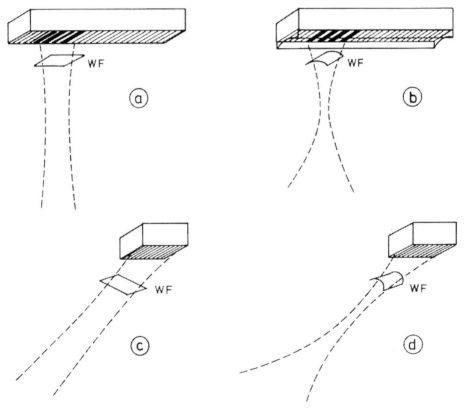

Figure 9.3. Principles of ultrasonic beam formation, scanning, steering and focusing by means of multi-element transducer arrays. Typical positions of wave fronts (WF) are indicated. See text for discussion

the relative phasing between different elements on both transmit and receive, and some fixed lens focusing in the orthogonal plane also may be provided. In a phased array (Figures 9.3c and 9.3d), the full array aperture is available for use on both transmit and receive, and both beam steering and in-plane focusing are implemented by appropriate phase adjustment. With both linear and phased arrays it is possible to move the position of the receive focus progressively outwards in step with the source of the returning echoes. On occasion there may be little to distinguish between a linear and a phased array, the naming convention being somewhat arbitrary as, for example, when adjustment of relative phase between elements is used with long arrays to achieve linear scanning with a wide aperture or when used to steer a linear scanned beam for purposes of compound image formation (see below). A disadvantage of arrays compared with single element-transducers is the occurrence of additional, and in general deleterious, components in their diffraction patterns. Any regularly spaced array constitutes, as in optics, a diffraction grating with the positions of grating lobes determined by wavelength and element spacing. At the same time individual elements express their own diffraction patterns, in turn determined by wavelength and element width. In practice, substantial suppression of grating lobes can be achieved by ensuring that they are positioned near the 'zero' of the element diffraction patterns. The construction of arrays becomes increasingly difficult at higher frequencies, in which situation single-element transducers may still need to be the technology of choice (Passman & Emmert 1996; Foster *et al.* 2000).

An apparently attractive line of development of array technology is to two-dimensional arrays and their use for two-dimensional focusing and for three-dimensional data acquisition. Substantial experimental work in this area has been reported but has not yet achieved widespread commercial implementation. The development of two-dimensional arrays has been inhibited by their potential cost and particularly the requirement to provide a separate electronic channel for each active element of the array. Help in this situation is available, however, from the use of 'sparse' arrays (e.g. Austeng & Holm 2002) and from an integrated circuit technology in which an electronic channel is formed to be integral with each element (e.g. Erikson *et al.* 1997). A practical compromise design is the '1.5-dimensional array', which can be visualised as a one-dimensional array in which each element is separated into a small number (say 3–5) of sub-units, thus allowing limited dynamic focusing in the thickness dimension of the scan plane (Rizzatto 1999).

Three-dimensional data acquisition has been accomplished for many years by mechanically moving a complete one-dimensional or 1.5-dimensional array. Following the discussion surrounding equation (9.2) and assuming again that unsophisticated pulse and beam-forming methods are employed, the time required for a volume echo data acquisition of 100×100 lines at 10 cm maximum depth using this method would be about 1.3 s. Although fast by comparison with other medical imaging modalities, this remains too slow for desired application to moving objects, particularly the heart. The year 2000, or thereabouts, saw the beginning of the availability of real-time volume ultrasound imaging systems based on two-dimensional arrays (Takuma *et al.* 2000; Espinola-Zavaleta *et al.* 2002). An acceptable frame rate may be achieved, with some loss of lateral resolution, by dividing the proposed number of image lines into groups and emitting a sequence of broad transmit beams, each steered and focused to cover a group of lines of sight to be imaged. Parallel-receive beam-forming electronics may then be used simultaneously to steer and focus the directional sensitivity pattern of the transducer's receiving elements along the originally proposed lines of sight within each group. This technique is an extension of a method first known as 'exploso-scanning' (Shattuck *et al.* 1984). In a practical device of, for example, 16:1 parallelism in the ratio of the number of imaged lines for each transmit beam, a volume of 10 cm maximum depth could be scanned by an array of 64×64 image lines in about 33 ms, making it feasible to achieve volume frame rates of the order of 20–30 Hz. The eventual extrapolation of this approach is not to focus on transmit at all, but to flood-illuminate the object and carry out all receive beam-forming in parallel. Such an approach was taken by Sandrin *et al.* (1999), who were able to achieve a two-dimensional real-time acquisition frame rate of at least 4000 frames per second, albeit for off-line beam forming and image reconstruction. This was employed for the observation of propagating shear-stress waves (see Chapter 10). With two-dimensional arrays such rates are achievable for scanning entire volumes, which would permit, for example, rapid volume scanning of extended fields of view by moving the two-dimensional array or full quantification of the velocity vector associated with fast-moving structures.

Three-dimensional data acquisition is, in effect, already a normal part of everyday practice: the clinical investigator commonly sweeps a transducer in a direction normal to its scan plane, the so-called elevational direction, and thereby builds up a three-dimensional mental picture of the examined anatomy. One of the remaining apparent attractions of engineered three-dimensional data acquisition is therefore the potential for reformatting data in any required set of planes (analogously to practice in CT and MRI). One such 'view' that is of interest, in the sense that it corresponds to that familiar in the plane X-ray and gamma-camera radioisotope images, is the so-called C-scan, representing planes normal to the ultrasonic beam axis. An early example of a set of such scans, taken with a purpose-built scanning device,

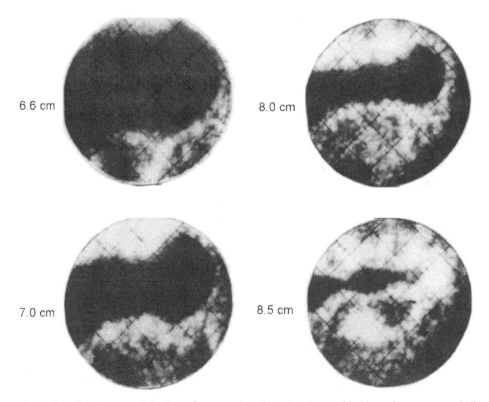

Figure 9.4. Set of constant-depth or C-scans taken through a human bladder, using a purpose-built scanner, at indicated depths below the abdominal skin surface. *Source*: From Hill and Carpenter (1976), reproduced by permission of the British Institute of Radiology

is reproduced in Figure 9.4. The C-scan plane is also proving very useful in other areas: improved demonstration of the malignant spiculations associated with some breast cancers; and high-frequency imaging of the skin, which is inherently layered in a manner that suits sectional imaging parallel to the surface and where such images have the appeal of direct and easy comparison with the visual appearance of the skin surface (Figure 9.5). The ability to acquire and process three-dimensional echo data sets, particularly in combination with the technique of speckle tracking discussed below, makes possible the presentation of image data in any selected scan plane, of which the C-scan is simply a special case. A conventional one-dimensional array may be scanned in an elevational direction and the frame-to-frame motion estimated from the degree of speckle decorrelation between images (Tuthill *et al.* 1998; Prager *et al.* 2003). This method is used in a number of commercial three-dimensional imaging systems, requiring only a software modification to the scanner with no external position sensor, but it suffers from lack of quantification of the distance moved in the elevational

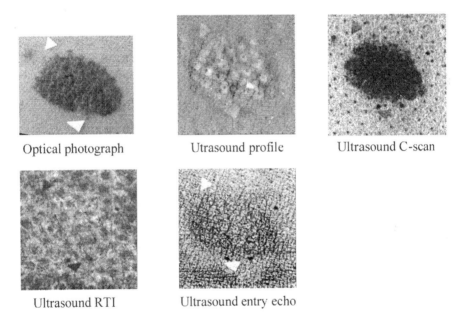

| Optical photograph | Utrasound profile | Ultrasound C-scan |

| Ultrasound RTI | Ultrasound entry echo |

Figure 9.5. Examples of C-scans derived from a three-dimensional echo data set of a human skin tumour (benign naevus) *in vivo*, in the form of a C-scan at the skin surface (labelled 'entry echo image'), a C-scan through the centre of the lesion (labelled 'C-scan') and a relative attenuation, or shadow, image (known as a 'reflex transmission image' and labelled 'ultrasound RTI') formed by integrating the echo magnitude from a large range of depths situated in the broad beam region beyond the focus of an $F0.95$ transducer. These images were made possible by first applying an echo tracking algorithm to automatically detect, and correct for, the distance of the skin surface (entry) echo from the transducer, so that the constant depth associated with a C-scan represented constant distance below the skin surface. A by-product of such tracking is the skin surface profile image also shown. Finally, scale and orientation registration of the ultrasound images with the optical photograph was achieved using the small triangular paper makers that are clearly visible on both ultrasound and optical images. The total image size of the ultrasound images is 22.4 × 22.4 mm. The method of ultrasound image acquisition is described by Bush *et al.* (2004) and that of image registration by Dickson (2003)

direction, which is due to the effects on the rate of decorrelation of acoustic field complexity and lack of knowledge of the tissue's backscatter impulse response function (see a related discussion by Bamber & Bush, 1996). An improvement, that also does not require an external transducer position sensor, involves a development of the 1.5-dimensional array concept; a conventional one-dimensional array is supplemented with two smaller one-dimensional arrays, one at each end of and orthogonal to the main imaging array. All three arrays are mounted in the same probe housing in a so-called 'I-beam' configuration (Hossack *et al.* 2002), which permits measurement of both elevational motion and change of transducer orientation by tracking the speckle in the images formed by each of the smaller arrays.

9.2.3 THE NATURE OF THE TRANSFER FUNCTION

The foregoing has provided an outline of the practicalities of launching, steering and echo-detecting the wave packets used in pulse–echo interrogation of tissues, and we can now consider the acoustic physics of the 'interrogation' process: in imaging parlance, the nature of the transfer function by which the system interprets an object as a set of image data. An exact description of the situation that we need to model here would entail a three-dimensional, scattering-ensemble object interrogated through an inhomogenous and non-linear propagation medium. For illustrative purposes, however, we shall consider here simply, in the linear approximation, a two-dimensional set of data $f(x, y)$ in object space being translated to a two-dimensional image $g(x, y)$ as a result of a particular system transfer function $h(x, y)$, where:

$$g(x, y) = f(x, y)*h(x, y) \tag{9.3}$$

where * indicates a convolution and where, in the spatial frequency domain, there is a corresponding relationship of the form:

$$G(u, v) = F(u, v) \cdot H(u, v) \tag{9.4}$$

In the following paragraphs the concept of the system transfer function will be used, in rather general terms, as a framework around which to discuss the process of ultrasonic pulse–echo image formation. In this, however, the qualifications noted in Chapter 8 concerning the validity of transfer function analysis in the present context should be borne in mind.

Real biological objects are generally complex and not amenable to exact mathematical analysis, but it can be informative nonetheless to consider the situation for more tractable objects (the spherical chicken, much beloved by physicists!). As has been pointed out already in analysing the process of formation of B-scans, one needs to consider separately transfer functions across and along the ultrasonic beam axis.

9.2.3.1 Point Targets

It is convenient analytically to discuss medical ultrasonic beams in terms of the field due to a perfect circular piston source. As has been discussed in Chapter 2, this is often a good first approximation but it must be borne in mind that actual beams will depart from this model because of inevitable phase and amplitude variations across the source and also, very commonly, because transducers are not circular. The field pattern due to a focused, ideal circular source has been described in Chapter 2, Section 2.5 where for the radial dependency in particular it was shown that the full width, d, at half-maximum of the intensity distribution in the region of the focus of a transducer of aperture radius a and radius of curvature A (approximating to the focal length l) is given by:

$$d = 2r \approx Z l \lambda / \pi a \tag{9.5}$$

for: $4Z^{-2} J_1^2(Z) = 0.5$, and thus $Z \approx 1.62$, we have:

$$d \approx 0.5 \, l \lambda / a \tag{9.6}$$

Thus, on this measure, the beam width of a 3 MHz transducer ($\lambda \approx 0.5$ mm) of 10 mm aperture radius at a focal distance of 100 mm, is some 2.5 mm. (Note that it also follows from the treatment of Section 2.5.1 that the value for d as given here is 0.45 times that of the diameter of the 'Airy disk', commonly quoted in optics, that measures the beam width out to the first intensity null.)

In frequency domain analysis the corresponding measure of resolution commonly used is the diffraction-limited spatial frequency:

$$v_D = a/\lambda \text{ cycles per radian} \tag{9.7}$$

In some situations none of these may be the most appropriate measure of lateral resolution (see Section 9.2.6), but they nevertheless give useful guidance as to the limiting values of this aspect of imaging performance, bearing in mind particularly that some degradation may be expected as a consequence of the coherence of the radiation.

In discussing and comparing focused acoustic systems a useful parameter is the focusing strength, defined as the ratio between the theoretical far-field distance and focal length (or radius of curvature of a focusing transducer element):

$$\gamma = a^2 / \lambda r_0 \tag{9.8}$$

When using fixed-focus transducers, different imaging modes will require correspondingly different values for focusing strength. C-Scanning, where only a small depth of focus is necessary, is best done with a rather strongly focused transducer ($\gamma = 10$–15), whereas for B-scanning, where the reverse situation holds, focusing strength must generally be kept below a value of 3 in order to maintain at least moderately good resolution over the complete depth range of interest. This compromise is of course overcome by the use of electronic focusing with arrays, but it remains applicable to the fixed lens focusing in the elevational direction of a one-dimensional array.

Resolution in the axial dimension in a pulse–echo system is determined primarily by the effective duration of the echo from a point target and thus, in turn, by the effective duration of the transmitted interrogating pulse. In practice, it is fairly easy, without undue loss in system sensitivity, to achieve a resolution in this dimension that is considerably better than that lateral to the beam. For the case quoted above, for example (which is fairly typical of beams used in abdominal contact scanning), axial resolution better than the 2.5 mm achieved laterally implies transmitted and echo pulse lengths of less than 5 mm in tissue (equivalent to 3.5 µs or 10 cycles at 3 MHz), which compares with typical values of 2–3 cycles practically employed.

As will be seen subsequently, it is important to bear in mind that the true physical point-spread function (PSF) of a B-scan system results from an r.f. waveform and thus contains negative values (which, strictly, exclude it from treatment by conventional imaging theory). Examples of computed PSFs for B-scan imaging, both before and following a rectification and filtering process, are given in Figure 9.6. Various methods of deconvolving this function from the recorded image have been considered but, although axial deconvolution may be relatively easy under limited circumstances, the real need is to improve lateral resolution, and this is difficult.

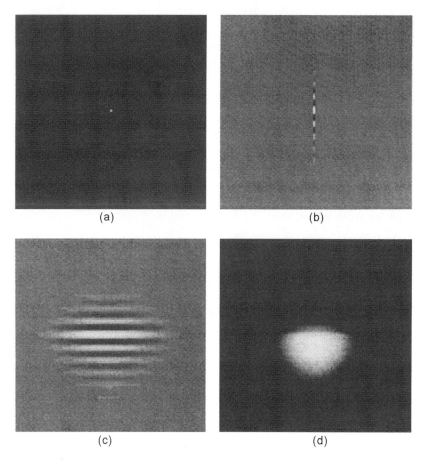

(a)   (b)

(c)   (d)

Figure 9.6. Illustration of the development of a point spread function in a B-mode image (the dimensions given below are in pixels and the full image is 100 × 100 pixels): (a) single-point object; (b) image after convolution with a sound pulse (wavelength = 6, pulse rise time = 7, pulse fall time = 8); (c) image after convolution with a beam profile (FWHM = 30); (d) image after full wave detection and smoothing (filter response time = 9). *Source*: From Bamber and Dickinson (1980)

9.2.3.2 Distributed Targets

Although a single-point scatterer model has been used above for illustrative convenience, many of the important targets for medical ultrasonics constitute some kind of three-dimensional distribution of scatterers. However, as discussed in Chapter 6 and in spite of information that is starting to emerge from acoustic microscopy (Chapter 11), we still do not have detailed knowledge of the nature of these acoustic scattering matrices. From what we do know it seems that, rather than simply an array of point scatterers, a more satisfactory model for some purposes would be based on the inhomogeneous continuum (Chapter 6) in which local values of the medium density and compressibility exhibit semi-random spatial variations around certain mean values. It is such a model that is now generally preferred for work in this field: such an approach can be very informative and can show in particular how, in a B-scan of an organ such as a liver, anatomical information can be strongly modulated by a coherent radiation artefact, giving rise to a characteristic speckled effect (Figure 9.7). In the special case of echoes backscattered from a distributed target exhibiting no structure that is resolvable at the interrogating frequency (e.g. blood at frequencies below about 100 MHz), the then 'fully

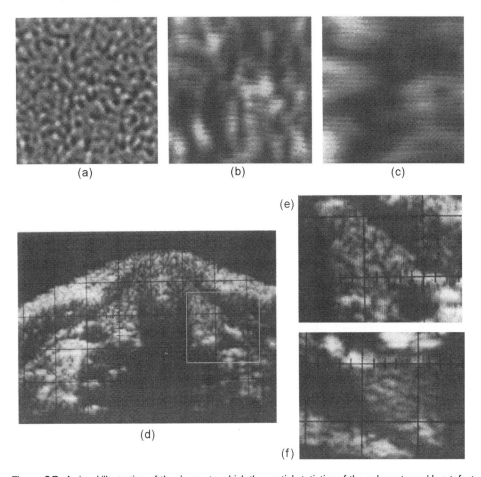

(a)   (b)   (c)

(e)

(d)

(f)

Figure 9.7. A visual illustration of the degree to which the spatial statistics of the coherent speckle artefact are characteristic of the imaging system, rather than the target, when scanning distributed targets that possess little resolvable structure (see also Chapter 6). A randomly inhomogeneous continuum with a Gaussian autocorrelation function of width 4 pixels (a) was scanned in simulation, first using a beam width of 10 pixels and a pulse length of 8 pixels (b), and again using a beam width of 30 pixels and a pulse length of 14 pixels; the wavelength was 6 pixels for both of the scans and all images were 100 × 100 pixels (from Bamber & Dickinson, 1980). Note that the image obtained when the system had poor spatial resolution (c) was not simply a smoothed version of that obtained when it had superior resolution (b) but scanned an identical target. Image (d) is an early water-bath scan of the human neck in cross-section. Detail indicated by the white box, and showing the left lobe of the thyroid gland and carotid artery, is expanded in (e) and (f) for scans of the same person's neck using different transducers of centre frequencies 5 MHz and 6 MHz, respectively. The appearance of the thyroid is also shown in Figure 9.13 and, despite the use of current state-of-the-art imaging technology, one may note the dominance of the speckle modulation throughout the non-compounded image

developed' speckle pattern becomes an artefact whose spatial statistics are characteristic solely of the interrogating system and independent of the target.

The factors affecting spatial resolution of a distributed target against a contrasting background have been discussed in Chapter 8 and it will be seen in Section 9.2.6 that coherent radiation speckle may act, in this context, as an important source of image noise.

9.2.3.3 Extended Interface Targets

There are a number of biological targets, particularly organ boundaries, that, because their lateral extent constitutes an appreciable number of acoustic wavelengths, might be expected to act as specular reflectors. Historically, the perception that this type of echo might be used to yield outline images of organ boundaries dominated much of the design and use of the 1960s' generation of B-scanners: they were built to be used in 'compounding' mode (deriving and superimposing echoes from a range of aspect angles within the scanning plane) and to provide a bi-stable (line diagram with no grey scale) display. This practice, abandoned in the 1970s, subsequently attracted renewed interest, as described below, but there has still been surprisingly little systematic study of the acoustic echo directionality of common anatomical structures. In the extreme case of the thoracic diaphragm, strong specular reflection has indeed been observed, giving rise to 'artefactual' images of actual structures within the liver that appear to lie within the lung (Cosgrove *et al.* 1978). Such investigations of specularity that have been carried out have shown that the surfaces responsible may be somewhat rough acoustically, resulting in diffusion of a reflected ray through a range of angles around the reflected direction (Chiang *et al.* 1994; Hokland & Kelly 1996).

9.2.4 PROPAGATION MEDIUM AND PROPAGATION NON-LINEARITY

The various aspects of acoustic wave propagation have been treated in previous chapters and it is only necessary to point out here that properties of the propagation medium, particularly those of tissues overlying the structures of interest, may contribute in a significant way to the image transfer function in a pulse–echo system.

Acoustic attenuation of tissue is a major factor and, as mentioned above, an approximate correction for this is made in practical imaging systems by the use of time-gain compensation (TGC: automatic progressive increase of receiver gain with time after initiation of each acoustic pulse). Because, however, a conventional pulse–echo imaging system has no knowledge of the actual attenuation coefficients of the propagation media, such compensation can only be approximate and cannot lead to image data that are quantitative in the sense of being referrable to any absolute standard of measurement. The tissue attenuation process also acts as a low-pass filter, selectively attenuating the higher frequency components of the transmitted frequency band.

An additional complexity arises as a result of finite amplitude ('non-linear') propagation effects (Chapters 1, 4 and 5). A substantial amount of commercial diagnostic equipment employs pulses of sufficient amplitude to experience significant non-linearity – a phenomenon that is itself medium dependent. This results, on the one hand, in the transfer of energy from fundamental to harmonic frequencies, with consequent increase in effective attenuation of the beam and, related to this, some diffractive narrowing of the beam. Such behaviour gives rise to both problems and opportunities. On the one hand, in the absence of detailed knowledge of properties of the media, it is impossible accurately to predict the influence of these phenomena on imaging behaviour. On the plus side, however, it opens up the possibility of deriving images from detected harmonics of the fundamental of a projected beam, with potential advantages in both tissue contrast and spatial resolution (Tranquart *et al.* 1999; Whittingham 1999; Desser *et al.* 2000). Figure 9.8 provides a practical example of such advantages in the context of abdominal imaging. In the image obtained at 4.0 MHz for transmit and receive (Figure 9.8a), clutter echoes have reduced the contrast resolution at depth and thus obscured detail in both the liver and gall bladder. Beam width also appears to have been degraded rapidly with depth in this image. On the other hand, in the image obtained by filtering to pass the received second harmonic of the fundamental (Figure 9.8b), contrast and spatial resolution are better than in (a) despite the lower transmit frequency of 3.0 MHz. The stone in the gall bladder and its acoustic shadow are seen more clearly in image (b). On close inspection of the fine structure of the images, particularly at the focal depth (indicated by the ' > ' sign at the left of the images), it may be seen that the bandwidth reduction needed to select the harmonic at 6.0 MHz has lengthened the effective imaging pulse (in b), worsening the axial resolution relative to (a), but with an improved beam width. Discussion of these images continues below.

A further important factor in the propagation process is inhomogeneity in sound speed (and thus in refractive index) within tissues. This can give rise to phase distortion, or loss of spatial coherence, in the acoustic wavefront and thus variable beam deflection, beam broadening and anomalous variation in attenuation (Foster & Hunt 1979; Tabei *et al.* 2003). Similar effects can also occur when there is inhomogeneity in acoustic absorption. They can become particularly important for heterogenous organs such as the breast, or when imaging through an aberrating layer such as the skull or an abdominal wall that contains many fat/muscle interfaces, and will determine the optimum value of the focusing strength of a transducer for a particular application. The phenomenon also provides an important extra reason why harmonic imaging (mentioned above) may be beneficial. Returning to the discussion of the images in Figure 9.8, it is hypothesised that in addition to the intrinsically narrower beam associated with the (higher) harmonic frequency the complex structure of the abdominal wall, which interestingly seems to be shown with better fidelity by the fundamental image (a) than the harmonic image (b), has acted as an aberrating layer that reduced the spatial coherence and hence the focusing properties of the projected wavefront. The harmonic components, however, do not build up until after the wave has propagated some distance into the body (see Chapters 1 and 4), i.e. once it has passed beyond the aberrating layer of fat and muscle, and furthermore are formed from that part of the propagating wave that has retained most of its spatial coherence. This would mean that the beam used to form the harmonic image in (b) suffers less from the beam-broadening and other degrading effects of these superficial inhomogeneities. Finally, reverberations in the fat/muscle layers at the abdominal wall, which may have generated clutter echoes, would have occurred before the harmonic components had formed and would thus be removed by the narrow band filter used to create the harmonic image. Thus, although the textural detail at the transmit focal depth is finer in (a) than in (b), this detail is likely to be largely characteristic of the speckle artefact associated with aberration (Smith *et al.* 1988), which is similar to that in the near-field of a large incoherent source (Bamber *et al.* 2000a), and with the presence of clutter echoes, and should not be taken to indicate better spatial resolution than the apparently coarser detail in (b) (see also Section 9.2.8, *spatial resolution*).

9.2.5 RECEPTION AND MANIPULATION OF ECHO SIGNALS

The general nature of the raw echo signals generated by a pulse–echo system will be evident from the previous discussion. In principle they will have encoded on them a rich set of information relating not only to the gross anatomy of the interrogated region but also to both

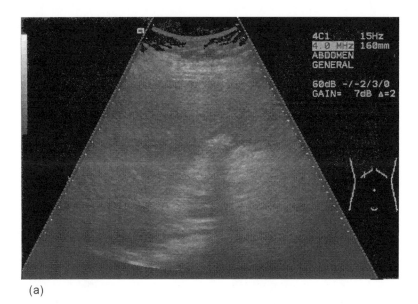

(a)

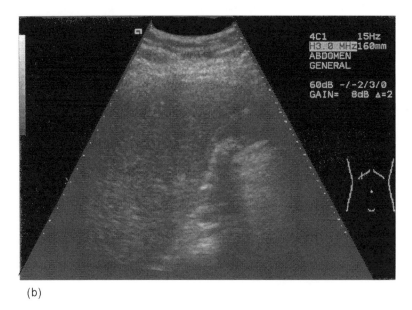

(b)

Figure 9.8. Demonstration of the improved quality that may be obtained by deriving images from detected harmonics of the fundamental of the projected beam. See text for discussion. *Source*: Images are courtesy of D. Cosgrove

local tissue structure – histology – and to kinetic behaviour in response to stress – rheology. At the same time, however, echo signals will have become corrupted by a number of factors: in particular, the effects of tissue attenuation and inhomogeneity, and the presence of noise and clutter. A vital function of the transmitter–transducer–receiver system is thus to compensate for or minimise the corrupting influences while optimising the potential for extracting useful information.

As already mentioned, a crucially important determinant of the quality of the recovered information is the electro-mechanical response characteristic of the transducer, taken together with the shape and amplitude of the excitation pulse. In a well-designed system these, together with the receiver frequency response, will address a requirement for tissue penetration up to a specified depth that will be determined by the intended application (e.g. abdominal, ophthalmological, etc.) and with echo signal levels above the noise. In practice, this seems to be done almost entirely on an empirical basis but, as should be evident from other chapters of this book, a more scientific approach is feasible in which it is possible to combine basic data to provide appropriate design criteria (Moran 1991).

Transducer arrays give rise to a parallel set of signal trains corresponding to the set of array elements. Referring to Figure 9.9, in the receiver these sets of signals will be combined eventually in the process of *beam-line formation*, but not until some pre-processing has taken place in the *individual receive channels*. In some systems, *beam-line processing* may be followed by a stage of processing involving *multiple beam-line data sets*. Finally will come the stages of *scan conversion* and *post-processing*. In the past, much of this processing has been carried out using analogue circuitry but, with its rapidly increasing availability and cost-effectiveness, the trend is towards predominant or total use of digital technology.

Receive channel-level processing, at a routine level, entails the application of time delays for beam steering and/or focusing purposes and of apodisation amplitude functions for side-lobe reduction. Further, more ambitious schemes for intervention at this stage can be implemented using feedback of information from the processed image data. In particular, rather than the use of a fixed, preset value of sound speed in focusing, one may use either an iterative guessing procedure based on some measure of image sharpness or more direct methods (Anderson & Trahey 1998). A similar approach has been used in attempting to compensate for the degradations arising, in spatial and contrast resolution, from phase aberrations due to propagation medium inhomogeneities. Methods studied for deriving the phase correction functions (the acoustic equivalent to 'adaptive optics') have included the use of image-derived geometrical information combined with knowledge of sound speeds (Carpenter *et al.* 1995), and a wide range of channel signal alignment algorithms that aim to maximise a spatial coherence measure, either at the channel level (e.g. Behar 2002; Karaman *et al.* 1993) or by analysing the beam-formed speckle (e.g. Freiburger & Trahey 1997), although there are equivalences between these domains of measurement and account may need to be taken of the shape of the spatial coherence function (Bamber *et al.* 2000b; Lacefield *et al.* 2002; Li & Li 2003). These methods tend to work best for the situation when the wave-front distortions can be modelled as having arisen from a thin aberrating layer close to the receiver, and their implementation is likely to be more successful when highly populated two-dimensional arrays eventually become available. Difficulties arise when a distributed aberrator is present, or when aberration has already broadened the transmit beam and a distributed incoherent scattering target such as soft tissue is being imaged. Methods have been under consideration for dealing with the former problem (e.g. Ng *et al.* 1997) and transmit beam aberration by a near-field thin screen is alleviated by harmonic imaging, as mentioned above. The time reversal technique (Fink & Dorme 1997; Tabei *et al.* 2003) appears to have the potential to cope with all situations and there may be ways to generate the reference targets required by the method

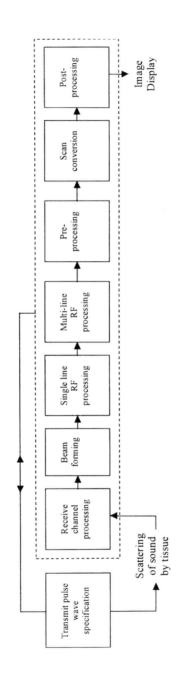

Figure 9.9. Stages of processing in ultrasonic image formation. *Source:* Adapted from Bamber (1999)

(Kripfgans *et al.* 2002) or to use structures already present in the tissue. Finally, channel-level signal processing has been investigated as a means of removing clutter, for example by the use of the so-called velocity-guided median filter that was first described in seismological signal processing (Szabo & Burns 1997).

The detailed nature of the signal-to-noise relationship in pulse–echo systems is outlined below, but an important component of this originates in the early stages of the receiver, where low-noise amplification thus needs to be provided. In a well-designed system, the level of incoherent noise should be determined primarily at the circuit position of the lowest signal, which in a pulse–echo system should be at the transducer terminals and should correspond approximately to the theoretical r.m.s. noise level determined by bandwidth Δf (Hz) and electrical impedance Z (ohms). For normal ambient temperature this is given by:

$$V_n = 1.25(Z \cdot \Delta f)^{0.5} \times 10^{-10} \text{ volts} \tag{9.9}$$

Single-line R.F. processing is carried out following combination of the signals from the set of array-element channels. The combined signal is amplified and subjected to TGC (or swept gain) to compensate for the effects of attenuation and diffraction on echo signal amplitude. A number of both simple and more complex TGC algorithms are in use, some of which attempt to improve the cosmetic appearance of images by using some averaged measure of backscattered signal amplitude as a gain control criterion.

Noise reduction and other benefits are achieved by bandpass filtering linked to the centre frequency and to the bandwidth of the transmitted pulse. Rejection of lower frequencies can be particularly important because the unwanted resonance modes of a transducer tend to fall in this region. The frequency dependence of tissue attenuation results, however, in a downshift of the centre frequency of returned echoes and some systems use dynamic adjustment of the filter frequency both to correct for and track this effect. Filtering is also used to detect in the echo signal the presence of harmonics of the transmitted frequency. This approach has enabled improvements to the signal-to-clutter ratio in the detection of microbubble contrast media (Section 9.2.7), and also improved imaging of tissues following propagation through reverberation- and aberration-inducing media, as described above.

In a well-designed system the echo signals seen at the transducer will cover a large dynamic range: echoes from a strong interface such as bone/soft tissue, if unattenuated, may be 100 dB above noise. This is greatly in excess of the 20 dB or so that can be handled directly by common display devices. Thus conventional signal processing also includes some form of dynamic range compression, such as logarithmic amplification, to allow for this. The final stages will generally effect some edge enhancement, prior to eventual demodulation to detect the envelope of the echo signal, with rejection of low-level signals and noise. In manipulating echo signals in this way, however, it will be important to bear in mind the possibility of adverse effects on their information content: compression of signals, for example, may have a significant influence on their statistical properties (Kaplan & Ma 1994).

As discussed in some detail in Section 9.4, there are several types of potentially valuable information that may be derived from the basic echo set, in addition to an echo amplitude image, and it is at this single line processing stage that much of such information may be extracted by appropriate processing (although some potential has been shown for deriving useful object-specific information from channel-level processing). Examples include algorithms to measure:

(a) the average attenuation coefficient and its frequency dependence (either from frequency downshifts or from echo decay with depth, as described in Chapter 4);

(b) properties such as scatterer size (from the frequency dependence of the scattering coefficient, as described in Chapter 6);
(c) flow velocity (by tracking displacements with time or measuring echo fluctuation rate, as in the Doppler technique, and as described in Chapter 10);
(d) tissue elasticity information (by tracking the displacements induced by some external force, as described in Chapter 10);
(e) local sound speed variations such as induced by localised temperature changes (again by displacement tracking, see Chapter 10).

Speckle noise reduction also has been applied at this level, both using frequency compounding and using algorithms that aim to estimate the envelope of the echo signal that would have existed had destructive interference not occurred (see the review by Bamber 1993).

Multi-line processing records and exploits correlations between data sets arising from two or more in a series of consecutive beam lines. Interpolation between such lines, prior to demodulation or other non-linear signal processing, may be applied in order to improve image quality and reduce the risk of aliasing in the lateral direction. Many variations on such processing are possible and some may be likened to that of a second stage of beam forming, perhaps paving the way for synthetic aperture imaging. Spatial compounding, in which correlation is made between two or more full-image data sets after amplitude demodulation, obtained from the same object plane observed from different observation points, again achieves improved signal-to-noise ratio and image quality, as illustrated in Figure 9.13.

A related procedure here is that of speckle tracking, which records and exploits two- (or three-) dimensional features of the image speckle pattern. The application of this procedure to tissue movement analysis will be taken up in the next chapter but it also has potentially powerful 'static' applications. In two dimensions it has been shown to enable the development of panoramic or 'extended field of view' images, as illustrated and explained in Figure 9.10. An extension of this approach to data sets acquired in three spatial dimensions allows the

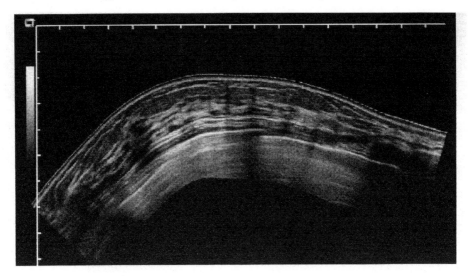

Figure 9.10. Panoramic scan through the breast for which position coordinates have been mapped progressively by use of a speckle tracking technique. Spatial (angle) compounding has also been employed for speckle reduction. A cyst is shown but the main benefit is the display of normal breast architecture over the extended field of view. *Source*: Images are courtesy of D. Cosgrove

reconstruction of images with good geometric conformity in any chosen set of image planes, such as the 'C-scan' plane that was illustrated in Figure 9.5.

A *scan conversion* step is necessary in order to transpose from a polar or other set of coordinates in which an image data set has been acquired to a conventional video standard raster. The particular algorithm chosen for this procedure can be an important determinant of final image quality.

Post-processing, following scan conversion, includes a function whose importance has been underlined in Chapter 8: the translation of echo amplitude values to a scale of display brightness or colour appropriate to human visual perception, taking into account ambient light conditions. In particular, it is important to optimise in this respect the overall receiver/display device gain characteristic and so enable a balanced perception of low, medium and high amplitude signals. This is commonly implemented through a user-selectable look-up table. The observer/investigator will normally carry out his or her interpretive work directly from the monitor screen but considerable use is also made of photographic records and, for this reason, knowledge of the properties of the photographic recording process in this context is of importance (Harder 1981; Neary 1981). Another facility often provided at this stage is frame averaging, as an attempt to improve contrast discrimination by speckle reduction, albeit at the expense of motion degradation of spatial resolution.

Largely because signals are more readily accessible at this than at earlier processing stages, a number of attempts have been made here at signal manipulation. Among these are systems for speckle reduction, employing adaptive spatial or temporal filtering, that have yielded worthwhile results albeit constrained by effects of the preceding stages of processing. Similarly, attempts to extract new information at this stage, for example via image texture analysis, have also suffered from this constraint but have been quite successful in some cases.

9.2.6 SIGNAL-TO-NOISE RATIO ENHANCEMENT IN PULSE–ECHO SYSTEMS

In Chapter 8 we discussed the nature and origins of noise in echographic systems, and emphasised the important and often dominating role of coherent radiation speckle – a phenomenon that is an inherent consequence of the particular nature of the transfer function in coherent imaging systems (Section 9.2.3). A striking illustration of the impact of such speckle noise on imaging performance is provided in Figure 9.11, which shows the experimental results of observer performance in detecting the presence of computer-generated 'lesions' within a contrasting background, with and without the presence of simulated speckle. Here, for a given lesion/background contrast, the presence of speckle increased the linear size of a detectable lesion by a good order of magnitude. Considered, for example, as the size of the 'smallest detectable tumour', this would be a difference of enormous practical significance. Central questions in the achievement of good echographic image quality (assuming, of course, appropriate transducer design and engineering of r.f. circuitry) are thus whether, how and to what degree the adverse effects of coherent speckle can be suppressed. Detailed consideration of these questions has been given by Bamber (1993), who discusses three lines of approach taken to the problem: compounding, adaptive filtering and signal reconstitution.

The most straightforward way to decrease the degree of coherence in an image data set is to substitute it for the average of a number of equivalent, but not coherently correlated, data sets: a procedure often referred to as compounding. In principle, this approach could be expected to increase the speckle signal-to-noise ratio in proportion to the square root of the number of such data sets employed for averaging. In practice its potential is more limited. In the first

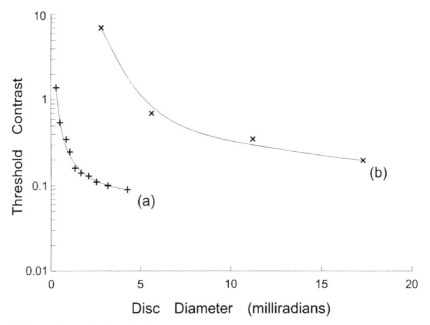

Figure 9.11. Experimentally determined contrast thresholds for visual detection of uniform disks against uniform backgrounds (a) and when both disks and backgrounds are modulated by a typical speckle pattern (b). *Source*: From Lowe *et al.* (1988) and Bamber (1993)

place there will always be a strict limit to the selection of truly decorrelated data sets available for averaging. Secondly, the subsequent averaging process will, in practice, lead to some loss of spatial resolution, in part because no two such data sets will be precisely equivalent geometrically but also because to create uncorrelated data sets of the same region of an object one must form each set using a restricted range of a variable such as bandwidth or aperture size. The latter compromise may not always be apparent in published images of angle compounding because a fair comparison has rarely been possible, and indeed largely requires further technological progress; in the majority of examples of angle compounding coherent image formation, using the whole of the available aperture has not been available, in which case the comparison becomes one of wide-aperture partially coherent imaging with narrow-aperture coherent imaging. In the 1960s most scanners were designed for angle compounding (albeit with a rationale of collecting supposed 'specular' reflections from organ boundaries, rather than for averaging out speckle) and, in the limited number of machines possessing sufficient display dynamic range, some useful signal-to-noise ratio enhancement seems to have been achieved (Figure 9.12). The rather elegant way of implementing such angle compounding by multi-line processing, and enabling display of the compound image at useful real-time frame rates (as mentioned above), is illustrated in Figure 9.13.

Two related procedures are spatial and temporal compounding. In the former, spatial averaging is performed over images obtained by translating the scan plane (Foster *et al.* 1981) – a technique that would only seem to be useful for anatomic structures, such as the neck or limbs, that vary rather slowly across that plane. Temporal compounding, which relies on either physiological tissue movement or operator-induced probe motion for what is again strictly spatial decorrelation compounding, but which permits a high degree of user control of

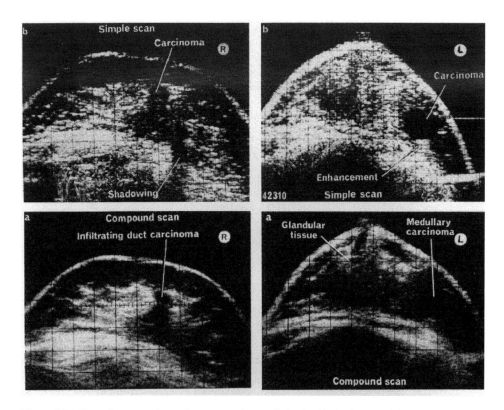

Figure 9.12. Examples comparing early compound scans (below) with simple scans (above) obtained with a water-bath breast scanner. It was recognised early in the development of these systems that compound and simple scanning had a degree of complementarity; the benefits of compounding – better outlining, specularly reflecting boundaries and improved contrast resolution through speckle reduction – were sometimes at the expense of other information such as acoustic shadowing or 'enhancement'. *Source*: Images are from Hill *et al.* (1978), courtesy of J. Jellins

the trade-off between speckle reduction and loss of spatial resolution, has proved sufficiently successful that many manufacturers have incorporated it in their equipment as a variable 'persistence' or 'temporal processing' feature.

Arguably, a more intelligent and powerful approach to speckle reduction is to exploit the fact that 'fully developed' speckle patterns, i.e. patterns generated in the absence of resolvable object structure, are statistically highly reproducible and specific to the particular imaging system. A filter can thus, in principle, be constructed that will carry out local adaptive smoothing of the image if, and only if, the unfiltered image data are consistent with that specific pattern (Bamber & Daft 1986). Preliminary clinical trials have indicated that this procedure can measurably improve the ability to interpret echograms in a variety of applications (Massay *et al.* 1989; Crawford *et al.* 1992) and reduce the thresholds for lesion detectability (Bamber *et al.* 1994b). According to Bamber (1993), this form of adaptive processing may be used to control any of the previously mentioned compounding methods, and temporal compounding in particular is shown to be substantially improved by using it.

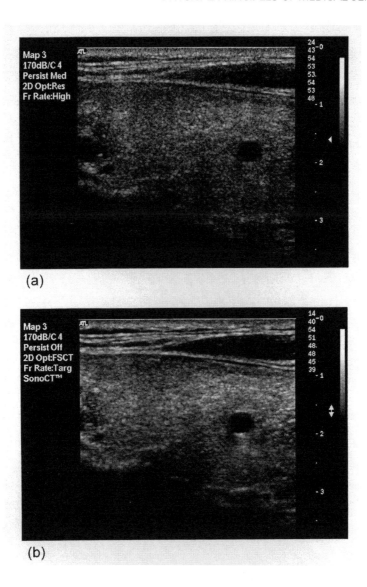

Figure 9.13. Example of real-time compounding by multi-line processing (b) in comparison with the simple scan in (a); even though the image in (a) is somewhat speckle reduced due to the use of moderate persistence (frame averaging), in (b) there is better display of a cyst, detail in the subcutaneous layers and muscle, and abnormal thyroid echo architecture associated with multi-nodular goitre. *Source*: Images are courtesy of D. Cosgrove

Over the years a number of attempts have been reported to use colour as a means of enhancing perceptibility of sonographic information. There seem to be a number of reasons why these have generally been unsuccessful, particularly the presence of high levels of speckle noise combined with the use of 'unnatural' colour scales. However, combined use of speckle reduction together with an appropriate natural scale, e.g. the heated-object or temperature-colour scale (Milan & Taylor 1975; Pizer & Zimmerman 1983), can lead to usefully enhanced perceptibility, particularly at the extremes of the display characteristic and for displays in high ambient light levels (Massay *et al.* 1989).

Finally, a number of ideas have been pursued in the area of signal reconstitution, in which the aim is to make good at least some of the artefacts that have been imposed on the image by the particular nature of the imaging system transfer function. An interesting example here is envelope reconstruction, which attempts to make use of instantaneous phase discontinuities in the A-line to recognise, and thus compensate for, local occurrences of destructive interference (Leeman & Seggie 1987; Forsberg 1991).

Clutter and wave aberration, both discussed above, can have a pronounced effect on the signal-to-noise ratio and, as was seen in Figure 9.8, substantial improvements may be obtained by taking advantage of non-linear propagation effects. New beam-forming methods such as adaptive beam-forming and velocity guided median filtering (mentioned above under receive channel-level processing) should also eventually have a considerable impact in reducing noise. Care must be taken, however, in interpreting numerical values of the B-mode image signal-to-noise ratio, conventionally defined as the ratio of the mean echo signal to its standard deviation. Firstly, inclusion of clutter with signal may of course lead to an erroneously high signal-to-noise ratio by this definition, despite reduced contrast resolution due to the incorrect positions of the clutter echoes. Secondly, because the process of beam-forming an incoherent wave produces a signal with similar first-order statistics to speckle, a method that successfully improves the spatial coherence of the received wave should show no great change in image signal-to-noise ratio for a completely incoherent scattering medium, but when there is a potentially resolvable structure present the signal-to-noise ratio is expected to decrease as focusing is improved (Bamber *et al.* 2000b). These predictions are consistent with the visual appearances of images such as those in Figure 9.8.

9.2.7 USE OF CONTRAST MEDIA

One of the characteristics of sonography that make it particularly attractive in clinical use is its non-intrusiveness: patient preparation is very simple and atraumatic and generally without the need for injection or ingestion procedures. There are, however, some clinical problems for which it has been found beneficial to include, as part of the investigative procedure, the administration of a 'contrast agent'. The objective here is usually either to enhance the echogenicity of blood, particularly for flow studies, or to achieve improved contrast for tissue differentiation. An example of the latter situation would be uptake of a colloidal material into the Kupfer cells that are present in normal liver but not in a tumour. The proposed use of contrast agents as vehicles for the delivery and release of therapeutic agents to targeted pathology (e.g. Unger 1999) and the measurement of their transit-time through vasculature (Kedar *et al.* 1996) provide further important motivations for their study and development.

For the majority of applications the physical requirements for a satisfactory contrast agent are that, within reasonable limits, it should be stable with time and should have a particle size that is uniform and small enough to pass through pulmonary capillaries. With these constraints it has been found possible to obtain the required acoustic contrast broadly in two ways: microbubbles of gas incorporated within either a sugar matrix or human albumin; and suspensions of colloidal particles of particular perfluorochemicals (whose combination of high density and low acoustic velocity leads to an acoustic impedance value, Z, some 75% of that of water and soft tissue). This is a subject on which there is a substantial and rapidly growing literature: see, for example, Dawson *et al.* (1999), Goldberg (1993), Nanda *et al.* (1997) and Thomsen *et al.* (1999).

The behaviour of microbubbles in an acoustic field constitutes the subject of *cavitation*, discussed in Chapter 12, although some aspects of the acoustic behaviour of microbubbles have been mentioned in Chapters 4, 5 and 6. An interesting, and serendipidous, observation in the present context is that, if a diagnostic ultrasound pulse train is interrupted for a few seconds, the echoes occurring in the first frame following recommencement can be some 20 dB higher than the preceding, or following, steady level. This so-called 'flash-echo' phenomenon (Kamiyama *et al.* 1998) has evident advantage in enhancement of the signal-to-noise ratio, and appears to be a consequence of the tendency of the microbubbles to be disrupted by steadily continued insonation. In another variant of the flash-echo technique the interruption of the pulse train is replaced by a period where the pulses are of low acoustic pressure, to minimise bubble destruction, followed by a brief insonation at high amplitude. For some microbubbles the shells tend to be disrupted by insonation at high acoustic pressures, releasing free gas bubbles that momentarily exhibit stronger resonant scattering than the encapsulated bubbles, before they disappear by dissolution or fragmentation. The concentration and amplitude dependence of backscattering for these agents suggest that at any given moment two populations of bubbles exist, one encapsulated and the other as free bubbles (Sboros *et al.* 2002), and innovative pulse-sequences have been designed to take advantage of the signal-to-noise ratio enhancement potential of such changes of confinement of the gas (Frinking *et al.* 2001).

In effect, the real challenge for signal-to-noise ratio improvement using microbubbles is to distinguish them from tissue and thus enhance the ability to image and measure them when they are stationary or only very slowly moving. Further progress here is being made by utilising knowledge of ultrasound scattering from microbubbles to create new modes of imaging. Second harmonic imaging (Burns *et al.* 1992) was the earliest example of this but suffered from the fact that, as seen early in this chapter, tissue also scatters substantial amounts of the second harmonic component of the sound field produced during the process of non-linear propagation of the projected sound beam, which is itself enhanced by the presence of the contrast agent in intervening tissue. The situation is improved by the use of higher harmonics (Bouakaz *et al.* 2002), and the pulse-inversion method, also known as wideband harmonic imaging and mentioned in Section 9.2.1, provides considerable improvement in bubble specificity of the image, having now reached the stage of widespread commercial implementation (Bauer *et al.* 1997a; Chapman & Lazenby 1997; Hwang & Simpson 1998). Another method that has been implemented commercially is one that makes use of the disappearance, through either fragmentation or dissolution, of microbubbles when the incident acoustic field is of sufficiently high pressure (e.g. Bauer *et al.* 1997b; Blomley *et al.* 1997). In fact this seems to occur at levels of insonation normally used for diagnostic purposes, and systems with low acoustic outputs have had to be built if bubble destruction is to be avoided. The method has been known variously as 'stimulated acoustic emission', 'sonoscintigriphy' and 'loss of correlation' imaging. A strong, if not the entire, contribution to the signature is the random change in phase in the received scattered wave that occurs if one or more bubbles disappear from within the resolution cell of the pulse–echo system, and this will be detected easily by typical Doppler-shift processing. When bubble destruction occurs, this effect also contributes to the signal detected by other processing schemes, such as pulse-inversion processing. Finally, bubbles undergoing resonant vibration in a sound field, unlike tissue, will emit subharmonic acoustic vibrations (Chapter 12). These too have been suggested as having potential for bubble-specific parametric imaging (Shi *et al.* 1999). Many of the methods mentioned above will receive further discussion in Chapter 10.

9.2.8 TESTING AND ASSESSMENT OF PERFORMANCE

There are many situations where it is desirable to be able to make objective measurements of the performance of pulse–echo systems: in developing and manufacturing new equipment, in assessing equipment for purchase, in preventive maintenance testing and in communicating research results. Development of suitable measurement procedures has therefore been the subject of work by a number of individuals and specialist groups. Much of this work, including a substantial set of standards and recommendations, is available in the published literature (AIUM/NEMA 1989; AIUM 1991; Insana & Hall 1993; Zagzebski 1996; ICRU 1999). Here we shall limit ourselves to a brief discussion of the subject.

Central to this topic is the concept of technical quality in investigative performance. Much of the background material relevant to this has been covered in earlier sections of this book, particularly that concerning the nature of the transfer function (Section 9.2.3), and more general discussion of performance criteria is taken up in Section 9.3.

Technical performance quality can be considered usefully as the result of a set of objectively quantifiable factors, several of which are interdependent and many of which are additionally dependent on spatial position in the interrogated field. For the present purposes, these may be considered individually as follows:

Spatial resolution. This is a measure of the minimum linear separation between a pair of point or line targets that, under specified conditions, the system can just distinguish as separate. It is limited by the size of the PSF, which in the dimensions lateral to the beam axis is determined primarily by echo beam width and longitudinally by echo pulse length, e.g. as measured at -6 or $-20\,dB$. Under appropriate conditions (discussed below), it is also expressed as the spatial density of the 'fully developed' speckle pattern that is characteristic of the system (Section 9.2.3.2 and Chapter 6). The measurement of spatial resolution is often, however, oversimplified. It cannot, for example, be separated from the issue of target contrast (see below) and, related to this, no single measure of echo beam width or pulse length is able to provide a complete characterisation of system spatial resolution. A good example of this may be noted from past attempts to develop very wide aperture focusing systems for water-bath breast imaging based on conically converging waves (Bamber *et al.* 1981; Foster *et al.* 1981). These were designed to maintain a very strong focus, and hence a very narrow beam, over a large depth without employing electronic focusing. It was indeed found, for example, that a $-6\,dB$ lateral PSF width of 0.6 mm could be maintained over a depth range of 8 cm for a 3.5 MHz single element transducer (Clarke *et al.* 1983). Unfortunately the first side lobe occurred at about $-11\,dB$, below which the beam width was far worse than that for the equivalent spherically focused aperture. Hence spatial resolution could appear to be excellent for high contrast targets of similar echo magnitude, such as points or wires in water, where system dynamic range could be restricted to display them as separated, but it was very poor for more realistic distributed targets where a wide display dynamic range is required. Related to this, spatial resolution is also dependent on the extent to which non-linear signal processing such as compression amplification is employed (Bamber & Phelps 1977).

Care must also be taken in what is meant by 'appropriate conditions' for the above statement concerning the equivalence between resolutions as measured using point targets and the spatial density of speckle. An analysis of the texture of a speckle image from a distributed scattering phantom has been studied with a view to creating a simple-to-use automated method of system performance characterisation (Bamber *et al.* 1994a) and it was noted that good correlation between the resolution assessed in this manner and that assessed using a conventional single wire target occurs only at the focal region of the imaging system. Outside of the focal region the two alternative measures are *inversely* related, the speckle method providing an incorrectly more favourable impression of resolution. This phenomenon has been broadly explained using the van Cittert–Zernike theorem (Bamber *et al.* 2000b); it is due to the fact that outside of the focal zone the receiving aperture is no longer in the Fraunhofer zone (far field) of the scattering volume, which acts as an incoherent source of relatively large size. As a result, the receive beam-forming process must integrate over a scattered wave that possesses poor spatial coherence, producing speckle statistics that are similar to those found when wave aberration is present (Section 9.2.4) but vary systematically with depth.

Contrast resolution. This is a measure of the minimum relative difference in mean echo amplitude, as between two specified regions of an imaged field that the system can just distinguish as being of different echo amplitude. This is determined by a number of factors, including characteristics of the ultimate observer (whether human or machine), and is specifically related, through the spatial density of the speckle pattern, to spatial resolution, bearing in mind the caveat at the end of the paragraph above and mentioned again below. It can also be influenced, to an important extent, by the side-lobe (including grating lobe) structure of the beam because this constitutes a source of inappropriate signal energy: effectively, noise. In the absence of such additional noise or clutter, an analytically rigorous definition that has been proposed for low-contrast detectability (Smith *et al.* 1983) is the 'lesion signal-to-noise ratio' SNR_l:

$$SNR_l = SNR_0 \, E_l (S_l/S_c)^{0.5} \tag{9.10}$$

where S_l and S_c are the areas, respectively, of the lesion and of a speckle spot in the far field, E_l is the echogenicity of the lesion relative to its background and SNR_0 is the signal-to-noise ratio for a point in the image, with a value of 1.91 (see Chapter 6) for linear, i.e. uncompressed, B-scan images. It turns out that the condition that the speckle spot, and hence also the lesion, should be in the 'far field' is exactly that specified above (under *spatial resolution*) as being required to maintain the spatial coherence of the received wave. Hence, equation (9.10) should only be valid in the focal region(s) of an imaging system (or of course in the far field of an unfocused transducer).

Sensitive range. This is a measure of the maximum depth through overlying anatomy from which, under specified conditions, informative echoes can be detected and exploited by the system. It is primarily determined by two factors: the effective acoustic centre frequency (i.e. allowing for low-pass acoustic filtering by tissue) and r.f. *sensitivity* (where this is defined as the ratio, or decibel difference, between transmitted signal amplitude and corresponding receiver noise level). In practice it can be considered to correspond to the distance out to the point of transition, illustrated in Figure 8.5, between speckle-dominated and r.f.-dominated noise regions.

Acoustic output. This is a set of measures of the acoustic power and stress to which a patient may be exposed in the course of an examination. Appropriate measurement techniques have been described in Chapter 3 (Section 3.8) and the biological implications of such exposures will be discussed in Chapter 14.

Geometrical conformity. This is a set of factors that express the accuracy with which spatial features of a target are reproduced in an image: on the one hand, the extent of any spatial distortion and, on the other, of particular practical importance, the accuracy with which linear distances and areas are reported.

The tools needed for assessing performance on the above measures are broadly of two kinds: hydrophones (Chapter 3) and test objects. A high-sensitivity, broad-band miniature hydrophone is usually the device of choice for fully characterising interrogating fields, including their side-lobe structure, as also for determining acoustic centre frequency and spectrum. The design of test objects that will enable realistic assessment of the performance of a system in imaging typical human anatomy and pathology has proved surprisingly difficult. A number, particularly of the early designs of resolution objects, were based on grids of wires or filaments that gave excessively strong echoes and, even for the more sophisticated 'tissue mimicking' objects, or 'phantoms', it has been very difficult to create materials that are, at the same time, both stable and possessed of scattering and attenuating properties that are reasonably representative of human soft tissues. Thus, although a number of such objects and phantoms are well established in commercial availability, their behaviour and relevance to clinical investigative situations still need to be examined somewhat critically.

9.2.9 FIELDS OF APPLICATION

There are few significant regions of the body that are technically inaccessible for ultrasonic investigation. Clinical practice has advanced hand-in-hand with general imaging technology and there can be a variety of considerations, perhaps not always totally objective, governing decisions to use ultrasound for tackling any particular investigative problem.

Foremost among these should be considerations of technical performance, preferably along lines such as those discussed in the next section but in common practice less rigorously determined. Ultrasound, as basically a tomographic imaging procedure, has much in common with both X-ray CT and NMR imaging ('MRI'), with which it is fairly readily open to comparison. Although excellently suited for visualising fluid-filled structures, such as cysts and the pregnant uterus, ultrasound, even with the use of microbubble contrast media, is generally inferior to MRI in contrast discrimination for some applications, e.g. tumour investigation; and both CT and MRI, but generally not ultrasound, can provide full cross-sectional visualisation, which can be vitally important for applications such as the planning of radiotherapy treatments.

There are then many considerations of cost-effectiveness, convenience and patient acceptability. Both CT and MRI are very costly, not only in equipment and space but also in labour and other running costs, so ultrasound will generally entail a much lower cost per investigation. It thus tends to be much more generally available, for example in small clinics and peripheral hospitals, where CT/MRI may not be affordable. Even in specialist hospitals it will often be the method of choice for many applications, e.g. in obstetrics and in a number of cardiological and paediatric applications, but it will also be used widely in the preliminary examination of cases that may then need to be referred on for CT or MRI for more definitive investigation. Patterns of use may differ for good reasons, as between different communities, and the World Health Organization has been very concerned that the perceived 'prestige' associated with CT and MRI should not unduly distort the deployment of limited medical funding resources in developing countries: they have published recommendations on the cost-effectiveness in deploying ultrasound, as against CT/MRI equipment (WHO 1990). A valuable feature of ultrasound, particularly in contrast to X-ray methods, is its apparent freedom from hazard (see Chapter 14), which can be of particular importance not only in obstetrics but also in programmes of well-person screening.

Rather fundamental, physics-related restrictions on use are imposed where bone and air spaces are present. Somewhat ironically (but for the very good reason that it is an important organ that was essentially invisible to alternative, pre-CT investigative techniques) the brain was the subject of a substantial proportion of early ultrasonic development work. What this did not take into account, however, was the nature of the adult human skull as an acoustically very complex, triple-layer sandwich that not only reflects back, and/or mode-converts, a high proportion of incident sound but seriously distorts even the transmitted component. In spite of this, however, impressive efforts have been reported in adaptive signal processing aimed at compensating for such distortion. Application of related processing methods also can substantially reduce the impact of reflection/refraction artefacts originating from other parts of the skeleton or from air spaces such as lung and bowel gas. The essentially uncalcified neonatal skull does not present such problems, thus allowing the routine use of ultrasound in paediatric neurology.

The wide variety of clinically worthwhile applications has its counterpart in the variety of specialised instruments that have been developed in response to such interest. Many of these are designed for external, skin-contact scanning, some for use through water-baths and an increasing number and variety for endoscopic examination. Typical operating centre frequencies are from around 3 MHz for abdominal and obstetric contact scanners up to 30 MHz or more for some skin and endoscopic devices.

9.3   A BROADER LOOK: PERFORMANCE CRITERIA

In the introductory section of this chapter it was pointed out that, historically, the development of echography, highly successful although it has been, took place to a large extent empirically, rather than being science-led. At the same time, much of this development took place in parallel with that of other imaging modalities: X-ray computed tomography (CT) was first described in 1972, shortly to be followed by nuclear magnetic resonance imaging (MRI) and, in a commercial form, positron emission tomography (PET). All of these techniques, apart from providing anatomical images, offered interesting prospects for supplying specific information related to tissue type and/or physiological function. Such prospects had, indeed, already been of interest to some workers in the ultrasound field, who then proceeded to investigate the possibilities for so-called ultrasonic tissue characterisation, or 'telehistology' (Chivers & Hill 1973). With time the emphasis here has moved towards attempting to present, in tomographic image format, specific, ultrasonically derived parametric data related to tissue type and physiology: an enterprise for which a more appropriate term seems to be 'parametric imaging'.

At this point, therefore, it should be helpful to take stock, to pose some questions and to attempt to suggest some answers. What is 'ultrasonic investigation' trying to achieve? How well is it succeeding? Particularly considering the enormous advances in supporting technology over the past 50 years, is conventional pulse–echo imaging the optimum technique? How does ultrasound compare, by objective criteria, with other modalities for addressing particular clinical problems? And what are the set of objective criteria that one might use in seeking answers to such questions? Discussion of such issues has been the subject of a paper by the present authors (Hill et al. 1990), from which the following text has been adapted.

As already discussed in the context of conventional pulse–echo imaging, the three particularly important aspects of performance of an ultrasonic or indeed any other tomographic system designed for tissue-specific imaging would seem to be: 'contrast resolution', 'spatial resolution' and 'presentation speed'. Although these concepts need to be separately defined and considered, it must be clear that they are, in practice, strongly interdependent and their application may need to be considered in the contexts of particular clinical investigative problems rather than necessarily being universal.

9.3.1 CONTRAST RESOLUTION

A vital attribute of any technique for parametric imaging is that it should discriminate well between different tissue types. This is a general requirement that may manifest itself in a number of different forms. Firstly, it may be desirable to locate a boundary between two adjacent tissue regions (e.g. extent of tumour invasion into a host tissue): in this case contrast is required as a component of an essentially conventional imaging procedure, where the contrast may be thought of as being provided parametrically (i.e. on the basis of measures of one or more quantities that are themselves useful but indirect indicators of tissue type). Secondly, it may be required to make a differential diagnosis between two or more possible histopathological identities of a particular tissue region, e.g. on a space-occupying lesion within an organ such as the liver. Again, thirdly, one may want to record the time course, extent and direction of any histopathological change occurring within a tissue region, as for example in response to an attempted therapeutic procedure. In each case it will be seen that the underlying need is to achieve differentiation, or 'contrast resolution', between two or more different tissue conditions.

In practical terms the achievement of good contrast resolution can be considered as a signal-to-noise problem, where the signal arises as a separation between the two mean values of a parameter that characterises two tissues of interest. Noise, in its general sense, will arise from several sources, which will include both biological variability and technical measurement uncertainty.

Quantitatively, we may suppose that the procedure for differentiation is based on numerical measures, P, of some underlying physical property (or mathematical combination of several properties) of the interrogated tissue and that, for each value of P, the technique will generate a corresponding signal of value S. For example, P might correspond to acoustic attenuation coefficient and S to 'frequency–distance slope' (see Section 9.4). For the purposes of the following discussion it is assumed that S is linearly dependent on P, i.e.:

$$dS/dP = k \text{ (constant)} \tag{9.11}$$

However, the general argument will remain valid provided that the relationship is monotonic.

The general requirement for a technique to be effective in differentiating between two tissue types, denoted by 1 and 2, could be expressed as:

$$\Delta P = (P_1 - P_2) \gg U \tag{9.12}$$

where P_1 and P_2 are the values of P for the two tissues and U is the numerical uncertainty (or 'noise') of the system. Evidently, this relationship is an oversimplification and includes implicitly the following specific factors:

(a) The relative nominal separation of 'property values', P_i/P_j, between two tissue types that it is required to differentiate. If multiple differentiation is to be undertaken, the parameter relevant to performance assessment may be the separation between the two closest P values.
(b) The 'biological' variance $s^2(P_b)$ in the value of P corresponding to nominally identical tissue types. In practice it may be appropriate to distinguish two forms of this variance, corresponding respectively to that arising within a given subject ('intrinsically': $s^2(P_{bi})$) and that between different subjects ('extrinsically': $s^2(P_{be})$). Related variances, $s^2(S_b)$ etc., will occur for the corresponding signals.
(c) The technical precision with which the technique transforms the numerical property measure, P, into a signal, S. This can be expressed as a variance in S, $s^2(S_t)$, for a given P, which in turn is the resultant of four contributions corresponding, respectively, to:

(i)   instrumental (stochastic) noise ($s^2(S_{ts})$);
(ii) 'intrinsic' variations (due to drift, etc.) as between measurements made on a given tissue with the same machine ($s^2(S_{ti})$);
(iii) 'extrinsic' variations, again as between measurements made on a given tissue (P value) but using a different machine ($s^2(S_{te})$);
(iv) and 'propagation loss' uncertainty ($s^2(S_{tp})$).

This last component arises because the quantitative relationships used to derive values for one parameter of tissue type (e.g. backscattering coefficient) commonly entail, explicitly or otherwise, terms dependent on some other parameter (e.g. attenuation coefficient, μ) and, although a first-order correction for this dependency can be made (e.g. by assuming that μ is constant throughout the tissue regions being examined), uncertainty will generally arise because of departures from this assumed condition. An example of the impact of this propagation loss uncertainty has been referred to above in relation to the provision of time-gain compensation in a conventional B-scanner.

If we assume that the variances will add incoherently, the effective standard deviation (noise level) of the system will be:

$$\sigma = [s^2(S_b) + s^2(S_t)]^{1/2} \tag{9.13}$$

and the 'differential signal' or 'contrast'-to-noise ratio, ψ_1, for a single measurement will be:

$$\psi_1 = \Delta S/\sigma \tag{9.14}$$

where ΔS is the difference in signal corresponding to the separation ΔP in property value. Correspondingly, if the complete procedure entails making N uncorrelated measurements, we have (but only approximately for small N):

$$\psi_N = (\Delta S/\sigma)N^{1/2} \tag{9.15}$$

It follows that we may define a figure of merit for the procedure as the contrast-to-noise ratio for a given fractional change in 'property value', P, between two tissues:

$$\Gamma = \psi_N/(\Delta P/P_i) = (dS/dP)P_iN^{1/2}/\sigma \tag{9.16}$$

This expression is, of course, simply a special example of the general formula for statistical variance (cf. Student's t-test) and is similar in form to a relationship derived by Edelstein et al. (1983) for comparing the performance of various pulse sequences in obtaining precise values of NMR relaxation times for clinical MRI. It should have value here in providing a basis for assessing the comparative effectiveness of various possible approaches, ultrasonic or otherwise, to the differentiation of specific tissue types.

We are now in a position to suggest performance criteria for parametric imaging procedures in achieving contrast discrimination. Firstly, in relation to the ability of a given procedure to contribute to the solution of a given diagnostic problem, it will be necessary that ψ_N is no less than unity and preferably considerably larger if several different tissue types are to be discriminated separately. It will, of course, be important to define the conditions of application sufficiently carefully that the appropriate set of variances can be used in the calculation. And, secondly, if comparison is to be made between the contrast discrimination achievable from different approaches to measuring the same property value, P, then this can be made objectively in terms of the above figure of merit.

9.3.2 SPATIAL RESOLUTION

The potential applications of parametric imaging methods are many and varied but, in almost all cases, it is desirable to localise the interrogated region(s) rather precisely. It is thus useful to define the spatial resolution of a particular procedure as 'the linear distance, L, (e.g. in mm) between the centres of two regions from which it is possible to derive separate and independent signals, S_a and S_b, relating to corresponding tissue property values, P_a and P_b'.

For any technique there will probably be a limiting minimum value of L set, for example, by fundamental laws of diffraction and by refractive index inhomogeneity within the propagation medium, as discussed above in Section 9.2.4, but practically useful values of L may also be set by signal-to-noise considerations (e.g. as reflected in the averaging provision included in equation (9.15)). This question of the trade-off between contrast and spatial resolution has been discussed by Lopez et al. (1987) and Wagner et al. (1987), who point out that the ultrasonic inverse scattering problem is 'ill-posed' and that parametric imaging techniques must be based on statistical methods working at low resolution. We shall discuss below some practical examples of this trade-off.

A useful approach to setting a performance criterion for spatial resolution in the present context may be to relate it to the maximum attainable anatomical resolution achievable, e.g. the point-target resolution obtainable in the conventional B-scan display of a pulse–echo image. Generally, it will not be possible to match this resolution while obtaining worthwhile contrast information: a factor of 3 linearly (9 in area) might be acceptable but a factor of 10 would often be unsatisfactory.

9.3.3 SPEED OF PRESENTATION

If an investigative test provides unique information that is expected to have decisive influence on patient management, a substantial delay in presenting its results may be acceptable. However, there is generally a high premium on rapidity of response, particularly in imaging related methods where the investigator needs to be sure that procedures are satisfactorily completed whilst the patient is present. With ultrasound techniques, the sheer ability to carry out investigations in so-called 'real time', facilitating as it does an interactive procedure, makes it desirable that supplementary information, such as that on tissue characterisation, should be provided sufficiently rapidly as to contribute to that interaction.

Thus a third important performance criterion in assessing image parameterisation techniques will be the speed at which data can be derived and presented to the investigator. Two quantitative measures of performance in this respect ('parameterisation rates') would seem to be useful: the reciprocals of the times taken (i.e. in s^{-1} or Hz) to acquire and display tissue characterising data, firstly from a single region of interest and, secondly from a complete parametric image with spatial resolution as defined above. Higher rates will clearly be the better, but there will often be particular value in being able to operate in 'real time' (practically, the rate required to achieve effectively flicker-free image viewing: approximately 10 Hz; see Chapter 8).

High speed will generally only be achievable at some cost, both financial and technical. The technical cost follows directly from the N term in equations (9.15) and (9.16), because without technical complexity multiple, uncorrelated measurements will generally need to be made sequentially. It is of relevance here that, under conditions of real time imaging, a limited degree of averaging of serially repeated measurement values will be made by the eye-and-brain system, which has an effective integration time constant in the region of a few tenths of a second.

9.4   FURTHER PROSPECTS FOR ULTRASONOLOGY AND IMAGE PARAMETERISATION

It is timely now to re-visit our earlier comment on the apparent arbitrariness of the choice of pulse–echo backscatter amplitude imaging as the basis for so much of the historical development of clinical investigative ultrasound. A unique feature of this approach, however, was that it could be taken without the need to rely on powerful digital processing. Clinical ultrasonic systems commonly generate information at data rates that are typically in the region of 10 MHz or more; this is substantially higher than that from CT, MRI or PET systems and, until the 1980s, thus placed it beyond the range of useful digital processing technology. With current access to such technology, however, a much wider technical variety of investigative methods can be implemented. These can be seen as arising in two ways: (a) derivation from backscattered echo signal data of information on a number of additional tissue 'properties'; and (b) derivation of signals from non-backscatter geometry (e.g. transmission and non-π scattering). Many studies have been carried out and reported in the 'tissue characterisation' literature on such possibilities (Greenleaf 1986; Dunn *et al.* 1996). Here we can only briefly refer to some of these and comment, where appropriate, on how they might be seen in relation to the scheme of performance criteria discussed in the previous section.

9.4.1 ACOUSTIC ATTENUATION AND SPEED OF SOUND

The first recorded thoughts in the whole field of medical ultrasonic imaging were those of the Dussiks (1947) who, in the 1930s, attempted to make shadow images of the human head that, similarly to the plain X-ray, purported to be 'ray-attenuation' maps. In the event, refraction and reflection artefacts totally obscured any real anatomical information and, for most parts of the human anatomy, such artefacts have constituted a practically insoluble barrier to this approach. The principal exception here is the female breast where Carson *et al.* (1977), inspired by the concept of X-ray CT, were able to make transmission reconstruction images of the attenuation coefficient. The transmission reconstruction approach also lends itself to the derivation of pulse transit times, and hence sound speed, leading Greenleaf and Bahn (1981) to report some interesting double parameter images (colour coded for both attenuation and sound speed). This approach performs well in the sense of exploiting contrast mechanisms different from those of backscatter amplitude. Speed of sound in particular (see Chapter 5) distinguishes well between fatty and watery (e.g. tumour) breast tissue and, moreover, is closely related mechanistically to NMR chemical shift (Sehgal & Greenleaf 1986). The approach is, however, very demanding on data processing resources and, although by using a hollow cylindrical transducer array it might be possible to approach real-time acquisition, it is questionable whether such a system would be economically worthwhile for such a limited, albeit clinically important, application, especially when the established breast imaging method, X-ray mammography, already provides excellent contrast for fat versus other tissues.

The apparent attenuating effect of a tissue region, manifested by posterior shadowing (positive or negative), is widely used as a diagnostic criterion in conventional pulse–echo imaging. Although of unquestionable value, the mechanism responsible for such shadowing may not always be clear but probably arises from local anomalies in both attenuation coefficient and sound speed, with the latter causing some refraction of the beam. Posterior shadowing, however, occurs in a highly system-dependent manner, being more or less apparent depending on factors such as strength and type of focusing, type of scan pattern and distance of the attenuation object from the transducer. Variations in such factors between one imaging system and another may well have been one of the things that accounted for differences of opinion that have been expressed over the years with regard to the diagnostic value of acoustic shadowing of breast masses. On the other hand, it provided Green and Arditi (1985) with the opportunity to design an imaging system for which shadow contrast, and shadow contrast-to-noise ratio, were maximised. The resulting method, which they called reflex transmission imaging (RTI) and is described in Chapter 4, Section 4.4.1.3, was later shown to hold promise for imaging tissue that has been thermally coagulated (Malcolm 1997; Baker & Bamber 2003). As shown above (Figure 9.5) RTI also provides a useful way of taking advantage of three-dimensional echo data for parametric imaging of the skin surface. Finally, although commercial one-dimensional arrays are not ideal for this form of imaging, studying the performance behaviour of an RTI system based on them provides considerable enlightenment with regard to the conditions under which one should expect current commercial scanners to provide useful B-mode posterior shadowing (Baker & Bamber 2002).

A somewhat more rigorous but still relatively simple approach to estimation of the tissue attenuation coefficient is to measure the rate of decrease with range of either the amplitude of echoes, or their average frequency, returning from a supposedly uniform region of tissue, such as the liver (see Chapter 4, Section 4.4.1.3). Such measurements can be relatively easily carried out using a conventional scanner but, in practice, substantial system and object-dependent bias may exist because of the difficulty of adequately correcting for the effects of the transducer diffraction field (causing sometimes large extrinsic technical variation, $s^2(S_{te})$) and, even with the use of multiple sampling ($N > 1$), an inherently large stochastic technical variance, $s^2(S_{ts})$, means that adequate precision for tissue differentiation seems to require sample lengths in excess of some 20 mm, thus rather limiting the range of applicability of the technique.

Indirect measurements of sound speed have also been achieved using modifications of conventional pulse–echo systems (Robinson *et al.* 1984; Bamber *et al.* 1989). More such methods were reviewed in Chapter 5 (Section 5.2.1.4). However, a substantial signal-to-noise limitation on spatial resolution arises here (as also with the transmission reconstruction approach) because of the rather low property contrast, ΔP, that is no more than some 5% even between 'fatty' and 'watery' tissue volumes. Because the time of flight across a 1 mm tissue layer is some 700 ps, the resulting ΔS has a value of around 35 ps, which has to be measured against the noise resulting from multiple propagation paths through the (inhomogenous) organ.

As mentioned below in Sections 9.4.2 and 9.4.5, substantially improved performance in ultrasonic image parameterisation may be achieved, through reduction of various uncertainties, by taking advantage of differencing techniques. One of the applications where this is possible is in visualising localised changes in sound speed due to focal hyperthermia. Because the propagation path inhomogeneities referred to above are reasonably constant from one image to the next, the high relative precision of time-of-flight estimation may be taken full advantage of by comparing the apparent positions of r.f. echoes in images taken before and during heating (Seip *et al.* 1996; Bamber *et al.* 1997; Miller *et al.* 2002a, 2003). This approach is illustrated and explained further in Figure 9.14. An interesting limitation of this technique, particularly with regard to the present discussion of performance criteria, is that equation (9.11) is only valid over limited regions of the property range, P (temperature); not only do the signals (change in sound speed and thence echo strain) vary non-linearly with P but the relationship, as seen in Chapter 5 (Figure 5.5), is not monotonic for most types of tissue. This restricts the highest contrast that can be achieved (Miller *et al.* 2002a).

(a)

(b)

(c)

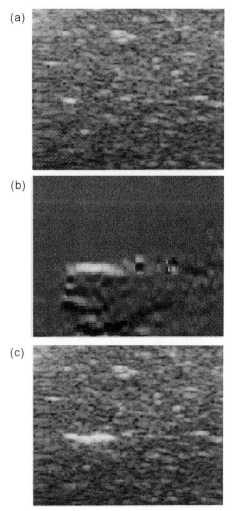

Figure 9.14. Demonstration of parametric imaging based on a difference of sound speed generated by localised hyperthermia. (a) Region (approximately 4.7 × 3.8 cm) of a B-mode image of *ex vivo* bovine liver that was briefly heated using a 1.7 MHz high-intensity focused ultrasound source positioned to the left of the image and with its acoustic axis horizontal in the imaging plane. (b) Image of the same region of tissue constructed by tracking the apparent axial displacement of r.f. echoes caused by heating (baseline temperature ∼ 24°C, spatial peak rise in temperature ∼ 10°C) and displaying apparent axial strain (contraction) of the echo structure as increasing brightness. Note the excellent signal-to-noise ratio; the spatial peak in measured echo strain was ∼ 0.8% and the strain noise anterior to (above) the heated (bright) region was ∼ 0.01%. Posterior to (below) the hot spot may be seen noise whose pattern is characteristic of the shape of the heated region and is believed to be due in part to refraction of the imaging beam, the heated region acting as a 'thermal lens'. (c) Another B-mode image of the same region, but created after the image in (b) was made and after a further rise in temperature, enough to cause irreversible tissue coagulation (∼ 60°C). A bright region in this image, caused by reflections from bubbles due to cavitation in the focal region of the high-intensity source, may be seen to correspond approximately in size and position to the hot spot in image (b). Note also the strong correlation between tissue echo texture and speckle elsewhere in the image, between images (c) and (a). Adapted from Miller *et al.* (2003)

9.4.2 PROPAGATION NON-LINEARITY PARAMETER

A number of authors have explored the possibility that tissue-specific differences in non-linearity parameter, B/A, could be exploited as an imaging contrast mechanism. In particular, Bjorno and Lewin (1986) suggested measuring the second harmonic pressure amplitude at a source distance x, $P_2(x)$, and thus deriving B/A from the approximate relationship:

$$B/A \approx KP_2(x)\exp(2\alpha x) - 2 \tag{9.17}$$

where K is a rather medium-independent constant at a given fundamental frequency and α is the absorption coefficient for the tissue at the fundamental frequency. However, the observed range of values for B/A in non-fatty human tissues is some 6.0–8.0 (Chapter 5; Law *et al.* 1985; Sehgal *et al.* 1986) and the above expression is very sensitive to the value of α, to the extent that an uncertainty of only 2% in its value (at 3 MHz and 10 cm path length) will constitute a 'propagation loss uncertainty' [equations (9.12)–(9.15)] in excess of the above range of B/A.

A very different approach to exploiting this contrast mechanism is to transmit successively, in the same beam position, two pulses of differing amplitude and consequent non-linearity, and then, by comparison of echoes, to infer values of B/A for preceding segments of the beam (Fatemi & Greenleaf 1996). This would seem to overcome the above problem of propagation loss uncertainty. Yet another approach to the exploitation of propagation non-linearity, previously explored in high-frequency acoustic microscopy (Chapter 11) and discussed in several sections above, is that of harmonic imaging, in which the receiving transducer is tuned to a harmonic of the (high amplitude) transmitted pulse. An illustration of the application of this technique was given above in Figure 9.8.

9.4.3 FEATURES OF ACOUSTIC SCATTERING

As has already been discussed, the conventional pulse–echo image maps a parameter that constitutes a backscatter cross-section modified to an uncertain extent by attenuation in the propagation path. For very many practical purposes a sufficiently good guess can be made in compensating for such attenuation that the resulting ('parametric') image can be used reliably for tissue differentiation. Indeed, historically again, it was Wild's attempts in 1952 to use this approach for objective differentiation of malignant and benign breast lesions that initiated the whole subject of ultrasonic parametric imaging (Wild 1978).

Speckle noise (Section 9.2.6) is a major limitation in this context and performance can be enhanced to some degree by processes such as adaptive filtering (Bamber 1993), which in turn open up the possibility of thresholding and optimisation of display conditions with respect to observer perception (Chapter 8), possibly also involving intelligent use of colour display (Pizer & Zimmerman 1983; Massay *et al.* 1989). Even when adopting such measures, however, this approach has its limitations: significant contrast between adjacent tissues or pathologies can only be achieved in a limited number of situations and absolute tissue identification is seldom possible, partly for the reasons mentioned above (see Recchia & Wickline 1993; Noritomi *et al.* 1997).

There has therefore been much interest in trying to exploit other features of the backscatter signals, particularly those that carry information about the structural properties of the scattering matrix: spatial density of the scattering centres, possible regularities in their spatial arrangement, shapes of large scatterers or of clusters of small ones. Such information may be expressed in a variety of signal forms, for example in the frequency spectra of backscattered energy, which is in principle able to extract some summary properties of tissue structure on a scale smaller than the resolution determined by the PSF of the imaging system or in quantifiable features of image texture. This general approach, which will be seen to have some conceptual relationship to x-ray crystallography, was first proposed some time ago (Hill 1974) and has the interesting feature of being relatively insensitive to acoustic propagation effects. There is a limitation on this approach, however, that might be termed the 'flashlight problem' (Bamber 1979). The unfortunate car driver who, on a dark night, drops his keys in the mud will only have a chance of retrieving them if he can point his flashlight at the appropriate patch of ground. Similarly, particular features of the mechanical structure of a tissue will be revealed only if the spectrum of the interrogating ultrasonic beam includes wavelengths capable of interacting with those features.

Possibly for this reason, some the most successful work in frequency spectroscopy was carried out for many years at the relatively high frequencies and bandwidths that can be used in the eye and orbit (Lizzi *et al.* 1983, 1986; Sigel *et al.* 1990; Silverman *et al.* 1995). The procedure here entails digitally recording, from a predetermined region of interest, a series of r.f. A-scan data sets, computing their Fourier transforms and then calculating values for particular features of the resulting spectrum (e.g. spectral slope and zero frequency intercept). The authors then use a physical model that enables them to calculate, from these data, values for 'absolute' physical properties of the tissue, such as mean scatterer strength and size and effective scatterer separation (Lizzi *et al.* 1987). A further observation of oscillations (or 'resonances') in the spectra from some tissues is found to correspond to the presence in those tissues of relatively large-scale, spatially periodic structure. In the orbit (for which acoustic access is through the eye, where propagation loss uncertainty is likely to be small), and also to some extent in the liver, the technique has been shown to be capable of good contrast resolution adequate to enable its implementation in the form of parametric imaging (Kuc 1986; Yaremko *et al.* 1987).

Alternative signal processing schemes, based on fitting the predictions of tissue models such as the inhomogeneous continuum to measured frequency dependences of the backscattering coefficient, have also been developed (Chaturvedi & Insana 1997; Mercer 1998) and the method has been successfully applied in various applications, including characterisation of the structure of the human kidney (Hall *et al.* 1996) and skin tumours (Mercer *et al.* 1997), and classification of plaque in coronary arteries using intravascular ultrasound (Nair *et al.* 2002). Problems may, however, be encountered due to large propagation loss uncertainty from a poorly known frequency-dependent attenuation coefficient for the intervening tissue, and to large extrinsic technical variation arising from difficulties in implementing adequate diffraction correction.

The information on which frequency spectrum analysis is based – groups of adjacent A-scan data sets – is, of course, the raw material of pulse–echo imaging. An alternative method of characterising the ensemble of returned echoes from a particular region, but admittedly one that largely aims to characterise resolved tissue architecture, is thus to derive quantitative features of the 'texture' of the corresponding two-dimensional image. Image texture analysis was originally developed for other applications, including aerial surveillance, but has been found to lend itself well to ultrasound work. The technique has been fully described by Nicholas *et al.* (1986) and has been shown, particularly in relation to pathologies of the liver, myocardium and breast, to be capable of useful contrast resolution (e.g. Räth *et al.* 1985; Schlaps *et al.* 1985; Chandrasekaran *et al.* 1986; Hart *et al.* 1986; Insana *et al.* 1986; Wagner *et al.* 1986; Fitzgerald *et al.* 1987; Oosterveld *et al.* 1991; Goldberg *et al.* 1992; Garra *et al.* 1993; Momenan *et al.* 1994; Valckx & Thijssen 1997; Zheng *et al.* 1997). It has also been shown, in work with tissue-mimicking phantoms, that, provided sufficient averaging is carried out, reliable and useful texture features may be extracted from very small two-dimensional image areas approaching the resolution cell that is inherent to the basic imaging system. But there is a trade-off, with implications for presentation speed, between contrast resolution (measured as classification accuracy) and spatial resolution, that is consistent with the effect of the N term in equations (9.14) and (9.15) (Bamber & Nassiri 1987). Furthermore, this is again a method that possesses substantial propagation loss and extrinsic technical uncertainties, for similar reasons to those encountered in spectrum analysis, making it difficult to compare or pool results from different research centres. However, the type of data processing required here is closely related to that needed for speckle reduction by adaptive filtering, which has been the vehicle for demonstrating two important points relevant to this section. Firstly, the development of three-dimensional sonographic imaging will benefit the trade-off between contrast and spatial resolution in this form of parametric imaging (and many others); the availability of an accurate third dimension of echo data permits a substantial reduction in the area needed within any single image plane for feature extraction whilst maintaining the same texture classification accuracy (Bamber *et al.* 1992). Secondly, texture classification of this type was shown to be capable of implementation at video frame rate (Loupas *et al.* 1989; Bamber & Phelps 1991) and has since appeared in related form on commercial scanning systems. This approach to parametric imaging therefore should be effective in principle and also technically feasible.

9.4.4 SHEAR ELASTIC MODULUS: ELASTOGRAPHY

A particularly interesting conclusion that emerged from the material presented in Chapter 7 was that, considered as 'property values' in the context of the discussion in Section 9.3.1, the relative range of values between different soft tissues for the shear elastic modulus is several orders of magnitude greater than that for the bulk modulus, which is the principal fundamental quantity responsible for conventional echo contrast. This is the scientific basis for an approach to parametric imaging that has come to be termed 'elastography' (Ophir *et al.* 1996).

Manual palpation – sensing through the finger-tips for abnormal hard lumps or soft cavities in a patient's anatomy – is one of the oldest clinical examination techniques. Elastography is essentially a method of remote palpation in which consecutive series of ultrasonic echo signals are analysed to quantify the mechanical displacement experienced by tissue structures in response to some kind of mechanical stress, which may be either artificially applied or physiological (e.g. as cardiac or respiratory motion). From the stress–strain relationship obtained in this way it is then possible, in principle, to deduce the regional values of shear modulus that were responsible for the observed behaviour. In its simplest form, and in the initial work in this field, determinations were made of the time rate of decorrelation between successive, co-linear A-scans taken through the region of interest (Dickinson & Hill 1982; Tristam *et al.* 1988). More recent developments of the technique have brought it into close relationship with the other main approach to movement quantification and imaging – Doppler processing – and demonstrated similar suitability for real-time display. These two are therefore considered together and discussed in more detail in the following chapter but it is appropriate to emphasise here that elastography is an outstanding example of a parametric imaging technique that has achieved substantial practical application. This theme is briefly expanded below, prior to its more detailed discussion in Chapter 10.

9.4.5 IMAGING TIME-DEPENDENT PHENOMENA

As parametric imaging methods, the parallel between elastography and colour Doppler blood flow imaging may be broadened to include other techniques that are based on the detection of time-dependent properties of ultrasonic echoes. This thought is worthy of consideration because, in addition to the benefit of imaging entirely new tissue properties, these two methods are outstanding success stories when considered in the light of the above discussion of performance criteria for image parameterisation; spatial resolution and presentation speed for each come close to those of echo imaging, and contrast resolution for the parameter being imaged (a component of tissue strain in the case of elastography and, for colour Doppler, a component of average flow velocity) is not only excellent but can be far superior (easily by more than an order of magnitude) to that for the original echo image from which the time-dependent parameters were derived. This latter fact, beautifully illustrated by the *in vitro* prostate elastogram of Figure 9.15, is perhaps surprising when first realised but derives in part from taking advantage of the fact that speckle structure remains unchanged (correlated) when tissue or blood structure moves in an appropriate manner (such as a sufficiently short distance) and such that it too remains correlated. As a result, the noise becomes limited not by the multiplicative coherent speckle that dominates the fixed ratio of $S/s^2(S_{ts})$ (Section 9.3.1) for echo-magnitude imaging (see also Chapters 6 and 8), but rather by the fundamental ability of a similarity measure, such as the correlation coefficient, to detect phase change or locate the position of an echo structure in the presence of additive electronic noise (Belaid *et al.* 1994; Walker & Trahey 1994, 1995; Cespedes *et al.* 1995). This is entirely consistent with the fact that from the earliest days of Doppler ultrasound it seems to have been noted often that what is effectively the same process, in the form of frequency demodulation, allows the Doppler shift from erythrocytes moving in arteries to be measured when the echoes that these scatterers produce are below the limit of visual detectability in a simple B-scan. The signal and noise become additive, enabling the signal-to-noise ratio to be increased simply by increasing the signal, until a limit is reached determined by the maximum signal (tissue displacement) that

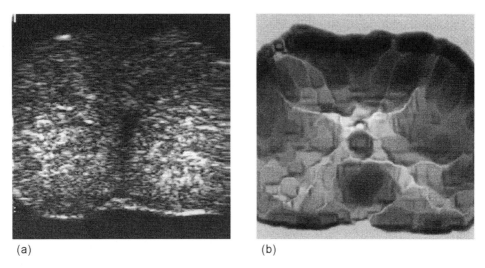

(a)   (b)

Figure 9.15. Illustration of the superior contrast resolution achievable, and its effect in also improving spatial resolution, by processing ultrasound echoes to detect and display a parameter (axial strain) that derives from a signal characteristic (tissue position) that is time dependent, rather than displaying instantaneous echo amplitude. The images show an elastogram (axial strain image) of a canine prostate *in vitro* (b) and the original sonogram (a) corresponding to one of the echo data sets from which the elastogram was computed. See text for discussion. *Source*: Image is courtesy of J. Ophir

can occur without significant decorrelation of the echo structure. This maximum is system, object and parameter dependent, but the ensuing decorrelation ultimately leads to a decrease in signal-to-noise ratio. A plot of signal-to-noise ratio against S will then depict new performance measures such as the smallest signal that can be measured (sensitivity), the peak signal-to-noise ratio reached and the dynamic signal range that the system can pass. Ophir and co-workers seem to have been the first to define such a curve, doing so for elastography and calling it the 'strain filter' (see Varghese *et al.* 2002). Clearly, at the high and low signal extremes of such a filter the relationship between physical property value, P, and signal value, S, will become less favourable until $\mathrm{d}S/\mathrm{d}P = 0$, i.e. no change in signal can be detected whatever the change in physical property. However, for elastography in particular, even within the signal-pass range of the system, S and P are related in a highly non-linear manner. This is due both to the reciprocal relationship between elastic modulus and strain (Miller & Bamber 2000) and to the manner in which stress may or may not be transmitted from a stiff region of tissue to a soft region, or vice versa. There is thus a difference in behaviour of equation (9.11) and hence equation (9.16), for the detection of positive and negative contrast objects. In elastography the study of the relationship of ΔS and ΔP has come to be known as that of 'contrast transfer efficiency' (Varghese *et al.* 2002). There are of course, in any new imaging method, new sources of variance or noise, and for strain imaging such sources include the strain pattern that is due to the object-dependent distribution of stress and the confounding influence of other variables, such as Poisson's ratio, stress–strain non-linearity or viscosity, which may not be accounted for and represent both intrinsic ($s^2(S_{ti})$) and propagation loss ($s^2(S_{tp})$) uncertainties in the context of the discussion of Section 9.3.1. As with other imaging methods, the branch of the subject that deals with inverse reconstruction, among other objectives, aims to correct for such uncertainties (Doyley *et al.* 2000; Barbone & Bamber 2002).

As was implied at the outset of this brief section, much of the above discussion ought to be extendable to other parametric imaging methods that process ultrasonic echoes to detect changes in echo position or changes in the echo structure at a point. Earlier examples were seen in this chapter, in the forms of relative temperature imaging (relying on changes in sound speed) and discriminating microbubbles from tissue by methods such as pulse-inversion, loss of correlation or flash-echo imaging. In both of these examples one finds again that under the right circumstances performance can be outstanding, with high spatial resolution, fast presentation and with potential for signal-to-noise ratio and contrast resolution that are superior to conventional sonography.

9.5   SUMMARY AND CONCLUSIONS

Ultrasound now plays an important and often vital role in almost every branch of clinical investigation, with a range of applications that continues to grow. Much of the technology, however, has developed in an empirical manner and thus, in many instances, may not yet have experienced the full benefit of recent advances in our understanding of the underlying scientific phenomena. At the same time, it is outstanding among medical 'imaging' technologies for the high information rates that it is, in principle, capable of providing, to the extent that in general practice it probably has not benefited yet to the full from even current fast data processing methods.

This chapter, with others in the book, has thus set out to document current knowledge of the underlying principles of the subject, in the hope that this may help to stimulate ideas for future advances in the technology and accelerate their implementation.

REFERENCES

AIUM (1991). *Standard Methods for Measuring Performance of Pulse–Echo Ultrasound Imaging Equipment*. American Institute of Ultrasound in Medicine, Rockville, MD.

AIUM/NEMA (1989). *Acoustic Output Measurement and Labeling Standard for Diagnostic Equipment*. American Institute of Ultrasound in Medicine, Rockville, MD.

Anderson, M.E. and Trahey, G.E. (1998). The direct estimation of sound speed using pulse-echo ultrasound. *J. Acoust. Soc. Am.* **104**, 3099–3106.

Anglesen, B.A.J. (2000). *Ultrasound Imaging: Waves, Signals and Signal Processing*. Emantec, Norway.

Austeng, A. and Holm, S. (2002). Sparse 2-D Arrays for 3-D phased array imaging – Design methods and Experimental validation. *IEEE Trans. Ultrason. Ferroelectr. Freq. Control* **49**, 1073–1086, 1087–1093.

Baker, L.A.S. and Bamber, J.C. (2002). Effect of dynamic receive focusing on reflex transmission imaging (RTI). *Proc. 2002 IEEE Ultrasonics Symposium*. Vols 1 and 2, D.E. Yuhas, S.C. Schneider (eds), ISBN 0-7803-7582-3, IEEE, Piscataway, NJ, pp. 1581–1584.

Baker, L.A.S. and Bamber, J.C. (2003). Reflex transmission imaging (RTI) of ex vivo bovine liver treated with focused ultrasound surgery (FUS). *Proceedings of the British Medical Ultrasound Society 34th Annual Scientific Meeting*, BJR Congress Series, ISBN 0-905749-51-0, British Institute of Radiology, London, p. 3.

Bamber, J.C. (1979). Theoretical modelling of the acoustic scattering structure of human liver. *Acoust. Lett.* **3**, 114–119.

Bamber, J.C. (1993). Speckle reduction. In *Advances in Ultrasound Techniques and Instrumentation*, P.N.T. Wells (ed.). Churchill Livingstone, New York, pp. 55–67.

Bamber, J.C. (1999). Medical ultrasonic signal and image processing. *Insight* **41**, 14–15.

Bamber, J.C. and Bush N.L. (1996). Freehand elasticity imaging using speckle decorrelation rate. In *Acoustical Imaging*, Vol. 22, P. Tortoli and L. Masotti (eds). Plenum Press, New York, pp. 285–292.

Bamber, J.C. and Daft, C. (1986). Adaptive filtering for reduction of speckle in pulse-echo images. *Ultrasonics* **24**, 41–44.

Bamber, J.C. and Dickinson, R.J. (1980). Ultrasonic B-scanning: a computer simulation. *Phys. Med. Biol.* **25**, 463–479.

Bamber, J.C., Clarke, R.L., Hill, C.R. and Wankling, P.F. (1981). Mirror axicons for improved ultrasonic imaging. *Br. J. Radiol.* **54**, 549.

Bamber, J.C., Cosgrove, D.O., Page, J. and Abbott, C. (1989). Simple and economical approaches to in-vivo measurement of average speed of sound in human liver. In *Ultrasonic Tissue Characterisation and Echographic Imaging*, J. M. Thijssen (ed.). CEC, Luxembourg, pp. 139–154.

Bamber, J.C., Eckersley, R.J., Hubregtse, P., Bush, N.L., Bell, D.S. and Crawford, D.C. (1992). Data processing for three-dimensional ultrasound visualization of tumour anatomy and blood flow. In *Visualization in Biomedical Computing*, SPIE Vol. 1808, R.C. Robb (ed.). Society of Photo-Optical Instrumentation Engineers, Bellingham, pp. 651–663.

Bamber, J.C., Meaney, P., Doyley, M.M., Clarke, R.L. and ter Haar, G.R. (1997). Non-invasive temperature imaging using ultrasound echo strain: preliminary simulations. In *Acoustical Imaging*, Vol. 23, S. Lees and L. Ferrari (eds). Plenum Press, New York, pp. 25–33.

Bamber, J.C., Mucci, R.A., Orofino, D.P. and Thiele, K. (2000a). B-mode speckle texture: the effect of spatial coherence. In *Acoustical Imaging*, Vol. 24, H. Lee (ed.). Kluwer Academic/Plenum Press, New York, pp. 141–146.

Bamber, J.C., Mucci, R.A. and Orofino, D.P. (2000b). Spatial coherence and beamformer gain. In *Acoustical Imaging*, Vol. 24, H. Lee (ed.). Kluwer Academic/Plenum Press, New York, pp. 43–48.

Bamber, J.C. and Nassiri, D.K. (1987). Spatial resolution and information content in echographic texture analysis. *IEEE 1986 Ultrasonics Symposium*, IEEE Cat. No. 86 CH 2375-4, pp. 937–940.

Bamber, J.C. and Phelps, J.V. (1977). The effective directivity characteristic of a pulsed ultrasound transducer and its measurement by semi-automatic means. *Ultrasonics* **15**, 169–174.

Bamber, J.C. and Phelps, J.V. (1991). A real-time implementation of coherent speckle suppression in B-scan images. *Ultrasonics* **29**, 218.

Bamber, J.C., Sakhri, Z. and Bell, D.S. (1994a). Assessment of ultrasound scanner performance using speckle. *Br. J. Radiol.* **67**, 710.

Bamber, J.C. and Tristam, M. (1988). Diagnostic ultrasound. In *The Physics of Medical Imaging*, S. Webb (ed.). IoP Publishing, Bristol, pp. 319–388.

Bamber, J.C., Wong, K.Y. and Crawford, D.C. (1994b). Visual detectability of simulated ultrasound lesions: methods and preliminary results. *Ultrasound Med. Biol.* **20**(Suppl.1), S87.

Barbone, P.E. and Bamber, J.C. (2002). Quantitative elasticity imaging: what can and cannot be inferred from strain images. *Phys. Med. Biol.* **47**, 2147–2164.

Bauer, A., Hauff, J. and Lazenby, J. (1997a). Wideband harmonic imaging with Levovist. *Eur. J. Ultrasound* **6**(Suppl. 2), 34.

Bauer, A., Schlief, R., Zomack, M., Urbank, A. and Niendorf, H-P. (1997b). Acoustically stimulated microbubbles in diagnostic ultrasound: properties and implications for diagnostic use. In *Advances in Echo Imaging using Contrast Enhancement* (2nd edn), N.C. Nanda *et al.* (eds). Kluwer Academic, Dordrecht, pp. 669–684.

Behar, V. (2002). Techniques for phase correction in coherent ultrasound imaging systems. *Ultrasonics* **39**, 603–610.

Belaid, N., Cespedes, I., Thijssen, J.M. and Ophir, J. (1994). Lesion detection in simulated elastographic and echographic images – a psychophysical study. *Ultrasound Med. Biol.* **20**, 877–891.

Bjorno, L. and Lewin, P.A. (1986). Measurement of non-linear acoustic parameters in tissue. In *Tissue Characterisation with Ultrasound*, Vol 1, J.F. Greenleaf (ed.). CRC Press, Boca Raton, pp. 141–163.

Blomley, M.J.K., Albrecht, T., Cosgrove, D.O., *et al.* (1997). Stimulated acoustic emission with the echo-enhancing agent Levovist: a reproducible effect with potential clinical utility. *Radiology* **205**, 278.

Bouakaz, A., Frigstad, S., Ten Cate, F.J. and de Jong, N. (2002). Improved contrast to tissue ratio at higher harmonies. *Ultrasonics* **40**, 575–578.

Burns, P.N., Poers, J.E. and Fritzsch, T. (1992). Harmonic imaging: a new imaging and Doppler method for contrast enhanced ultrasound. *Radiology* **185**, 142.

Bush, N.L., Bamber, J.C. and Symonds-Tayler, R. (2004). A clinical ultrasound scanner developed for imaging the relative surface attenuation, reflectivity and profile of skin lesions. In *Acoustical Imaging*, Vol. 27, Kluwer Academic/Plenum Press, New York (in press).

Carpenter, D.A., Kossoff, G. and Griffiths, K.A. (1995). Correction of distortion in US images caused by subcutaneous tissues – results in tissue phantoms and human-subjects. *Radiology* **195**, 563–567.

Carson, P.L., Oughton, T.V., Hendee, W.R. and Ahuja, A.S. (1977). Imaging of soft tissue through bone with ultrasound transmission by reconstruction. *Med. Phys.* **4**, 302–309.

Cespedes, I., Insana, M. and Ophir, J. (1995). Theoretical bounds on strain estimation in elastography. *IEEE Trans. Ultrason. Ferroelectr. Freq. Control* **42**, 969–972.

Chandrasekaran, K., Cha, A., Nimmagada, R.R., Greenleaf, J.F., Seward, J.B. and Tajik, A.J. (1986). Texture analysis of intracardiac masses. *Ultrason. Imag.* **8**, 38.

Chapman, C. and Lazenby J. (1997). Ultrasound imaging system employing phase inversion subtraction to enhance the image. *US Patent No. 5632277.*

Chaturvedi, P. and Insana, M.F. (1997). Bayesian and least squares approaches to ultrasonic scatterer size image formation. *IEEE Trans. Ultrason. Ferroelectr. Freq. Control* **44**, 152–160.

Chiang, E.H., Adler, R.S., Meyer, C.R., Rubin, J.M., Dedrick, D.K. and Laing, T.J. (1994). Quantitative assessment of surface roughness using backscattered ultrasound – the effects of finite surface curvature. *Ultrasound Med. Biol.* **20**, 123–135.

Chivers, R.C. and Hill, C.R. (1973). An approach to telehistology: ultrasonic scattering by tissues. *Br. J. Radiol.* **46**, 567.

Clarke, R.L., Bamber, J.C., Hill, C.R. and Wankling, P. (1983). Recent developments in axicon imaging. In *Acoustical Imaging*, Vol. 12, E. Ash and C.R. Hill (eds). Plenum Press, New York, pp. 339–350.

Cosgrove, D.O., Garbutt, P. and Hill, C.R. (1978). Echoes across the diaphragm. *Ultrasound Med. Biol.* **3**, 385–392.

Crawford, D.C., Cosgrove, D.O., Tohno, E., *et al.* (1992). The visual impact of adaptive speckle reduction on ultrasound B-mode images. *Radiology* **183**, 555–561.

Dawson, P., Cosgrove, D.O. and Grainger, R.G. (1999). *Textbook of Contrast Media.* Isis Medical Media, Oxford.

Desser, T.S., Jedrzejewicz, T. and Bradley, C. (2000). Native tissue harmonic imaging: basic principles and clinical applications. *Ultrasound Quart.* **16**, 40–48.

Dickinson, R.J. and Hill, C.R. (1982). Measurement of soft tissue motion using correlation between A-scans. *Ultrasound Med. Biol.* **8**, 263–271.

Dickson, M. (2003). Combining information from ultrasound and optical images to distinguish between benign and malignant skin lesions. PhD Thesis, University of London.

Donald, I. (1974). Sonar – the story of an experiment. *Ultrasound Med. Biol.* **1**, 109–117.

Dowsett, D.J., Kenney, P.A. and Johnston, R.E. (1998). Ultrasound principles, and ultrasound imaging. In *The Physics of Diagnostic Imaging*. Chapman & Hall, London, pp. 413–465.

Doyley, M.M., Meaney, P.M. and Bamber, J.C. (2000). Evaluation of an iterative reconstruction method for quantitative elastography. *Phys. Med. Biol.* **45**, 1521–1540.

Duck, F.A., Baker, A.C. and Starrit, H.C. (1998). *Ultrasound in Medicine*. IoP Publishing, Bristol.

Dunn, F., Tanaka, M., Ohtsuki, S. and Saijo, Y. (1996). *Ultrasonic Tissue Characterisation*. Springer, Tokyo.

Dussik, K.T., Dussik, F. and Wyt, L. (1947). Auf dem Wege zur Hyperphonographie des Gehirnes. *Wien Med. Ochenschr.* **97**, 425–429.

Edelstein, W.A., Bottomley, P.A., Hart, H.R. and Smith, L.S. (1983). Signal, noise and contrast in nuclear magnetic resonance (NMR) imaging. *J. Comput. Assist. Tomogr.* **7**, 391–401.

Erikson, K., Hairston, A., Nicoli, A., Stockwell, J. and White, T. (1997). A 128×128 (16k) ultrasonic transducer hybrid array. In *Acoustical Imaging*, Vol. 23, S. Lees and L. Ferrari (eds). Plenum Press, New York, pp. 485–494.

Espinola-Zavaleta, N., Vargas-Baron, J., Keirns, C., *et al.* (2002). Three-dimensional echocardiography in congenital malformations of the mitral valve. *J. Am. Soc. Echocardiogr.* **15**, 468–472.

Fatemi, M. and Greenleaf, J.F. (1996). Real-time assessment of the parameter of nonlinearity in tissue using 'nonlinear shadowing'. *Ultrasound Med. Biol.* **22**, 1215–1228.

Fink, M. and Dorme, C. (1997). Aberration correction in ultrasonic medical imaging with time-reversal techniques. *Int. J. Imag. Syst. Technol.* **8**, 110–125.

Fitzgerald, P.J., Magnuson, J.A. James, D.H. and Strahbehn, D.W. (1987). Ultrasonic texture analysis to discriminate between normal, ischemic and infarcted myocardium. *Ultrason. Imag.* **9**, 52.

Forsberg, F. (1991). Assessment of hybrid speckle reduction algorithms. *Phys. Med. Biol.* **36**, 1539–1549.

Foster, F.S. and Hunt, J.W. (1979). Transmission of ultrasound beams through human tissue – focusing and attenuation studies. *Ultrasound Med. Biol.* **3**, 257–268.

Foster, F.S., Patterson, M.S., Arditi, M. and Hunt, J.W. (1981). The conical scanner: a two-transducer ultrasound scatter imaging technique. *Ultrason. Imag.* **3**, 62–82.

Foster, F.S., Pavlin, C.J., Harasiewicz, K.A., Christopher, D.A. and Turnbull, D.H. (2000). Advances in ultrasound biomicroscopy. *Ultrasound Med. Biol.* **26**, 1–27.

Freiburger, P.D. and Trahey, G.E. (1997). Parallel processing techniques for the speckle brightness phase aberration correction algorithm. *IEEE Trans. Ultrason. Ferroelectr. Freq. Control* **44**, 431–444.

Frinking, P.J.A., Cespedes, E.I., Kirkhorn, J., Torp, H.G. and de Jong, N. (2001). A new ultrasound contrast imaging approach based on the combination of multiple imaging pulses and a separate release burst. *IEEE Trans. Ultrason. Ferroelectr. Freq. Control* **48**, 643–651.

Garra, B.S., Krasner, B.H., Horii, S.C., Ascher, S., Mun, S.K. and Zeman, R.K. (1993). Improving the distinction between benign and malignant breast-lesions – the value of sonographic texture analysis. *Ultrason. Imag.* **15**, 267–285.

Goldberg, B.B. (1993). Ultrasound contrast agents. In *Advances in Ultrasound Techniques and Instrumentation*, P.N.T. Wells (ed.). Churchill Livingstone, New York, pp. 35–45.

Goldberg, V., Manduca, A., Ewert, D.L., Gisvold, J.J. and Greenleaf, J.F. (1992). Improvement in specificity of ultrasonography for diagnosis of breast tumors by means of artificial intelligence. *Med. Phys.* **19**, 1475–1481.

Green, P.S. and Arditi, M. (1985). Ultrasonic reflex transmission imaging. *Ultrason. Imag.* **7**, 201–214.

Greenleaf, J.F. (1986). *Tissue Characterisation with Ultrasound*. CRC Press, Boca Raton.

Greenleaf, J.A. and Bahn, R.C. (1981). Clinical imaging with transmissive ultrasonic computerised tomography. *IEEE Trans. Biomed. Eng.* **BME-28**, 177–185.

Hall, T.J., Insana, M.F., Harrison, L.A. and Cox, G.G. (1996). Ultrasonic measurement of glomerular diameters in normal adult humans. *Ultrasound Med. Biol.* **22**, 987–997.

Harder, D. (1981). Performance parameters of photographic imaging. In *Medical Ultrasonic Images: Formation, Display, Recording and Perception*, C.R. Hill and A. Kratochwil (eds). Excerpta Medica, Amsterdam, pp. 86–92.

Hart, R., Angermann, C.H., Zwehl, W., Kemkes, B., Reichenspurner, H. and Gokel, M. (1986). 2D-Echocardiographic tissue characterisation of the myocardium by analysis of radiofrequency signals. *Ultrason. Imag.* **8**, 37–38.

Hill, C.R. (1974). Interactions of ultrasound with tissues. In *Ultrasonics in Medicine*, M. de Vlieger *et al.* (eds). Excerpta Medica, Amsterdam, pp. 14–20.

Hill, C.R. (1993). History – now and then. In *Abdominal and General Ultrasound*, Vol. 1, D. Cosgrove *et al.* (eds). Churchill Livingstone, Edinburgh, pp. 1–11.

Hill, C.R.; Bamber, J.C. and Cosgrove, D.O. (1990). Performance criteria for quantitative ultrasonology and image parameterisation. *Clin. Phys. Physiol. Meas.* **11**(Suppl. A), 57–73.

Hill, C.R. and Carpenter, D.A. (1976). Ultrasonic echo imaging of tissues: instrumentation. *Br. J. Radiol.* **49**, 238–243.

Hill, C.R., McCready, V.R. and Cosgrove, V.R. (1978). *Ultrasound in Tumour Diagnosis*. Pitman Medical, Tunbridge Wells.

Hokland, J.H. and Kelly, P.A. (1996). Markov models of specular and diffuse scattering in restoration of medical ultrasound images. *IEEE Trans. Ultrason. Ferr.* **43**, 660–669.

Hossack, J.A., Sumanaweera, T., Napel, S. and Ha, J. (2002). Quantitative 3D diagnostic ultrasound imaging using a modified transducer array for an automated image tracking technique. *IEEE Trans. Ultrason. Ferroelectr. Freq. Control* **49**, 1029–1038.

Hwang, J.J. and Simpson, D.H. (1998). Ultrasonic diagnostic imaging with harmonic contrast agents. *US Patent 3640271.*

ICRU (1999). *Tissue Substitutes, Phantoms and Computation Modelling in Medical Ultrasound*, Report No. 61. International Commission on Radiation Units and Measurements, Bethesda, MD.

Insana, M.F. and Hall, T.J. (1993). Quality management of ultrasound diagnosis. In *Advances in Ultrasound Techniques and Instrumentation*, P.N.T. Wells (ed.). Churchill Livingstone, New York, pp. 161–181.

Insana, M.F., Wagner, R.F., Garra, B.S., Brown, D.G. and Shawker, T.H. (1986). Analysis of ultrasound image texture via generalized rician statistics. *Opt. Eng.* **25**, 743–748.

Kamiyama, N., Moriyasu, F., Mine, Y. and Goto, Y. (1998). Analysis of flash-echo from contrast agent for designing optimal ultrasound diagnostic systems. *Ultrasound Med. Biol.* **25**, 411–420.

Kaplan, D. and Ma, Q.L. (1994). On the statistical characteristics of log-compressed rayleigh signals – theoretical formulation and experimental results. *J. Acoust. Soc. Am.* **95**, 1396–1400.

Karaman, M., Koymen, H., Atalar, A. and O'Donnell, M. (1993). A phase aberration correction method for ultrasound imaging. *IEEE Trans. Ultrason. Ferroelectr. Freq. Control* **40**, 275–282.

Kedar, R.P., Cosgrove, D.O., McCready, V.R., Bamber, J.C. and Carter, E.R. (1996). Microbubble contrast agent for color Doppler US: effect on breast masses. *Radiology* **198**, 679–686.

Kripfgans, O.D., Fowlkes, J.B., Woydt, M., Eldevik, O.P. and Carson, P.L. (2002). *In vivo* droplet vaporization for occlusion therapy and phase aberration correction. *IEEE Trans. Ultrason. Ferroelectr. Freq. Control* **49**, 726–738.

Kuc, R. (1986). Employing spectral emission procedures for characterising diffuse liver disease. In *Tissue Characterisation with Ultrasound*, J.F. Greenleaf (ed.). CRC Press, Boca Raton.

Lacefield, J.C. and Waag, R.C. (2002). Spatial coherence analysis applied to aberration correction using a two-dimensional array system. *J. Acoust. Soc. Am.* **112**, 2558–2566.

Law, W.K., Frizzel, L.A. and Dunn, F. (1985). Determination of the non-linearity parameter, B/A, of biological media. *Ultrasound Med. Biol.* **11**, 307–318.

Leeman, S. and Seggie, D.A. (1987). Speckle reduction via phase. In *Pattern Recognition and Acoustical Imaging*, L. Ferrari (ed.). SPIE Publ. 768. Society of Photo-Optical Instrumentation Engineers, Bellingham, p. 173.

Li, P.C. and Li, M.L. (2003). Adaptive imaging using the generalized coherence factor. *IEEE Trans. Ultrason. Ferroelectr. Freq. Control* **50**, 128–141.

Lizzi, F.L., Feleppa, E.J. and Coleman D.J. (1986). Ultrasonic ocular tissue characterisation. In *Tissue Characterisation with Ultrasound*, Vol. 2, J.F. Greenleaf (ed.). CRC Press, Boca Raton, pp. 41–60.

Lizzi, F.L., Feleppa, E., Yaremko, M., Rorke, M., Hui, J. and King, D. (1987). Applications of acoustic parameter images of liver. *Ultrason. Imag.* **9**, 61–62.

Lizzi, F.L., Greenbaum, M., Feleppa, E.J., Elbaum, M. and Coleman, D.J. (1983). Theoretical framework for spectrum analysis in ultrasonic tissue characterisation. *J. Acoust. Soc. Am.* **73**, 1366–1373.

Lopez, H., Loew, M.H., Butler, P.F. and Hill, M.H. (1987). A clinical evaluation of contrast-detail analysis of ultrasound images. *Ultrason. Imag.* **9**, 49–50.

Loupas, T., Allen, P.L. and McDicken, W.N. (1989). Clinical evaluation of a digital signal-processing device for real-time speckle suppression in medical ultrasonics. *Br. J. Radiol.* **62**, 761.

Lowe, H., Bamber, J.C., Webb, S. and Cook-Martin, G. (1988). Perceptual studies of contrast, texture and detail in ultrasound B-scans. In *Medical Imaging II*, R.H. Schneider *et al.* (eds). SPIE Publ. 914. Society of Photo-Optical Instrumentation Engineers, Bellingham, pp. 40–47.

Malcolm, A.L. (1997). An investigation into ultrasonic methods of imaging the tissue ablation induced during focused ultrasound surgery. PhD thesis, University of London.

Massay, R.J., Logan-Sinclair, R.B., Bamber, J.C. and Gibson, D.G. (1989). Quantitative effects of speckle reduction on cross sectional echocardiographic images. *Br. Heart J.* **62**, 298–304.

Mercer, J. (1998). Ultrasound scatterer size imaging of skin tumours – potential and limitations. PhD thesis, University of London.

Mercer, J.L., Bamber, J.C., Bell, D.S., Bush, N.L. and Mortimer, P.S. (1997). Ultrasound scatterer size imaging of skin tumours. *Skin Res. Tech.* **3**, 201.

Milan, J. and Taylor, K.J.W. (1975). The application of the temperature-colour scale to ultrasonic imaging. *J. Clin. Ultrasound* **3**, 171–173.

Miller, N.R. and Bamber, J.C. (2000). Thresholds for visual detection of Young's modulus contrast in simulated ultrasound image movies. *Phys. Med. Biol.* **45**, 2057–2079.

Miller, N.R., Bamber, J.C. and Meaney, P.M. (2002a). Fundamental limitations of noninvasive temperature imaging by means of ultrasound echo strain estimation. *Ultrasound Med. Biol.* **28**, 1319–1333.

Miller, N.R., Bamber, J.C. and ter Haar, G.R. (2003). Noninvasive temperature imaging by means of ultrasound echo strain estimation: preliminary in vitro results. *Ultrasound Med. Biol.* (in press).

Momenan, R., Wagner, R.F., Garra, B.S., Loew, M.H. and Insana, M.F. (1994). Image staining and differential-diagnosis of ultrasound scans based on the Mahalanobis distance. *IEEE Trans. Med. Imag.* **13**, 37–47.

Moran, C.M. (1991). Theoretical basis for optimum frequency in backscatter imaging. In *The Physical Basis for Ultrasonic Investigation of Human Skin*. PhD thesis, University of London, Chapt. 5.

Nair, A., Kuban, B.D., Tuzcu, E.M., Schoenhagen, P., Nissen, S.E. and Vince, D.G. (2002). Coronary plaque classification with intravascular ultrasound radiofrequency data analysis. *Circulation* **106**, 2200–2206.

Nanda, N.C., Schlief, R. and Goldberg, B.B. (1997). *Advances in Echo Imaging Using Contrast Enhancement* (2nd edn). Kluwer Academic, Dordrecht.

Neary, R.J. (1981). Photographic imaging from CRT monitors. In *Medical Ultrasonic Images: Formation, Display, Recording and Perception*, C.R. Hill and A. Kratochwil (eds). Excerpta Medica, Amsterdam, pp. 77–85.

Ng, G.C., Freiburger, P.D., Walker, W.F. and Trahey, G.E. (1997). A speckle target adaptive imaging technique in the presence of distributed aberrations. *IEEE Trans. Ultrason. Ferroelectr. Freq. Control* **44**, 140–151.

Nicholas, D., Nassiri, D.K., Garbutt, P. and Hill, C.R. (1986). Tissue characterisation from ultrasound B-scan data. *Ultrasound Med. Biol.* **12**, 135–143.

Noritomi, T., Sigel, B., Swami, V., Justin, J., Gahtan, V., Chen, X.L., Feleppa, E.J., Roberts, A.B. and Shirouzu, K. (1997). Carotid plaque typing by multiple-parameter ultrasonic tissue characterization. *Ultrasound Med. Biol.* **23**, 643–650.

Oosterveld, B.J., Thijssen, J.M., Hartman, P.C., Romijn, R.L. and Rosenbusch, G.J.E. (1991). Ultrasound attenuation and texture analysis of diffuse liver disease: methods and preliminary results. *Phys. Med. Biol.* **36**, 1039–1064.

Ophir, J., Cespedes, I., Maklad, N. and Ponnekanti, H. (1996). Elastography: a method for imaging the elastic properties of tissue *in vivo*. In *Ultrasonic Tissue Characterisation*, F. Dunn *et al.* (eds). Springer, Tokyo, pp. 95–123.

Passmann, C. and Ermert, H. (1996). A 100-MHz ultrasound imaging system for dermatologic and ophthalmologic diagnostics. *IEEE Trans. Ultrason. Ferr.* **43**, 545–552.

Pizer, S.M. and Zimmerman, J.B. (1983). Colour display in ultrasoniography. *Ultrasound Med. Biol.* **9**, 331.

Prager, W.R., Gee, A.H., Treece, G.M., Cash, C.J.C. and Berman, L.H. (2003). Sensorless freehand 3-D ultrasound using regression of the echo intensity. *Ultrasound Med. Biol.* **29**, 437–446.

Räth, U., Zuna, I., Schlaps, D., Lorenz, A.L., *et al.* (1985). Image texture of normal and pathological ultrasonic liver B-scan: role of histomorphological tissue structure. *Ultrason. Imag.* **7**, 81.

Recchia, D. and Wickline, S.A. (1993). Ultrasonic tissue characterization of thrombosis with a clinical vascular integrated backscatter imaging system. *Clin. Res.* **41**, A287.

Rizzatto, G. (1999). Evolution of ultrasound transducers: 1.5 and 2D arrays. *Eur. Radiol.* Suppl. 9, S304–S306.

Robinson, D.F., Chen, C.F. and Doust, B. (1984). Sound speed determination by pulse-echo methods: accuracy assessment and clinical results. *Ultrason. Imag.* **6**, 226–227.

Sandrin, L., Catheline, S., Tanter, M., Hennequin, X. and Fink, M. (1999). Time-resolved pulsed elastography with ultrafast ultrasonic imaging. *Ultrason. Imag.* **21**, 259–272.

Sboros, V., Ramnarine, K.V., Moran, C.M., Pye, S.D. and McDicken, W.N. (2002). Understanding the limitations of ultrasonic backscatter measurements from microbubble populations. *Phys. Med. Biol.* **47**, 4287–4299.

Schlaps, D., Rath, U., Zuna, I., Volk, J.F., *et al.* (1985). On-line ultrasonic tissue characterisation using B-mode and RF data analysis. *Ultrason. Imag.* **7**, 80–81.

Sehgal, C.M., Brown, G.M., Bahn, R.C. and Greenleaf, J.F. (1986). Measurement and use of acoustic nonlinearity and sound speed to estimate composition of excised livers. *Ultrasound Med. Biol.* **12**, 865–874.

Sehgal, C.M. and Greenleaf, J.F. (1986). Correlative studies of properties of water in biological systems using ultrasound and magnetic resonance. *Magn. Reson. Med.* **3**, 978–985.

Seip, R., VanBaren, P., Cain, C. and Ebbini, E.S. (1996). Noninvasive real-time multipoint temperature control for ultrasound phased array treatments. *IEEE Trans. Ultrason. Ferroelectr. Freq. Control* **43**, 1063–1073.

Shattuck, D.P., Weinshenker, M.D., Smith, S.W. and von Ramm, O.T. (1984). Explososcan – a parallel processing technique for high-speed ultrasound imaging with linear phased-arrays. *J. Acoust. Soc. Am.* **75**, 1273–1282.

Shi, W.T., Forsberg, F., Hall, A.L., Chiao, R.Y., Liu, J-B., Miller, S., Thomenius, K.E., Wheatley, M.A. and Goldberg, B.B. (1999). Subharmonic imaging with microbubble contrast agents: initial results. *Ultrason. Imag.* **21**, 79–94.

Shiina, T., Nitta, N., Ueno, E. and Bamber, J.C. (2002). Real time tissue elasticity imaging using combined autocorrelation method. *J. Med. Ultrason.* **29**, 119–128.

Sigel, B., Feleppa, E.J., Swami, V., Justin, J., *et al.* (1990). Ultrasonic tissue characterization of blood clots. *Surg. Clin. N. Am.*, **70**, 13–29.

Silverman, R.H., Rondeau, M.J., Lizzi, F.L. and Coleman, D.J (1995). Three dimensional, high frequency parameter imaging of anterior segment pathology. *Ophthalmology* **102**, 837–843.

Smith, S.W., Trahey, G.E., Hubbard, S.M and Wagner, R.F. (1988). Properties of acoustical speckle in the presence of phase aberration. 2. Correlation lengths. *Ultrason. Imag.* **10**, 29–51.

Smith, S.W., Wagner, R.F. Sandrik, J.M. and Lopez, H. (1983). Low-contrast detectability and contrast/detail analysis in medical ultrasound. *IEEE Trans.* **SU-30**, 164.

Szabo, T.L. and Burns, D.R. (1997). Seismic signal processing of ultrasound signal data. In *Acoustical Imaging*, Vol. 23, S. Lees and L.A. Ferrari (eds). Plenum Press, New York, pp. 131–136.

Tabei, M., Mast, T. D. and Waag, R.C. (2003). Simulation of ultrasonic focus aberration and correction through human tissue. *J. Acoust. Soc. Am.* **113**, 1166–1176.

Takuma, S., Cardinale, C. and Homma, S. (2000). Real-time three-dimensional stress echocardiography: a review of current applications. *Echocardiography* **17**, 791–794.

Thomsen, H.S., Muller, R.N. and Mattrey, R.F. (1999). *Trends in Contrast Media.* Springer Verlag, Berlin.

Tranquart, F., Grenier, N., Eder, V. and Pourcelot, L. (1999). Clinical use of ultrasound tissue harmonic imaging. *Ultrasound Med. Biol.* **25**, 889–894.

Tristam, M., Barbosa, D.C., Cosgrove, D.O., Bamber, J.C. and Hill, C.R. (1988). Application of Fourier analysis to clinical study of patterns of tissue movement. *Ultrasound Med. Biol.* **14**, 695–707.

Tuthill, T., Krucker, J., Fowlkes, J. and Carson, P. (1998). Automated 3-D US frame positioning computed from elevational speckle decorrelation. *Radiology* **209**, 575–582.

Unger, E.C. (1999). Targeting and delivery of drugs with ultrasound contrast agents. In *Trends in Contrast Media,* H.S. Thomsen *et al.* (eds). Springer Verlag, Berlin, pp. 406–412.

Valckx, F.M.J. and Thijssen, J.M. (1997). Characterization of echographic image texture by co-ocurrence matrix parameters. *Ultrasound Med. Biol.* **23**, 559–571.

Varghese, T., Ophir, J., Konofagou, E., Kallel, F. and Righetti, R. (2002). Tradeoffs in elastographic imaging. *Ultrason. Imag.* **23**, 216–248.

Wagner, R.F., Insana, M.F. and Brown, D.G. (1986). Unified approach to the detection and classification of speckle texture in diagnostic ultrasound. *Opt. Eng.* **25**, 738–742.

Wagner, R.F., Insana, M.F., Brown, D.G. and Smith, S.W. (1987). Fundamental statistical physics of medical ultrasonic images. *Ultrason. Imag.* **9**, 49.

Walker, W.F. and Trahey, G.E. (1994). A fundamental limit on delay estimation using partially correlated speckle signals. *IEEE Trans. Ultrason. Ferroelectr. Freq. Control* **42**, 301–308.

Walker, W.F. and Trahey, G.E. (1995). A fundamental limit on the performance of correlation-based phase correction and flow estimation techniques. *IEEE Trans. Ultrason. Ferroelectr. Freq. Control* **41**, 644–654.

Wells, P.N.T. (1993). *Advances in Ultrasound Techniques and Instrumentation.* Churchill Livingstone, New York.

Whittingham, T.A. (1999). Tissue harmonic imaging. *Eur. Radiol.* **9**(Suppl. 3), S323–S326.

WHO (1990). *Effective Choices for Diagnostic Imaging in Clinical Practice*, Technical Report Series No. 795. World Health Organization, Geneva.

Wild, J.J. (1978). The use of pulse-echo ultrasound for early tumour detection: history and prospects. In *Ultrasound in Tumour Diagnosis,* C. R. Hill *et al.* (eds). Pitman Medical, Tunbridge Wells, pp. 1–16.

Yaremko, M., Lizzi, F.L., Feleppa, E.J., Coleman, D.J. and King, D.L. (1987). Two dimensional power spectrum analysis for ultrasonic tissue characterisation. *IEEE Trans. Ultrason. Ferroelectr. Freq. Control* **UFFC-34**, 405.

Zagzebski, J.A. (1996). *The Essentials of Ultrasound Physics.* Mosby-Year Book, St Louis.

Zheng, Y., Greenleaf, J.F. and Gisvold, J.J. (1997). Reduction of breast biopsies with a modified self-organizing map. *IEEE Trans. Neural Networks* **8**, 1386–1396.

10

Methodology for Imaging Time-Dependent Phenomena

R. J. ECKERSLEY[1] and J. C. BAMBER[2]

[1]Imperial College School of Medicine, London, UK and [2]Institute of Cancer Research, Royal Marsden Hospital, UK

10.1 INTRODUCTION

This chapter continues to explore the theme of methodology for clinical investigation, as introduced in Chapter 9, by extending the subject to a more detailed consideration of the fourth dimension of time. As such, it follows directly from the penultimate section of Chapter 9 (Section 9.4.5). By using signal processing to extract characteristics of the temporal dependence of one-, two- or three-dimensional ultrasonic echo signals it is possible to measure, and image, fluid flow and tissue movement. The latter may be extended to determine the, potentially very informative, elastic characteristics of solid tissues (Chapter 7), as well as other properties that generate apparent echo distortion, such as change in temperature (again, see Chapter 9). Temporal processing can also be utilised to locate and study contrast media that exhibit time-dependent echo properties, for example due to instability of ultrasonic echoes from microbubbles.

One of the most significant developments in the field of medical ultrasound has been the combination of real-time two-dimensional ultrasound B-mode images with real-time two-dimensional displays of motion information. Flow imaging was first demonstrated by Reid and Spencer (1972). The first commercial combined B-mode real-time colour flow system was launched by the Aloka Co. Ltd (Japan) in 1982, based on signal processing developed by Kasai *et al.* (1985). Over the 20 years since this first system, colour flow imaging has found widespread use in clinical diagnosis and is now provided as a standard feature on nearly all commercial ultrasound systems. Typically these implementations are based on the Doppler processing described by Kasai *et al.* (1985), although fast cross-correlation-based tracking algorithms also have been introduced (e.g. Bonnefous & Pesque 1986; Trahey *et al.* 1987). Colour flow imaging systems initially found their application in cardiology (Switzer & Nanda 1985), although their utility in the study of both superficial and deep blood vessels has also been demonstrated and they are now firmly established in a wide range of applications (Taylor *et al.* 1988; Evans & McDicken 2000).

As explained in Chapter 9, this is not intended to be a 'user handbook' and the reader is once again referred to other texts that deal with aspects of the subject, particularly Doppler

Physical Principles of Medical Ultrasonics, Second Edition. Edited by C. R. Hill, J. C. Bamber and G. R. ter Haar.
© 2004 John Wiley & Sons, Ltd: ISBN 0 471 97002 6

methods, at the practical level (e.g. Bamber & Tristam 1988; Wells 1993; Zagzebski 1996; Dowsett *et al.* 1998; Duck *et al.* 1998; Anglesen 2000; Evans & McDicken 2000). In this chapter the principles of ultrasound-based motion detection and estimation are introduced and the signal processing methods explained. To avoid unnecessary replication of standard texts on Doppler methods, where we cover Doppler techniques the main emphasis will be on colour flow imaging, which in the didactic literature has received less attention than it deserves. A thorough awareness of basic Doppler methods is, however, necessary to understand colour flow imaging. Much of the material in this chapter was drawn from Kasai *et al.* (1985), Wells (1994) and Ferrara and DeAngelis (1997).

In reviewing the various methods for velocity estimation, an attempt has been made to bring together the apparently disparate approaches using a more unified treatment of the underlying principles than one tends to find in the literature.

10.2   THE PRINCIPLES OF ULTRASOUND MOTION DETECTION

10.2.1 *SIMPLE CONTINUOUS WAVE MOTION DETECTION*

In the simple case of a single reflector sited in a continuous sinusoidal ultrasound field (Figure 10.1) the measured echo signal will have both an amplitude related to the strength of the reflection and an associated phase-offset given by the frequency and time of flight of the sound wave. If the reflector is stationary, both the amplitude and phase of the returning signal will remain constant relative to the transmitted signal. As soon as the target moves, depending on the direction of the motion relative to the ultrasound beam, the characteristics of the returned signal will change. The general wisdom is that if a component of the motion is axial, directed along the sound beam, the phase of the detected signal will vary. Over time this change of phase is perceived by the detector as a shift in frequency (or Doppler shift) of the returned signal relative to the original. If a component of the motion is lateral, or perpendicular to the beam axis, there will be a change in the amplitude of the echo signal as the target passes through the ultrasound beam. Note, however, that a phase change may also occur as a target moves laterally across a sound beam even when there is no axial component to the motion.

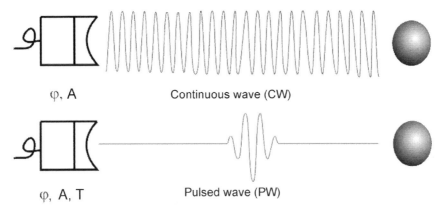

φ, A   Continuous wave (CW)

φ, A, T   Pulsed wave (PW)

Figure 10.1. Continuous wave (CW) and pulsed wave (PW) ultrasound fields; a target moving through the beams can cause variation in both amplitude (A) and phase (φ) of the reflected signal. In the PW case the time of flight (T) of the echo signal is also affected

This is due to the fact that the phase of the sound field from any diffracting aperture, even at a fixed axial distance, may vary with lateral position. Only when the target trajectory exactly follows the shape of the wavefront would no phase change be expected. Such a trajectory may actually require a small amount of axial motion.

10.2.2 SIMPLE PULSED-WAVE MOTION DETECTION

Pulsed wave (PW) operation of ultrasound equipment adds depth range capabilities as described in Chapter 9. If the transducer is excited in short repetitive bursts it is possible to measure the time of flight of the returned echoes and, using knowledge of the speed of sound in the intervening media, the depth of the reflecting target can be obtained. Again each echo will have an associated amplitude and phase, as in the continuous wave (CW) case, and in the situation where the target moves, these characteristics will change. In addition, the time of flight of the echoes will be affected if the target moves with a component of its motion along the beam axis.

10.3 TECHNIQUES FOR MEASURING TARGET VELOCITY

The simple description above suggests a number of possibilities for detecting the motion of scatterers moving within an ultrasound field using changes in phase, amplitude or the time of flight of the reflected signals (note that it also suggests an interaction between the effects of these three variables that could lead to measurement uncertainties not unlike those discussed in Chapter 9). There are two discrete approaches that can be used to extract the motion information using these parameters. Firstly, the motion may be obtained by measuring changes in the phase or amplitude of the echoes at a fixed position within the reflected sound signal. Techniques that work along these lines will be termed *fluctuation techniques* in the subsequent discussion. The commercially prevalent Doppler processing techniques fall into this category. Secondly, using the time shift associated with the changing time of flight from one pulse–echo to the next, both phase information and amplitude information can be tracked and the target motion again extracted. These techniques will be termed *tracking techniques*.

Depending on whether phase information or envelope detected (amplitude) information is used in the measurement process, these two categories can each be subdivided into phase and envelope techniques, as shown in Figure 10.2. All four methods, and in fact combinations of methods, have at some point been employed for both blood flow and tissue displacement (and hence strain) measurement, although blood flow velocimetry has most commonly been accomplished with the phase fluctuation (Doppler) technique. In the following sections the theory, limitations and signal processing associated with each technique are presented. In doing so the effects of diffraction on either phase or time shift will be ignored, i.e. the conventional simplistic viewpoint will be taken that axial motion corresponds to the direction of wave propagation and lateral motion corresponds to a direction along the wavefront.

10.4 PHASE FLUCTUATION (DOPPLER) METHODS

10.4.1 POINT SCATTERERS (HYPOTHETICAL)

Phase fluctuation velocimetry, usually labelled Doppler shift detection, measures the rate of change of phase in the signal reflected from a moving target relative to the transmitted signal

Velocity / Displacement Estimation Techniques

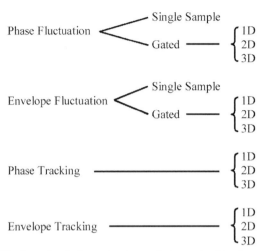

Figure 10.2. Classification of velocity estimation techniques. In this chapter only the simplest one-dimensional implementations are considered

(Figure 10.3). In the simple CW case described above, the velocity of the wave relative to the moving target is given by

$$c' = c + V \tag{10.1}$$

where c is the speed of the sound in the transmitting medium and V is the axially directed component of the velocity of the target. The frequency of the sound perceived by the target, f', is then given by

$$f' = \frac{c'}{\lambda} = \frac{1}{\lambda}(c + V) \tag{10.2}$$

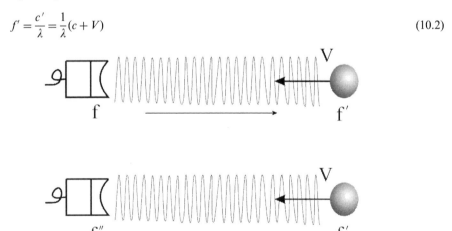

Figure 10.3. The frequency shift arising from reflection of a wave from a moving target is in fact a double shift. Firstly, a signal emitted from a stationary source impinges on a moving observer (the reflector) and, secondly, the reflector acts as a moving source and the echo signal is detected at the stationary transducer

$$f' = f + \frac{V}{\lambda} \tag{10.3}$$

$$f' = f\left(1 + \frac{V}{c}\right) \tag{10.4}$$

The wave is then re-emitted by the target (now a moving source) with frequency f' and is incident on the stationary transducer. The wavelength of the emitted signal is given by

$$\lambda'' = \lambda' - \delta\lambda \tag{10.5}$$

where

$$\delta\lambda = \frac{V}{f'} \text{ and } \lambda' = \frac{c}{f'} \tag{10.6}$$

therefore

$$\lambda' - \delta\lambda = \frac{c}{f'} - \frac{V}{f'} = \frac{1}{f'}(c - V)$$

$$\rightarrow \frac{c}{f''} = \frac{1}{f'}(c - V) \tag{10.7}$$

which gives

$$f'' = \frac{f'c}{c - V} \tag{10.8}$$

$$f'' = \frac{f'}{\left(1 - \frac{V}{c}\right)} \tag{10.9}$$

Using the expansion

$$\frac{1}{(1 - x)} = 1 + x + \frac{x^2}{2} \cdots \tag{10.10}$$

with $x = V/c$, and ignoring all terms higher than the first order since $V \ll c$, then

$$f'' = f' + f'\frac{V}{c} \tag{10.11}$$

Substituting the result for f' obtained in equation (10.4) gives

$$f'' = f\left(1 + \frac{V}{c}\right) + f\frac{V}{c}\left(1 + \frac{V}{c}\right) \tag{10.12}$$

Again discarding the second-order term gives

$$f'' = f + 2f\frac{V}{c} \tag{10.13}$$

The frequency shift between transmitted and received signals is therefore

$$\delta f = f'' - f = 2f\frac{V}{c} \tag{10.14}$$

The above derivation deals with the case of CW ultrasound. If a PW technique (Figure 10.4) is employed to provide good depth resolution, the pulse is typically too short (2–3 cycles) to measure accurately the induced Doppler shift. The intervening time between pulses is relatively large, however, and in this situation the rate of change in the phase of the reflected signal is measured by comparing the phase of the reflections of successive pulses. If one pulse in a sequence of pulses is reflected from a target at depth z_a, then the phase φ_a of the reflection is

$$\varphi_a = f \frac{2z_a}{c} \tag{10.15}$$

Similarly, if the target is moving in an axial direction, then the subsequent consecutive pulse will be reflected from point z_b with phase

$$\varphi_b = f \frac{2z_b}{c} \tag{10.16}$$

The rate of change of this phase is given by

$$\frac{\delta \varphi}{\delta t} = \frac{2f(z_b - z_a)}{c} \frac{1}{T} \tag{10.17}$$

where T is the time between consecutive pulses. Thus the frequency change induced is given by

$$\delta f = \frac{2fV}{c} \tag{10.18}$$

where V is the velocity of the reflector, given by $(z_b - z_a)/T$. As defined above, V is the axially directed component of the target velocity. Any non-axial target motion will cause a breakdown, or decorrelation, of the backscattered signal over time. This will result in an increase in the noise component of velocity or displacement estimates generated using phase fluctuation processing.

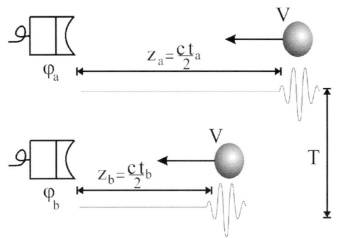

Figure 10.4. In the PW case the phase of the echo φ is related to the time of flight t of the signal. The rate of change of this phase with respect to time is the Doppler shift signal

10.4.2 DISTRIBUTED SCATTERERS (MORE REALISTIC)

The above description deals with the simplified situation of a single scatterer. In real situations the signals will be scattered from multiple targets, with a variety of velocities. In these circumstances it is no longer practical to think of the returning signal as simply shifted by a single Doppler frequency. Instead, the returned signal will contain a spectrum of frequencies. This range of frequencies, or spectral broadening, is induced by a number of processes (Figure 10.5). These include the amplitude modulation of the returned signal as the target moves through the volume of interest, defined by the length of the pulse and the width of the sound beam, and the effect of multiple scatterers moving with different speeds and directions. In the PW case even the original signal is inherently broadband. These factors contribute to create a complex, time-varying, frequency-shifted signal. In addition, scattering from an ensemble of randomly positioned scatterers will generate an interference pattern resulting in spatial (and hence temporal) fluctuations in the amplitude and phase of the signal measured by the transducer (see Chapter 9, Section 9.2.3.2). Finally, if the scatterers in this ensemble do not move as a whole but change their positions relative to each other as they move (e.g. by a shear strain or by a random component of motion), then echo decorrelation and loss of velocity or displacement signal-to-noise ratio occur in addition to that mentioned in the previous paragraph as being due to off-axis (lateral) motion.

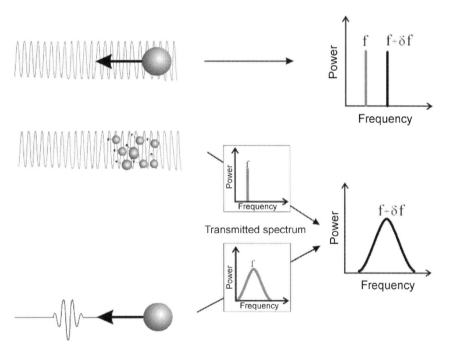

Figure 10.5. A single scatterer in a CW field will produce a single uniform Doppler shift in the reflected signal (top). Typical real systems involve non-uniform scatterer motion, multiple scatterers and pulsed wave signals, all of which contribute to the broad range of frequencies usually present in a typical Doppler signal

10.4.3 SIGNAL PROCESSING FOR PHASE FLUCTUATION (DOPPLER) METHODS

The processing of such signals for the extraction of velocity of motion via the phase fluctuation (Doppler shift) information is essentially a two-stage process: demodulating the returned signal to extract a Doppler shift signal and estimation of the frequency and spectral properties of this signal. The following sections deal with these stages in detail.

10.4.3.1 Doppler Demodulation

The simplest technique for the extraction of frequency-shifted Doppler signals from the returned wave is coherent demodulation as used in CW flow-meters (e.g. Baker 1970; Atkinson & Woodcock 1982). Coherent demodulation involves mixing the returned r.f. signal with one having the original oscillator frequency (Figure 10.6).

If

$$S_t(t) = A_t \cos(\omega t) \tag{10.19}$$

is the transmitted signal, where ω $(= 2\pi f)$ is the angular frequency and A_t is the signal amplitude, then the reflected signal is given by

$$S_r(t) = A_r \cos(\omega t + \delta\omega t + \varphi) \tag{10.20}$$

where A_r is the reflected signal amplitude, $\delta\omega$ is the Doppler shift frequency and φ is the phase difference. Multiplying the two signals together gives

$$S_d(t) = \frac{A_t A_r}{2}[\cos(2\omega t + \delta\omega t + \varphi) + \cos(\delta\omega t + \varphi)] \tag{10.21}$$

Low-pass filtering to remove the higher (2ω) frequency components gives

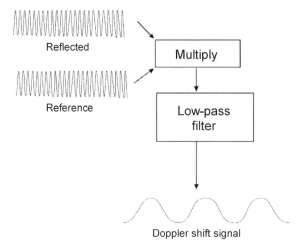

Doppler shift signal

Figure 10.6. Simple coherent demodulation. The reflected signal is multiplied by a reference signal with the frequency of the originally transmitted signal, to produce a signal beating at the Doppler frequency. Low-pass filtering then yields the pure Doppler signal

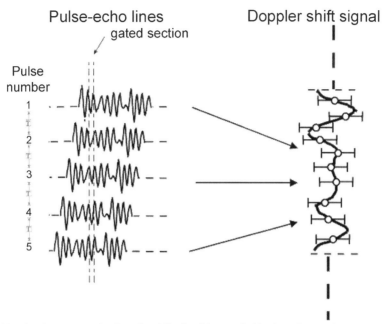

Figure 10.7. In PW systems the Doppler shift signal is sampled in time. Each pulse generates a single sample of the Doppler shift signal. To avoid misrepresentation or aliasing of the signal the pulses must be sufficiently frequent

$$S_{d\_filtered}(t) = \frac{A_t A_r}{2}\cos(\delta\omega t + \varphi) \qquad (10.22)$$

The resulting signal contains the motion-induced Doppler shift frequency. Although this analysis is based on CW signals, similar logic can be applied for the PW case where, instead of a continuous oscillation, the transmitted signal consists of short bursts separated by time T (Figure 10.7). In this case the reference oscillator for mixing during demodulation may be derived from the previous pulse, as opposed to the system oscillator; this may aid in reducing effects due to frequency-dependent attenuation and scattering (Holland *et al.* 1984).

10.4.3.1.1 Phase Quadrature Detection

Although the above demodulation process will successfully isolate the frequency-shifted components of the returned signal, in order to preserve information concerning the direction of the scatterers (whether towards or away from the transducer) a form of complex demodulation is required. A number of techniques have been devised (Coghlan & Taylor 1976), and the most general example is that of phase quadrature demodulation (Atkinson & Woodcock 1982). This technique, an extension of the simple demodulation described above, processes the received signal via two channels: one mixing the r.f. signal with the standard reference as described above and the other mixing a $\pi/2$ phase-shifted reference with the r.f. signal (Figure 10.8). After low-pass filtering the two outputs have the standard Doppler shift frequency, but the phase relationship between the two channels now contains information relating to the direction of the original target motion.

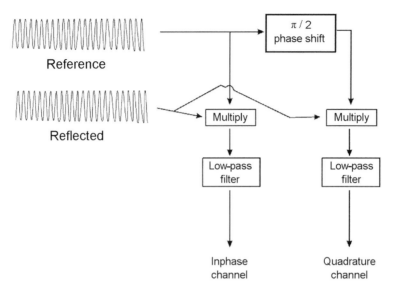

Figure 10.8. Principle of phase quadrature demodulation. This system generates a complex signal from which directional information concerning the target motion may be obtained. Each channel is a simple coherent demodulator, with the only difference lying in the $\pi/2$ phase shift of the quadrature channel reference

If the reflected r.f. signal is given by

$$S_r(t) = A_F \cos(\omega t + \delta\omega_F t + \varphi_F) + A_R \cos(\omega t + \delta\omega_R t + \varphi_R) \qquad (10.23)$$

where $\delta\omega_F$ and $\delta\omega_R$ are the respective forward and reverse Doppler shift frequency components, then demodulation with $\cos(\omega t)$ and $\sin(\omega t)$ in two channels gives

$$S_i(t) = \frac{1}{2}[A_F \cos(\omega_F t + \varphi_F) + A_R \cos(\omega_R t - \varphi_R)] \qquad (10.24)$$

and

$$S_q(t) = \frac{1}{2}[A_F \sin(\omega_F t + \varphi_F) - A_R \sin(\omega_R t - \varphi_R)] \qquad (10.25)$$

Rearranging equation (10.25) gives

$$S_q(t) = \frac{1}{2}\left[A_F \cos\left(\omega_F t + \varphi_F - \frac{\pi}{2}\right) - A_R \cos\left(\omega_R t - \varphi_R + \frac{\pi}{2}\right)\right] \qquad (10.26)$$

where $S_i(t)$ and $S_q(t)$ are the in-phase and quadrature channels of the demodulator. Once the in-phase and quadrature signals have been extracted, they can be processed in a number of ways (described below) to determine velocity components in both forward and reverse directions along the ultrasound axis. The associated processing represents the second stage of the velocity estimation procedure.

As in the simple demodulation case, in PW systems the reference signal can be derived from previously received pulse echoes, although in this case a quadrature $\pi/2$ reference must be produced. If the ratio of the sampling rate to the carrier frequency is known, a quadrature reference may be generated by delaying one channel by an appropriate number of samples relative to the other. However, as discussed in Section 10.4.2, the signals involved are typically broadband in nature and the selective phase shifting of the signal with respect to the carrier frequency alone will increase the signal decorrelation from one pulse to the next. An alternative approach for obtaining a quadrature signal is to employ a Hilbert transform (Bracewell 1986). The Hilbert transform

$$F_{HI} = \frac{1}{\pi} \int_{-\infty}^{+\infty} \frac{S(t)\mathrm{d}t}{t - t'} \tag{10.27}$$

induces a $\pi/2$ phase change on all the frequency components in the signal $S(t)$ without affecting the signal amplitude.

10.4.3.2 Doppler Frequency-shift Estimation Strategies

The following section describes the final stage of the Doppler, or phase fluctuation, processing system. There are several methods for estimating the frequency shift associated with demodulated Doppler shifted echoes from moving targets; again these can be broken down into two categories. *Spectral estimators* provide information on all frequencies contained within the input signal. The mean or maximum frequency and the associated variance then can be calculated from the spectrum. *Instantaneous frequency estimators* provide an immediate estimate of both the mean frequency and variance of the input Doppler shift signal.

10.4.3.2.1 Spectral Estimation Techniques

The Fourier periodogram. The Fourier periodogram provides a mathematical tool through which the frequency components of a signal may be analysed. The discrete Fourier transform, $F(\omega)$, of a time-varying signal $S(t)$ is given by

$$F(\omega) = \sum_{t=0}^{t=N-1} S(t) \exp\left(\frac{-i\omega t}{N}\right) \tag{10.28}$$

where N is the number of available samples from the input. Note that the functions $F(\omega)$ and $S(t)$ in this equation are sampled at discrete intervals in frequency and time, respectively (more precisely the variable t represents tT, where T is the time interval between consecutive samples).

The power spectrum $P(\omega)$ is given by

$$P(\omega) = |F(\omega)|^2 \tag{10.29}$$

The mean frequency of the signal is then obtained from

$$\bar{\omega} = \frac{\displaystyle\sum_{k=0}^{k=\omega_{\max}} kP(k)}{\displaystyle\sum_{k=0}^{k=\omega_{\max}} P(k)} \tag{10.30}$$

where $\omega_{\max}$ is the maximum frequency defined by

$$\omega_{\max} = \pm\frac{\pi}{\Delta} \tag{10.30a}$$

Detailed accounts of the background, application and limitations of the discrete Fourier transform are numerous; two useful and practical sources of reference used by the authors are those of Bracewell (1986) and Press *et al.* (1988).

Alternative spectral estimation techniques. Although the Fourier periodogram is an efficient and generally reliable technique for spectral analysis, it does suffer from several inherent performance limitations. These are primarily due to the fixed frequency resolution, which is inversely proportional to the time sampling interval of the available data and the windowing of the data that occurs when selecting a section of signal for analysis. When analysing short data records these limitations can be particularly troublesome. In a detailed tutorial on spectral analysis Kay and Marple (1981) examine and compare a number of alternative spectral estimation techniques that have been proposed to overcome such limitations. One area in which extensive research has been carried out is termed autoregressive estimation. Techniques involving autoregression are based on a parametric modelling approach. Instead of assuming that the data values outside the sampled segment are periodic, as in the Fourier periodogram, these modelling techniques use knowledge available from the actual data and assume a time series model using the data to determine the parameters. It may be possible to obtain a better spectral estimate with these techniques. In general there are three stages involved: firstly, to select a suitable time series model; secondly, to estimate the parameters using the known data; and thirdly, to obtain the spectral estimate by substituting the estimated parameters into the model. Techniques based on these principles have been applied to Doppler processing (Kaluzynski 1987; Vaitkus & Cobbold 1988; Vaitkus *et al.* 1988; Schlindwein & Evans 1989). One example of such a technique is the autoregressive maximum entropy method (MEM) (Press *et al.* 1988). The MEM technique is based on the approximation of the power spectrum:

$$P(\omega) \approx \frac{a_0}{\left|1 + \sum_{k=1}^{M} a_k z^k\right|^2} \tag{10.31}$$

where

$$z^k = \exp(i\omega k) \tag{10.32}$$

and $a_0 \ldots a_k$ are coefficients of the series and M is the order of the model. The Wiener-Khinchin or autocorrelation theorem equates the autocorrelation function of a signal to the Fourier transform of its power spectrum. This allows us to rewrite equation (10.31) as

$$\sum_{t=0}^{M} r(t)z^t = \frac{a_0}{\left|1 + \sum_{k=1}^{M} a_k z^k\right|^2} \tag{10.33}$$

where $r(t)$ is the autocorrelation of the input signal at lag-time t. The autocorrelation can be calculated over the measured range of the signal and the coefficients of the right-hand side can be solved for, providing a continuous estimate for the power spectrum.

Advantages of using autoregressive techniques over Fourier periodogram techniques include a greater stability in the estimates obtained when processing a limited data segment and the finer frequency obtainable, because there is no trade-off between the sampling interval and the frequency resolution as in the Fourier technique. If low-order autoregressive models are used, the computational demands of this technique are also much less than those required for fast Fourier transform analysis. Autoregressive techniques will be mentioned again in the following section because their ability to evaluate specific features of the spectrum also makes them suitable for implementation as real-time instantaneous frequency estimators (Loupas & McDicken 1990). Autoregressive techniques are just one example of specialist spectral estimation techniques. It is beyond the scope of this work to provide further details, although many more may be found elsewhere (Kay & Marple 1981; Evans & McDicken 2000).

10.4.3.2.2 Instantaneous Frequency Detectors

The demand for a fast, computationally efficient, frequency estimator for real-time imaging has led to the development of a number of approaches. These are explained and compared in this section. The signal output $S_d(t)$ after phase quadrature detection can be represented by the complex signal

$$S_d(t) = S_i(t) + iS_q(t) \tag{10.34}$$

where $S_i(t)$ and $S_q(t)$ are the in-phase and quadrature signals (Figure 10.8). The phase of the signal $\varphi(t)$ is given by

$$\varphi(t) = \tan^{-1}\left[\frac{S_q(t)}{S_i(t)}\right] \tag{10.35}$$

The instantaneous frequency at time t is given by the rate of change of this phase with respect to time, thus differentiating both sides with respect to time gives

$$f(t) = \frac{d\varphi(t)}{dt} = \frac{S_i(t)\dot{S}_q(t) - \dot{S}_i(t)S_q(t)}{2\pi[S_i(t)^2 + S_q(t)^2]} \tag{10.36}$$

This in turn can be approximated with a first-order difference equation to give

$$f(t) = \frac{S_i(t-1)S_q(t) - S_i(t)S_q(t-1)}{2\pi[S_i(t)^2 + S_q(t)^2]} \times \frac{1}{T} \tag{10.37}$$

Alternatively

$$f(t) = \frac{\varphi(t) - \varphi(t-1)}{2\pi T} \tag{10.38}$$

where T is the time between consecutive pulses. The mean frequency measured over N pulses is

$$\bar{f}(t) = \frac{1}{2\pi NT} \sum_{i=0}^{i=N-1} \tan^{-1}\left[\frac{S_q(t+i)}{S_i(t+i)}\right] - \tan^{-1}\left[\frac{S_q(t+i-1)}{S_i(t+i-1)}\right] \tag{10.39}$$

from equation (10.35) above.

The autocorrelator. The autocorrelator technique (Kasai *et al.* 1985) is a further example of instantaneous frequency estimation. The technique has been well described and documented in the literature. Implementation of this technique requires complex multiplication followed by integration. The in-phase and quadrature signals, obtained by phase quadrature sampling the returned r.f. pulses, are used as the real and imaginary input to the complex autocorrelator. The multiplication and integration of the autocorrelator circuit are very similar in essence to the demodulation (mixing and low-pass filtering) used in actually extracting the Doppler shifted waveform (but the two stages of processing are not to be confused). The autocorrelator technique provides a relatively fast and reliable estimate for both the mean and variance of the frequency of the quadrature-demodulated signals. It can be implemented easily in both serial and parallel Doppler processing systems and is often used in commercially available Doppler colour flow imaging equipment. The underlying principle is described below.

If $P(\omega)$ is the power spectrum of the Doppler shift signal, then the mean frequency is given by

$$\bar{\omega} = \frac{\int_0^\infty \omega P(\omega)\mathrm{d}\omega}{\int_0^\infty P(\omega)\mathrm{d}\omega} \tag{10.40}$$

Similarly, the variance of the frequency is

$$\sigma^2 = \frac{\int_0^\infty (\omega - \bar{\omega})P(\omega)\mathrm{d}\omega}{\int_0^\infty P(\omega)\mathrm{d}\omega} = \overline{(\omega^2)} - (\bar{\omega})^2 \tag{10.41}$$

Again we make use of the Wiener-Khinchin theorem, which relates the autocorrelation of a signal $r(t)$ to the Fourier transform of the power spectrum of the signal

$$r(t) = \int_0^\infty P(\omega)\exp(i\omega t)\mathrm{d}\omega \tag{10.42}$$

Combining the above equations gives

$$i\bar{\omega} = \frac{\dot{r}(0)}{r(0)} \tag{10.43}$$

for the mean frequency, and

$$\sigma^2 = \left[\frac{\dot{r}(0)}{r(0)}\right]^2 - \left[\frac{\ddot{r}(0)}{r(0)}\right] \tag{10.44}$$

The autocorrelation of a function can be represented in complex form as

$$r(t) = |r(t)|\exp[i\varphi_r(t)] \tag{10.45}$$

where $\varphi_r(t)$ is the phase of the complex autocorrelation signal (not the demodulated frequency shift signal). Substituting for r ($t = 0$) in the equations above gives

$$\bar{\omega} = \frac{\varphi_r(T)}{T} \tag{10.46}$$

and

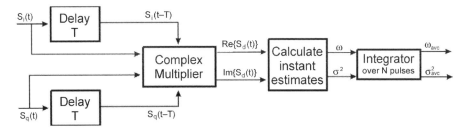

Figure 10.9. The autocorrelator generates the complex autocorrelation of the signal obtained from a phase quadrature demodulator. The phase and magnitude of this quantity can be used to calculate the mean frequency of the Doppler shift signal and associated variance

$$\sigma^2 = \frac{2}{T^2}\left[1 - \frac{|r(T)|}{r(0)}\right]$$
(10.47)

The variable T again denotes the time between consecutive ultrasound pulses. The processing required to generate the complex autocorrelation signal is shown in Figure 10.9.

Using similar notation to that of the direct phase detection techniques presented in the preceding section, the signal from the phase quadrature demodulator is

$$S_d(t) = S_i(t) + iS_q(t)$$
(10.48)

The complex multiplier performs the following calculation

$$S_d'(t) = S_d(t) \times S_d^*(t - T)$$
(10.49)

where $S_d^*(t - T)$ is the time-delayed complex conjugate of $S_d(t)$. In terms of $S_i(t)$ and $S_q(t)$, the output from the complex multiplier is

$$S_d'(t) = S_i(t)S_i(t - \Delta) + S_q(t)S_{qi}(t - \Delta) + i[S_q(t)S_i(t - \Delta) - S_q(t - \Delta)S_i(t)]$$
(10.50)

The integrators serve to perform time averaging over a number of pulses. Thus, from the phase of the autocorrelation the mean frequency after N pulses is

$$\bar{\omega} = \frac{1}{NT}\tan^{-1}\sum_{t=1}^{N}\left[\frac{S_q(t)S_i(t - T) - S_q(t - T)S_i(t)}{S_i(t)S_i(t - T) + S_q(t - T)S_q(t)}\right]$$
(10.51)

This result also can be arrived at by considering

$$\bar{\omega} = \frac{\varphi(t) - \varphi(t - T)}{T}$$
(10.52)

and

$$\tan[\varphi(t) - \varphi(t - T)] = \frac{\sin[\varphi(t) - \varphi(t - T)]}{\cos[\varphi(t) - \varphi(t - T)]}$$
(10.53)

where $\varphi(t)$ represents the phase of the demodulated quadrature signals and the derivation proceeds from the instantaneous phase detectors as described above.

A low-order autoregressive instantaneous estimator. Autoregressive techniques were introduced earlier in this chapter as a means of estimating the Doppler shift signal spectrum. Other researchers (e.g. Loupas & McDicken 1990) have suggested low-order autoregressive techniques as a possible alternative approach for calculating instantaneous frequency information.

Considering the autoregressive model [equation (10.31)], the first-order approximation is given by

$$P(\omega) \approx \frac{a_0}{|1 + a_1 \exp(i\omega T)|^2} \tag{10.54}$$

The maximum value of $P(\omega)$ will result at the pole when

$$a_1 \exp(i\omega T) = -1 \tag{10.55}$$

Now from the Yule-Walker equations (Kay & Marple 1981) it can be shown that

$$r(t) = -\sum_{k=1}^{M} a_1 r(t-k) \tag{10.56}$$

where M is the order of the autoregression. Therefore, for a first-order process

$$a_1 = \frac{r(T)}{r(0)} \tag{10.57}$$

Combining equations (10.55) and (10.57) gives

$$r(T) = -r(0) \exp(-i\bar{\omega}T) \tag{10.58}$$

and the phase of this complex signal is given by

$$\bar{\omega}T = \tan^{-1}\left\{\frac{\text{Im}[r(T)]}{\text{Re}[r(T)]}\right\} \tag{10.59}$$

This result shows the first-order MEM autoregressive approach to be exactly the same as the instantaneous Kasai autocorrelator described above, and agrees with the theoretical and experimental results obtained by Loupas and McDicken (1990).

10.4.4 INHERENT LIMITATIONS OF PHASE FLUCTUATION METHODS

Although phase fluctuation techniques for extracting flow information from the backscattered echo signals have been demonstrated both theoretically and experimentally, there are a number of inherent limitations associated with this approach (Figure 10.10).

10.4.4.1 Angle Dependence

Only the axial component of the target velocity is measured. Vessels containing flow perpendicular to the line of interrogation will be underestimated or missed altogether (Figure 10.10a).

10.4.4.2 Aliasing

When using PW, the complex Doppler shift signal is sampled at the pulse repetition frequency (PRF) of the pulse sequence. The Nyquist theorem states that if this frequency is less than

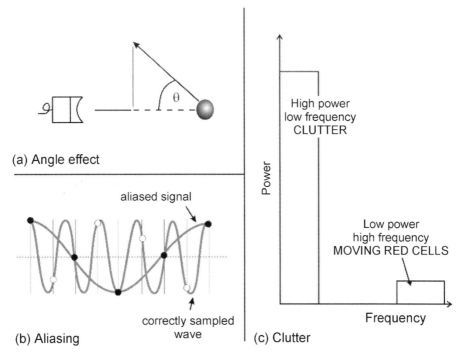

Figure 10.10. The inherent limitations of phase fluctuation velocimetry: (a) angle dependence; (b) aliasing and the compromise between depth and velocity; (c) high-amplitude, low-frequency clutter signals from tissue moving within the sample volume, which has on occasion been somewhat colourfully referred to as 'bloody noise' (unpublished, but believed to be credited to P. Atkinson)

double the frequency of the highest component of the Doppler spectra (as in the case of the solid sample dots in Figure 10.10b) then aliasing will occur. The maximum unambiguously detectable velocity V_{max} is defined in terms of the pulse repetition frequency (PRF) by

$$V_{max} \leqslant \frac{c\text{PRF}}{4f} \leqslant \frac{\left(\frac{\lambda}{4}\right)}{T} \tag{10.60}$$

Aliasing leads to wrongly classified velocity values. In direction-sensitive complex systems, aliased high positive velocities may be presented as high negative velocities. This problem, together with the finite time of flight of the ultrasound pulses in the tissue, results in a maximum detectable target velocity for a given depth, unless one is prepared to accept the spatial ambiguity that would result from using a PRF higher than the reciprocal of the time for the pulse travel to and from the maximum depth of interest, Z_{max}. The relationship between depth and velocity is given by

$$V_{max} \leqslant \frac{2c\lambda}{Z_{max}} \tag{10.61}$$

10.4.4.3 Spectral Clutter

The backscattered echoes from red cells moving through the sample volume of the ultrasound beam are weaker (by around 40 dB) than echoes from surrounding tissue structure. Slowly moving solid tissues will introduce a high-amplitude low-frequency component into the Doppler shift spectrum (Figure 10.10c). Clutter rejection filters, their design and optimisation are an important area of development in ultrasound flow imaging. Filtering strategies that have been applied to this area include finite impulse response (simple delay-line cancellation), infinite impulse response and regression filters (Rajaonah *et al.* 1994; Kadi & Loupas 1995; Tysoe & Evans 1995). A recent review can be found in Evans and McDicken (2000). The reverse process, of displaying only the low-frequency high-amplitude velocity components associated with moving soft tissue, is easier from the point of view of the signal-to-noise ratio and has come to be known as Doppler tissue imaging. Evans and McDicken also review this technique, its main application being in the context of research for methods to study myocardial disease.

10.5   ENVELOPE FLUCTUATION METHODS

The amplitude of ultrasonic echoes backscattered by blood fluctuates with time, due to movement through the acoustic sample volume of red cells whose pattern of distribution is random but remains fixed, or correlated (see Section 10.4.2), over the time scale of observation (Atkinson & Berry 1974; Yuan and Shung 1987). For fast moving blood or a large sample volume (resolution cell), where the blood structure can be assumed to be an incoherent source of scattered waves, the rate of this fluctuation has been shown to depend only on the dimensions of the resolution cell and the velocity of the scatterers. It has been shown theoretically (Atkinson 1975) that, under these conditions and when the medium retains its structural correlation as it moves, the mean velocity of the medium V can be calculated from f_c, the rate of fluctuation of the echo level, after envelope detection, about its mean value. The two quantities are related by the equation

$$V \approx \frac{f_c R_b}{0.32} \tag{10.62}$$

where R_b is the beam width of the sample volume. Equation (10.62) is derived for motion in a direction transverse to the ultrasound beam and relies on accurate perpendicular alignment of the transducer and the vessel to within 5°. As the beam-vessel angle decreases, the axial component of the velocity will introduce additional fluctuation components and the ratio in the above equation will become more complex. If a symmetrical resolution cell can be generated (pulse length = beam width) the method should provide an estimate of the magnitude of the velocity independent of the direction of flow. For slowly moving blood, where aggregates of red cells (rouleaux) can form, and for small resolution cells the assumption of an incoherent scattering source may break down and move a little towards the situation that is predominant for most solid tissues, for which the acoustic scattering impulse response of the tissue would also ideally need to be known and incorporated in equation (10.62) (Bamber & Bush 1996). Nevertheless, the method has provided a reasonable means of monitoring soft tissue relative displacement (e.g. Dickinson & Hill 1982; Tristam *et al.* 1988) and, as was mentioned in Chapter 9, measurement of elevational probe motion for reconstructing three-dimensional ultrasound images from freehand scans (Tuthill *et al.* 1998; Prager *et al.* 2003).

10.5.1 INHERENT LIMITATIONS

As in the previous discussion regarding phase fluctuation processing, the angle between the direction of motion and the ultrasound beam is again a consideration, although this is primarily a consequence of the typically asymmetric nature of the ultrasound sample volume. Also, clutter signals will introduce error in the estimator output. This technique actually can be considered to be a special case of the phase fluctuation technique already described; the processing and limitations are primarily the same. One consequence arising from the use of envelope-detected signals as opposed to the r.f. phase information may be the ability to measure larger velocities or displacements, because the velocity limit for the more slowly fluctuating envelope signals will be much higher. In addition, the nature of the limit is different, reaching a situation where greater displacement or velocity is indistinguishable from the limiting value rather than appearing as an incorrect but apparently measurable value, which is the consequence of aliasing. The converse may, however, also be true, i.e., the much faster rate of fluctuation of the phase of the echo enables much smaller displacements or velocities to be measured with high precision for a given echo signal-to-noise ratio.

Preliminary parametric colour flow images, showing the pattern of flow speed in large veins such as the inferior vena cava, against the echo anatomy of the liver, were made as long ago as 1988 (Bamber *et al.* 1988). The method suffers, however, from very poor performance in conditions of low signal to noise ratio or large amounts of clutter, making it difficult to apply to observation of arterial blood flow and smaller vessels. However, the availability of ultrasound contrast agents that enhance the ratio of the blood echo signal to noise and clutter (see below) may provide a timely opportunity to return to examine the potential benefits of envelope fluctuation methods (Rubin *et al.* 1999).

Both envelope and phase methods will be influenced by the random nature of the echo signal interference (speckle). However, the possibility that small amounts of structural decorrelation of the medium (Section 10.4.2) may have less of an effect on the envelope than on the phase, combined with the above-mentioned ability to observe larger displacements using the envelope, was in part responsible for the method being the first to be studied for application to freehand elastography, where induced displacements are likely to be large and difficult to control (Bamber & Bush 1996). It appears, however, that there are advantages in combining envelope and phase methods; the large displacement measurement capability of envelope techniques may provide the information that enables the phase ambiguity (aliasing) to be overcome so that, even when the displacement between consecutive pulses is large, full advantage may be taken of the high precision associated with the phase of the signal (Shiina *et al.* 2002).

10.6 PHASE TRACKING METHODS

This class of motion detectors relies on the signal processing technique of cross-correlation to match specific reflections in consecutive pulse echoes. As noted in Section 10.2.1, when using PW techniques the time delay of the reflected signal provides information related to the depth of the scatterer in the medium. If, by comparison of two echo signals, the echoes associated with a particular scatterer or group of scatterers can be matched from one signal to the next, then the time shift between these echoes may be found. The axial velocity V of the scatterer is then given by

$$V = \frac{\delta tc}{2T} \tag{10.63}$$

where δt is the time shift between matching echoes in successive signals (see Figure 10.11.). A comprehensive review of the development of time domain techniques for the measurement of tissue movement and blood flow imaging was provided by Hein and O'Brien (1993a). The application of such techniques to blood flow imaging initially generated much interest (Bonnefous & Pesque 1986; Bohs *et al.* 1993; Hein & O'Brien 1993b) but has achieved only limited and transient commercial application, being somewhat overshadowed by the more established Doppler-based techniques. On the other hand, for tissue motion and elasticity imaging research there tends to be strong interest in the use of tracking methods, but this may be due simply to the difficulty that researchers encounter in arranging for control of the pulse sequencing of commercial ultrasound scanners. As a result, one must make do with a pulse repetition rate along a given line that is one per ultrasound frame, meaning that tracking methods may be preferred to cope with large tissue displacements between consecutive frames.

Phase fluctuation and phase tracking techniques can be related through the process of cross-correlation (Figure 10.12). Both approaches require a stage that is equivalent to pulse-to-pulse correlation. In the phase fluctuation techniques the demodulation stage through which the complex Doppler shift signal is generated is simply a measure of the correlation coefficient at zero time shift of each pulse-to-pulse or pulse-to-reference correlation. The zero shift correlation coefficient is proportional to the change in phase between consecutive pulses, $\delta\varphi$, in Figure 10.12b. The rate of change of this phase yields the Doppler shift signal. The phase tracking technique, as mentioned above, measures the time shift δt of the peak in the pulse-to-pulse correlation coefficients. The target velocity is calculated directly from this time shift.

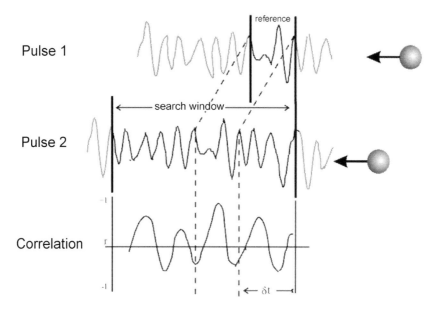

Figure 10.11. The motion of scatterers between pulse 1 and pulse 2 causes a time shift δt in the corresponding echo signal. Taking a reference section of pulse 1 and correlating this with a search window in the reflected data from pulse 2 enables target movement to be measured. The situation for a single scatterer was illustrated in Figure 10.4

Reflected rf echoes from distributed moving scatterers

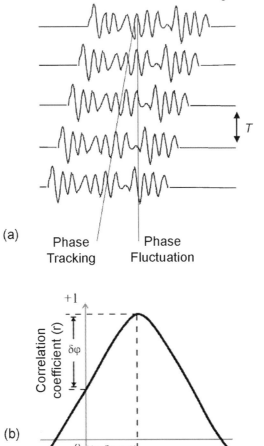

(a)   Phase   Phase
        Tracking   Fluctuation

(b)

Figure 10.12. The relationship between phase fluctuation and phase tracking techniques demonstrated through the pulse-to-pulse correlation of backscattered signals. The Doppler shift frequency is the rate of phase fluctuation $\delta\varphi/T$ along the vertical line in (a), and may be estimated from the time-varying value of the correlation coefficient at zero shift δt in propagation time, as shown in (b). This is then related to the axial component of target velocity via the ultrasonic frequency and propagation speed. Phase tracking, on the other hand, measures the rate of change of axial target position in propagation time, shown as the diagonal line in (a), by directly determining the time shift δt that maximises the correlation coefficient, as seen in (b)

10.6.1 SIGNAL PROCESSING FOR PHASE TRACKING

In order to track a signal, an initial reference data segment must be defined. Search areas are then defined in subsequent data and a best match is found by calculating correlation coefficients throughout the search area. Typically, tracking algorithms are based on standard cross-correlation techniques. The normalised coefficient of correlation between a time segment W of a reference signal $x(t)$ with a similar data segment $y(t)$ from the search signal is given by

$$r_{xy} = \frac{\sum_W [x(t) - \bar{x}][y(t) - \bar{y}]}{\sqrt{\sum_W [x(t) - \bar{x}]^2 \sum_W [y(t) - \bar{y}]^2}} \tag{10.64}$$

where $\bar{x}$ and $\bar{y}$ are the mean values of x and y. Each summation is performed for the number of samples contained within the reference data segment. The correlation coefficients range from $+1$ for identical signals, through zero for no correlation and to -1 for identically opposite signals. To enhance the computational efficiency of the standard cross-correlation calculation the above equation can be rearranged as

$$r_{xy} = \frac{\sum_W x(t)y(t) - \dfrac{\sum_W x(t) \sum_W y(t)}{N}}{\left[\left[\sum_W x(t)^2 - \dfrac{\left[\sum_W x(t) \right]^2}{N} \right] \left\{ \sum_W y(t)^2 - \dfrac{\left[\sum_W y(t) \right]^2}{N} \right\} \right]^{0.5}} \tag{10.65}$$

Although this formulation appears more complex, calculation time is reduced by removing the necessity for calculating $\bar{x}$ and $\bar{y}$ prior to the main correlation procedure. The correlation coefficient is not the only similarity measure, and alternatives that have been used in this context are mentioned below.

10.6.2 INHERENT LIMITATIONS OF PHASE TRACKING

Without interpolation the minimum detectable velocity is limited by the sampling interval of the digitised r.f. signals. If the time shift resulting from the target motion is smaller than the sampling interval of the r.f. signals, it may not be detectable. Finer sampling, signal interpolation or interpolation of the correlation function can be implemented to overcome this problem, with different performance and artefacts depending on the type of interpolation employed (Cespedes *et al.* 1995). More generally the velocity resolution of this technique is governed by the echo signal-to-noise ratio and pulse bandwidth (Cespedes *et al.* 1995; Walker & Trahey 1995).

The limit on the maximum detectable velocity is defined by the search range of the algorithm and the distance over which the arrangement of the scatterers remains unchanged as they move. However, as the search range is increased above a single wavelength $(+\pi/2)$, detection of the wrong correlation peak in the presence of noise becomes a possibility. This is due to the *cyclic* nature of the signals generating correlation side lobes. It is possible to restrict the search region to avoid these erroneous peaks, although by doing this the maximum measurable time shift is

$$\delta t = \frac{\left(\dfrac{\lambda}{2} \right)}{c} \tag{10.66}$$

Substituting this into equation (10.63) gives

$$V_{\max} \leqslant \frac{\left(\frac{\lambda}{4}\right)}{T} \qquad (10.67)$$

which is exactly the same as the aliasing limit of the phase fluctuation estimators. There are a number of possible solutions to this problem, for example, *a priori* knowledge of the target motion may be used to select the search region (Jensen 1993) or envelope information may be used to guide the search (Shiina *et al.* 2002). Alternatively, increasing the size of the reference segment may improve the correlation but at the expense of spatial resolution, and would only help as long as the arrangement of the scatterers remains constant at large distances, which is unlikely to be true, for example, when there is a flow profile or when tissue strains occur.

Temporal averaging of velocity estimates obtained from a series of pulses may also be used to improve the velocity estimate, both in the presence of noise and when searching above the aliasing limit. This can also be performed in conjunction with non-linear filtering to reject errors arising from incorrect correlations. This is discussed in detail by Eckersley (1996). The use of a series of pulses to produce more than a single velocity estimate also provides an instantaneous and quantitative estimator for the standard deviation or reliability of the estimate, a parameter that is produced in similar fashion by fluctuation processing.

Cross-correlation is a computationally intensive process and a number of alternative algorithms have been suggested. For example, Bonnefous and Pesque (1986) demonstrated the utility of a simple one-bit cross-correlator and Bohs *et al.* (1993) have demonstrated a simple sum absolute difference technique, which was also the similarity measure employed by a neural network used for flow tracking (Bamber *et al.* 1991). In this technique the similarity estimate e, which serves the same purpose as the correlation coefficient in the above description of tracking techniques, is the sum over the reference segment of the absolute difference between the reference data and corresponding values in the search data segment. Thus

$$e = \sum_W |[x(t) - y(t)]| \qquad (10.68)$$

For a perfect match $e = 0$; the larger the difference between the reference and search data, the greater the value of e.

10.7 ENVELOPE TRACKING TECHNIQUES

10.7.1 SIGNAL PROCESSING FOR ENVELOPE TRACKING

Envelope tracking techniques use the same basic principles as phase tracking, with the addition of an envelope detection stage in the signal processing. Envelope detection is an integral part of B-mode imaging and in real-time imaging sequences it is possible to see by eye the motion of image structure and speckle. In general these time-domain tracking techniques measure the physical displacement of the speckle pattern associated with the reflected sound from target volumes within the sound beam. It has been shown that, with the exception of large displacements between pulses, the motion of the underlying scatterers is generally reproduced by the speckle pattern motion (Trahey *et al.* 1986).

10.7.2 INHERENT LIMITATIONS OF ENVELOPE TRACKING

The limitations associated with this technique are principally the same as for phase tracking. As in the earlier discussion of envelope and phase fluctuation techniques, the primary difference between envelope tracking and phase tracking arises due to the more slowly varying envelope signals. This means that correlation can be performed over a wider range before the chance of a wrongly matched peak occurs. However, the substantially reduced bandwidth compared with the r.f. signal greatly reduces the velocity or displacement resolution, and in order to perform accurate correlation of noisy echo signals a larger reference window section would be required to contain sufficient signal structure.

10.8 CONSIDERATIONS SPECIFIC TO COLOUR FLOW IMAGING

The combination of B-mode anatomical information and velocity information to produce two-dimensional colour flow images has been a key stage in the development of clinical diagnostic ultrasound. This has been made possible by the development of fast instantaneous velocity estimators such as those described in this chapter. In addition to the signal processing presented above there are a number of further processing stages that are not specific to the velocity estimation strategy employed. The clutter rejection filter (or wall filter), briefly mentioned above, is an example of this. It is an integral part of any colour flow imaging system, enabling the removal of echoes due to slow-moving tissue structures from the r.f. signals prior to processing. In connection with this, at the post-processing stage, the imaging system must decide for each resolution cell in the image whether to display colour flow information or grey-scale B-mode information. The logic applied in this situation is a further part of the clutter rejection filtering and is typically based on user-definable thresholds involving backscatter power, velocity magnitude and velocity reliability. Further post-processing is also possible and includes interpolation between velocity estimates to allow an increase in frame rate at the expense of spatial resolution and persistence of velocity estimates, which may be included to provide temporal averaging from one colour flow image to the next.

The velocity estimation algorithms are able to provide estimates of the mean velocity, the standard deviation of the velocity estimate and the signal power associated with the moving scatterers. In a colour flow system there is a choice of which parameter, or parameters, to display. For example, either the mean velocity or the power provides direct indicators of the presence of flow, and can be viewed as qualitative indices of the tissue vascularisation, whereas the variance of the velocity can yield valuable information on the haemodynamics.

10.9 ANGLE-INDEPENDENT VELOCITY MOTION IMAGING

The velocity estimation techniques presented in this chapter have, without exception, been presented as one-dimensional approaches. The information generated by each algorithm is derived from one-dimensional projection of the true velocity vector along the line of the ultrasound beam. For many applications the one-dimensional projection will result in incomplete and potentially misleading displayed information. A good example of this would be tumour vasculature, where the vessel structure is typically a complex three-dimensional network. Techniques for overcoming the angle dependence are the subject of much research and involve either multiple-beam compounding or extension of the velocity estimation technique to two or more dimensions. As was pointed out above (Section 10.5), it has also been suggested that, with appropriate design to control beam and pulse shape, to obtain a symmetrical resolution cell, a correlation measure of the echo envelope fluctuation may provide a simple non-directional angle-independent measure of displacement or flow speed. However, one simple approach that is widely available is to display only the backscattered power of the detected moving scatterers.

10.9.1 POWER MODE IMAGING

In power mode imaging (also known as colour angiography or colour Doppler energy imaging) the power of the Doppler shift signal is calculated and displayed as a two-dimensional colour map. The resulting information is proportional to the backscattered signal strength arising from moving scatterers. This is equivalent to introducing a binary discrimination to identify moving scatterers from stationary scatterers on a standard B-scan image. The primary justification for the introduction of this display modality is that it overcomes ambiguities in the final image due to both beam angle and aliasing of the data. Figure 10.13 shows an idealised Doppler shift spectrum. If the scatterers that gave rise to this spectrum were to undergo a reduction in velocity, the position of the spectrum would shift relative to the frequency axis while the area under the spectrum, the backscattered power, would remain unchanged. The direction of flow should therefore have no effect on the calculated power. At higher velocities when aliasing occurs the spectrum wraps around and, although mean velocity calculations break down in these conditions, the power is less affected.

The provision of this facility in a modern colour flow system is straightforward and involves direct implementation of the Wiener-Khinchin principle [equation (10.36)]. Using this, it is evident that taking the zero time lag of the autocorrelation function will yield the integrated power of the Doppler shift spectrum

$$r(0) = \int_{-\infty}^{+\infty} P(\omega) \mathrm{d}\omega \tag{10.69}$$

In discrete processing terms the complex un-normalised autocorrelation at zero time lag is given by

$$r(0) = \sum_{n=1}^{N} S_i(n)^2 + S_q(n)^2 \tag{10.70}$$

In fact, $r(0)$ is calculated as part of the standard autocorrelation processing technique applied in most scanners (see Section 10.4.3.2.2). In theory the power of the signal is independent of the magnitude of the target velocity, and images generated using this information will appear less dependent on the angle between the ultrasound and the vessel, while low-flow regions will be more clearly represented. The thresholds presented in Figure 10.13, which are necessary to remove the effects of clutter and noise, will re-introduce a degree of angle dependence. A further key advantage to this approach arises from the manner in which noise affects the results. In a standard velocity detection system, as the gain is increased to image a low signal and the noise consequently emerges above the threshold (Figure 10.13c) for analysis, the mean velocity estimation fails and a random and quickly varying colour noise that may take any velocity value is displayed on the image. In power mode, however, this low amplitude noise is displayed as a relatively constant additive low-noise signal. This difference, combined with appropriate post-processing for optimal display, means that it is possible in power mode to visualise lower power signals, closer to the noise floor of the system, than with velocity mode.

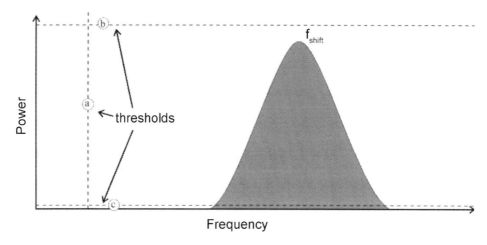

Figure 10.13. The power spectrum of the Doppler shift signal. The area under the curve is the total power of the signal. Arbitrary thresholds may be used to reduce signals associated with: (a) slow moving or stationary structures; (b) strongly reflecting structures; and (c) background noise

The power mode imaging technique and its clinical application have been discussed further by Rubin *et al.* (1994).

10.10   TISSUE ELASTICITY AND ECHO STRAIN IMAGING

The concept of elastography, where images are formed of parameters such as the tissue strain induced by an applied stress, was introduced in Chapter 9 (Sections 9.4.4 and 9.4.5). A related imaging method was also mentioned: that of backscatter imaging of relative temperature, in which the displayed quantity is the apparent echo strain that results from the change in sound speed induced by localised heating. Examples of images produced by these methods were also provided. There are now a number of reviews of elastography (e.g. Ophir *et al.* 1999, 2003; Gao *et al.* 1996; Bamber 1999; Bamber *et al.* 2002), as well as an extensive and growing literature, so the present brief discussion will be restricted to a few comments that are relevant to the discussion of motion estimation described above.

   A great many alternative schemes exist for creating elasticity images with ultrasound: the method of applying the stress may be mechanically-controlled, freehand, using modulated radiation force from another sound source or even taking advantage of naturally occurring pulsations of the heart and blood vessels; the loading of the tissue may be at the body surface or deep within the tissue; the applied stress or strain may be static, dynamically vibrating or an impulse; one may apply an initially compressive or a shear loading; the observation may be of a static strain, a dynamic strain (continuous wave), or a propagating shear wave (burst); one may attempt to solve the inverse problem for any of these forms of deformation. This is not a complete list, even of all the possibilities that have already been investigated, but the one thing they all have in common is the need to employ pulse-echo methods to estimate the displacement or strain induced. Temperature imaging is less well developed as yet but a similar statement can be made.

For both elastography and backscatter temperature imaging, a strain measurement may in principle be obtained either from the echo signal directly or by taking the spatial gradient of measured displacement. An intriguing, and potentially valuable, apparent difference between elastography and blood flow measurement is that whilst, as noted in Section 10.4.1, an ultrasound imaging pulse is too short to allow an accurate direct measurement of the (Doppler shift) distortion induced by scatterers moving through it (making it necessary to observe the shift by sampling over a number of acoustic pulses), the echo signal distortion induced by mechanical strain of tissue is sufficient to be observed directly. Direct strain estimators that have been studied involve observing the shift, induced by tissue deformation, in the centroid of the power spectrum of a short window of the echo signal, or using cross-correlation to detect the shift in the whole spectrum, although the latter was found to be more sensitive to small strains (Konofagou *et al.* 2000; Varghese *et al.* 2000). Direct strain estimators are said to suffer less from decorrelation noise than estimators that first require the measurement of displacement, described below. One can imagine that many other direct strain estimators may be conceived; for example, the spectral and instantaneous frequency estimators discussed in Sections 10.4.3.2.1 and 10.4.3.2.2 might be applied advantageously to this problem.

As mentioned above, indirect estimation of strain involves measuring the spatial gradient of tissue displacement that has first been detected using any one of, or a combination of, the fluctuation and tracking estimators described in Sections 10.4 to 10.7. The relative advantages and disadvantages of these were mentioned in each of the four sections, although it is perhaps worth mentioning here that strain imaging may be a good example, because of the need to maintain high spatial resolution, where it is valuable to retain the advantage that tracking techniques have over fluctuation techniques in that there is no conflict between the B-mode imaging and displacement measurement components when bandwidth is altered; increasing bandwidth improves both accuracy and precision of the displacement estimates (Eckersley 1996). Finally, it is interesting to note that taking the spatial derivative of tissue velocity, perhaps from a Doppler tissue image for example, has been proposed as a method of imaging of tissue 'strain rate' (Torp *et al.* 2002).

10.11 PERFORMANCE CRITERIA

Section 9.3 introduced a number of key concepts in terms of performance criteria that should be useful for assessing and comparing image parameterisation methods, namely contrast resolution, spatial resolution and speed of presentation (which here is termed temporal resolution). Definitions were provided for these quantities that are directly transferable to the methods discussed in this chapter. Furthermore, Section 9.4.5 described how in many respects, and by many of these criteria, images such as those of blood flow, tissue elasticity, temperature and contrast agents, which make use of time-dependent phenomena, perform extremely well relative to many other parametric imaging techniques, and even relative to the B-mode method of displaying echo information.

The inherent physical limitations of the velocity and displacement estimation processing techniques were presented in Sections 10.4–10.7. Under practical (*in vivo*) operational conditions the limit to the accuracy and reliability of these methods will be dictated by the amount of signal corruption due to the various forms of noise that were also discussed above.

10.12   USE OF CONTRAST MEDIA

10.12.1 PERFORMANCE ENHANCEMENT DUE TO INCREASED SIGNAL

The introduction of stable, safe echo-enhancing contrast agents has opened up a new range of possibilities for ultrasound imaging. An important property of ultrasonic contrast agents is that they increase the strength of the backscattered signal from blood (Ophir & Parker 1989; Schlief 1991). This increase in backscattered power enables the detection of both smaller vessels and regions of slow flow. Ultrasound contrast media were also discussed in Chapter 9 (see Section 9.2.7), where references were provided from a number of recent and comprehensive textbooks dealing with the subject. A comprehensive overview of contrast ultrasonography can also be found in Burns and Becher (2000) and Goldberg *et al.* (2001). In this section we will comment on the effects of the agents on colour flow imaging. In Section 10.12.2 we mention the development of signal processing techniques for detecting the time-dependent behaviour of the acoustic response of the microbubbles. The following brief remarks are based on the more detailed discussion given by Eckersley (1996) but it is interesting to note that, at the time of writing, commercial systems have yet to provide the user with facilities that will allow full advantage to be taken of the potential to control the specific nature of system performance enhancement that contrast media are capable of providing, even in the fundamental (linear) imaging mode.

10.12.1.1 Enhancement of Velocity Resolution (Signal-to-Noise Ratio)

The most direct benefit arising from the increased signal-to-noise ratio is an improvement in the accuracy of the velocity estimation process. This in turn provides the opportunity to detect previously undetected vessels with slower flows and, for non-imaging Doppler applications, to make more accurate quantitative measurements.

10.12.1.2 Enhancement of Temporal and Spatial Resolution

The enhancement caused by the microbubbles can be employed in other ways as well. For example, if the velocity resolution is acceptable prior to enhancement then the extra signal strength might be used to reduce the number of imaging pulses per scan line. The temporal resolution of the measurement is thus improved by the higher frame rate. Alternatively, the spatial resolution might be improved by using higher frequencies, or shorter pulses. Once again the improved echo strength is used to maintain an acceptable velocity resolution.

10.12.2 SIGNATURE RECOGNITION

The improvements afforded by microbubbles as described above all depend on the straightforward increase in the backscattered signals from blood. These allow the signal processing to be tuned to improve the velocity, temporal or spatial resolutions of the resulting information. However, owing to the corresponding increase in attenuation of the ultrasound due to the agent, there is a limit to the amount of improvement available (Uhlendorf 1994). This limitation is particularly problematic in organs containing large concentrations of blood such as the heart or liver. In addition, simply boosting the backscattered signal strength is often not enough to allow visualisation of small vessels containing slow flow within the tissue background, because the strong tissue echoes are inseparable from the echoes of the microbubbles. In order to overcome these limitations, and indeed to detect and measure stationary contrast agents that may have been targeted to a specific organ or tissue type, a general reduction of the background tissue signals must be achieved.

A number of techniques have been proposed and implemented, and these are described below (some have already been mentioned in Chapter 9, Section 9.2.7). In each case, use is made of the difference in acoustic behaviour of the bubbles compared with the background tissues.

10.12.2.1 Frequency Dependence of Attenuation and Scattering (Linear)

The frequency dependence of the attenuation due to microbubbles has been shown to be highly specific, with peaks in attenuation corresponding to particular frequencies and sizes of bubbles (Bleeker *et al.* 1990). This behaviour is characteristic of resonant behaviour, which was discussed more extensively in Chapter 4 (Sections 4.3.9 and 4.4.2.5). A simplified theory (Ophir & Parker 1989) can be used to predict the resonant frequency of bubbles with a particular radius. For example, a 3 µm radius free air bubble in water resonates at 3 MHz. This combination is perfectly suited for diagnostic ultrasound, because a 3 µm bubble can circulate freely throughout the vascular network and 3 MHz is the centre frequency widely used for both cardiac and abdominal imaging applications. Arditi has, for example, explored the use of multiple frequencies to turn such properties into a bubble signature imaging technique (Arditi *et al.* 1997), but high bubble concentrations and a very wide measurement bandwidth are likely to be needed if the frequency dependence of attenuation or scattering from perfused tissue is to be modified to a detectable degree by the presence of contrast agent.

10.12.2.2 Amplitude Dependence of Scattering and Generation of Harmonics (Non-linear)

As the transmitted ultrasound field strength is increased, the resonating microbubbles respond in a highly non-linear manner. One consequence of this is that differences arise in the compression and expansion phases of the bubble oscillation. As a bubble is compressed at high pressures it becomes stiffer, whereas during the low-pressure half-cycle the bubble enlarges more freely. This asymmetry gives rise to harmonic overtones in the received echoes (Schrope & Newhouse 1993). By combining this harmonic behaviour with colour Doppler imaging, further improvements in signal-to-noise ratio can be achieved. In particular, harmonic power mode imaging has been used to demonstrate flow in vessels as small as 40 µm and can be used to image flow in the myocardium (Villanueva & Kaul 1995; Burns 1996). There are still limitations with this approach, because the tissues through which the ultrasound propagates also contribute a non-linear harmonic component due to effects of wave propagation (see Chapters 1, 4 and 9). Furthermore, the filtering process required to detect the narrowband harmonic component (at twice the fundamental) restricts the resolution of the final image. This limitation results in a familiar compromise between spatial resolution and image contrast. To counter this, multiple pulse detection sequences, which make use of the non-linear response of the bubble while enabling wideband detection of the echoes, have been devised (Burns & Simpson 1998; Hope Simpson *et al.* 1999). As was mentioned in Chapter 9, with these approaches the phase or amplitude of consecutive pulses is changed. The echoes from successive pulses are combined arithmetically such that linear reflections are cancelled while non-linear reflections are preserved. Again, the detection process is compromised by non-linear propagation and, because multiple pulses are employed, tissue motion may be a problem. For non-stationary microbubbles these problems can be overcome by combining the signal processing with a motion detection strategy. This technique has been used successfully *in vivo* to detect flow in the myocardium at real-time rates (Tiemann *et al.* 1999).

10.12.2.3 Instability Effects

As the ultrasound field strength is increased, the bubbles can be forced to fracture, fragment or perhaps dissolve. This can lead to a rapid disappearance of the reflected signal, especially for air-filled microbubbles. This effect has been used in two differing imaging applications: by using a brief excitation at high incident acoustic pressure to disrupt the bubbles in the imaging plane and subsequent imaging with a non-destructive (low pressure) non-linear detection approach (as described above) to measure the refill rates within the scan plan (Wei *et al.* 1997, 1999); and a real-time flow system that works at high acoustic pressures can be used both to produce and image this destruction process (Blomley *et al.* 1999). Microbubbles in the scan plan give rise to a wideband random velocity estimate because their sudden disappearance between one imaging pulse and the next will dramatically influence the phase of the scattered acoustic wave at the transducer. The resulting rapid loss of correlation of the echo waveform will therefore be interpreted as random motion by any of the four detection strategies described in this chapter. Harvey *et al.* (2001) have shown that the same effect can be achieved using high-power pulse-inversion sequences. Provided that the ultrasound energy can be deposited uniformly throughout the region of interest, and the effects of attenuation can be compensated for, this technique may produce an estimate of the total vascular volume of the tissues. The fact that the bubbles are destroyed by the imaging process is, of course, a disadvantage for applications such as when the bubbles are targeted to localise at a specific site, where they are not quickly refreshed.

10.13 CONCLUDING REMARKS

It was concluded in Chapter 9 that ultrasound is outstanding amongst medical clinical investigative technologies in the high information rates that it is, in principle, capable of providing. In many respects major advances in capability can be anticipated to follow simply from developments in the technologies for flexible control and reception of acoustic fields, and for rapid data processing. This chapter has set out to supplement Chapter 9 in documenting in more detail current knowledge of the underlying principles of how the time-dependence of echoes, i.e., echo motion or echo fluctuation, may be imaged.

We have largely ignored the vast subject of Doppler techniques and their applications, in favour of attempting to bring together what may have seemed, because of their separate description in the literature, disparate approaches to the problem of displacement and velocity estimation. These were classified as fluctuation and tracking methods, both employing the phase and the envelope of the signal but being related through measurement of echo similarity using, for example, the correlation coefficient. Each has advantages and disadvantages, and indeed, there are substantial benefits to be gained from combining them.

In many respects, the evolution noted in Chapter 9 of technology towards real-time 3D ultrasonic echo data acquisition is what motion and fluctuation processing has been waiting for, enabling a volumetric assessment and the measurement of all components of the displacement or velocity vector. This should, for example, provide opportunities for methods such as flow imaging and elastography to become more quantitative, and will pave the way for practical automated motion-compensation devices in ultrasound-guided interventional procedures.

REFERENCES

Anglesen, B.A.J. (2000). *Ultrasound Imaging: Waves, Signals and Signal Processing*. Emantec, Norway.

Arditi, M., Brenier, T. and Schnieder, M. (1997). Differential contrast echography. *Ultrasound Med. Biol.* **23**, 1185–1194.

Atkinson, P. (1975). An ultrasonic fluctuation velocimeter. *Ultrasonics* **13**, 275–278.

Atkinson, P. and Berry, M.V. (1974). Random noise in ultrasonic echoes diffracted by blood. *J. Phys. A* **7**, 1293–1302.

Atkinson, P. and Woodcock, J.P. (1982). Doppler flowmeters. In *Doppler Ultrasound and its Use in Clinical Measurement*. Academic Press, London, pp. 22–74.

Baker, D.W. (1970). Pulsed ultrasonic blood-flow sensing. *IEEE Trans. Son. Ultrason.* SU17, 170–185.

Bamber, J.C. (1999). Ultrasound elasticity imaging: definition and technology. *European Radiology* **9**(Suppl. 3), S327–S330.

Bamber, J.C., Barbone, P.E., Bush, N.L., Cosgrove, D.O., Doyley, M.M., Fuechsel, F.G., Meaney, P.M., Miller, N.R., Shiina, T. and Tranquart, F. (2002). Progress in freehand elastography of the breast. *IEICE Trans on Information and Systems* **85-D**(1), 5–14.

Bamber, J.C. and Bush, N.L. (1996). Freehand elasticity imaging using speckle decorrelation rate. In *Acoustical Imaging*, Vol. 22, P. Tortoli and L. Masotti (eds). Plenum Press, New York, pp. 285–292.

Bamber, J.C. and Tristam, M. (1988). Diagnostic ultrasound. In *The Physics of Medical Imaging*, S. Webb (ed.), IoP Publishing, Bristol, pp. 319–388.

Bamber, J.C., Dance, C., Bell, D.S. and Bush, N.L. (1991). Imaging flow and shear by speckle tracking with a neural network. *Br. J. Radiol.* **64**, 651.

Bleeker, H., Shung, K., *et al.* (1990). On the application of ultrasonic contrast agents for blood flowmetry and assessment of cardiac perfusion. *J. Ultrasound Med.* **9**, 461–471.

Blomley, M.J.K., Albrecht, T., *et al.* (1999). Stimulated acoustic emission to image a late liver and spleen-specific phase of Levovist((R)) in normal volunteers and patients with and without liver disease. *Ultrasound Med. Biol.* **25**, 1341–1352.

Bohs, L.N., Friemel, B.H., *et al.* (1993). Real-time system for angle-independent ultrasound of blood-flow in 2 dimensions – initial results. *Radiology* **186**, 259–261.

Bonnefous, O. and Pesque, P. (1986). Time domain formulation of pulse-doppler ultrasound and blood velocity estimation by cross-correlation. *Ultrason. Imag.* **8**, 73–85.

Bracewell, R.N. (1986). *The Fourier Transform and its Applications*. McGraw-Hill, New York.

Burns, P.N. (1996). Harmonic imaging with ultrasound contrast agents. *Clin. Radiol.* **51**, 50–55.

Burns, P.N. and Becher, H. (2000). *Handbook of Echocardiography*. Springer Verlag, Berlin.

Burns, P.N. and Simpson, D.H. (1998). Pulse inversion doppler: a new ultrasound technique for nonlinear imaging of microbubble contrast agents and tissue. *Radiology* **209**, 190.

Cespedes, I., Huang, Y., *et al.* (1995). Methods for estimation of subsample time delays of digitized echo signals. *Ultrason. Imag.* **17**, 142–171.

Coghlan, B.A. and Taylor, M.G. (1976). Directional Doppler techniques for detection of blood velocities. *Ultrasound Med. Biol.* **2**, 181–188.

Dickinson, R.J. and Hill, C.R. (1982). Measurement of soft tissue motion using correlation between A-scans. *Ultrasound Med. Biol.* **8**, 263–271.

Dowsett, D.J., Kenney, P.A. and Johnston, R.E. (1998). Ultrasound principles, and ultrasound imaging. In *The Physics of Diagnostic Imaging*. Chapman & Hall, London, pp. 413–465.

Duck, F.A., Baker, A.C. and Starrit, H.C. (1998). *Ultrasound in Medicine*. IoP Publishing, Bristol.

Eckersley, R.J. (1996). Potential and limitations of ultrasound for imaging tumour vasculature. PhD thesis, University of London.

Evans, D.H. and McDicken, W.N. (2000). *Doppler Ultrasound; Physics, Instrumentation and Signal Processing* (2nd edn). John Wiley, Chichester.

Ferrara, K. and DeAngelis, G. (1997). Color flow mapping. *Ultrasound Med. Biol.* **23**, 321–345.

Gao, L., Parker, K.J., Lerner, R.M. and Levinson, S.F. (1996). Imaging of the elastic properties of tissue – a review. *Ultrasound Med. Biol.* **22**, 959–977.

Goldberg, B.B., Raichlen, J.S., *et al.* (2001). *Ultrasound Contrast Agents.* Martin Dunitz, London.

Harvey, C.J., Blomley, M.J., *et al.* (2001). Improved detection of liver metastases with pulse inversion mode during the liver-specific phase of microbubble Levovist (SHU 508A) in colorectal cancer. *Radiology* **221**, 268–269.

Hein, I.A. and O'Brien, W.D. (1993a). Current time-domain methods for assessing tissue motion by analysis from reflected ultrasound echoes – a review. *IEEE Trans. Ultrason. Ferroelectr. Freq. Control* **40**, 84–102.

Hein, I.A. and O'Brien, W.D. (1993b). A real-time ultrasound time-domain correlation blood flowmeter. 2. Performance and experimental verification. *IEEE Trans. Ultrason. Ferroelectr. Freq. Control* **40**, 776–785.

Holland, S.K., Orphanoudakis, S.C., *et al.* (1984). Frequency-dependent attenuation effects in pulsed Doppler ultrasound – experimental results. *IEEE Trans. Biomed. Eng.* **31**, 626–631.

Hope Simpson, D., Chin, C.T., *et al.* (1999). Pulse inversion Doppler: a new method for detecting nonlinear echoes from microbubble contrast agents. *IEEE Trans. Ultrason. Ferroelectr. Freq. Control* **46**, 372–382.

Jensen, J.A. (1993). Range velocity limitations for time-domain blood velocity estimation. *Ultrasound Med. Biol.* **19**, 741–749.

Kadi, A.P. and Loupas, T. (1995). On the performance of regression and step-initialized air clutter filters for color Doppler systems in diagnostic medical ultrasound. *IEEE Trans. Ultrason. Ferroelectr. Freq. Control* **42**, 927–937.

Kaluzynski, K. (1987). Analysis of application possibilities of autoregressive modeling to Doppler blood-flow signal spectral-analysis. *Med. Biol. Eng. Comput.* **25**, 373–376.

Kasai, C., Namekawa, K., *et al.* (1985). Real-time two-dimensional blood-flow imaging using an auto-correlation technique. *IEEE Trans. Son. Ultrason.* **32**, 458–464.

Kay, S.M. and Marple, S.L. (1981). Spectrum analysis – a modern perspective. *Proc. IEEE* **69**, 1380–1419.

Konofagou, E.E., Varghese, T. and Ophir, J. (2000). Spectral estimators in elastography. *Ultrasonics* **38**, 412–416.

Loupas, T. and McDicken, W.N. (1990). Low-order complex AR models for mean and maximum frequency estimation in the context of Doppler color flow mapping. *IEEE Trans. Ultrason. Ferroelectr. Freq. Control* **37**, 590–601.

Ophir, J., Alam, S.K., Garra, B.S., Kallel, F., Konofagou, E., Krouskop, T.A., Merritt, C.R.B., Righetti, R., Souchon, R., Srinivasan, S. and Varghese, T. (2003). Elastography: imaging the elastic properties of soft tissues with ultrasound (review article). *J. Med. Ultrasonics* **29**, 155–171.

Ophir, J., Alam, S.K., Garra, B., Kallel, F., Konofagou, E., Krouskop, T. and Varghese, T. (1999). Elastography: ultrasonic estimation and imaging of the elastic properties of tissues. Proceedings of the Institution of Mechanical Engineers Part H. *J. Eng. Med.* **213**, 203–233.

Ophir, J. and Parker, K.J. (1989). Contrast agents in diagnostic ultrasound. *Ultrasound Med. Biol.* **15**, 319–333.

Prager, W.R., Gee, A.H., Treece, G.M., Cash, C.J.C. and Berman, L.H. (2003). Sensorless freehand 3-D ultrasound using regression of the echo intensity. *Ultrasound Med. Biol.* **29**, 437–446.

Press, W.H., Flannery, B.P., *et al.* (1988). *Numerical Recipes.* Cambridge University Press, Cambridge.

Rajaonah, J.C., Dousse, B., *et al.* (1994). Compensation of the bias caused by the wall filter on the mean Doppler frequency. *IEEE Trans. Ultrason. Ferroelectr. Freq. Control* **41**, 812–819.

Reid, J. M. and Spencer, M.P. (1972). Ultrasonic Doppler technique for imaging blood vessels. *Science* **176**, 1235–1236.

Rubin, J.M., Bude, R.O., *et al.* (1994). Power Doppler ultrasound – a potentially useful alternative to mean frequency-based color Doppler ultrasound. *Radiology* **190**, 853–856.

Schlief, R. (1991). Ultrasound contrast agents. *Curr. Opin. Radiol.* **3**, 198–207.

Schlindwein, F.S. and Evans, D.H. (1989). A real-time autoregressive spectrum analyzer for Doppler ultrasound signals. *Ultrasound Med. Biol.* **15**, 263–272.

Schrope, B.A. and Newhouse, V.L. (1993). 2nd-Harmonic ultrasonic blood perfusion measurement. *Ultrasound Med. Biol.* **19**, 567–579.

Shiina, T., Nitta, N., Ueno, E. and Bamber, J.C. (2002). Real time tissue elasticity imaging using combined autocorrelation method. *J. Med. Ultrason.* **29**, 119–128.

Switzer, D.F. and Nanda, N.C. (1985). Doppler color flow mapping. *Ultrasound Med. Biol.* **11**, 403–416.

Taylor, K.J.W., Burns, P.N., *et al.* (1988). *Clinical Applications of Doppler Ultrasound.* Raven, New York.

Tiemann, K., Lohmeier, S., *et al.* (1999). Real-time contrast echo assessment of myocardial perfusion at low emission power: first experimental and clinical results using power pulse inversion imaging. *Echocardiogr. J. Cardiovasc. Ultrasound Allied Tech.* **16**, 799–809.

Torp, H., Olstad, B., Heimdal, A. and Bjaerum, S. (2002). Method and apparatus for providing real-time calculation and display of tissue deformation in ultrasound imaging. US Patent No. 6,352,307 B1.

Trahey, G.E., Smith, S.W. and von Ramm, O.T. (1986). Speckle pattern correlation with lateral aperture translation – experimental results and implications for spatial compounding. *IEEE Trans. Ultrason. Ferr.* **33**, 257–264.

Trahey, G.E., Allison, J.W., *et al.* (1987). Angle independent ultrasonic detection of blood-flow. *IEEE Trans. Biomed. Eng.* **34**, 965–967.

Tristam, M., Barbosa, D.C., Cosgrove, D.O., Bamber, J.C. and Hill, C.R. (1988). Application of Fourier analysis to clinical study of patterns of tissue movement. *Ultrasound Med. Biol.* **14**, 695–707.

Tuthill, T., Krucker, J., Fowlkes, J. and Carson, P. (1998). Automated 3-D US frame positioning computed from elevational speckle decorrelation. *Radiology* **209**, 575–582.

Tysoe, C. and Evans, D.H. (1995). Bias in mean frequency estimation of Doppler signals due to wall clutter filters. *Ultrasound Med. Biol.* **21**, 671–677.

Uhlendorf, V. (1994). Physics of ultrasound contrast imaging – scattering in the linear range. *IEEE Trans. Ultrason. Ferroelectr. Freq. Control* **41**, 70–79.

Vaitkus, P.J. and Cobbold, R.S.C. (1988). A comparative study and assessment of Doppler ultrasound spectral estimation techniques. 1. Estimation methods. *Ultrasound Med. Biol.* **14**, 661–672.

Vaitkus, P.J., Cobbold, R.S.C., *et al.* (1988). A comparative study and assessment of Doppler ultrasound spectral estimation techniques. 2. Methods and results. *Ultrasound Med. Biol.* **14**, 673–688.

Varghese, T., Konofagou, E.E., Ophir, J., Alam, S.K. and Bilgen, M. (2000). Direct strain estimation in elastography using spectral cross-correlation. *Ultrasound Med. Biol.* **26**, 1525–1537.

Villanueva, F.S. and Kaul, S. (1995). Assessment of myocardial perfusion in coronary artery disease using myocardial contrast echocardiography. *Coron. Artery Dis.* **6**, 18–28.

Walker, W.F. and Trahey, G.E. (1995). A fundamental limit on the performance of correlation-based phase correction and flow estimation techniques. *IEEE Trans. Ultrason. Ferroelectr. Freq. Control* **41**, 644–654.

Wei, K., Skyba, D.M., *et al.* (1997). Interactions between microbubbles and ultrasound: *in vitro* and *in vivo* observations. *J. Am. Coll. Cardiol.* **29**, 1081–1088.

Wei, K., Thorpe, J. *et al.* (1999). Quantification of total and regional renal blood flow using contrast ultrasonography. *Circulation* **100**, 921.

Wells, P.N.T. (1993). *Advances in Ultrasound Techniques and Instrumentation.* Churchill Livingstone, New York.

Wells, P.N.T. (1994). Ultrasonic colour flow imaging. *Phys. Med. Biol.* **39**, 2113–2145.

Yuan, Y.W. and Shung, K.K. (1987). Fluctuation rate of ultrasound backscattered from blood. *IEEE Trans. Ultrason. Ferroelectr. Freq. Control* **34**, 402.

Zagzebski, J.A. (1996). *The Essentials of Ultrasound Physics.* Mosby-Year Book, St Louis.

11

The Wider Context of Sonography

C. R. HILL

Institute of Cancer Research, Royal Marsden Hospital, UK

11.1 INTRODUCTION

This book is focused on the various roles of ultrasound in biology and medicine. It may be useful, however, briefly to stand back at this point and recall that investigative methods based on ultrasound have wide and varied applications outside this field, and that from some of these we may be able to derive useful ideas for our own work. Part of the purpose of this chapter is to take a quick look at such possibilities. At the same time we shall briefly outline a number of technical approaches that, having been developed for medical and biological purposes and although interesting in themselves, have not progressed to widespread usefulness.

In a manner that may seem to be somewhat arbitrary we shall consider these approaches in two groups: *macroscopy* and *microscopy*. The first of these includes methods and ideas that have been described as working at acoustic frequencies that allow appreciable penetration through human organs: roughly the range 1–30 MHz. Acoustic microscopy is generally thought of as predominantly a laboratory technique, operating at frequencies above this range and running up to some 3 GHz. Inevitably there is overlap: as previously described, for example (Chapter 9), clinical skin and interstitial approaches are reportedly working at frequencies up to some 100 MHz.

11.2 MACROSCOPIC TECHNIQUES

11.2.1 PLAIN TRANSMISSION IMAGING

Historically, the first medical ultrasonic images to be made were acoustic analogies of the plain X-ray: transmission shadowgraphs. These were trans-skull views of the human brain, using quartz crystals as projector and receiver, and were claimed at the time to demonstrate the outlines of the ventricles (Dussik *et al.* 1942, 1947). It is now known, however, that there are two major sources of artefact that arise in this type of imaging, and that the Dussiks' valiant efforts were dominated by these. In the first place (and a problem that is particularly acute in trans-skull work), velocity inhomogeneity between different tissues gives rise to refraction artefacts. This problem can now, to some extent, be overcome by recording only the first arrival signal at each point in the image, thus discriminating against non-rectilinear ray paths.

Physical Principles of Medical Ultrasonics, Second Edition. Edited by C. R. Hill, J. C. Bamber and G. R. ter Haar.
© 2004 John Wiley & Sons, Ltd: ISBN 0 471 97002 6

The second problem is the familiar one of coherent radiation speckle and here, to a greater extent than with pulse–echo imaging, it is possible to achieve substantial improvement in image clarity by arranging the irradiating source of ultrasound to be both spatially and temporally incoherent (Havlice *et al.* 1977).

Mainly because of interest in transmission imaging for industrial applications, there have been attempts to develop acoustic versions of a television camera. This idea was pioneered by Sokolov in Russia. A version of this due to Brown *et al.* (1975), together with a transmission image obtained with it, is illustrated in Figure 11.1.

11.2.2 TRANSMISSION RECONSTRUCTION IMAGING

The concept of 'computerised axial tomography' using X-rays, first described by Hounsfield in 1972, stimulated interest in the development of analogous acoustic techniques. We have already described how parametric images of attenuation coefficient and sound speed can be obtained in this way (see Chapter 9, Section 9.4.1), and examples of the kind of image that result are shown in Figure 11.2.

It is of interest here to note how the term 'axial tomography' was put to use in the context of digital reconstruction methods, generally without explicit recognition that it applies equally well to the pulse–echo ultrasound (analogue) reconstruction imaging that in fact pre-dated it by some 20 years.

11.2.3 BACKSCATTER DIGITAL RECONSTRUCTION

The comment has also been made in Chapter 9 that pulse–echo imaging, as conventionally used, is essentially unquantitative in the sense that observed echo amplitude is a resultant of two quantities, attenuation coefficient and backscattering coefficient, that are not separated by the technique.

The potential to separate such variables is inherent in the 'reconstruction imaging' process and, provided that adequate and appropriate sampling is carried out, the concept can be extended readily from transmission to the use of backscattered signals. The practical feasibility has been demonstrated for such an approach, thus offering the twin prospects of, on the one hand, true gain compensation of the pulse–echo image (which thus becomes quantitative and repeatable in the extent to which a particular display amplitude level correlates with histology, regardless of location) and, on the other, an independent attenuation image (Duck & Hill 1979a, b). A related but more ambitious approach, theoretical principles for which have been outlined in Chapter 6, is that of so-called *diffraction tomography*. This attempts to reconstruct, again from appropriate samples of scattered ultrasound, spatial distributions of mechanical quantities such as density and compressibility modulus (Mueller *et al.* 1978; Mueller 1980).

11.2.4 ACOUSTICAL HOLOGRAPHY

The concept of *holography* is well known in the optical context, where the term was proposed by Gabor, with connotation of the *whole picture* providing information not just on amplitude but also on phase. In optics the development of a method by which such a complete set of image information could be recorded readily and then exploited for image reconstruction was a major achievement and this soon led to thoughts that similar techniques might be developed in acoustics. Commencing in about 1965 a considerable amount of work

339

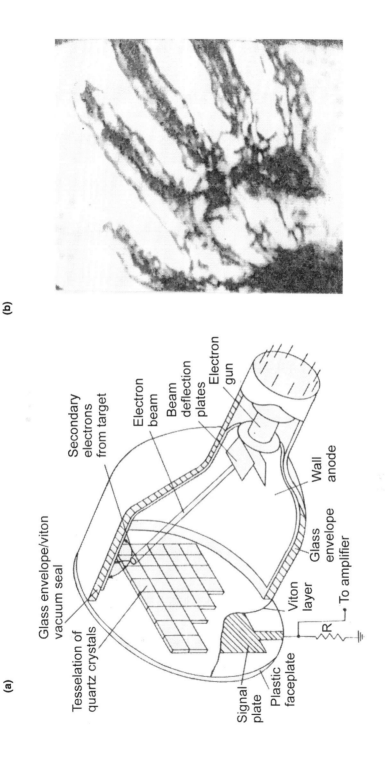

(a)

(b)

Figure 11.1. (a) Schematic arrangement of an ultrasonic image camera. The inner tube face is covered with piezoelectric material and charge distribution on its surface is sampled by means of a scanned electron beam. (b) Transmission image obtained by placing a hand over the face of the camera. *Source:* From Brown *et al.* (1975), published by IPC Science and Technology Press

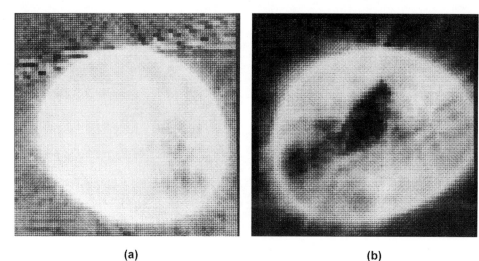

(a)   **(b)**

Figure 11.2. Tomographic *in vivo* breast images obtained by reconstructing the speed of sound from time-of-arrival data. Increasing speed of sound is indicated by a grey-scale shift in the direction white to black. (a) Normal, post-menopausal breast; (b) breast with large fibroadenoma. *Source*: From Glover (1977), reproduced by permission of Elsevier

was carried out in this direction and reported in the literature: see, for example, the review by Chivers (1977).

The logic of transposing the holography concept to acoustics needs careful examination. A major contrast with optics is that in acoustical imaging there is generally no fundamental difficulty in acquiring and recording phase information alongside amplitude, because sampling within the relevant range of acoustical frequencies is straightforward; it is merely simpler and cheaper to sample in amplitude only. In fact, a number of the methods under trial or proposed for parametric imaging (Chapter 9) use fairly conventional techniques for acquiring and using such 'holographic' data sets.

Such methods, however, entail appreciable instrumental complexity and so highlight a second contrast with optical holograms, which are normally formed relatively simply as interferograms between modulated and reference beams in the plane of a photographic emulsion. A practical acoustical analogy to this approach is to record, by scanned laser interferometry, the spatial patterns of liquid elevation resulting from local variations in acoustic radiation pressure that occur at an acoustic impedance interface on which a modulated ultrasonic beam is incident. An alternative is to scan the wavefront directly with an acousto-electric transducer (singly, or as an array) and to use an electrical signal for the phase reference. Both of these approaches have been used in acoustic microscopy and will be referred to below in more detail.

A problem arises in any attempt to reconstruct acoustical holograms. Whereas the image of an optical hologram can be reconstucted using radiation (visible light) of wavelength similar to that used for its formation, an acoustical hologram reconstructed using visible light will generally entail a wavelength shift by a factor of some 100–1000, with a consequent foreshortening of the image by the same proportion. The possibility remains, of course, to record an image in three dimensions and subsequently to display individual, selected planes. Even this approach, however, can be adversely affected by the inevitable contribution of out-of-plane signals to image noise, on which is superimposed a level of coherent radiation speckle that is accentuated by the requirement for narrow bandwidth operation.

Thus, although acoustical holography is an intriguing concept, appearing to offer some possibility for three-dimensional visualisation of human internal anatomy, its direct analogy to its optical counterpart is qualified by a number of major physical limitations. Its real value in medicine in the future seems more likely to be in the rather broader interpretation of the concept of joint exploitation of phase and amplitude information.

11.3 ACOUSTIC MICROSCOPY

11.3.1 BACKGROUND

The familiar, frequency-determined trade-off between spatial resolution and penetration depth has led to much interest in developing high-definition imaging devices for specialist clinical applications. As an example, Pavlin *et al.* (1991) have used frequencies up to 100 MHz for imaging corneal and other anterior structures of the eye. At the same time, there are several reasons for interest in using ultrasonic methods to study the fine-scale mechanical properties of biological tissues both *in vivo* and *ex vivo*: acoustic contrast will arise from very different mechanisms to, and thus may be expected to complement, optical microscopy; detailed information on the acoustic characteristics of tissues may also be able to guide developments in clinical parametric imaging.

Thus has grown up the subject that might be termed *biomedical acoustic microscopy*. This occupies a frequency range whose lower end is somewhat ill-defined, say between 20 and 50 MHz, and thus at present is around the upper frequency limit for transducer array technology. For most purposes a practical upper limit for microscopy is set by the properties of water as a transmission medium, because its absorption coefficient has a frequency-squared dependence and at 1 GHz has a value of 88 dB mm^{-1}.

Acoustic microscopy has so far found its main usefulness in materials science, where its application has largely been in the investigation of solid structures (see reviews by: Lemons & Quate 1979; Briggs *et al.* 1989; Kessler 1989). The idea was first investigated by Sokolov, in 1936, using a version of the ultrasonic image camera referred to above. Another approach, using a fine-wire thermocouple as a scanned detector, was subsequently described by Dunn and Fry (1959) but neither of these methods could provide a satisfactory combination of sensitivity and spatial resolution, and substantial developments only commenced after about 1970.

11.3.2 TECHNIQUES

There are several tried and successful approaches to acoustic microscopy, all of which are based on a scanning process. The two main classes of technique place the object being scanned respectively in the *far field* and *near field* of the acoustic transducer. In the former arrangement the beam is raster-scanned relative to the object (generally, for convenience, the object moves and the heavier transducer is fixed): hence the term *Scanning Acoustic Microscope* (*SAM*). In the near-field system the beam, having been amplitude- and phase-modulated by traversing the object, strikes the underside of a plane, liquid–solid surface whose resulting pattern of elevation (caused by radiation pressure of the beam) is sensed using a rapidly scanned laser beam: the *Scanned Laser Acoustic Microscope* (*SLAM*).

11.3.3 FAR-FIELD MICROSCOPIES: SAM

The basic arrangement of a scanning acoustic microscope is illustrated in Figure 11.3. An irradiating plane wave is lens-focused onto a resolution element of a thin object and the modulated energy is collected by an identical lens in the receiving system. Imaging is carried out by scanning the object in its own plane and recording the corresponding values of phase and amplitude. In a simple variant of this basic design, a single transducer/lens assembly is used for both transmission and reception and a plane reflector is placed immediately behind the object. Alternatively this single-transducer configuration can be used in backscatter instead of transmission mode. In this arrangement (previously referred to in Chapter 9 as a *C-scan*), echo signals returned from a thin layer of an extended object are selectively recorded by means of a time gate in the receiver: a system sometimes referred to in the literature as a *C-mode Scanning Acoustic Microscope (C-SAM)*.

A feature of immediate interest in the 'optics' of this type of acoustical instrument is that it is possible to build a system in which the lens and propagation fluid have very different propagation velocities (e.g. an acoustical speed ratio of 0.135 for water/sapphire; *cf.* a typical optical ratio of 0.66 for glass/air), a situation that gives negligibly low spherical aberration even at high relative apertures. This provides the prospect of very high resolving power, the

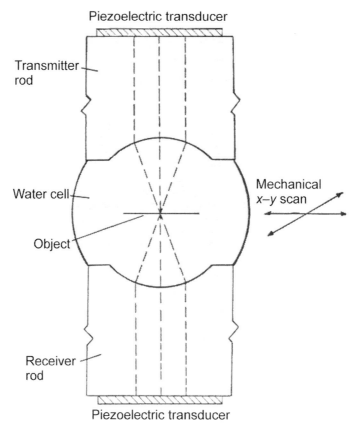

Figure 11.3. Principle of a scanning acoustic microscope (SAM), operating here in simple transmission mode. Transmission–reflection, stereo, dark-field and C-mode are other configurations potentially available

practical limit to which is imposed by the attenuation coefficient and sound speed of the propagation fluid. In fact it has been found useful to define a figure of merit, M, for a given propagation fluid (normalised to water) that is indicative of the potential resolving power of an instrument of given geometry and acousto-electrical properties, such that:

$$M^2 = [c_w^2 \cdot (\alpha/f^2)_w]/[c^2 \cdot (\alpha/f^2)]$$

where c_w and c are the propagation speeds in water and the fluid, respectively, and $(\alpha/f^2)_w$ and (α/f^2) are the corresponding values for attenuation coefficient per frequency squared.

For most molecular liquids M values are less than unity but higher values can be obtained with mercury (1.89), liquid nitrogen (2.1) and liquid helium (3.6) (Lemons & Quate 1979). Values of up to 5 can be obtained by working with compressed noble gasses: xenon at 4 MPa (40 bar), for example, has been predicted to enable resolution of 170 nm at 740 MHz, thus considerably exceeding the limit achievable with conventional optical microscopes (Petts & Wickramasinghe 1980).

The basic scanning acoustic microscope that has been described here is capable of a variety of modes of operation. The backcatter mode has been mentioned already but alternatively, in the two-transducer arrangement, if the axes of the transducers are mutually offset by some 10–20° while they remain confocal, dark-field imaging is achieved in which only forward-scattered energy is recorded. It is also possible to exploit the phenomenon of *harmonic pumping* (Chapter 1, Section 1.8.2): by irradiating at one frequency (e.g. 450 MHz) and tuning the receiving transducer to the second harmonic (900 MHz), an image representing spatial variations of the non-linearity parameter within the object is recorded (Lemons & Quate 1979). Examples of acoustic transmission micrographs, together with a corresponding harmonic image, are shown in Figure 11.4. Finally, using a single-transducer arrangement with a modified measurement procedure, it is possible to make rather accurate spot measurements of the attenuation coefficient and sound speed in a thin specimen placed on the surface of a plane reflector. Values of these quantities are extracted from the pattern of variation of the transducer-received signal output voltage, V, observed as the transducer is

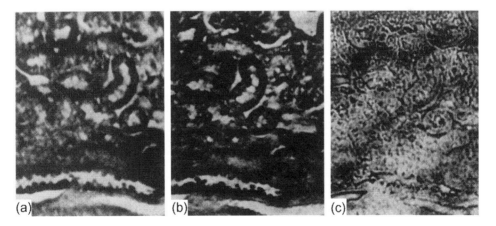

Figure 11.4. Acoustic transmission micrographs of a section of kidney tissue obtained with a scanning acoustic microscope: (a, b): images obtained at 450 and 900 MHz, respectively; (c) harmonic image obtained with a 450 MHz projector and a 900 MHz receiver. *Source*: From Lemons and Quate (1979), reproduced by permission of Elsevier

moved in the axial (z) direction relative to the object and reflector. This so-called $V(z)$ signal thus records the complex relationship that results from mode conversion of the incident compression-wave energy, subsequent radial propagation of surface waves at the reflector/ object interface and eventual re-radiation as compression waves (Weglein 1979). An extension of this technique that enables measurement of anisotropy in properties of the specimen is to use a line-focus transducer.

11.3.4 NEAR-FIELD MICROSCOPES: SLAM

In this class of instrument, illustrated in Figure 11.5, the modulated acoustic field is sensed through its radiation-pressure-induced displacement pattern in an optically reflecting surface (Kessler 1989). The specimen is immersed in a fluid, such as water, whose upper boundary is in contact with an optically flat and semi-reflecting surface of a solid transparent block. The amplitudes of displacements of this surface will be related to the attenuation coefficient in underlying regions of the object, and can be sensed as deflection of a scanned laser beam. The beam may be scanned in a standard video raster, thus permitting derivation and display of an image in 'real time'. Another useful feature of the arrangement is that a corresponding optical absorption image of the object can be obtained simultaneously by the use of a photodiode (placed as indicated in the figure).

The relative aperture, and thus the effective resolving power of this type of system at a given frequency, are limited by the critical angle for acoustic reflection at the optically reflecting

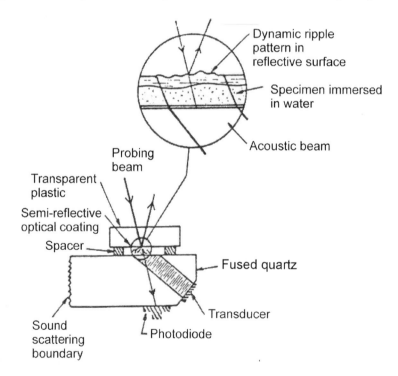

Figure 11.5. Principle of operation of a scanned laser acoustic microscope. *Source*: From Kessler (1989), reproduced by permission of ASM International

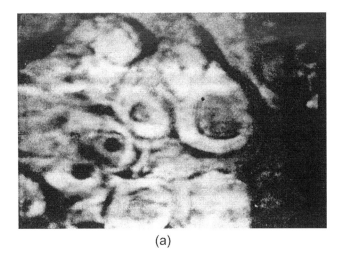

(a)

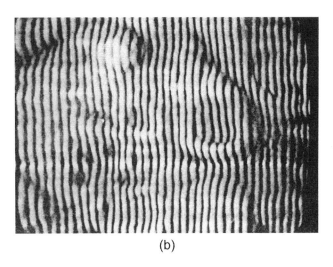

(b)

Figure 11.6. Acoustic micrographs of a 0.5 mm thick, unstained section of a human metastatic adenocarcinoma in the liver, obtained using a 100 MHz scanned laser acoustic microscope: (a) absorption micrograph showing collagenous septae surrounding groups of tumour cells, some of which have necrotic centres and appear to be the more strongly absorbing to ultrasound (darker in the image); (b) interference micrograph of the same section showing fringes whose lateral shift is proportional to the speed of sound in the specimen. *Source*: Courtesy of Dr R. Waag, University of Rochester and Dr L.W. Kessler, Sonoscan Inc

surface. Thus it is desirable to arrange for the ratio of sound speeds in the fluid and solid materials to be close to unity, and an appropriate plastic material is therefore chosen for the overlying block. An operating frequency range extending up to 500 MHz has been claimed, with achievable resolution corresponding to about one wavelength in the object material (e.g. 3 μm in water). Phase information (indicative of local values of sound speed in the specimen) can be derived in the form of an interferogram by appropriately mixing the received signals with an electronic reference signal. In a modification of the standard system, the acoustic angle of incidence at the reflecting block is set to coincide with the critical angle, thus achieving a dark-field image. Examples of acoustical absorption and phase-interferogram images obtained with a SLAM system are shown in Figure 11.6.

11.3.5 CONCLUSION

Although high spatial resolution is in itself an attractive prospect for acoustic microscopes, a more important role may prove to lie in their ability to provide information complementary to that given by optical microscopes. Contrast in an acoustical microscope arises from differences in the mechanical properties of materials and, although little systematically seems to be known about high-frequency properties of biological materials, it already appears that actual degrees of contrast found in acoustical images can be much greater than those seen in optical images, certainly in the absence of staining. Thus acoustical micrographs may prove to provide new information and also prove to be useful for examination of living cells and tissues (Bereiter-Hahn *et al.* 1989). They should also provide useful information about the nature of the acoustic inhomogeneities that give rise to the acoustic scattering processes (Chapter 6), which in turn provide the basis for many forms of clinical ultrasonic imaging (Chapter 9). In this context, the emphasis in acoustical microscopy may need to be not so much in high spatial resolution as in more quantitative assessment of the spatial patterns of variation of the mechanico-elastic properties of different tissues.

REFERENCES

Bereiter-Hahn, J., Litniewski, J., *et al.* (1989). What can scanning acoustic microscopy tell about animal cells and tissues? In *Acoustical Imaging*, Vol. 17. Plenum Press, New York, pp. 27–38.

Briggs, G.A.D., Daft, C.M.W., *et al.* (1989). Acoustic microscopy of old and new materials. In *Acoustical Imaging*, Vol. 17. Plenum Press, New York, pp. 1–16.

Brown, P.H., Randall, R.P., Fiyer, R.F. and Wardley, J. (1975). A high resolution, sensitive ultrasonic image converter. In *Ultrasonics International 1975 Conference Proceedings*. IPC Science and Technology Press, Guildford, pp. 73–79.

Chivers, R.C. (1977). Acoustical holography. In *Recent Advances in Ultrasound in Biomedicine*, Vol. 1, D.N. White (ed.). Research Studies Press, Forest Grove, pp. 217–251.

Duck, F.A. and Hill, C.R. (1979a). Mapping true ultrasonic backscatter and attenuation distribution in tissue: a digital reconstruction approach. In *Ultrasonic Tissue Characterisation II*, M. Linzer (ed.). NBS Special Publication No. 525. US Government Printing Office, Washington, DC, pp. 247–251.

Duck, F.A. and Hill, C.R. (1979b). Acoustic attenuation reconstruction from backscattered ultrasound. In *Computer Aided Tomography and Ultrasonics in Medicine*, J. Raviv *et al.* (eds). North Holland, Amsterdam, pp. 137–149.

Dunn, F. and Fry, W.J. (1959). Ultrasonic absorption microscope. *J. Acoust. Soc. Am.* **31**, 632–633.

Dussik, K.T. (1942). Über die Möglichkeit hochfrequente mechanische Schwingungen als diagnostisches Hilfsmittel zu verweten. *Z. Neurol. Psych.* **174**, 153–168.

Dussik, K.T., Dussik, F. and Wyt, L. (1947). Auf dem Wege zur Hyperphonographie des Gehirnes. *Wien Med. Ochenschr.* B97, 425–429.

Glover, G.H. (1977). Computerised time of flight ultrasonic tomography for breast examination. *Ultrasound Med. Biol.* **3**, 117–127.

Havlice, J.F., Green, P.S., Taenzer, J.C. and Mallen, W.F. (1977). Spatially and temporally varying insonification for the elimination of spurious detail in acoustic transmission imaging. In *Acoustic Holography*, Vol. 7, L.W. Kessler (ed.). Plenum Press, New York, pp. 291–305.

Kessler, L.W. (1989). Acoustic microscopy. In *Metals Handbook* (9th edn), Vol. 17. ASM International, Materials Park, OH, pp. 465–482.

Lemons, R.A. and Quate, C.F. (1979). Acoustic microscopy. In *Physical Acoustics*, Vol. 14, W.P. Mason and R.N. Thurston (eds). Academic Press, New York, pp. 1–91.

Mueller, R.K. (1980). Diffraction tomography I: the wave equation. *Ultrason. Imag.* **2**, 213–222.

Mueller, R.K., Kaveh, M. and Iverson, R.D. (1978). A new approach to acoustic tomography using diffraction techniques. In *Acoustical Imaging*, Vol. 8, A. Metherell (ed.). Plenum Press, New York, pp. 615–628.

Pavlin, C.J., Harasiewicz, K., Sherar, M.D. and Foster, F.S. (1991). Clinical use of ultrasound microscopy. *Ophthalmology* **98**, 287–295.

Petts, C.R. and Wickramasinghe, H.K. (1980). Acoustic microscopy in gasses. *Electron. Lett.* **16**, 9–11.

Weglein, R.D. (1979). *Appl. Phys. Lett.* **34**, 179–181.

12

Ultrasonic Biophysics

GAIL R. TER HAAR

Institute of Cancer Research, Royal Marsden Hospital, UK

12.1 INTRODUCTION

Ultrasonic biophysics is the branch of science that attempts to seek logical and quantitative understanding of a series of observations in which exposure to ultrasound is found to lead to various specific modifications in living cells and tissues. Historically, the first such observations seem to have been those of Langevin, in about 1917, who observed damage to fish in the course of his experimental development of high-power underwater ultrasonic transmitters intended for submarine detection. This observation stimulated the very remarkable biophysical research of Wood and Loomis (1927), which in turn led to a considerable body of observations, by numerous authors, much of which was unfortunately devoid of serious attempt at scientific understanding. In the present chapter we examine a variety of physical phenomena that are known, or thought, to account for the various types of link between ultrasonic exposure and biological effect.

Broadly speaking, such links can be classified as either 'thermal' or 'non-thermal'. In an empirical sense this distinction can be seen as one in which observed changes are, or are not, due primarily to an increase in temperature consequent on absorption of ultrasonic energy. A more physically satisfactory view, however, is gained by considering that the absorption of acoustic energy results largely from interaction at the molecular or macromolecular levels of a biological tissue, causing the molecules or parts of them to vibrate or rotate. If the molecules are relatively small and the system is fluid, the vibrational or rotational energy causes no specific chemical or biological change but is rapidly converted into heat. The absorption process may then be described as 'thermal'. In systems that are less fluid or contain giant molecules, or both, there is a possibility of 'non-thermal' specific effects. A somewhat quantitative appreciation of the situation can be gained by comparing some measure (e.g. velocity) of the motion of molecules that results from acoustic and thermal vibration (Clarke 1969). In a progressive, plane wave acoustic field the particle velocity, v_a, is given by [Chapter 1, table 1.1]

$$v_a = (2I/\rho_0 c)^{1/2} \tag{12.1}$$

and thus, for example, an intensity of $10\,\mathrm{W\,cm^{-2}}$ in water would correspond to a value of $v_a \approx 37\,\mathrm{cm\,s^{-1}}$.

By contrast, the mean particle velocity in thermal vibration modes is given classically by

Physical Principles of Medical Ultrasonics, Second Edition. Edited by C. R. Hill, J. C. Bamber and G. R. ter Haar.
© 2004 John Wiley & Sons, Ltd: ISBN 0 471 97002 6

$$v_t = (kT/m)^{1/2} \tag{12.2}$$

where T is absolute temperature, k is Boltzmann's constant and m is particle mass. Particle velocity here is dependent on mass and for a water molecule and a DNA molecule of molecular weight 10^7 we find $v_t = 3.8 \times 10^4$ and $52 \, \text{cm s}^{-1}$, respectively (at 37°C).

It might be of interest to examine the above situation using a more sophisticated analysis, but this simplistic approach serves to illustrate the general point that 'non-thermal' mechanisms in this context are likely to occur, if at all, in systems involving large molecular structures.

The above discussion has been concerned with systems having linear behaviour, in the sense that strain in the medium can be assumed to be linearly dependent on applied acoustic stress. Another class of mechanism is that in which non-linear behaviour is a critical factor, and in particular where oscillatory acoustic energy is transformed ('rectified') into a non-oscillatory energy form. In a strict sense the generation of heat by acoustic absorption is one example of such a situation, but other examples can be considered non-thermal. Of these, the phenomenon of cavitation is of particular importance and is dealt with in some detail later in this chapter. Here, as will be seen, acoustic energy may be transformed both into the energy of a steady-state fluid shear stress field and into the energy of reactive chemical species.

12.2 THERMAL MECHANISMS

12.2.1 THEORETICAL

The energy transported by an ultrasonic beam is attenuated as it passes through any viscous medium. If the intensity of a plane travelling wave is I_0 at the point of origin $x = 0$, it has reduced intensity $I(x)$ at a distance x from the origin, given by the expression

$$I(x) = I_0 e^{-\mu x} \tag{12.3}$$

where μ is the intensity attenuation coefficient (see Chapter 4). Thus, the energy lost from a unit cross-section of the primary sound beam in travelling the unit distance dI/dx is given by μI. As has been discussed in Chapter 4, Section 4.2, the attenuation coefficient μ is made up of two components: that due to absorption, μ_a, and that due to scattering, μ_s. Energy scattered out of the main beam may be absorbed elsewhere in the tissue.

To obtain an estimate of the temperature rise that may occur in tissue due to the attenuation of an ultrasonic beam, let us assume that all the energy removed from the primary beam leads to local tissue heating, i.e. we assume that attenuation is entirely due to absorption. (This may be a reasonable approximation because quoted values for μ_a in soft tissues vary between 0.6 and 0.9.) The rate of heat deposition per unit volume, $\dot{Q}$, is given by the equation

$$\dot{Q} = \mu I \tag{12.4}$$

If no heat is lost from this volume by conduction, convection or radiation

$$\dot{Q} = \rho C \frac{dT}{dt} \tag{12.5}$$

where ρ is the density of the medium, C is heat capacity and dT/dt is the rate of temperature rise. Figure 12.1 shows the way in which the rate of heat deposition varies with depth into homogeneous tissue for different frequencies, assuming an absorption coefficient of $1 \, \text{dB cm}^{-1} \, \text{MHz}^{-1}$.

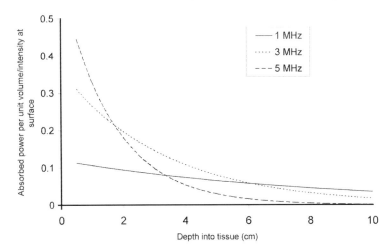

Figure 12.1. Graph showing the variation of heat deposition with depth travelled into homogeneous tissue for frequencies of 1, 3 and 5 MHz. An absorption coefficient of 1 dB cm^{-1} MHz^{-1} is assumed

Consider, for example, a substance for which $\mu = 0.2$ nepers cm^{-1}, $\rho = 1$ g cm^{-3} and $C = 4.18$ J g^{-1} °C^{-1}. These are approximate values for liver at room temperature at 1 MHz. Using these values and for an intensity of 1 W cm^{-2} the rate of temperature rise dT/dt is 0.048°C s^{-1} (2.88°C min^{-1}).

It is possible to estimate the effect that the thermal conductivity of the medium has on the final temperature achieved at equilibrium. Nyborg (1975) has shown that the temperature difference maintained at equilibrium between the centre of a highly absorbing sphere of radius R (at a temperature T_0) and its surrounding (T_∞) can be given by

$$\Delta T = \frac{\mu I}{2k} \cdot R^2 \tag{12.6}$$

where k is the thermal conductivity. From equation (12.4), $\dot{Q} = \mu I$ and thus

$$T_0 - T_\infty = \Delta T = \frac{\dot{Q}R^2}{2k} \tag{12.7}$$

For $I = 1$ W cm^{-2}, $\Delta T = 22.7\, R^2$°C ($k = 4.4\ 10^{-3}$ W cm^{-1}°C^{-1}; *cf.* Table 12.1). Thus, the centre of an absorbing sphere of radius 1 cm will maintain a temperature difference of 22.7°C above its surroundings, whereas a sphere of 1 mm will only maintain a temperature difference of 0.23°C. The characteristic time for the system to reach equilibrium, τ, is of the order R^2/D, where D is the thermal diffusivity ($D = k/\rho C$). For $R = 1$ cm, $\tau \sim 700$ s, for $R = 1$ mm, τ is 7 s.

Using simple heat diffusion equations, it is possible to calculate the temperature rise that would be expected in a tissue composed of a variety of tissue types. The advantage of such mathematical modelling is that it allows one to predict the influence of ultrasonic and tissue parameters on the temperature profiles that can be obtained.

The temperature distribution within the tissue is given by the equation

$$\frac{dT}{dt} = D\nabla^2 T \tag{12.8}$$

Table 12.1. Representative values of thermal conductivity, heat capacity, attenuation coefficient and thermal diffusivity for water, blood, bone and soft tissues

Parameter	Symbol	Water	Soft tissue	Bone	Blood	Units
Thermal conductivity	k	6×10^{-3}	4.4×10^{-3a}	$2.9\text{–}5.0 \times 10^{-3c}$	5×10^{-3c}	$W\,cm^{-1}C^{-1}$
Heat capacity	C	4.18	3.36^b	1.3^c	3.84^c	$J\,g^{-1}C^{-1}$
Attenuation coefficient (at 1 MHz)	μ	0.2×10^{-3}	$0.17\text{–}0.33^b$	$2.5\ (\text{skull})^c$ $1.44\ (\text{long bone})$	2.4^c	neper cm^{-1}
Thermal diffusivity	D	1.44×10^{-3}	1.2×10^{-3a}		1.2^c	$cm^2\,s^{-1}$

[a]Chan *et al.* (1973).
[b]Nassiri *et al.* (1979) (values for skeletal muscle).
[c]Duck (1990).

where D is the diffusion constant (diffusivity).

The temperature rise in a system for which there is both a source of heat (of power deposition rate per unit volume, $\dot{Q}$) and a mechanism for cooling may be described by the transient heat transfer equation

$$\rho_t C_t \frac{\partial T}{\partial t} = k_t \nabla^2 T - A(x, y, z, t) + \dot{Q} \tag{12.9}$$

where ρ_t, C_t and k_t are the density, specific heat and thermal conductivity of the tissue (Pennes 1948). The absorbed power per unit volume, $\dot{Q}$, is given by $\dot{Q} = \mu_a I$. (Electromagnetic heating sources are often described in terms of their specific absorption rate, SAR, which is the time derivative of the incremental energy absorbed by an incremental mass: $\dot{Q} = \text{SAR} \times \rho_0$).

The cooling term $A(x, y, z, t)$ depends on thermal conductivity and blood flow to the region, and is thus dependent on both ambient temperature and position. In general, to a good approximation, $A(x, y, z, t)$ may be written as

$$A(x, y, z, t) = W_b C_b (T - T_b) + [G(T - T_b)^2 f(t)] \tag{12.10}$$

where W_b, C_b and T_b are the perfusion, specific heat and temperature of the blood, respectively, and G is a constant. The function $f(t)$ is an appropriate function of time that takes into account, for example, the cooling due to vasodilation that is triggered when a threshold is exceeded. Commonly the squared term is taken to be negligible and the cooling term is reduced to

$$A(x, y, z, t) = W_b C_b (T - T_b) \tag{12.11}$$

This describes tissue cooling by blood perfusion. It is assumed that blood enters the volume at the temperature of arterial blood (core temperature) and leaves at the temperature of heated tissues.

Equation (12.9) may be solved numerically using either a finite difference or finite element method (Crank 1967; Wu & Nyborg 1992; Kolios *et al.* 1996; Meaney *et al.* 1998). Chan *et al.* (1973) have shown that good agreement is achieved between theory and experiment using these equations. Figure 12.2a shows the intensity distribution for a focused bowl transducer (10 cm diameter, 15 cm focal length, 1.7 MHz) incident on tissue. The effect of tissues of different attenuation coefficient values in the central layer of the tissue sandwich is seen. Figure 12.2b shows the absorbed energy distribution for the same beam and tissue geometry. These figures are used to illustrate the difficulties encountered in predicting the temperature distributions that may be achieved with a specified ultrasonic beam when the acoustic

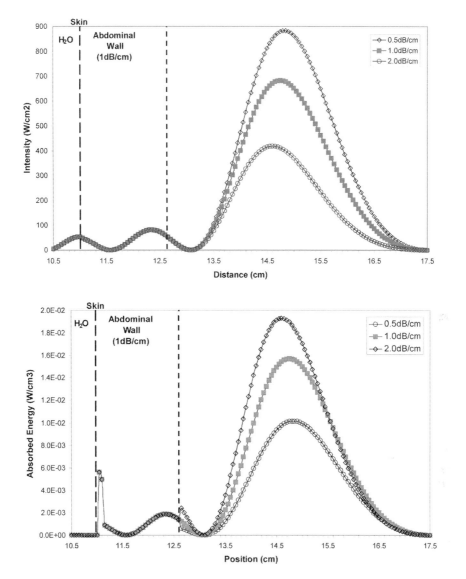

Figure 12.2. (a) Intensity distribution in layered tissues from a focused bowl transducer such as is used for focused ultrasound surgery (see Chapter 13, Section 13.5). Abdominal wall is assumed to overlie a homogeneous soft tissue layer of attenuation 0.5, 1.0 or 2.0 dB cm^{-1}. (Bowl diameter 10 cm; focal length 15 cm; frequency 1.7 MHz.) (b) Absorbed energy distribution for the beam and tissue geometry shown in (a) *Source*: Courtesy of Dr I. Rivens

properties of the tissue are not known accurately. The spread of attenuation coefficients illustrated reflects that measured for different orientations of skeletal muscle fibres (Nassiri *et al.* 1979). Similar variations in temperature profiles may be seen when the blood flow in the modelled tissue volume is altered slightly (Hynynen *et al.* 1981).

Figure 12.3 shows the temperature distributions that result from exposure of liver to the focused ultrasound beam illustrated in Figure 12.2. This type of beam is used in high-intensity focused ultrasound surgery (see Chapter 13, Section 13.5). Figure 12.3a shows the temperature distribution immediately after a 2 s exposure (spatial peak intensity $I_{SP} = 1220\,\text{W cm}^{-2}$) and Figure 12.3b shows the temperature 3 s later. It can be seen that, over this time scale, the peak temperature in the field drops but conduction broadens out the heated region.

The temperature rise induced in tissue by diagnostic probes is of particular interest to those concerned with the safety aspects of ultrasound. There have been a number of models designed to address this topic for both focused and unfocused beams (Nyborg & Steele 1983; Thomenius 1990; Wu & Nyborg 1992; Wu *et al.* 1992; NCRP 1992; AIUM/NEMA 1992; Bly *et al.* 1992; Filipczinski *et al.* 1993; Wojcik *et al.* 1999). The NCRP model estimates the 'worst case' (i.e. the highest) steady-state temperature that is ever to be expected in tissue as a result of exposure to a given ultrasonic field. This is different from the AIUM/NEMA predictions that estimate the temperatures that are 'not expected' to be exceeded in the majority of ultrasound examinations. This type of model is often referred to as 'reasonable worst case'. The differences in the models result from the choice of geometry and the acoustic properties ascribed to the tissues lying in the beam path. The AIUM Bio-effects Committee has compared the results from these two models in homogeneous soft tissues and showed that there may be as much as a factor of 3 difference in the estimated temperature rise (AIUM 1994). Duck *et al.* (1989) have made some measurements showing that there may be significant electrical heating of the transducer front surface. The maximum temperature rise was found in pulsed Doppler mode where a surface temperature rise of 50°C was recorded for a transducer operating in air. Wu *et al.* (1992) introduced the effects of transducer heating into their calculations of temperatures achieved in tissue and showed that this may be the dominant source of tissue heating near the transducer.

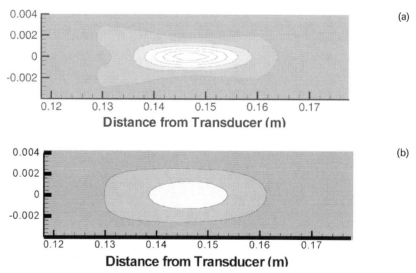

Figure 12.3. Temperature distributions resulting from the exposure of liver to the intensity distribution shown in Figure 12.2a. (a) The distribution after 2 s as the sound is switched off. (b) The distribution 3 s after the sound is switched off. The calculation is for a spatial peak intensity of 1220 W cm^{-2}. *Source:* Courtesy of Dr P. Meaney

As has been discussed in earlier chapters, transverse (shear) waves are very strongly absorbed in soft tissues. Thus, where they are launched into such a tissue, as may happen at a bone surface (as a result of 'mode conversion' or otherwise), there can be a very high rate of heating close to that surface. In particular, this may be experienced as heating of the periosteum – a region rich in nerve endings. If the temperature rise is sufficiently great, pain may be felt and permanent damage is possible.

Bly *et al.* (1992) used the NCRP model to calculate maximum temperature rises in the fetus during trans-abdominal pulsed Doppler fetal applications. They based their calculations on the maximum outputs from pulsed Doppler equipment used in Canada. Although they estimated that the majority of exposures during the first trimester would give temperature rises below 1°C, they calculated that the maximum would be 1.6°C. It has been estimated that at the FDA maximum derated intensity limit of I_{SPTA} (720 mW cm^{-2}) (see Chapter 14, Section 14.2) the maximum temperature rise at the conceptus would be 2°C (AIUM 1994). There is considerable discrepancy in calculated temperature rises later in pregnancy when there is bone present. Bly *et al.* (1992) used the Canadian output data from diagnostic ultrasound equipment to calculate a maximum of 8.7°C, whereas Patton *et al.* (1994) used output data from equipment approved by the US FDA between 1990 and 1991 and estimated the maximum to be 5.9°C. The accuracy of these predictions is, in part, determined by the choice of acoustic parameters used for bone. For example, the attenuation coefficient of bone varies with degree of mineralisation (and therefore with gestational age) (Drewniak *et al.* 1989; Bosward *et al.* 1993).

12.2.2 EXPERIMENTALLY DETERMINED TEMPERATURE DISTRIBUTIONS

The complex nature of the dependence of tissue temperature rise on ultrasonic, environmental and tissue parameters that has been discussed in Section 12.2.1 means that it can be difficult to predict temperature distributions with any accuracy. The published literature contains very little information about experimentally determined temperature distributions *in vivo*. Early published data were concerned primarily with therapeutic ultrasound exposure conditions.

As discussed in Section 12.2.1 above, the temperature distributions that are achieved in an irradiated volume of soft tissue can be modified greatly if that volume contains or overlies bone. Bender *et al.* (1953) have described the effect of ultrasonic irradiation on dog femora into which thermocouples had been implanted. They used 800 kHz ultrasound for 2 min, with 5 W of power being emitted from a 5 cm^2 irradiating area. Temperature measurements were made in the bone cortex, in bone marrow and in the soft tissue lying between the transducer and the femur. Data from their paper are shown in Figure 12.4. The greatest temperature rise was found in the cortical bone. Similar differential heating has been described by Lehmann *et al.* (1967a).

Lehmann *et al.* (1967b) have indicated that heating at bone interfaces (presumably due to mode conversion as discussed above) may define the pain tolerance limits for ultrasonic treatment. They showed that patients with less than 8 cm of soft tissue cover over bone reached their pain tolerance limit more quickly (in terms of treatment time at a given intensity) than those with more soft tissue cover.

In a comparative study of the effects of short-wave, microwave and ultrasonic diathermy for the treatment of hip joints, it has been found that short-wave and microwave heating (at the maximum tolerated dose) gave rise to first-degree burns in skin and subcutaneous tissue without appreciable heating of the hip joint. Ultrasound, however, produced an adequate temperature rise at the bone without skin heating (Lehmann *et al.* 1959).

Very little information is available as to heating patterns obtained in soft tissues in the absence of bone, as might be important in diathermy applications. ter Haar and Hopewell

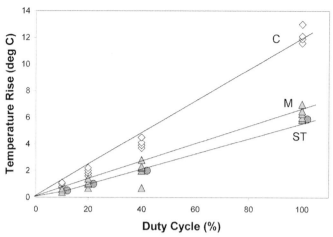

Figure 12.4. Temperature rise measured in dog femora, 800 kHz, 1 W cm^{-2}, 2 min. ST: soft tissue; M: marrow; C: cortex. *Source*: Adapted from Bender *et al.* (1953)

(1982) have studied temperatures in the pig thigh muscle. Figure 12.5 shows the results of these measurements. The normal resting temperatures in the pig thigh measured down to a depth of 4 cm are shown. The data are averaged over six experimental animals. Also shown is the temperature distribution obtained following 0.75 MHz ultrasonic irradiation at 2.0 W cm^{-2}. A normal physiological response to elevated temperatures is a change in blood flow. Volume blood flows in heated muscle, calculated from the cooling curves obtained when the ultrasound is switched off in the work described above, show a 2–3-fold enhancement over the basal value when the temperature is raised to 40–45°C. Paul and Imig (1955) also found that ultrasonic heating of tissue to temperatures of 42–44°C increased the flow in dog femoral arteries.

Rosenberger (1950) showed that when the sciatic nerves of experimental animals were irradiated *in situ* with 2 W cm^{-2} of 0.8–1 MHz ultrasound, the sciatic nerve showed a greater temperature rise than the surrounding tissues (see Figure 12.6). This has also been seen by Gersten (1959). Herrick (1953) has shown in the rat that ultrasonic irradiation (0.8–1 MHz) that gives rise to no observable histological change in muscle surrounding nerve fibres may lead to degeneration of the nerve fibres themselves. The damage seen is similar to that produced by excessive heating.

The debate about diagnostic ultrasound safety has led to several studies of temperature rises induced by clinical beams incident on tissue *in vitro* and, more importantly, *in vivo*. A 5 MHz mechanical sector scanner with $I_{SPTA} = 2$ W cm^{-2} (beam width 1.9 mm) gave a maximum temperature increase in fresh pig liver of 1.9°C after 2 min (ter Haar *et al.* 1989); similar equipment gave a maximum temperature rise in freshly excised sheep brain of 2.5°C after 5 min (WFUMB 1992). *In vitro* exposure of guinea pig brain to a 3.2 MHz ($I_{SPTA} = 2.95$ W cm^{-2}, 2.5 mm beam width) simulated pulsed Doppler beam led to a maximum temperature rise of 2.5°C (Bosward *et al.* 1993).

The majority of studies have concentrated on heating of bone by pulsed Doppler beams and in particular, because of the potential of thermal damage to the central nervous system, heating at the interface between bone and the fetal brain has been a focus for interest. Temperatures of 5°C have been recorded in the guinea pig fetal brain close to the parietal bone (Bosward *et al.* 1993; Horder *et al.* 1999). Duggan *et al.* (1995) recorded a temperature rise of 1.7°C in the cerebral cortex of sheep fetuses exposed *in utero* to 0.3 W cm^{-2} (I_{SPTA}) for 120 s. Tarantal *et al.* (1993)

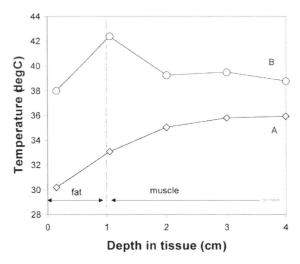

Figure 12.5. Temperature distributions in pig thigh: (A) resting temperatures in the thigh; (B) temperature achieved using 0.75 MHz ultrasound at a spatial average intensity of 2.0 W cm^{-2} (see text for details)

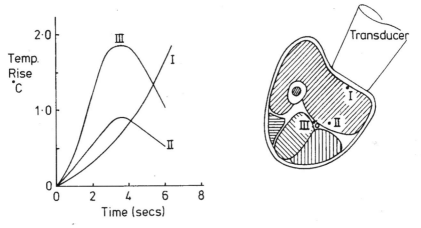

Figure 12.6. Temperatures measured in mouse sciatic nerve (III), muscle (II) and subcutaneous tissue (I) following ultrasonic radiation. *Source*: Adapted from Rosenberger (1950)

measured intracranial temperatures in monkeys. They found that the greatest temperature they could measure 3.6–4.6 cm deep in the brain was 0.6°C (72–54 mW cm^{-2} I_{SPTA} in water). A number of people have shown that the temperature rise achieved in the fetus increased with gestational age (and thus degree of bone mineralisation) (Drewniak *et al.* 1989 – in human femora; Carstensen *et al.* 1990b – in mice; Bosward *et al.* 1993 – in guinea pig brain; Horder *et al.* 1998 – in guinea pigs; Doody *et al.* 1999 – in human vertebrae). Doody *et al.* (1999) showed that the temperature rise resulting from a 50 mW pulsed Doppler beam incident on human fetal vertebrae *in vitro* ranged from 0.6°C after 295 s in the 14-week gestational age samples to 1.8°C in 39-week samples. Horder *et al.* (1998) recorded a peak temperature rise of 4.9°C at the skull/brain interface in guinea pig fetuses of gestational age 57–61 days and 4.3°C for the same beam in

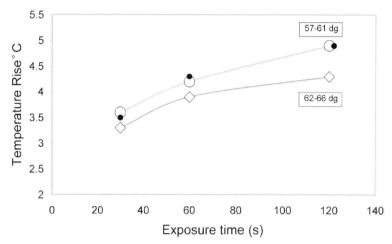

Figure 12.7. Temperature rises recorded at the skull/brain interface in guinea pig fetuses at 57–61 days' gestation and 62–67 days' gestation during exposure to beams typical of pulsed Doppler examinations: (○) 57–61 day gestation live fetuses; (◇) 62–66 day gestation live fetuses; (●) dead fetuses. *Source:* Adapted from Horder *et al.* (1998)

fetuses aged 62–67 days' gestation (see Figure 12.7). There was a 9% difference in temperature between perfused (live) and unperfused tissue for the older fetuses but only a 2% difference for the younger, and so they attributed this to the more substantially developed cerebral vasculature in the older fetuses.

Thus, although it is a well-known fact that absorption of ultrasonic energy by tissue leads to a rise in temperature, sufficient scientific investigation of this effect has not yet been undertaken to allow accurate prediction of heating profiles in tissue. It is known, however, that bony or gaseous inclusions in irradiated soft tissue volumes can give rise to local 'hot spots' because of mode conversion, reflection of the ultrasound beam or cavitation effects (see Section 12.3). Thus, special attention should be given to the nature of the irradiated tissue structure when thermal effects are either specifically desired or are to be avoided. The thermal index (*TI*) that is displayed on modern diagnostic ultrasound scanners is designed to help the user make an informed decision about the thermal risk associated with an ultrasound scan (see Chapter 12, Section 12.7, and Chapter 14, Section 14.6).

12.3 CAVITATION

Much of the literature reporting chemical and biological effects of ultrasound has been without adequate evidence to enable the identification of an operative mechanism. Much of the work that has been carried out has been under conditions (particularly that where liquid media are exposed) for which the occurrence of cavitation as a predominant mechanism would have been a strong possibility, whereas the basis for extrapolating the results to conditions applying in intact mammalian tissues has generally been unclear. In this situation a good understanding of the phenomenon of cavitation and of the factors that determine and limit its operation will be essential for any thorough comprehension of the subject of ultrasonic biophysics. The present section therefore takes up the study of this phenomenon in some detail.

12.3.1 DEFINITION

Many definitions of cavitation are to be found in the literature. Neppiras (1980a) defines cavitation as occurring 'whenever a new surface is created in the body of a liquid'. This broad definition includes boiling and effervescence. Apfel (1980) defines cavitation as the 'formation of one or more pockets of gas (or "cavities") in a liquid', whereas Coakley and Nyborg (1978) think of cavitation as being the term used to describe 'the activities, simple or complex, of bubbles or cavities containing gas or vapour, in liquids or any media with liquid content'.

In this section, attention is concentrated on *acoustic cavitation*, which is defined here as the formation and activity of gas- or vapour-filled cavities (bubbles) in a medium exposed to an ultrasonic field.

Common terminology distinguishes two types of bubble activity, namely *inertial* (formerly known as collapse or transient) and *non-inertial* (formerly referred to as stable) cavitation. Inertial cavitation occurs when a gas-filled cavity in a liquid expands during part of an acoustic cycle and then collapses very rapidly to a small fraction of its initial volume. The bubble's inertia controls its motion during collapse, hence the name (Flynn 1964). High temperatures and pressures are generated at the position of the bubble's minimum volume, and these may have important practical consequences of energy transfer to such forms as emission of light and the formation of reactive chemical species (as discussed below). Gaitan and Crum (1990) have shown that under some circumstances the bubble may remain intact after collapse and may repeat the expansion–contraction cycle indefinitely in a continuous sound field. Under other conditions, the bubble may collapse asymmetrically and disintegrate into small fragments.

Non-inertial cavitation is the term used to describe the activities of a range of gas-filled bodies in an ultrasonic field. The gas may be in bubbles in a liquid or may, for example, be contained within channels in plant tissues or in an animal's lung. The activities include translational motion, surface distortions, growth by rectified diffusion or other means and microstreaming.

Figure 12.8 shows radius–time curves to demonstrate the difference in bubble behaviour between inertial and non-inertial cavitation activity.

12.3.2 FORMATION OF CAVITIES

The origin of cavities that grow and become active under the action of an externally applied acoustic field has been the subject of some controversy. A detailed discussion of this complex topic is contained in Leighton (1994).

Large bubbles of radius R will rise in a fluid at a velocity, defined by Stokes' viscous drag and the buoyant force, given by

$$v = \frac{2\rho_0 g\, R^2}{9\eta} \tag{12.12}$$

where ρ_0 is the liquid density and η is the liquid viscosity. A $10\,\mu m$ bubble in water, for example, rises at the rate of $\sim 0.2\,\mathrm{mm\,s^{-1}}$. Smaller bubbles, on the other hand, may dissolve. Consider a bubble of radius R with internal pressure p_b. If the hydrostatic pressure in the liquid is p, the difference in pressure across the bubble surface is given by

$$p_b - p = \frac{2\sigma}{R} \tag{12.13}$$

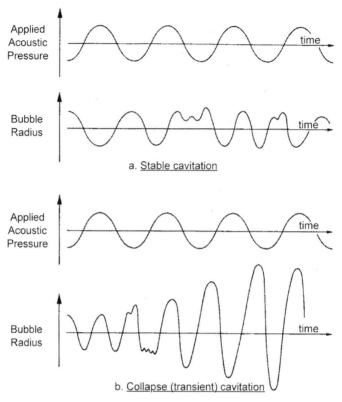

Figure 12.8. Radius–time curves for cavitating bubbles in an ultrasonic field: (a) non-inertial cavitation – the cavity exists for a considerable number of acoustic cycles, oscillating about an equilibrium radius; (b) inertial cavitation – the cavity oscillates in an unstable fashion, grows rapidly and collapses violently

where σ is the surface tension. It is seen that the excess pressure within the bubble increases with decreasing bubble radius. For bubbles of radius 1 μm in a liquid for which $\sigma = 80$ dyne cm^{-1}, the excess pressure is ~ 1.5 atmospheres.

For an unsaturated liquid, the pressure of the dissolved gas, p_g, is less than the hydrostatic pressure p. It therefore follows that the pressure of gas within the bubble is greater than the gas pressure in the liquid ($p_b > p_g$) and gas will diffuse out of the cavity. In this way, small bubbles in a liquid will dissolve. It can be calculated (Epstein & Plesset 1950) that for water that is just saturated ($p_g = p_b$) a 10 μm bubble takes 7 s to dissolve.

Thus, because large bubbles rise up out of a liquid by buoyancy and small bubbles dissolve, it is necessary to provide some explanation for the existence of nuclei from which cavities are formed. Several theories have been put forward as to the way in which gas or vapour-filled nuclei may be stabilised.

It has been reported (Sette & Wanderlingh 1962) that cosmic rays, neutrons and heavy ions can create nuclei in a liquid such as water. Greenspan and Tschiegg (1967) describe artificial nucleation by neutrons and alpha particles.

Fox and Herzfeld (1954) have suggested that organic molecules may form a 'skin' on the bubble and that this could act as a barrier to gas diffusion out of the cavity. Another theory that has been put forward to account for stabilisation of microbubbles is that the bubble may carry a surface charge (Flynn 1964).

Crevices can exist on dust particles and impurities contained in fluids and also on the surfaces of the container. These crevices, known as motes, can trap gas. Apfel (1970) has discussed the role of motes in promoting cavitation. The excess pressure inside a mote is small (given by σ/R where R is the radius of the mote), but under the action of a sufficiently high intensity sound field gas may be pumped into it and the cavity may grow. It has been shown that the intensity of sound required to produce cavitation is markedly increased as the purity of the liquid is increased.

Small bubbles may grow by a process of 'rectified diffusion'. A simple explanation of this is that during the acoustic pressure cycle gas alternately diffuses into the bubble (during rarefaction) and out of the bubble (during compression). The net flow of gas is inwards, because the surface area is greatest during rarefaction and this leads to bubble growth. A more sophisticated explanation is given by Hsieh and Plesset (1961). In order for bubbles to grow by rectified diffusion, the acoustic pressure must exceed a threshold value. It is this diffusion threshold value that is thought to determine the threshold for cavitation occurrence.

12.3.3 CAVITATION THRESHOLDS

There has been recognition in the literature that several 'thresholds' may be involved in acoustic cavitation (see Figure 12.9). Neppiras (1980a, b) defines two thresholds.

Thresholds are usually described in terms of the parameters P_A (acoustic pressure amplitude), P_0 (ambient pressure), R_0 (initial bubble radius) and w (angular frequency of the ultrasonic radiation).

12.3.3.1 Non-inertial Cavitation Threshold

Hsieh and Plesset (1961) have shown that the rate at which gas flows into a bubble during rarefaction, dm/dt, is given by

$$\frac{dm}{dt} = \frac{8\pi}{3} DC_\infty R_0 \left(\frac{P_A}{P_0}\right)^2 \qquad (12.14)$$

where D is the diffusion constant and C_∞ is the gas concentration in the liquid in the absence of the bubble. This expression ignores surface tension effects. Surface tension may be included if the right-hand side is multiplied by (Neppiras 1980b)

$$\left(1 + \frac{2\sigma}{R_0 P_A}\right)$$

Similarly, the rate at which gas diffuses out of the bubble during compression is given by

$$\frac{dm}{dt} = -4\pi DC_\infty R_0 \left(1 + \frac{2\sigma}{R_0 P_0} - \frac{C_\infty}{C_0}\right) \qquad (12.15)$$

where C_0 is the saturation gas concentration in the liquid.

A threshold condition is reached when the flow of gas during both phases of the pressure cycle is equal. This condition is described by the equation

$$\left(\frac{P_A}{P_0}\right)^2 = \frac{3}{2}\left[1 - \frac{C_\infty}{C_0}\left(1 + \frac{2\sigma}{R_0 P_0}\right)^{-1}\right] \qquad (12.16)$$

Above this threshold bubbles can grow and may eventually achieve resonant size in the sound field. The equation applies only for bubbles very much smaller than resonant size.

Neppiras (1980b) has shown that the threshold is described more exactly by the condition

$$\left(\frac{P_A}{P_0}\right)^2 = \frac{3}{2}\left[1 + \frac{2\sigma}{R_0 P_0} - \frac{C_\infty}{C_0}\right]\left[1 + \frac{2\sigma}{R_0 P_0}\right]^{-1}[(1 - \beta^2)^2 + \beta\delta^2] \tag{12.17}$$

where

$$\beta^2 = \left(\frac{\omega}{\omega_0}\right)^2 = \frac{\rho R_0^2 \omega^2}{3\gamma P_0}$$

δ is the damping factor and ω and ω_0 are the imposed and resonant angular frequencies, respectively (Coakley & Nyborg 1978).

Derivation of equation (12.17) takes into account that the forced oscillation of a bubble in a liquid under the influence of an ultrasonic field is a resonant system. For frequencies up to 100 kHz, resonance occurs for

$$\omega_0 = \frac{1}{R_0}\left(\frac{3\gamma P_0}{\rho}\right)^{1/2} \tag{12.18}$$

(Minnaert 1933), where γ is the ratio of the specific heats for the gas inside the bubble.

Above 100 kHz, surface tension effects must be taken into account and resonance is defined by the equation

$$\omega_0 = \frac{1}{R_0}\left\{\frac{3\gamma}{\rho_0}P_0\left[1 + \frac{2\sigma(3\gamma - 1)}{3\gamma R_0 P_0}\right]\right\}^{1/2} \tag{12.19}$$

[*cf.* equation (4.31)].

At megahertz frequencies, the effective value of γ lies between 1 and 1.4. Figure 12.9 shows a graph of resonant bubble size plotted against frequency for a surface tension of 73 dyne cm^{-1} and $\gamma = 1$ (curve A) and $\gamma = 1.4$ (curve B), and also for zero surface tension with $\gamma = 1$ (Coakley & Nyborg 1978). It can be seen from equation (12.17) that the acoustic pressure required to produce cavitation exhibits a minimum at resonance frequency.

12.3.3.2 Inertial Cavitation Thresholds

Corresponding calculations have been made for the upper and lower thresholds that define the range of acoustic pressures over which inertial (collapse) cavitation may occur (see, for example: Noltingk & Neppiras 1950; Neppiras & Noltingk 1951; Neppiras 1980b).

For small bubbles (well below resonant size) the threshold for inertial cavitation is known as the 'Blake' threshold (Blake 1949). This is given by

$$P_T = P_0 + \frac{4}{3}\left\langle 2\sigma^3\left\{3 R_0^3\left(P_0 + \frac{2\sigma}{R_0}\right)\right\}^{-1}\right\rangle^{1/2} \tag{12.20}$$

(Neppiras 1980b). For bubbles greater than resonant size, this condition becomes

$$\frac{R_0}{R_r} = 0.46(p - 1)p^{1/2}\left[1 + \frac{2}{3}(p - 1)\right]^{-1/3} \tag{12.21}$$

where R_r is the resonant radius and $p = P_A/P_0$.

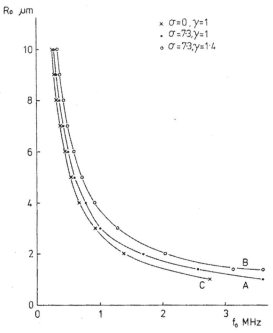

Figure 12.9. Graph of bubble radius at resonance as a function of frequency for three conditions (see text). (A) $\sigma = 7.3\,\mathrm{N\,m^{-2}}$, $\gamma = 1$; (B) $\sigma = 7.3\,\mathrm{N\,m^{-2}}$, $\gamma = 1.4$; (C) $\sigma = 0\,\mathrm{N\,m^{-2}}$, $\gamma = 1$

12.3.3.3 Cavitation Processes in Free Liquid

It is possible to describe the cavitation process in free liquid in terms of a pressure–radius diagram as shown in Figure 12.10. Curve A shows the stable cavitation threshold as defined by equation (12.17), curve B shows the Blake threshold described by equation (12.20) and curve C shows the threshold defined by equation (12.21).

Any bubble lying in region I will not grow but will dissolve into the liquid. Any bubble in region II undergoes unstable growth, collapse and possible disintegration into microbubbles of different sizes that may populate regions II and/or III. Bubbles in region II may also grow by rectified diffusion and undergo stable oscillation. Some bubbles (a) will grow into region III where they will collapse, and others (b) will remain in region II until they have grown sufficiently to allow them to rise out of the field through buoyancy. This process is known as degassing.

Thus, once nucleation for cavities has occurred, the formation of bubbles of suitable size to become active in an ultrasonic field becomes self-perpetuating.

12.3.4 BUBBLE MOTION

A bubble sitting in an ultrasonic pressure field undergoes non-linear oscillations. It is possible to formulate equations to describe the motion of a bubble in a time-varying field in an incompressible liquid. By equating kinetic energy to work done, one obtains

$$R\ddot{R}+\frac{3}{2}\frac{\dot{R}^2}{2}=\frac{1}{\rho}\left[\left(p_0+\frac{2\sigma}{R_0}-p_v\right)\left(\frac{R_0}{R}\right)^{3\kappa}+p_v-\frac{2\sigma}{R}-p_0-P(t)\right]$$

In reality, the effects of fluid viscosity must be taken into account. This gives the modified equation:

$$R\ddot{R}+\frac{3}{2}\frac{\dot{R}^2}{2}=\frac{1}{\rho}\left[\left(p_0+\frac{2\sigma}{R_0}-p_v\right)\left(\frac{R_0}{R}\right)^{3\kappa}+p_v-\frac{2\sigma}{R}-\frac{4\eta\dot{R}}{R}-p_0-P(t)\right]$$

This is known as the Rayleigh–Plesset equation (Rayleigh 1917; Plesset 1949; Neppiras & Noltingk 1951; Poritsky 1952; Leighton 1994). A number of simplifying assumptions have been made in these derivations (Leighton 1994). It is assumed that there is only a single bubble that remains spherical and is situated in an infinite liquid of high density and infinitesimally small compressibility compared with that of the gas contained within the bubble. The bubble radius is assumed to be small compared with the acoustic wavelength. A number of people have developed more sophisticated models that account for some of these assumptions (Gilmore 1952; Flynn 1964, 1975; Keller & Miksis 1980; Prosperetti *et al.* 1988). These models have been compared with experiment by Gaitan *et al.* (1992).

Figure 12.11 shows solutions to the Rayleigh–Plesset equation for three different sized bubbles (radii 0.2, 0.7 and 1.4 µm) driven at 4.5 MHz. At this frequency bubbles with radius 0.7 µm are resonant. Figure 12.12a also shows solutions to the Rayleigh–Plesset equation. Here, the changes in bubble size (R/R_0) are shown as a grey scale and are plotted against equilibrium radius and time. This form of presentation highlights the different frequencies of oscillation that may be induced when bubbles of different equilibrium sizes (R_0) are present in an acoustic field. Figure 12.12b shows the Fourier transform of this plot and shows the presence not only of the fundamental (driving) frequency of 4.5 MHz but also of the first subharmonic (2.25 MHz) and the second harmonic (9 MHz).

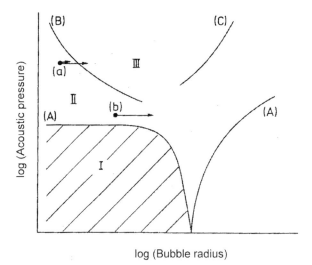

Figure 12.10. Schematic diagram showing non-inertial cavitation thresholds (B, C) and rectified diffusion threshold (A) for bubbles (see text for details)

12.3.5 CAVITATION MONITORING

Several methods are available for monitoring cavitation activity in fluids. These fall into three main categories: measurement of the acoustic emissions from cavitating bodies; analysis of chemical reactions produced within the medium; and direct imaging of bubbles. Discussion here is restricted to methods that are suitable for monitoring cavitation in biologically relevant systems.

12.3.5.1 Acoustic Emission

Cavitating bubbles act as secondary sources of sound, the emissions of which can be monitored and analysed. A hydrophone in the vicinity of cavitation activity can pick up the acoustic signals, which then may be displayed on a spectrum analyser or fed through frequency filters to select specific frequencies. This method has been used successfully to detect cavitation arising *in vivo* due to extracorporeal shock-wave lithotripsy pulses (Coleman *et al.* 1995, 1996). At low intensities (sub-threshold) only the drive frequency, f_0, is detected. As the intensity is increased, the emission spectrum from the medium becomes more complex.

Half-order subharmonic, $f_0/2$. Esche (1952) was the first author to describe the emission of the half-order subharmonic ($f_0/2$) from cavitating bubbles. This has now become a well-established indicator of bubble activity. The mechanism by which the subharmonic is produced has been discussed widely but still may not be fully understood (Neppiras 1968, 1969a, b, 1980a; Vaughan 1968; Eller & Flynn 1969; Coakley 1971; Lauterborn 1976; Leighton 1994).

Sporadic subharmonic emission is detected in non-inertial (stable) cavitation fields. Neppiras (1980a) has discussed the mechanism for this. Surface vibrations of a bubble may be at half the drive frequency, but the weak coupling of these to the fluid would mean that they would only be detected by a probe at the bubble surface. Bubbles of a size that would be resonant at half the driving frequency can be driven to emit their own resonant frequency. The threshold intensity for this can be chosen to be below the inertial cavitation threshold (Neppiras 1968). Under some conditions in a highly compressible, non-linear fluid, an $f_0/2$ signal can be detected due to parametric amplification in the absence of cavitation (Tucker 1965), but this is unlikely to be of significant magnitude where cavitating bubbles are present.

A second theory for subharmonic emission is that it may arise from the acoustic field acting on bubbles that have equilibrium radii larger than those of resonant bubbles at the driving frequency. Eller and Flynn (1969) have calculated the threshold acoustic pressure required to generate the subharmonic of a given drive frequency, and have demonstrated that this has a pronounced minimum for bubbles with radii close to twice that of resonant bubbles at that frequency (see Figure 12.12). However, Leighton *et al.* (1992, 1995) have shown that this theory is not adequate to explain subharmonic emissions because they have also been detected in the absence of these large bubbles.

A third explanation for the origin of subharmonic signals lies in chaotic oscillations of the bubbles. It may be possible to model bubble oscillation mathematically but, if a numerical solution is required, very slight changes in initial conditions can lead to errors that diverge rapidly with time. This means that one may only have confidence in the solution very close to the start of the calculation. This unpredictable behaviour is known as chaos. Chaos theory has been applied to bubble dynamics (Lauterborn & Cramer 1981; Lauterborn & Suchla 1984; Lauterborn 1986; Lauterborn & Parlitz 1988). Period doubling has been successfully predicted in this way (Parlitz *et al.* 1990). The reader is advised to turn to more detailed texts for an in-depth description of this highly complex field.

As the ultrasonic intensity is increased through the inertial cavitation threshold, the amplitude of the subharmonic signal rises rapidly. At these intensities, the subharmonic may arise from bubbles that take two pressure cycles to collapse. The amplitude of the subharmonic signal reaches a plateau as the intensity of the sound beam is increased (see Figure 12.13a).

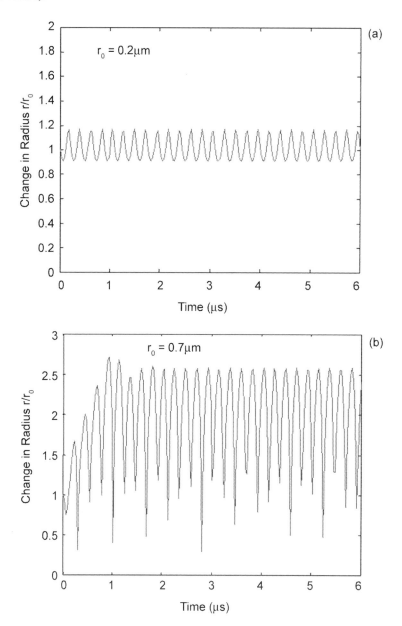

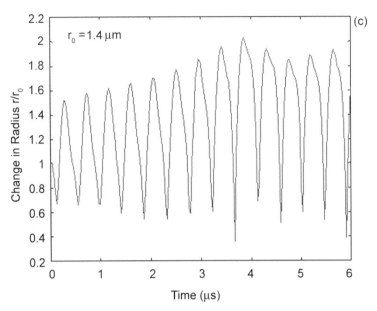

Figure 12.11. Solutions to the Rayleigh–Plesset equation for bubbles driven at 4.5 MHz: (a) bubbles of radius 0.2 μm (smaller than resonant size); (b) bubbles of radius 0.7 μm (resonant size); (c) bubbles of radius 1.4 μm (larger than resonant size). *Source*: Courtesy of Mr J. Austin

Morton *et al.* (1982) have shown that the extent of biological damage seen within cell samples irradiated *in vitro* correlates well with the total subharmonic energy detected from the sample during ultrasonic irradiation (Figure 12.13b). This is one of the very few examples yet to have been demonstrated of an acoustic quantity being a quantitative predictor of biological change.

Other harmonics. In non-inertial cavitation fields, the second harmonic $(2f_0)$ is the most prominent frequency. The $(2n + 1)f_0/2$ ultraharmonics are also seen.

As the inertial cavitation threshold is reached and exceeded, the received level of subharmonics and higher harmonics increases. The second harmonic remains the strongest of these, but signals at $3f_0/2$ are also detected. Neppiras and Coakley (1976) suggest that these may be due to interaction between drive frequency, f_0, and the half-order subharmonic, $f_0/2$.

Neppiras and Coakley (1976) and Neppiras (1980a) also describe the appearance of the $f_0/3$ subharmonic. This is probably generated in the same fashion as the $f_0/2$ half-order subharmonic.

Techniques that monitor second harmonic emissions have also been developed (Miller 1981). These have been used to detect bubbles arising from decompression (Christman *et al.* 1986), from ultrasound (Gross *et al.* 1985) and from lithotripsy (Williams *et al.* 1989). Second harmonic emission from gas-body contrast agents has also been used for blood perfusion measurement (Schrope & Newhouse 1993).

White noise. As the cavitation activity within an ultrasonic field builds up, the level of white noise increases. As the inertial threshold is reached, the level increases rapidly, and above this intensity the white noise increases linearly with excitation pressure (Neppiras 1980a) (see

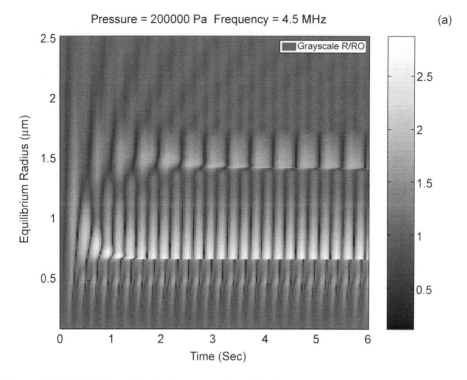

Figure 12.13c). White noise has been monitored both *in vitro* and *in vivo* (Neppiras *et al.* 1969a, b; Holland & Apfel 1990; Coleman *et al.* 1992).

Barger (1964) detected white noise as soon as bubble surface activity was observed. Neppiras and Coakley (1976) also found that white noise was emitted from the turbulence associated with the fast translatory motion of bubbles in a high-intensity field. The shock wave associated with the collapse of a transient cavity also contributes to the noise level.

Active cavitation detection. Active cavitation detection sends high-frequency tone bursts into tissue and monitors the signal scattered by cavitating microbubbles (Roy *et al.* 1990; Holland *et al.* 1996). In the system developed by Roy *et al.* (1990) a 30 MHz, 15 μs detector pulse was used. The scattered signal was sampled at 100 MHz. The duration of the received signal allowed discrimination between scatter from cavitation events, which occurred on the time scale of a single acoustic cycle or the length of the cavitation-inducing ultrasonic pulse (typically 1 μs) and from other quiescent scatterers, which lasted for the 15 μs of the detector pulse. This method has been used to provide direct evidence of cavitation induced *in vivo* in rats by diagnostic pulses of ultrasound.

Except in the case of the half-order subharmonics, no quantitative relationship has yet been demonstrated between the above phenomena and specific biological endpoints.

12.3.5.2 Impedance Change

As bubbles form in an irradiated fluid, the acoustic properties of that fluid are altered. The change in acoustic impedance of the medium reflects the amount of cavitation activity within

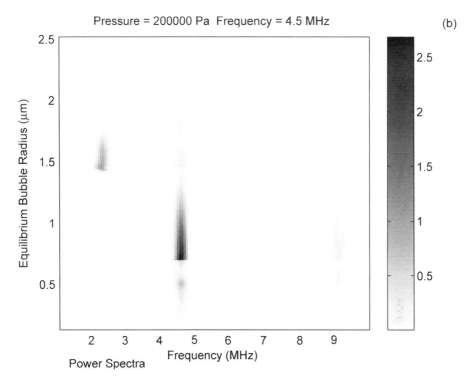

Figure 12.12. (a) Solutions to the Rayleigh–Plesset equation for bubbles driven at 4.5 MHz for which the ratio of bubble radius to equilibrium radius is presented as a grey scale and is plotted against equilibrium radius and time. (b) Fourier transform of (a) showing the presence of the fundamental, first subharmonic and second harmonic frequencies. *Source*: Courtesy of Mr J. Austin

it. Observation of the electric signals across the transducer allows measurement of the acoustic impedance into which the beam is propagating (Neppiras & Coakley 1976). The method provides a sensitive method of monitoring cavitation activity without needing to interfere with the ultrasonic field by the insertion of a probe of any kind. The impedance of water may decrease by as much as 60% in a high-intensity field (Rozenberg & Sirotyuk 1961). The signal seen at the transducer terminals is a frequency-modulated voltage. Specific frequencies may be monitored by the use of relevant filters. The pattern of harmonic and subharmonic emission observed is similar to that described in the previous section (Section 12.2.4).

12.3.5.3 Sonoluminescence

The phenomenon of sonoluminescence is the emission of light from media irradiated with ultrasound, and is generally thought to be an indicator of inertial (transient) cavitation activity, although the mechanism of light generation is still not fully understood.

Fogging of photographic plates as a result of ultrasonic irradiation was first described by Marinesco and Trillat in 1933, and the phenomenon was first attributed to ultrasonically induced light emission (sonoluminescence) by Frenzel and Schultes in 1934.

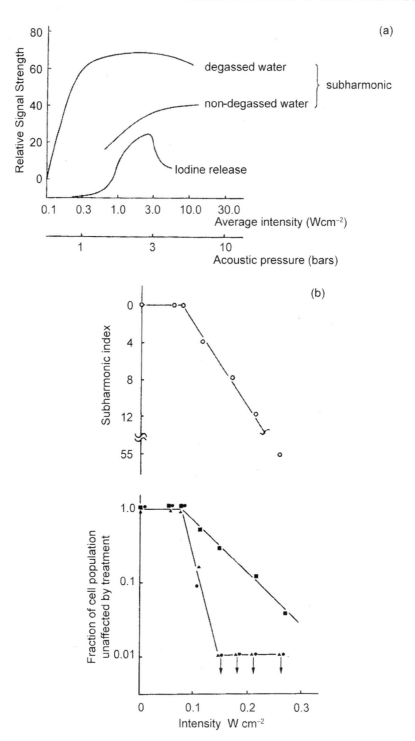

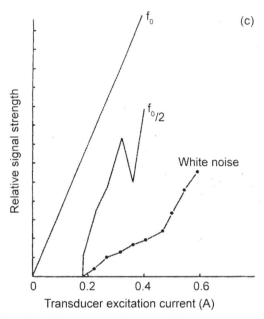

Figure 12.13. (a) Variation of cavitation level as a function of ultrasonic intensity for gassy and degassed water. Both subharmonic emission and iodine release methods of detection are shown. (b) The effect of ultrasonic intensity on subharmonic emission and cell damage: (■) intact cells, (●) undamaged cells (trypan blue assay), (Δ) surviving cells (clonogenic assay). (30 min irradiation at 1 MHz.) A correlation between subharmonic signal and cell damage can be seen. *Source*: Adapted from Morton *et al.* (1982). (c) Variation of acoustic emissions with transducer excitation current in freshly stirred, air-saturated water. The fundamental, first harmonic and white noise emissions are shown. *Source*: Adapted from Neppiras (1969b)

Early work on sonoluminescence involved observation of the light flashes by the 'dark adapted eye'. In tap water, the luminescence is just discernible but can be enhanced by the addition of carbon tetrachloride or by saturation with inert gases. More recent work has made use of sensitive photomultiplier tubes. The characteristics of the sonoluminescence signal are that it:

(a) decreases with increasing ultrasonic frequency and has not been observed at frequencies above 2 MHz (Finch 1963);
(b) appears at a definite threshold intensity and increases approximately linearly with increasing intensity (Griffing & Sette 1955; Parke & Taylor 1956) but may disappear completely if a sufficiently high intensity is reached (Negeshi 1961);
(c) decreases with increasing ambient pressure (Harvey 1939; Polotskii 1949);
(d) decreases with increasing ambient temperature.

Early theories for the production of sonoluminescence required the 'rupture' of a liquid to produce the effects seen. More recent theories rely on the growth of bubbles from nuclei within the field. These theories have been reviewed by Finch (1963). Mechanisms for sonolumines-cence occurrence include electrical theories (see, for example, Degrois & Baldo 1974) and thermal theories. Noltingk and Neppiras (1950) and Neppiras and Noltingk (1951) predict that the high temperatures and pressures associated with the adiabatic collapse of bubbles are sufficient to produce incandescence. The fact that many of the characteristics of the sonoluminescence signal described above can be explained by this model, and the observation of Negeshi (1961) that the light emission is associated with the bubble when it is at its minimum volume, lend weight to this theory. Griffing and Sette (1955) proposed a thermochemical mechanism requiring thermal dissociation of molecules followed by their recombination and chemiluminescence rather than incandescence. This requires less energy than the incandescence mechanism and is consistent with the observations of Saksena and Nyborg (1970) that luminescence may be associated with stable cavitation when surface wave activity on the bubble is eliminated.

Sonoluminescence has been detected by a number of investigators in systems *in vitro* (Negeshi 1961; Saksena & Nyborg 1970; Roy *et al.* 1985; Daniels & Price 1991; Coleman *et al.* 1993) but although it provides a useful method for studying the physics of collapse cavitation in liquids it is not suitable for the study of cavitation in opaque tissues, although studies have been carried out in the semi-transparent model of the human cheek (Leighton *et al.* 1990). This is a limitation of cavitation 'detection' techniques.

12.3.5.4 Sonochemistry

One indicator of cavitation activity within an irradiated sample is the occurrence of chemical reactions typical of the presence of energy-rich species such as ionised and excited molecules, ions and free radicals. These chemical reactions are thought to be indicative of collapse (inertial or transient) cavitation and are attributed to the electrical and thermal effects discussed in the previous section (Section 12.3.5.3). Although the chemistry is not understood completely, it is generally believed that, in the presence of acoustic cavitation, water undergoes the reaction

$$H_2O \leftrightarrow H^{\cdot} + OH^{\cdot} \hspace{3cm} \text{(Weissler 1959)}$$

A number of chemical consequences of this reaction are used to assess cavitation activity. These include:

1. The release of free iodine from potassium iodide. This is thought to be due to the action of the OH radical. If carbon tetrachloride is present, the yield of iodine is increased by the action of oxidising chlorine (Weissler *et al.* 1950). Iodine concentrations were estimated by titration against sodium thiosulphate, using starch as an indicator.
2. The oxidation of ferrous sulphate, as used in the Fricke ionising radiation dosimetry method. In simple terms, the reactions involved are thought to be (Fricke & Hart 1966)

$$Fe^{2+} + OH \rightarrow Fe^{3+} + OH^{-}$$
$$H + O_2 \rightarrow HO_2$$
$$Fe^{2+} + HO_2 \rightarrow Fe^{3+} + HO_2^{-}$$
$$HO_2^{-} + H^{+} \rightarrow H_2O_2$$
$$Fe^{2+} + H_2O_2 \rightarrow Fe^{3+} + OH + OH^{-}$$

Todd (1970) describes the application of this method to ultrasound. The yield of ferric sulphate was measured spectrophotometrically. The reduction of ferric sulphate to ferrous sulphate also may be used.
3. Other methods include monitoring of the formation of a highly fluorescent species when hydroxyl radicals react with terephthalate acid (McLean & Mortimer 1988; Miller &

Thomas 1993a; Price & Lenz 1993; Wang *et al.* 1993; Price 1998) and spin trapping (Makino *et al.* 1983).

Again, sonochemical techniques are useful for studying collapse cavitation *in vitro* but are in no way useful to *in vivo* investigations.

12.3.5.5 Direct Imaging Methods

12.3.5.5.1 Visual Observation

Visual observation of bubble fields was the earliest method used for the description of cavitation events. Before the advent of high-speed photography, bubble formation and surface wave activity were all that could be recorded. Collapse cavitation could only be studied in terms of its physical effects, such as microbubble formation. Transient events may have a lifetime of only a few pressure cycles (10–50 ms) and thus sophisticated fast photographic techniques are required to capture them on film.

Blake (1949), working at 60 kHz, observed bubbles and distinguished between two types of transient activity that he called 'gaseous' and 'vaporous'. Gaseous transients formed at discrete bubbles in the focal region, whereas vaporous transients, which appeared at higher intensities, formed 'streamers' and their collapse was heard as a snapping noise. [There is some confusion in the literature as to the use of the terms gaseous and vaporous cavitation. They are more usually used to describe the content of the bubbles (Flynn 1964; Neppiras 1980a).]

Willard (1953) used a fast-moving film and a frame rate of 24–1000 per second to demonstrate the breakdown of transient cavities in a cloud of microbubbles.

Lauterborn and his colleagues have used high-speed photography and pulsed laser holographic techniques to study the behaviour both of single, isolated bubbles (Lauterborn & Bader 1975) and of the bubble field (Lauterborn *et al.* 1972). Benjamin and Ellis (1966), Lauterborn *et al.* (1972) and Crum (1979) have described jet formation in collapsing cavities near boundaries.

Much of the above work has been carried out at comparatively low acoustic frequencies where resonant bubble sizes are sufficiently large to allow ready visualisation. At megahertz frequencies, detection can become difficult and is sometimes only practically possible for bubbles that have grown well beyond resonant size.

12.3.5.5.2 Ultrasonic Imaging

Optical detection of bubbles is a useful method of viewing cavitation in optically transparent liquids but is of no real use in opaque media such as biological tissues.

Bubble formation in tissues can be monitored using a pulse–echo ultrasonic imaging system. This technique was first investigated for decompression sickness studies by Rubissow and Mackay (1971) and more recently by Daniels *et al.* (1980). ter Haar and Daniels (1981) and ter Haar *et al.* (1982) have described the use of an 8 MHz imaging system to detect bubbles formed under the action of therapy intensity levels of ultrasound in mammalian tissue. The detection threshold diameter for gas microbubbles using this system was 10 μm.

12.3.5.6 Fibre Optic Methods

Fibre optic hydrophones, which can use ultrasonically induced refractive index changes in the propagation medium to allow the measurement of pressure, have been used both to detect cavitation *in vitro* and *in vivo* (Staudenraus & Eisenmenger 1988, 1993; Huber *et al.* 1994) and to measure acoustic pressures *in vivo* (Coleman *et al.* 1998). Huber *et al.* (1994) have used this technique in lithotripsy fields and demonstrated that the lifetime of a cavitation bubble in water varied between 250 and 750 μs as the energy in the ultrasonic pulse was increased, whereas in tumour tissue for the same pulse energy increase the lifetime varied from 100 to 220 μs.

12.3.5.7 Comparison of the Different Methods Available for Cavitation Monitoring

Table 12.2 attempts to compare the different methods of monitoring cavitation that have been discussed in Sections 12.3.4.1–12.3.4.6, and to indicate the different levels of activity for which signals are received. All the methods described show a strong response to inertial cavitation events, whereas only the acoustic emissions at the subharmonic and higher harmonics of the drive frequency are recorded from stable (non-inertial) cavitation fields.

Table 12.3 outlines the suitability of the different techniques for bio-effects studies. There have been several attempts in the literature to compare the various monitoring techniques within the same system and some of these reports are reviewed here:

1. De Santis et al. (1967), working in the frequency range 1–4 MHz, were able to detect $f_0/2$ subharmonic signals just before the optical appearance of bubbles. Neppiras (1968) observed the same thing. Both Neppiras (1968) working at 28 kHz, and Neppiras and Coakley (1976) working with a 1 MHz focused field, found that visual detection of bubbles and onset of white noise were simultaneous.
2. Eastwood and Watmough (1976) found that the sporadic half-order subharmonic signals, detected before sonoluminescence was seen, reached a constant level when the sonoluminescence threshold was crossed. Broadband noise was detected only in the presence of sonoluminescence. Saksena and Nyborg (1970) found that the sono-luminescence and white noise thresholds coincided, and observed occasional light flashes in non-inertial cavitation fields at 30 kHz.
3. Graham et al. (1980) found that at 1.5 MHz $f_0/2$ subharmonic emission always accompanied both iodine release, from potassium iodide in the presence of carbon tetrachloride, and sonoluminescence. The threshold intensities for all three were virtually coincident. Coakley and Sanders (1973) found that at 1 MHz, iodine was released at the same intensity as was required to produce a change in acoustic impedance as measured at the transducer electrodes. Hedges et al. (1977) reported that, although the intensity thresholds for the $f_0/2$ subharmonic emission and free iodine release were identical, the peak in ferric sulphate concentration occurred at a higher intensity.
4. Hill et al. (1969) looked at half-order subharmonic emission, free iodine release, DNA degradation to 50% of its original molecular weight and sonoluminescence in aqueous solutions irradiated with 1 MHz ultrasound. They found that although they could not detect sonoluminescence, the intensity thresholds for the other three effects were identical.

12.3.6 EXPERIMENTALLY MEASURED THRESHOLDS OF ACOUSTIC CAVITATION

The ultrasonic intensity at which acoustic cavitation will occur in a sample depends, among other things, on the purity of the sample, its gas content and previous ultrasonic and pressurisation history, sample viscosity, ambient temperature and pressure, ultrasonic frequency and pulsing characteristics and the configuration of the ultrasonic field within the sample. It is therefore meaningless to quote threshold values without qualification: Coakley (1978) points out that published values for cavitation thresholds in water at 1 MHz range from about 1 W cm^{-2} to 2.7×10^3 W cm^{-2}. Coleman et al. (1995) have suggested, using lithotripsy

Table 12.2. Sensitivities of various cavitation monitoring methods over the range of levels of cavitation activity

Acoustic pressure region	White noise	f_0 harmonics	$f_0/2$ subharmonics	Other subharmonics f_0/n	Impedance change	Sonoluminescence	Sonochemistry	Direct imaging (visual observation B-scan)
Transient cavitation events	Strong	Yes $2f_0$ and $3f_0/2$[e]	Strong	Yes	Yes	Yes	Yes	Yes microbubble formation can be seen
Threshold region	Level increases[a,c,f]	General increase in level	Rapid increase in level[a]	Increase[a,b]		Appears	Appears	Yes
Stable cavitation events	Present at low level[c]	Yes $2f_0$ strong[a,b,c,d]	Occasional appearance[a-f]	Sometimes seen: mostly at high f_0	Yes[d,e]	No (some indication in absence of surface waves)[g]	No	Yes[e]
Threshold region								Bubble growth
Subthreshold	Absent	Absent	Absent	Absent	Absent	Absent	Absent	No active bubbles

[a]Esche (1952).
[b]Negeshi (1961).
[c]Neppiras (1980a).
[d]Coakley (1971).
[e]Neppiras and Coakley (1976).
[f]Apfel (1980).
[g]Saksena and Nyborg (1970).

Table 12.3. Suitability of various cavitation monitoring techniques for bio-effects studies

Method	Suitable for *in vivo* studies?	Advantages	Restrictions
Acoustic emission	Yes	1. Sensitive indicator of cavitation activity 2. Quantitative measurements possible	Unsuitable for deep tissue volumes because emitted signals are attenuated
Impedance change	No	Sensitive indicator of cavitation activity	
Sonoluminescence	No	Quantitative measurements possible	Unsuitable for opaque media
Sonochemistry	No	Quantitative measurements possible	Unwanted chemical reactions may restrict use on biological samples
Optical imaging	No	Provides information on bubble location	1. Unsuitable for opaque media 2. Unsuitable for frequencies $\gtrsim 1\,\text{MHz}$
Ultrasonic imaging	Yes	1. Provides information on bubble location 2. Investigations may be carried out at raised ambient pressures	Only detects bubble presence; does not give information on activity

pulses, that the temporal peak negative pressure required to produce cavitation in tissue lies between 1.5 MPa and 3.5 MPa.

12.3.6.1 Variation of Cavitation Activity with Intensity

As the ultrasonic intensity within a sample is increased from zero, initially there is no indication of cavitation but as the intensity crosses a 'threshold' level, cavitation begins. As the intensity is increased further, the inertial (transient) cavitation threshold is passed and cavitation 'activity' becomes stronger. The level of cavitation activity reaches a plateau and may decrease at higher intensities.

Figure 12.11a shows data obtained by Hill (1972) indicating the way in which subharmonic signal and free iodine release vary as the average intensity of a 1 MHz beam is increased both in gassy and degassed water. Neppiras (1969b), for example, showed the way in which subharmonic and white noise signals build up with increasing intensity (Figure 12.13c).

Figure 12.13b shows the work of Morton *et al.* (1982) in which cells in suspension were irradiated with 1 MHz ultrasound and the sample was monitored for emissions at the first subharmonic. The total subharmonic energy emitted during a 30 min irradiation period was determined by integration of the signal. It was found that there was clearly a threshold intensity at which subharmonics appeared. This intensity was also found to be a threshold above which cell lysis was seen, membrane damage as indicated by the trypan blue assay was found and the cells began to lose their reproductive integrity as determined by a clonogenic assay (ter Haar *et al.* 1980).

12.3.6.2 Variation of Cavitation Intensity Threshold with Frequency

Hill (1972) has collated data on the behaviour of cavitation as a function of frequency. It can be seen that, in general, as the ultrasonic frequency is increased, a higher intensity is required to produce cavitation (Figure 12.14).

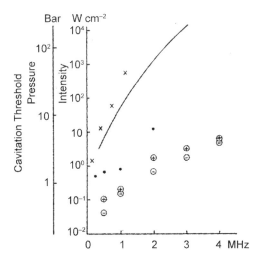

Figure 12.14. Frequency dependence of cavitation threshold in air-equilibrated water. Collated data from different sources, quoted by Hill (1972)

12.3.6.3 Variation of Cavitation Activity with Pulsing Conditions

Hill and Joshi (1970) have shown the build-up and decline of free iodine release from an aqueous solution as the duty factor of a pulsing regime is increased from 0.01 to 1.0 for pulse lengths in the range 0.03–10 ms at 2 MHz. The peak iodine release rate occurred for duty factors between 10% and 30%. These data are represented in Figure 12.15a. Figure 12.15b shows Hill and Joshi's data for the release of iodine as a function of increasing pulse length. It can be seen that at 1 MHz the maximum iodine release is obtained for 10 ms pulse lengths (the duty factor used was 0.1). This behaviour was thought to be related to the dynamics of the growth of bubbles and their maintenance at a resonant or near-resonant size.

12.3.6.4 Variation of Cavitation Intensity Threshold with Ambient Pressure

Hill (1972) showed that the peak acoustic pressure required to induce cavitation in air-saturated water increased with increasing ambient pressure (Figure 12.16a). A similar relationship was recorded by Galloway (1954).

Morton *et al.* (1983) have demonstrated the effect of ambient pressure on cavitation-associated loss in reproductive ability in cells irradiated with 1 MHz ultrasound in suspension (Figure 12.13b). Figure 12.16b shows the way in which increasing the ambient pressure by 0.5–3×10^5 Pa affects the threshold for loss of survival. The threshold was $0.1\,\mathrm{W\,cm^{-2}}$ at atmospheric pressure and $2.0\,\mathrm{W\,cm^{-2}}$ at 0.5×10^5 Pa above atmospheric pressure. At 2×10^5 Pa above atmospheric pressure, no loss in survival could be detected for intensities up to $3\,\mathrm{W\,cm^{-2}}$.

12.3.6.5 Variation of Cavitation Intensity Threshold with Gas Content of Irradiated Medium

Strasberg (1959) showed that the acoustic pressure required to produce cavitation in a liquid falls as the gas content of that fluid is increased (Figure 12.17).

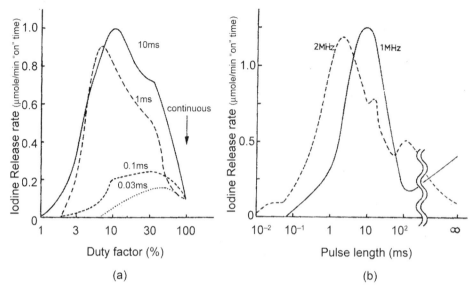

Figure 12.15. (a) Dependence of cavitation level (as measured by iodine release) on duty factor. (b) Dependence of cavitation level (as measured by iodine release) on pulse length for 1 MHz (spatial average intensity in the pulse 2.2 W cm^{-2}) and for 2 MHz (spatial average intensity in the pulse 4.7 W cm^{-2}). *Source*: Adapted from Hill and Joshi (1972)

12.3.6.6 Variation of Cavitation Intensity Threshold with Ambient Temperature

Connolly and Fox (1954) found a linear relationship between $\ln(P_C)$ and reciprocal temperature, where P_C is the acoustic pressure amplitude required to produce cavitation (Figure 12.18); P_C decreased as the temperature increased. Although there are few published data on the temperature dependence of cavitation, this same trend has been seen by several experimenters.

12.3.6.7 Variation of Cavitation Intensity Threshold with Medium Viscosity

The threshold acoustic pressure for cavitation increases with increasing viscosity. Briggs *et al.* (1947) found a linear relationship between ln(viscosity) and acoustic pressure threshold for cavitation, whereas Connolly and Fox (1954) found that the relationship between viscosity and acoustic pressure was nearly linear (Figure 12.19).

12.4 RADIATION PRESSURE, ACOUSTIC STREAMING AND 'OTHER' NON-THERMAL MECHANISMS

The physical mechanisms by which ultrasound interacts with tissue, outlined in Sections 12.2 and 12.3 (namely, heat and cavitation), have been widely investigated and there is abundant evidence that they can cause changes to biological systems.

In this section we discuss a class of phenomena that are non-thermal and non-cavitational in nature but may, nevertheless, be instrumental in producing bio-effects. In general the evidence for the biological consequences of these phenomena will be seen to be less well established than that described for heat and cavitation, and in some cases the evidence is still little more than

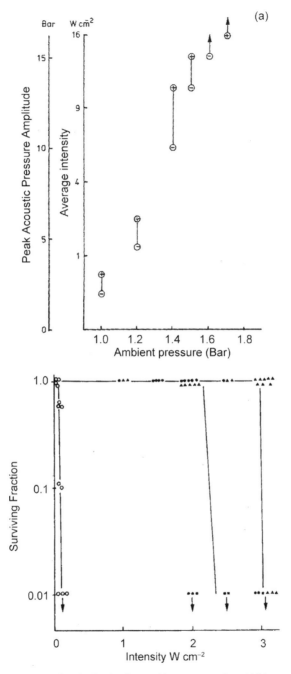

Figure 12.16. (a) Dependence of cavitation level on ambient pressure for a 1 MHz continuous wave beam. *Source*: Adapted from Hill (1972). (b) Intensity thresholds for cell damage (measured by clonogenic assay) obtained at atmospheric pressure (○) and at raised ambient pressures: (●) 1.5×10^5 Pa; (△) 3×10^5 Pa; (▲) 4×10^5 Pa (1 MHz; 30 min irradiation). *Source*: Adapted from Morton *et al.* (1983)

hypothetical. It will become evident in the subsequent chapters of this book, however, that such non-thermal, non-cavitational mechanisms of action of ultrasound may be of considerable importance in determining and controlling either the therapeutic and surgical actions of ultrasound or any possible damage that it may cause. Such considerations would be particularly important if, as is likely, the ultrasonic and environmental parameters that determine the different mechanisms are dissimilar.

12.4.1 RADIATION PRESSURE

An ultrasonic field will exert forces at the boundaries of the container of the propagation medium and also on any inhomogeneities lying within that field. These forces have two components – an oscillatory component having the same frequency as the sound beam and with a time average of zero, and a component that has a non-zero time average. This steady component is known as the radiation force and it arises from non-linearities in the sound field. This subject has been treated theoretically elsewhere in this book (see Chapter 1, Section 1.8).

Radiation force can be used to advantage for measuring spatially averaged intensities, by measuring the deflection caused by a beam impinging on a suitable target (see Chapter 1, Section 1.3 and Chapter 3, Section 3.4). It can be shown that the force on a perfectly reflecting target may be written as

$$F_{RP} = \frac{2IS}{c} \tag{12.22}$$

where S is the area that the target presents at right angles to the beam (Nyborg 1978b).

The force on a perfectly absorbing target may be written as

$$F_{RP} = \frac{IS}{c} \tag{12.23}$$

The radiation force on a sphere of radius a ($\gg \lambda$), in a plane ultrasonic field may be written [equation (3.21)] as

$$F_{RP} = \frac{\pi a^2 I}{c} Y_p \tag{12.24}$$

where Y_p is a constant.

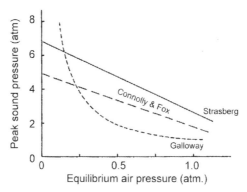

Figure 12.17. Variation of cavitation threshold with total air content in water. *Source*: Adapted from Strasberg (1959)

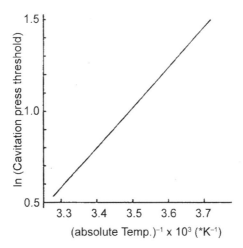

Figure 12.18. Variation of cavitation threshold with absolute temperature. *Source*: Adapted from Connolly and Fox (1954)

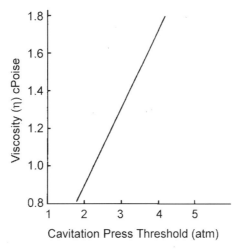

Figure 12.19. Variation of cavitation threshold with the viscosity of the cavitating liquid. *Source*: Adapted from Connolly and Fox (1954)

Similarly, an expression can be obtained for the radiation force on a rigid sphere that is small compared with a wavelength ($a \ll \lambda$). The general expression for the force on a small sphere in a field that is symmetrical in the immediate vicinity of that sphere is

$$F_R = V_0 \left(B \frac{\partial T}{\partial x} - \frac{\partial U}{\partial x} \right) + \Delta \qquad (12.25)$$

where V_0 is the sphere volume, T and U are second-order approximations to the time-averaged kinetic energy density and potential energy density, respectively, and B is given by $3(\rho - \rho_0)/$

$(2\rho + \rho_0)$, where ρ is the sphere density; Δ is a term that is important only when T and U are essentially uniform, as in a plane progressive wave (Nyborg 1967).

It can be shown that, in a standing wave field, equation (12.25) reduces to

$$F_R = V_0 B \frac{\partial T}{\partial z} \tag{12.26}$$

(ter Haar & Wyard 1978).

It is also possible to calculate the force on a compressible sphere (Yosioka & Kawasima 1955; Gor'kov 1962). It can be shown that the force on a compressible sphere is the sum of the force on a rigid sphere and the force due to its compressibility (Crum 1971). Eller (1968) has shown that the force due to the sphere compressibility is F_c, given by

$$F_c = \left\langle V(t) \frac{\partial p(x, t)}{\partial x} \right\rangle \tag{12.27}$$

where $\langle \rangle$ denotes time average, $V(t)$ is the instantaneous volume of the sphere and $p(x, t)$ is the pressure distribution along the x-axis.

The force on a compressible sphere due to radiation pressure in a standing wave field, F_{SW}, may be shown to be

$$F_{\mathrm{SW}} = \frac{V_0 P_A^2}{4\rho_0 c_0^2} k\sin(2kx) f(\rho/\rho_0) \tag{12.28}$$

where

$$f(\rho/\rho_0) = \left[\frac{\rho_0 c_0^2}{\rho c^2} - \left(\frac{5\rho - 2\rho_0}{3\rho + \rho_0} \right) \right]$$

(ter Haar 1977).

This force is periodic in half a wavelength and thus could be responsible for the phenomenon of blood cell stasis (Dyson *et al.* 1974; ter Haar *et al.* 1979) in which circulating erythrocytes in small blood vessels, when subjected to an acoustic standing wave field, are seen to clump into apparently static bands oriented to the normal field direction.

The direction in which particles move in a standing wave field depends on the sign of the function $f(\rho/\rho_0)$ (Yosioka & Kawasima 1955). In blood cell stasis, erythrocyte bands form at the pressure nodes (Gould & Coakley 1974).

12.4.2 ACOUSTIC STREAMING

Acoustic streaming is the unidirectional circulation that may be set up by an acoustic field in a fluid. This results from a transfer of momentum to the liquid as it absorbs energy from the acoustic field. The velocity gradients associated with this fluid motion may be quite high, especially in the vicinity of boundaries within the field, and the shear stresses set up may be sufficient to cause changes and/or damage.

If the instantaneous pressure, density and velocity at a point in a homogeneous, isotropic fluid are given by $p(x, y, z, t)$, $\rho(x, y, z, t)$ and $v(x, y, z, t)$ respectively, then the equation of motion may be written as

$$\frac{\delta v}{\delta t} + (v \cdot \nabla)v = -\frac{1}{\rho}\Delta p \tag{12.29}$$

or

$$F = \rho \left[\frac{\delta v}{\delta t} + (v \cdot \nabla)v \right]$$

where F is the net force per unit volume due to stresses within the fluid. For a fluid with bulk viscosity η' and shear viscosity η, it may be shown that

$$F = -\Delta p + \left(\eta' + \frac{4}{3}\eta \right) \nabla \nabla \cdot v - \eta \nabla \nabla v \qquad (12.30)$$

(Landau & Lifshitz 1966). Nyborg (1965) has used equation (12.30) to obtain the general streaming equation

$$\eta \nabla^2 v_2 = \nabla p_2 - F$$
$$- F = \rho_0 \langle v_1 \cdot \nabla \rangle v_1 \cdot \langle \nabla \cdot v_1 \rangle \qquad (12.31)$$

where v_1 is the first-order velocity and v_2 and p_2 are the second-order, time-dependent velocity and pressure, respectively.

It can be shown (Nyborg 1965) that the time-averaged torque exerted on a fluid element via viscous stresses associated with v_2 is $I\eta \nabla^2 (\nabla \wedge v_2)$, where I is the moment of inertia of the spherical volume element. Thus, a volume element in a non-linear sound field is subjected both to a translational force and to a torque. The torque is greatest at positions in which the velocity gradient is maximum, such as at the boundary between two different media. This can be demonstrated experimentally by observing the motion of polystyrene spheres in a glycerine–water mixture that is being irradiated with ultrasound (Jackson & Nyborg 1958).

The fluid motion associated with acoustic streaming exerts considerable stress at boundaries within the fluid because of the velocity gradients that exist. This is covered more fully in Section 12.4.3. Streaming may account for the increases in heat transfer, acceleration of rate processes and stripping of cell surfaces that can occur in biological tissues as a consequence of irradiation with ultrasound. These will be discussed in more detail in Sections 12.4.4 and 12.4.5.

Starritt *et al.* (1989) have measured the streaming produced in a water tank from commercial diagnostic ultrasound scanners. They reported flow rates up to $14\,\mathrm{cm\,s^{-1}}$ in pulsed Doppler beams, $5\,\mathrm{cm\,s^{-1}}$ in M-mode and $1\,\mathrm{cm\,s^{-1}}$ in B-mode. It is to be expected that in many biological fluids (e.g. amniotic fluid and urine) similar flows will be achieved, but these may be expected to be lower in blood where the ratio of absorption coefficient to viscosity is sufficiently greater than for water.

12.4.3 SHEAR STRESS

The development of unidirectional fluid circulation (streaming) in an ultrasonic field has been described in the previous section. Because the induced fluid velocity is spatially non-uniform, velocity gradients exist within the field. Objects within streaming fields are thus subjected to shear stress. Velocity gradients are highest near boundaries because the non-slip condition determines that the fluid velocity is zero at a boundary. The region in which the velocity varies between zero and the bulk velocity of the fluid is known as the boundary layer, whose thickness may be expressed as

$$\beta^{-1} = \left(\frac{2\eta}{\omega \rho} \right)^{1/2} \qquad (12.32)$$

where ω is the angular frequency of the sound field and ρ_0 and η are the density and shear viscosity of the fluid, respectively (Nyborg 1978a). As can be seen, the boundary layer thickness is inversely proportional to the square root of frequency. It is, for example, $\sim 0.56\,\mu m$ at 1 MHz in water.

Two types of velocity gradient are set up in a fluid. The velocity gradients due to acoustic streaming are 'steady' and relatively invariant with time. The periodic nature of the ultrasonic beam means that oscillatory velocity gradients exist at boundaries within the field. The shear stress, S, associated with a velocity gradient G is given by

$$S = \eta G \tag{12.33}$$

Nyborg (1978b) has calculated that this oscillatory stress is of the order of $200\,N\,m^{-2}$ for a 1 MHz field of intensity $1\,W\,cm^{-2}$ in water.

It can be shown that the oscillatory stress may be expressed as

$$S_{osc} = -\left(\frac{1}{2}\eta\omega^3\rho\xi\right)^{1/2} \tag{12.34}$$

where ξ is the particle displacement amplitude, and the steady stress exerted on a boundary due to unidirectional streaming around a spherical vibrating obstacle of radius b is

$$S_{steady} = \left(\frac{1}{2}\eta\omega^3\rho\frac{\xi^2}{b}\right)^{1/2} \tag{12.35}$$

(Rooney 1972). Although the steady stress may be an order of magnitude smaller than the oscillatory stress, it acts for a longer time at the boundary and is the more significant factor in producing cellular effects. The biological system that has been used most widely for the study of shear-induced bio-effects is that of haemolysis of red blood cells in suspension *in vitro* (e.g. Leverett *et al.* 1972; Rooney 1972). Not surprisingly, the critical stress necessary for haemolysis increases with decreasing stress duration. This is illustrated in Figure 12.20.

The high shear stresses produced by acoustic streaming may thus be instrumental in producing damage in biological materials. It has, for example, been suggested that the endothelial damage seen both in embryonic chick blood vessels (Dyson *et al.* 1974) and in mouse uterine blood vessels (ter Haar *et al.* 1979) was due in part to shear stress arising from acoustic streaming. This suggestion derives from the observation that damage occurred at the luminal aspect of the vessel wall, a site at which fluid is in contact with a membrane. The ground substance on the abluminal (i.e. external) aspect is also fluid but is more viscous than blood plasma, and thus the viscous stresses from acoustic streaming would be less significant.

12.4.4 ACOUSTIC MICROSTREAMING AROUND BUBBLES

The oscillations of bubbles in a sound field set up eddying motions of the fluid immediately around the bubble. Because of the small scale of the streaming it is called microstreaming. High velocity gradients can be set up and thus significant shear stresses may act on boundaries within the region. This can be an effective mechanism for the damage caused in a cavitation field.

Elder (1959) has described the streaming patterns obtained for different bubble oscillation amplitudes and fluid viscosities when the bubble is resting on a surface. Boundary layers and vortices exist around the bubble (see Figure 12.21). Streaming within cytoplasm can be seen when the gas spaces in plant leaves are excited with ultrasound (Martin & Gemmell 1979; Miller 1979a).

Biological molecules and cells situated near bubbles will be subjected to the shearing forces generated within these streaming fields (see Section 12.4.3). Rooney (1970) has shown that the shearing caused by bubble activity can lead to haemolysis when the oscillation amplitude exceeds a threshold value.

The velocity gradient, G around a vibrating bubble of radius R_0 with boundary layer b is given by

$$G = \frac{\omega \xi_0^2}{R_0 \beta}$$

where ξ_0 is the vibration amplitude of the bubble; thus the viscous stress is

$$S = \frac{\omega \eta \xi_0^2}{R_0 \beta}$$

(Nyborg 1978a, b).

12.4.5 'OTHER' NON-THERMAL EFFECTS

It is possible to envisage a number of types of force, related to the viscosity of the surrounding fluid, that may act on an object in an ultrasonic field. The force opposing the motion of a spherical object of radius a travelling at a velocity v in a medium of viscosity η (known as the Stokes' drag) is given by

$$F = 6\pi \eta a v \qquad (12.36)$$

For a disc, this is modified by a constant factor to

$$F = 6\pi \eta a K v \qquad (12.37)$$

If a disc is travelling broadside to the direction of movement, then $K = 0.85$; if it is travelling edgeways on, then $K = 0.57$ (Lamb 1945). If there is a velocity gradient in the fluid, the disc will also be subjected to a torque.

A force also exists because of the temperature dependence of viscosity. The temperature in a medium through which sound propagates varies during different phases of the pressure cycle. The associated changes in viscosity lead to a net time-averaged force. For a 'perfect' fluid, the resultant force is likely to be negligible because the viscosity is inversely proportional to the square root of absolute temperature; however, for a complex medium such as biological tissue a stronger temperature dependence may exist and the force may be significant.

Similarly, the sound velocity increases with the temperature of the propagation medium. This means that, in waves of finite amplitude, propagation becomes non-linear and the crest of the sound wave moves faster than the trough and can lead to wave distortion (*cf.* Chapter 1, Section 1.8). A sinusoidal wave may thus change to a sawtooth waveform. The rate of change of momentum of a particle will thus be greater at the leading edge than at the trailing edge, and the forces on that particle will be different. The resultant net force (known as the Oseen force) depends on the second harmonic content of the wave (Westervelt 1957) and thus is likely to be negligible in water but may be more significant in tissue (see Chapter 2, Section 2.9). As the sawtooth progresses, the higher frequencies will be attenuated most rapidly and the waveform reverts to a sinusoid.

12.4.6 INTER-PARTICLE FORCES

If two particles are in close proximity in an ultrasonic field, there will be an interactive force between them resulting from the interaction of each oscillating body with the sound field re-radiated by the other. Embleton (1962) considered the interaction between two spheres when the line joining their centres is parallel to the direction of a plane progressive wave field. The

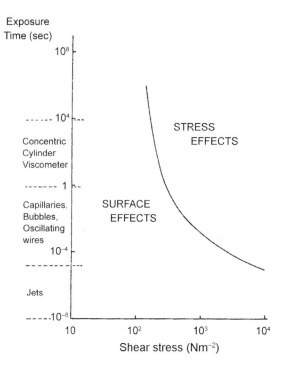

Figure 12.20. Graph demonstrating the way in which the critical stress necessary for haemolysis varies with exposure time. *Source*: Adapted from Leverett (1972)

force is proportional to the product of the sphere volumes and increases as the distance between the spheres decreases.

Gershoy and Nyborg (1973) extended the theory to consider two spheres with centres lying along a line with orientation perpendicular to the direction of propagation. They showed that there is a force of repulsion along the propagation direction and an attractive force in the perpendicular direction. The form of the force is given by

$$F_\theta = F_0 \sin 2\theta \tag{12.38}$$
$$F_r = F_0(\cos^2 \theta - 1)$$

where

$$F_0 = \frac{2\pi}{3} \left[\frac{(\rho - \rho_0)}{\rho_0} \right] \frac{a^3 b^3 v_0^2}{r^4}$$

and a and b are the sphere radii, r is their separation, v_0 is the velocity amplitude in the suspending medium and ρ_0 is its density. For touching erythrocytes in blood plasma, the maximum force is 10^{-13} N in a 1 W cm^{-2}/3 MHz beam ($a = b = 4\,\mu$m; $\rho/\rho_0 = 1.1/1.03$).

12.4.6.1 Radiation Forces Due to Gas Bubbles

If a bubble exists in an irradiated fluid it will oscillate with the field, thus acting as a secondary source that will interact with the particles around it. An attractive force of the same form as the

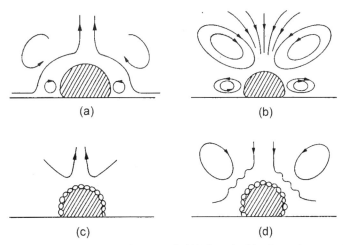

Figure 12.21. Four acoustic streaming regimes. The bubble is excited by the surface on which it sits. (a) Surface-contaminated bubble: low-amplitude oscillations in a liquid of low viscosity. (b) As (a) but with a wider range of amplitudes and viscosities. (c, d) Patterns obtained when surface modes occur: (c) when (b) breaks down; (d) when stable surface modes break down and regime returns to type (b). *Source*: Adapted from Elder (1959)

inter-particle force described in Section 12.4.5 will exist around the bubble. Because $\rho \gg \rho_0$ for a bubble in water or blood plasma, the force may be written [see equation (12.38)] as

$$F_\theta = F_0^1 \sin 2\theta \qquad (12.39)$$
$$F_r = F_0^1 (3 \cos^2 \theta - 1)$$

where

$$F_0^1 = \frac{2\pi}{3} \rho_0 \frac{a^3 R^3 v_0^2}{r^4}$$

Miller *et al.* (1979) have shown that, if blood platelets are irradiated in the presence of gas bubbles stabilised in the pores of treated filter papers, low intensities ($32\,\mathrm{mW\,cm^{-2}}$, spatial peak, temporal average intensity) are sufficient to produce platelet aggregates around the bubbles.

If gas bubbles are present in a standing wave field, those smaller than resonant size travel to the pressure antinodes (Crum & Eller 1970).

If the velocity of the bubble surface is $v_{1R} (= \omega \xi_0)$ when the radius is R, the velocity v_1 of the fluid at a point Q at distance d_1 is given by

$$v_1 = v_{1R} \frac{R^2}{d^2} \cos \omega t \qquad (12.40)$$

The force on a sphere of volume V_0 at the point Q is given by

$$\langle F \rangle = B V_0 \nabla \langle G \rangle \qquad (12.41)$$

where

$$\nabla \langle G \rangle = \frac{\partial}{\partial r} \langle G \rangle = \frac{\partial}{\partial r} \left[\frac{\rho_0}{4} v_{1R}^2 \frac{R^4}{d^4} \right]$$

Thus

$$\langle F \rangle = V_0 \frac{3(1 - \beta)}{(2 + \beta)} \rho_0 \omega^2 \xi_0^2 \frac{R^4}{d^5} \tag{12.42}$$

It can be shown (ter Haar & Wyard 1978) that

$$\left| \frac{\Delta V}{V_0} \right| = \left| \frac{P_A}{\gamma P_0} \right|$$

where ΔV is the change in volume under the action of a pressure wave of amplitude P_A when the ambient pressure is P_0. It can be calculated that for 3 MHz and 1 W cm^{-2} the force due to a 1 μm bubble is 10^{-9}N when the bubble and a 4 μm sphere are touching and 10^{-14}N when they are separated by 10 μm. The effect of bubbles in speeding up banding of red blood cells in a standing wave field due to this force has been described by ter Haar and Wyard (1978).

12.4.7 BIOLOGICAL SIGNIFICANCE OF THESE EFFECTS

There is anecdotal evidence that acoustic streaming occurs *in vivo* in clinical practice (Duck 1998). It has been seen in cysts in the breast, ovary and testicle and in liquefied vitreous humour. Although it seems unlikely that it presents a significant biological risk, it may be useful as a diagnostic indicator of a fluid-filled (as opposed to solid) lesion (Nightingale *et al.* 1995).

There is more, circumstantial, evidence for radiation pressure effects occurring in biological systems *in vivo*. Lizzi *et al.* (1981) reported transient blanching of rabbit eye choroid at high pulse amplitudes during work on the sealing of retinal tears with focused ultrasound surgery. This has also been reported by ter Haar (1977) in mouse uterine vessels. This has been attributed to radiation stress-induced compression of the blood vessels. There have been a number of reports that sensory receptors can be stimulated by ultrasound. Gavrilov (1984) reported stimulation of temperature and pain receptors. Dalecki *et al.* (1995) showed similar effects with pressure sensors on the skin. There have also been reports of stimulation of auditory response (Magee & Davies 1993).

It may also be constructive to look at three possible biological configurations and to consider which of the forces discussed above may be important:

(a) *Configuration 1*: a liquid confined within boundaries, e.g. blood within a blood vessel or cytoplasm within a plant cell. Where a fluid flows along a fixed boundary, a velocity gradient is set up and shear stresses may result. Where the ultrasonic intensity is adequate, acoustic streaming may occur within the fluid, which increases the velocity gradient and therefore the shear stress.

(b) *Configuration 2*: structures fixed within their surroundings, e.g. lysosomes and mitochondria. A structure that has a density different from that of its surroundings will be subjected to a cyclic displacement force that, for a spherical object, is equal to the product of its volume, the density difference and the acceleration. For most biological systems, structural inclusions have much the same density as that of their surroundings and the effect will be small. Where an object lies within a fluid while being attached to a liquid/solid boundary, it will be subject to shear stress and may move within the fluid if sufficiently 'floppily' bound.

(c) *Configuration 3*: structures free to move within a field, e.g. erythrocytes, platelets and bubbles. If a structure within a field has an acoustic impedance different from that of its surroundings, it may be moved by radiation pressure and is most likely to be pushed against a boundary. Similarly, if a gas bubble is in the vicinity, an attractive force may be set up that may draw the structure towards it.

12.5 NON-CAVITATIONAL SOURCES OF SHEAR STRESS

In an attempt to study the effects of acoustic streaming and associated shear stresses and velocity gradients, such as those set up around stable, oscillating bubbles, several different applicators designed to produce extremely localised vibrations have been devised. A commonly used applicator for this type of work has been the oscillating wire.

Several authors have described the use of a fine wire, tapering to 5–20 μm at the tip and driven longitudinally at frequencies around 25 kHz, to study acoustic streaming in plant cells (Dyer & Nyborg 1960a; Nyborg & Dyer 1960). For this type of study the wire is pressed against the outside of the cell wall. Different effects may be identified for different wire vibration amplitudes. In one experiment (Dyer & Nyborg 1960b) it was found that, for amplitudes of 1–2 μm, gentle but definite motion was seen; for amplitudes in the range 3–5 μm, orderly but high-speed motion was seen; and, for vibration amplitudes greater than 5 μm, chaotic violent motion that led to destruction was observed. Similar effects were seen when the wire was held as far as 10 μm from the cell wall.

Qualitatively similar results were seen by Wilson *et al.* (1966) when streaming was produced in the egg cells of marine invertebrates. In this case, 85 kHz ultrasound was produced from a stepped exponential horn. Dyer and Nyborg (1960b) have discussed the biophysics of the effects seen using these systems. They describe the eddying motions seen in fluids, and also the aggregation and rotation of particles within the fluids (see Section 12.4).

Williams *et al.* (1970) and Williams (1971) used a transversely oscillating wire (diameter 115 μm, frequency 20 kHz) to study the shear stresses required to produce haemolysis in suspensions of red blood cells. A threshold of 560 N m^{-2} was found (vibration amplitude 20 μm). When such a wire was placed in contact with a blood vessel *in vivo* (Williams 1977), platelet aggregates were seen for vibration amplitudes above 10 μm. For amplitudes in the range 5–8 μm, platelets were occasionally seen sticking to the endothelial surface of the vessel. Crowell *et al.* (1977) have used a similar system to study effects on white cells suspended in canine blood plasma. The threshold shear stress for white cell destruction was found to be lower than that for red blood cells.

Although the vibrating wire presents quite a good model for stable bubble oscillation, it is more instructive to use real bubbles. The problem has been to stabilise bubbles of resonant diameters in the ultrasonic field. Rooney (1970) overcame this problem by stabilising a hemispherical bubble at the end of a 260 μm tube driven at 20 kHz. He found a threshold stress for haemolysis of erythrocytes in suspension of approximately 450 N m^{-2}. This compares well with Williams' (1971) vibrating wire result.

Pritchard *et al.* (1966) have studied DNA degradation in solution. The macromolecules were irradiated using a plate, driven at 20 kHz, in which holes of 200 μm diameter (approximately the resonant diameter for air bubbles in water at that frequency) had been drilled to provide a stable, oscillating bubble field. Degradation of DNA was seen.

Subsequently attempts have been made to study the consequences of bubble activity at megahertz frequencies. Miller *et al.* (1979) have described a system in which a hydrophobically coated filter with pores of diameter in the range 0.1–10 µm can be irradiated in the presence of cell suspensions. Miller *et al.* (1978) describe the motion of platelets irradiated in this system as:

1. Particles near a hole tend to move towards it, the speed of inward motion increasing rapidly as the particle nears the centre. Small aggregates of particles are often seen near the holes after continued sonation for a short period. This motion is partly the result of radiation force.
2. Particles near a hole take part in an acoustic streaming motion similar to that known to occur near gas bubbles at lower frequencies. When a biological entity such as a blood platelet takes part in this motion, it is subjected to relatively high stresses when it traverses the boundary layer region near a hole and may experience damage.
3. Particles or cells that have collected near a hole may rotate continuously or tumble about in an irregular fashion. If the particles are not perfectly symmetrical, as is true for the disc-like red cell, a favoured orientation may be achieved in which the particle tends to remain. If several red cells collect at the same hole they interact in complex but interesting patterns of rotation and orientation.

These authors conclude that the intensity threshold for platelet aggregation lies in the range 32–64 mW cm^{-2} at 1 MHz. Williams and Miller (1980) have demonstrated ATP release (suggestive of membrane damage) in erythrocytes irradiated using this system at spatial peak intensities of 20–30 mW cm^{-2} at 1.6 MHz.

This type of experiment shows that the presence of stable oscillating bubbles may lead to disruption and in some cases damage in biological systems, in a manner apparently similar to that associated with cavitation in bulk liquid. Mechanisms of interaction can be isolated using these artificial studies where this would be more difficult using more complex systems.

12.6   EVIDENCE FOR NON-THERMAL EFFECTS IN STRUCTURED TISSUES

The main effort in the search for non-thermal effects has been aimed at the study of cavitation. Until recently, the available cavitation methods did not lend themselves to the study of opaque structured tissues (see Section 12.2.4, Tables 12.2 and 12.3). For this reason, much of the cavitation work reported on such tissues had either been carried out on plant tissues, in which direct observation has been possible, or has relied on circumstantial evidence from histological study of mammalian tissues that have been excised and fixed after irradiation.

It is extremely difficult to identify in a definitive manner effects that are caused by non-thermal, non-cavitational mechanisms, because it is difficult to isolate these effects when cavitation and/or heating is also present. Some such work has been done, however, and this is described in Section 12.6.2.

12.6.1 PLANT SYSTEMS

One of the earliest reports of non-thermal effects produced by ultrasound comes from Harvey (1930) who reported cell wall disruption, twisting and tearing of organelles from cell walls, and cytoplasmic movement in Spirogyra, Nitella and Elodea. These effects were diminished if the gas tension in the plants was reduced prior to irradiation. Although no gas bubbles were obvious to the observer, it would appear that the effects seen were due to acoustic cavitation and streaming.

Miller (1977) has identified three categories of response of Elodea leaves (which are known to contain natural gas vacuoles) to ultrasonic irradiation, namely: a slight perturbation (increase in cyclosis, changes in the chloroplast distribution), disruption of cellular organisation leading to cell death and homogenisation of the cellular contents. He found that the response of cells to 1 MHz irradiation conditions was highly non-uniform in any one leaf, the sensitivity of any one cell depending on its proximity to a gas body. An extensive study of threshold intensities showed that the ultrasonic intensity (SPTP) necessary to produce cell death was proportional to (irradiation time)$^{-0.29}$. The threshold intensities (SP) for cell death have been shown to be highly frequency dependent (Miller 1979a, b). Miller and Thomas (1993b) have developed a theoretical model to allow computation of the shear stresses generated when these cylindrically shaped gas bodies in Elodea leaves are driven by an ultrasonic field. They found that the acoustic pressure required to maintain a given shear stress increased as $f^{1/2}$ over the range 1–10 MHz. They also suggested a threshold for cell lysis of 1 MPa MHz^{-1} for 3 μs pulses (0.75–15 MHz). This was the threshold found by Carstensen *et al.* (1990a) for frequencies of 1–3 MHz.

Gershoy *et al.* (1976) found perturbations in cells near intercellular gas spaces at an average intensity of 350 mW cm^{-2} (1 MHz), although in some cells chloroplast rotations and streaming eddies could be detected at 35 mW cm^{-2}. Irreversible effects were not seen below intensities of about 3.5 W cm^{-2}. In plants devoid of intercellular gas spaces (such as Hydrodictyon) intensities of 35 W cm^{-2} were required to produce the slight perturbations seen at 350 mW cm^{-2} in Vicia faba roots, which contain such spaces. Goldman and Lepeschkin (1952) studied standing wave effects in plants. They found that ultrasonically induced damage was maximum at the pressure antinodes in both Spirogyra and Elodea. They attributed the effects to bubble activity in the medium containing the leaves.

Morris and Coakley (1978, 1980) have detected subharmonic emissions from plant roots during ultrasonic irradiation. They managed to show that the intensity at which the subharmonic appeared was the same as that required to produce growth inhibition in Vicia faba roots at 1 MHz. The subharmonic was first measured at 24 W cm^{-2} after an irradiation time of 70 s. A rapid temperature rise within the root was found to precede strong subharmonic emissions. Carstensen *et al.* (1979) have found a similar growth rate reduction in the roots of the pea (Pisum sativum).

12.6.2 MAMMALIAN SYSTEMS

12.6.2.1 Cavitation Events

It is very difficult to produce unequivocal evidence for cavitation events in mammalian tissues. Much of the existing literature relies on histological studies of tissue that has been excised and processed after irradiation with ultrasound. Among the earliest reports of 'holes' seen in tissue are those from Hug and Pape (1954), Lehmann and Herrick (1953) and Bell (1957).

Lehmann and Herrick (1953) studied petechial haemorrhages at the peritoneal surfaces in mice. At the frequency used (1 MHz) they found that increasing the ambient pressure reduced the incidence of haemorrhages. At an intensity of 2.5 W cm^{-2}, pressures of 3–4 atmospheres or 4–5 atmospheres were required. Histological study of the irradiated tissues revealed 'large empty spaces' that 'presumably might correspond to gas bubbles'.

Hug and Pape (1954) carried out histology on rat and mouse tissues after irradiation with 1 MHz ultrasound. Groups of 'bubbles' could be seen in the liver following 8 min of irradiation at 2.2 W cm^{-2}. Similar 'bubbles' were found to form in bands along the white matter/grey matter border. This 'bubble' formation is referred to by the authors as 'pseudocavitation'. It is extremely difficult to be certain that circular holes seen in tissue sections after processing for histology are truly due to the presence of gas bubbles present at the time of fixation. Bell (1957) has also reported 'pseudocavitation' holes in mouse livers. He found damage at 1 MHz, but not at

27 MHz. Although the damage seen was in some ways similar to that seen from excessive heating, pre-cooling of the tissue such that the tissue temperature remained at an acceptable level during ultrasonic irradiation still resulted in some damage. 'Holes' have also been seen in electromicrographs of irradiated mouse uterine tissues by ter Haar *et al.* (1979).

Hug and Pape (1954) measured the intensity transmitted through slabs of freshly excised tissue as a function of time. They found that, for some tissue types, after about 120 s of irradiation the intensity dropped appreciably. They attributed this to bubble formation within the slab preventing transmission through the tissue. This effect was found to be greatest in brain and liver (see Figure 12.22). In fat, the intensity first rose and then dropped to about 50% of the initial value. The initial rise was attributed to heating within the fat causing a decrease in absorption coefficient.

Martin *et al.* (1981) have studied the effects of 0.8, 1.5 and 3.0 MHz ultrasound on mouse livers exposed and irradiated through a contact medium. They found that at 0.8 MHz and 1.5 MHz, for intensities above 2 W cm^{-2}, highly localised damage was seen superficially on the incident surface of the liver. At intensities up to 10 W cm^{-2} no such damage could be seen at 3 MHz. The temperature rise was measured to be 7.5°C, and the intensity at which damage was first seen coincided with the intensity at which a subharmonic signal was first received from the system. Close investigation revealed that the effects seen were due to cavitation events within the contact medium. By use of a gel, or a thin membrane laid over the liver, the damage could apparently be prevented.

Diagnostic ultrasound imaging systems have been used to demonstrate the existence of bubbles in biological systems. Daniels *et al.* (1979) and Mackay and Rubissow (1978) showed bubble growth produced by decompression, ter Haar and Daniels (1981) and Hynynen (1991) demonstrated bubbles induced by therapy ultrasound, and Coleman *et al.* (1995) and Zeman *et al.* (1990a, b) reported bubbles resulting from lithotripsy. ter Haar and Daniels (1981) have

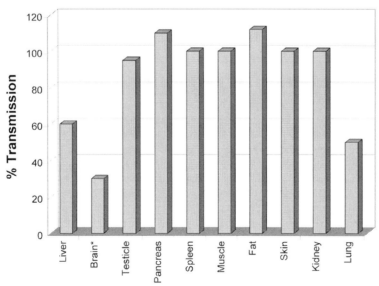

Figure 12.22. Diagram showing the drop in ultrasonic intensity transmitted through different tissues after 120 s of irradiation. The drop is thought to be due to bubble formation within tissues. *Source*: Adapted from Hug and Pape (1954)

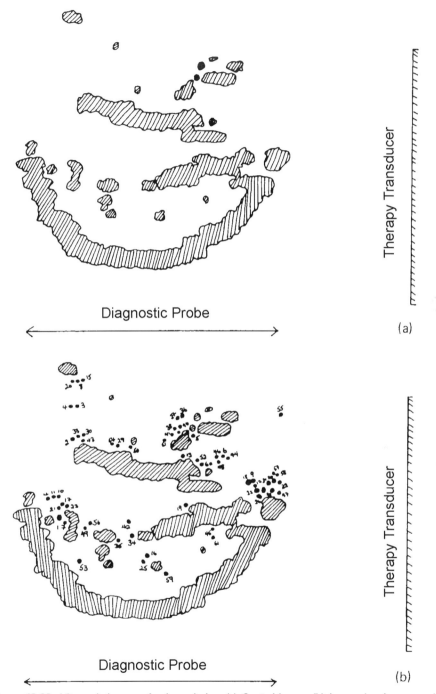

Figure 12.23. Ultrasonic images of guinea pig leg. (a) Control image. (b) Image showing new echoes attributed to bubbles within the leg, arising due to irradiation by 0.75 MHz/1.0 W cm^{-2} ultrasound

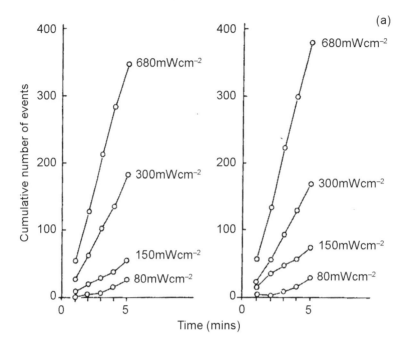

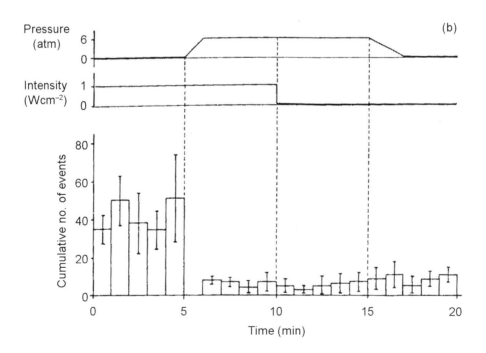

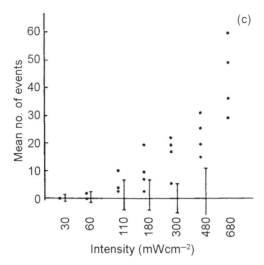

Figure 12.24. (a) Cumulative number of events (appearance of bubbles in guinea pig leg) plotted as a function of time for different intensities in two different animals. See text for details. *Source*: Adapted from ter Haar and Daniels (1981). (b) Variation of number of events with applied pressure. It can be seen that the appearance of bubbles is reduced when the ambient pressure is increased. *Source*: Adapted from ter Haar and Daniels (1982). (c) Number of events plotted against intensity. Data taken from four animals. Bars show spurious 'events' as registered in controls

used an 8 MHz ultrasonic imaging system to image bubble formation in the legs of anaesthetised guinea pigs. This system, developed for the study of decompression sickness, does not tell the observer anything about the activity of the bubble, once formed. At a frequency of 0.75 MHz, for 5 min exposure times, bubbles were first seen at an intensity of 80 mW cm^{-2}. Bubbles of diameter above 10 μm (i.e. rather greater than resonant size) could be detected using this method. In a later paper ter Haar *et al.* (1982) were able to demonstrate that increasing ambient pressure led to the disappearance of the bubbles. Figure 12.23 shows a schematic diagram of the 8 MHz ultrasonic image before (a) and during (b) 0.75 MHz irradiation. Some of the bubbles seen appeared to be positionally stable, whereas others were seen for a short time only. The bubbles appear largely on the side of the leg at which the 0.75 MHz beam is incident and seem to be associated with fat and with intermuscular fascia. If an event is defined as the new appearance of a bubble in the image, Figure 12.24 shows the way in which the total number of events varies with time for different intensities for two animals. Figures 12.24a, b, c show how the number of events varies with the ambient pressure and how it builds up with increasing ultrasonic intensity. In this way, a 'threshold' may be determined. This work has shown that quite low ultrasonic intensities (within the 'therapeutic' range; *cf.* Chapter 13) can give rise to bubble formation *in vivo*. It does not, however, tell us anything about the activity of bubbles, once formed. A different system is necessary to discover the way in which these bubbles behave under the action of an ultrasonic beam.

The finding that both the shock waves associated with lithotripsy and ultrasound pulses can lead to extravasation of blood cells in the lung (commonly referred to in the literature as lung haemorrhage) is thought to be a cavitation-like phenomenon (Child *et al.* 1990; Penney *et al.* 1993; Tarantal & Canfield 1994; Dalecki *et al.* 1997). Holland *et al.* (1996) have reported signs of cavitation activity in or near the rat lung using an active bubble detector. Leighton *et al.* (1995)

have investigated the behaviour of cylindrical bubbles contained in pulmonary capillaries. Spatial peak pressure thresholds for induction of this effect appear to be the same for focused and unfocused fields. Positive and negative pressures appear to have equally damaging effects (Bailey *et al.* 1996). This finding has been discussed in more detail in Chapter 14, Section 14.4.2.

Figure 12.25 shows a summary of published data from mammalian systems from which biological effects attributed to cavitation-related mechanisms have been reported.

12.6.2.2 Acoustic Streaming

Bell (1957) has described histological studies of mammalian tissues after irradiation with 1 MHz ultrasound. He observed that the walls of blood vessels were often damaged. Dyson *et al.* (1974) observed similar effects when they irradiated chick embryos with 3 MHz ultrasound. In some vessels, the luminal aspect of the plasma membrane was seen to be damaged. Similar results were obtained by ter Haar *et al.* (1979), who used electron microscopy to study the effect of 3 MHz ultrasound on the mouse uterus. Again, damage was seen at the luminal aspect of the plasmalemma, and rounded up membrane fragments were found within the vessel lumen. This type of damage was thought to be due to the high shear stresses associated with acoustic streaming of the blood plasma against the vessel wall.

12.6.2.3 Standing Waves

Goldman annd Lepeschkin (1952) have shown in plant cells that, in a standing wave, the biological effects they observed were associated with the pressure antinodes. Although similar experiments are difficult to carry out in mammalian tissues *in vivo*, some work has been done in studying the effects of standing waves on blood flow. Schmitz (1950) first demonstrated, in frogs, that if a sufficiently high intensity was used, the red cells would clump together to form bands at half-wavelength separation. Dyson *et al.* (1974) have demonstrated the same effect in 3.5-day-old chick embryos, and ter Haar and Wyard (1978) and ter Haar *et al.* (1979) have produced red blood cell banding in mammalian vessels. While the sound is on, the red cells are held stationary in bands but the plasma continues to flow along the vessel. The effect is usually reversible, with the bands relaxing into a parabolic profile corresponding to the flow velocity across the vessel when the sound is turned off.

12.7 THERMAL AND MECHANICAL INDICES

The only country to regulate acoustic output from diagnostic ultrasound scanners is the USA. The 'Standard for real-time display of thermal and mechanical indices on diagnostic ultrasound equipment' (AIUM/NEMA 1992), known colloquially as the ODS, has been adopted as a means of satisfying the 'track 3' path of the Food and Drug Administration's 510 000 requirement for acoustic outputs. The output indices that have been chosen are the thermal index (*TI*) and the mechanical index (*MI*).

Mechanical index. The mechanical index (*MI*) is designed to indicate the potential for mechanically induced bio-effects. These effects include those due to streaming and cavitation. The level of knowledge available about non-thermal effects is probably inadequate to be certain about the exact form the MI should take. The form chosen assumes the existence of cavitation nuclei of appropriate size to undergo acoustic excitation at the frequency of interest. It was not designed for pressures above the inertial cavitation threshold. However, it is generally accepted that the probability of producing bio-effects from these non-thermal

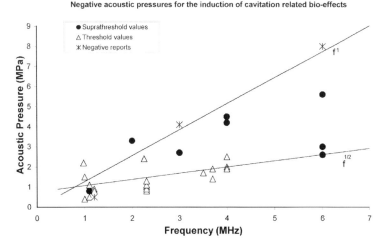

Figure 12.25. Summary of published data from mammalian systems from which biological effects attributed to cavitation-related mechanisms have been reported

mechanisms increases with rarefactional pressure and decreases with increasing ultrasonic frequency. Mechanical index has been defined as:

$$MI = p_{r, 0.3}/[CMI(f_{awf})]$$

where CMI is a normalising factor to ensure that MI is unitless and equals $1\,\text{MPa}\,\text{MHz}^{-1/2}$. Parameter $p_{r, 0.3}$ is the peak rarefactional acoustic pressure (in MPa) in tissue (*in situ*). This is calculated from free field (water) measurements assuming a uniform attenuation coefficient of $0.3\,\text{dB}\,\text{cm}^{-1}\,\text{MHz}^{-1}$. Parameter f_{awf} is the acoustic working frequency in MHz (f_{awf} is defined by IEC 61157 (1992) as the arithmetic mean of the frequencies f_1 and f_2 at which the amplitude of the spectrum of the acoustic signal first becomes $3\,\text{dB}$ lower than the peak amplitude).

There are a number of limitations to this index. The validity of the square-root frequency dependence has not been established unambiguously (Apfel & Holland 1991; WFUMB 1998). A more serious concern is that measurement of acoustic pressure in water followed by linear derating (calculation of an *in situ* value using a uniform attenuation coefficient) can lead to considerable underestimation of the actual *in situ* pressure amplitude. This is because diagnostic ultrasound beams propagate non-linearly in water, with energy being transferred from the fundamental frequency into its harmonics. This leads to peak pressures that are lower than would be measured under linear conditions (see Chapter 3). There is significantly less non-linear propagation in tissue.

Thermal index. In theory, heating should be an easier phenomenon for which to define an index than non-thermal effects. The relationship between the temperature rise and biohazard has been the subject of much research, although not for ultrasound as the source of heating. The majority of work on the embryo and fetus (the areas of most concern for diagnostic ultrasound safety) has been with whole-body heating using hot air or water. This is not entirely appropriate for ultrasonic heating where only a small fraction of the total volume is exposed. As pointed out by Abbott (1999), estimates of tissue temperature rise can be made using a combination of output power, temporal average intensity and spatial peak temporal average intensity. None of these parameters is sufficient on its own.

In general terms, the thermal index (*TI*) is defined by the equation:

$$TI = W_{\mathrm{P}}/W_{\mathrm{deg}}$$

where W_{P} is a power parameter defined within the ODS and W_{deg} is the estimated power needed to raise the target tissue by 1°C. W_{deg} is calculated for a number of different tissue models.

Clearly, predicting the temperature rise resulting from absorption of all the available different ultrasonic fields for all potential tissue geometries is an impossible task. Simplified models based on 'average' conditions have therefore been used. Three different thermal indices have been chosen. These are the soft tissue thermal index (*TIS*), used when there is no bone in the path, the bone thermal index (*TIB*), used when bone lies at the beam focus, and the cranial thermal index (*TIC*), used when bone lies near the surface. These are the indices that the user sees. Their derivation depends on aperture size and on whether the beam is scanned or unscanned.

Considerable effort is being made into assessing whether these indices provide good estimates of temperature rise that may actually be achieved in tissue. A major criticism is that knowledge of temperature rise alone is not sufficient to allow assessment of risk. It is also important to know for how long the elevated temperature is maintained. In addition, for the case of obstetric exposures, the maternal temperature must be taken into account.

12.8 CONCLUSION

The field of ultrasonic biophysics is a complex one. From the physicist's point of view it is not difficult to postulate a range of possible interaction mechanisms that may arise in biological tissues. It is, however, more difficult to isolate these mechanisms experimentally, to confirm their existence and to establish thresholds for their occurrence. For example, the intensities required to produce collapse cavitation will also produce significant heating in tissue. The mechanisms are in no way mutually exclusive.

Quantitative information has been noticeable by its absence in this chapter. The reason for this is simple – it is not available. Where it is available, the figures quoted strictly have relevance only to the experimental conditions used. It is more meaningful in this context to describe trends, and the dependence on acoustic variables such as frequency and intensity. The need for more rigorous experimentation is apparent.

In the following chapters in this book (Chapters 13 and 14), well-established biological effects are described and their relevance either for therapeutic benefit or to diagnostic 'hazard' is discussed. It is hoped that this chapter has provided adequate background to understand what ensues.

REFERENCES

Abbott, J.G. (1999). Rationale and derivation of MI and TI – a review. *Ultrasound Med. Biol.* **25**, 431–441.

AIUM (1994). *Bio-effects and Safety of Diagnostic Ultrasound.* American Institute of Ultrasound in Medicine, Laurel, MD.

AIUM/NEMA (1992). *Standard for Real-time Display of Thermal and Mechanical Acoustic Output Indices on Diagnostic Ultrasound Equipment.* American Institute of Ultrasound in Medicine, Rockville, MD.

Apfel, R.E. (1970). The role of impurities in cavitation – threshold determination. *J. Acoust. Soc. Am.* **48**, 1179–1186.

Apfel, R.E. (1980). Ultrasonics. In *Methods of Experimental Physics*, L. Marton (ed.). Academic Press, New York.

Apfel, R.E. and Holland, C.K. (1991). Gauging the likelihood of cavitation-threshold determination. *J. Acoust. Soc. Am.* **17**, 179–185.

Bailey, M.R., Dalecki, D., Child, S.Z., *et al.* (1996). Bioeffects of positive and negative acoustic pressures *in vivo. J. Acoust. Soc. Am.* **100**, 3941–3946.

Barger, J.E. (1964). *Thresholds of Acoustic Cavitation* (section 57). Acoustics Research Lab., Harvard Univ., Cambridge, MA.

Bell, E. (1957). The action of ultrasound on the mouse liver. *J. Cell Comp. Physiol.* **50**, 83–103.

Bender, L.F., Herrick, J.F. and Krusen, F.H. (1953). Temperatures produced in bone by various methods used in ultrasonic therapy. *Arch. Phys. Med. Rehab.* **34**, 424–433.

Benjamin, T.B. and Ellis, A.T. (1966). The collapse of cavitation bubbles and the pressures thereby produced against solid boundaries. *Philos. Trans. R. Soc. London. A* **260**, 221–240.

Blake, F.G. (1949). The onset of cavitation in liquids. 1. Cavitation threshold sound pressures in water as a function of temperature and hydrostatic pressure. *Tech. Mem. 12.* Acoustics Research Lab., Dept. of Engineering, Sciences and Applied Physics, Harvard University, Cambridge, MA.

Bly, S.H.P., Vlahovich, S., Mabee, P.R. and Hussey, R.G. (1992). Computed estimates of maximum temperature elevations in fetal tissues during transabdominal pulsed Doppler examinations. *Ultrasound Med. Biol.* **18**, 389–397.

Bosward, K.L., Barnett, S.B., Wood, A.K.W., Edwards, M.J. and Kossoff, G. (1993). Heating of guinea pig fetal brain during exposure to pulsed ultrasound. *Ultrasound Med. Biol.* **19**, 415–424.

Briggs, H.B., Johnson, J.B. and Mason, W.P. (1947). Properties of liquids at high sound pressure. *J. Acoust. Soc. Am.* **19**, 664.

Carstensen, E.L., Child, S.Z., Crane, C. and Parker, K.J. (1990a). Lysis of cells in *Elodea* leaves by pulsed and continuous wave ultrasound. *Ultrasound Med. Biol.* **16**, 167–173.

Carstensen, E.L., Child S.Z., Law, W.K., Horowitz, D.R. and Miller, M.W. (1979). Cavitation as a mechanism for the bioeffects of ultrasound in plant roots. *J. Acoust. Soc. Am.* **66**, 1285–1291.

Carstensen, E.L., Child, S.Z., Norton, S. and Nyborg, W.L. (1990b). Ultrasonic heating of the skull. *J. Acoust. Soc. Am.* **87**, 1310–1317.

Chan, A.K., Siegelmann, R.A., Guy, A.W. and Lehmann, J.F. (1973). Calculation by the method of finite differences of the temperature distribution in layered tissues. *IEEE Trans. Biomed. Eng.* **BME-20**, 86–90.

Child, S.Z., Hartman, C.L., McHale, L.A. and Carstensen, E.L. (1990). Lung damage from exposure to pulsed ultrasound. *Ultrasound Med. Biol.* **16**, 817–825.

Christman C.L., Catron P.W., Flynn, E.T. and Weathersby, P.K. (1986). *In vivo* microbubble detection in decompression sickness using a second harmonic resonant bubble detector. *Undersea Biomed. Res.* **13**, 1–18.

Clarke, P.R. (1969). Studies of the biological effects of ultrasound and of synergism between ultrasound and X-rays. PhD thesis, University of London.

Coakley, W.T. (1971). Acoustical detection of single cavitation events in a focused field in water at 1 MHz. *J. Acoust. Soc. Am.* **49**, 792–801.

Coakley, W.T. (1978). Biophysical effects of ultrasound at therapeutic intensities. *Physiotherapy* **64**, 166–169.

Coakley, W.T. and Nyborg, W.L. (1978). Methods and phenomena, Vol. 3. In *Ultrasound: Its Applications in Medicine and Biology Part I.* F.J. Fry (ed.). Elsevier Scientific Publishing, New York, pp. 77–159.

Coakley, W.T. and Sanders, M.F. (1973). Sonochemical yields of cavitation events at 1 MHz. *J. Sound Vib.* **28**, 73–85.

Coleman, A.J., Choi, M.J. and Saunders, J.E. (1996). Detection of acoustic emission from cavitation in tissue during clinical extracorporeal lithotripsy. *Ultrason. Med. Biol.* **22**, 1079–1087.

Coleman, A.J., Choi, M.J., Saunders, J.E. and Leighton, T.G. (1992). Acoustic emission and sonoluminescence due to cavitation at the beam focus of an electrohydraulic shock wave lithotripter. *Ultrason. Med. Biol.* **18**, 267–281.

Coleman, A.J., Draguioti, E., Tiptaf, R., Shotri, N. and Saunders, J.E. (1998). Acoustic performance and clinical use of a fibreoptic hydrophone. *Ultrason. Med. Biol.* **24**, 143–151.

Coleman, A.J., Kodama, T., Choi, M.J., Adams, T. and Saunders, J.E. (1995). The cavitation threshold of human tissue exposed to 0.2 MHz pulsed ultrasound: preliminary measurements based on a study of clinical lithotripsy. *Ultrason. Med. Biol.* **21**, 405–417.

Coleman A.J., Whitlock, M., Leighton, T.G. and Saunders, J.E. (1993). The spatial distribution of cavitation-induced acoustic emission sonoluminescence and cell lysis in the field of a shock-wave lithotripter. *Phys. Med. Biol.* **38**, 1545–1560.

Connolly, W. and Fox, F.E. (1954). Ultrasonic cavitation thresholds in water. *J. Acoust. Soc. Am.* **26**, 843–848.

Crank, J. (1967). *The Mathematics of Diffusion.* Clarendon Press, Oxford.

Crowell, J.A., Kusserow, B.K. and Nyborg, W.L. (1977). Functional changes in white blood cells after microsonation. *Ultrasound Med. Biol.* **3**, 185–190.

Crum, L.A. (1971). Acoustic force on a liquid droplet in an acoustic stationary wave. *J. Acoust. Soc. Am.* **50**, 157–163.

Crum, L.A. (1979). Surface oscillations and jet development in pulsating bubbles. *J. Phys.* **40**, C8–285.

Crum, L.A. and Eller, A. (1970). Motion of bubbles in a stationary sound field. *J. Acoust. Soc. Am.* **48**, 181–189.

Dalecki, D., Child, S.Z., Raeman, C.H. and Carstensen, E.L. (1995). Tactile perception of ultrasound. *J. Acoust. Soc. Am.* **97**, 3165–3170.

Dalecki, D., Child, S.Z., Raeman, C.H., *et al.* (1997). Thresholds for fetal haemorrhage produced by lithotripter fields. *Ultrasound Med. Biol.* **23**, 287–297.

Daniels, S., Davies, J.M., Paton, W.D.M. and Smith, E.B. (1980). The detection of gas bubbles in guinea pigs after decompression from air saturation dives using ultrasonic imaging. *J. Physiol.* **308**, 369–383.

Daniels, S., Paton, W.D.M. and Smith, E.B. (1979). An ultrasonic imaging system for the study of decompression induced gas bubbles. *Undersea Biomed. Res.* **6**, 197–207.

Daniels, S. and Price, D.J. (1991). Sonoluminescence in water and agar gels during irradiation with 0.75 MHz continuous-wave ultrasound. *Ultrasound Med. Biol.* **17**, 297–308.

Degrois, M. and Baldo, P. (1974). A new electrical hypothesis explaining sonoluminescence, chemical actions and other effects of gaseous cavitation. *Ultrasonics* **12**, 25–28.

Doody, C., Porter, H., Duck, F.A. and Humphrey, V.F. (1999). *In vitro* heating of human fetal vertebra by pulsed diagnostic ultrasound. *Ultrasound Med. Biol.* **25**, 1289–1294.

Drewniak, J.L., Carnes, K.I. and Dunn, F. (1989). *In vitro* ultrasonic heating of fetal bone. *J. Acoust. Soc. Am.* **88**, 26–34.

Duck, F.A. (1990). *Physical Properties of Tissue.* Academic Press, New York.

Duck, F.A. (1998). Acoustic streaming and radiation pressure in diagnostic applications: what are the implications? In *Safety of Diagnostic Ultrasound, Progress in Obstetrics & Gynecology Series*, S.B. Barnett and G. Kossoff (eds). Parthenon, New York, pp. 87–98.

Duck, F.A., Starritt, H.C., ter Haar, G.R. and Lunt, M.J. (1989). Surface heating of diagnostic ultrasound transducers. *Br. J. Radiol.* **62**, 1005–1013.

Duggan, P.M., Liggins, G.C. and Barnett, S.B. (1995). Ultrasonic heating of the brain of the fetal sheep *in utero*. *Ultrasound Med. Biol.* **21**, 553–560.

Dyer, H.J. and Nyborg, W.L. (1960a). Ultrasonically induced movements in cells and cell models. *IRE Trans. Med. Electron.* **ME–7**, 163–165.

Dyer, H.J. and Nyborg, W.L. (1960b). Characteristics of intracellular motion induced by ultrasound. *Proc. 3rd Int. Conf. Med. El.* Illiffe, London, pp. 445–449.

Dyson, M., Pond, J.B., Woodward, B. and Broadbent, J. (1974). The production of blood cell stasis and endothelial damage in the blood vessels of chick embryos treated with ultrasound in a stationary wave field. *Ultrasound Med. Biol.* **1**, 133–148.

Eastwood, L.M. and Watmough, D.J. (1976). Sonoluminescence, in water and in human blood plasma, generated using ultrasonic therapy equipment. *Ultrasound Med. Biol.* **2**, 319–323.

Elder, S.A. (1959). Cavitation microstreaming. *J. Acoust. Soc. Am.* **31**, 54–64.

Eller, A. (1968). Force on a bubble in a standing acoustic wave. *J. Acoust. Soc. Am.* **43**, 170–171.

Eller, A. and Flynn, H.G. (1969). The generation of subharmonics of order one half by bubbles in a sound field. *J. Acoust. Soc. Am.* **46**, 722–727.

Embleton, T.F.W. (1962). Mutual interaction between two spheres in a plane sound field. *J. Acoust. Soc. Am.* **34**, 1714–1720.

Epstein, P.S. and Plesset, M.S. (1950). On the stability of gas bubbles in liquid gas solutions. *J. Chem. Phys.* **18**, 1505–1509.

Esche, R. (1952). Untersuchung der Schwingungskavitation in Flüssigkeiten. *Akust. Beih.* **4**, 208.

Filipczynski, L., Kujawska, T. and Wojcik, J. (1993). Temperature elevation in focused Gaussian ultrasonic beams at various insonation times. *Ultrasound Med. Biol.* **19**, 667–679.

Finch, R.D (1963). Sonoluminescence. *Ultrasonics* **1**, 87–98.

Flynn, H.G. (1964). Physics of acoustic cavitation in liquids. In *Physical acoustics*, Vol. IB, W.P. Mason (ed.). Academic Press, New York, pp. 57–172.

Flynn, H.G. (1975). Cavitation dynamics. I. A mathematical formulation. *J. Acoust. Soc. Am.* **57**, 1379–1396.

Fox, F.E. and Herzfield, K.F. (1954). Gas bubbles with organic skin as cavitation nuclei. *J. Acoust. Soc. Am.* **26**, 984–989.

Frenzel, H. and Schultes, H. (1934). Lumineszenz im ultraschallbeschichteten Wasser. *Z. Physik. Chem.* **27B**, 421–424.

Fricke, H. and Hart, E.J. (1966). Chemical dosimetry. In *Radiation Dosimetry*, Vol. 11, F.H. Attrix and W.C. Roesch (eds). Academic Press, New York, pp. 167–239.

Gaitan, D.F. and Crum, L.A. (1990). Observation of sonoluminescence from a single cavitation bubble in a water/glycerine mixture. *Frontiers of Nonlinear Acoustics* (12th ISNA), M.F. Hamilton and D.T. Blackstock (eds). Elsevier, New York, p. 459.

Gaitan, D.F., Crum, L.A., Church, C.C. and Roy, R.A. (1992). An experimental investigation of acoustic cavitation and sonoluminescence from a single bubble. *J. Acoust. Soc. Am.* **91**, 3166–3183.

Galloway, W.J. (1954). An experimental study of acoustically induced cavitation in liquids. *J. Acoust. Soc. Am.* **26**, 849–857.

Gavrilov, L.R. (1984). Use of focused ultrasound for stimulation of nerve structures. *Ultrasonics* **22**, 132–138.

Gershoy, A., Miller, D.L. and Nyborg, W.L. (1976). Intercellular gas: its role in sonated plant tissue. In *Ultrasound in Medicine and Biology*, Vol. 2, D.N. White and R. Barnes (eds). Plenum Press, New York, pp. 501–510.

Gershoy, A. and Nyborg, W.L. (1973). Microsonation of cells under near threshold conditions. In *Ultrasonics in Medicine*, M. de Vlieger *et al.* (eds.). Excerpta Medica, Amsterdam, 1974, pp. 360–365.

Gersten, J.W. (1959). Temperature rise of various tissues in the dog on exposure to ultrasound at different frequencies. *Arch. Phys. Med.* **40**, 187–192.

Gilmore, F.R. (1952). *Hydrodynamics Laboratory Report 26–4*. California Institute of Technology.

Goldman, D.E. and Lepeschkin, W.W. (1952). Injury to living cells in standing sound waves. *J. Cell. Comp. Physiol.* **40**, 255–268.

Gor'kov, L.P. (1962). On the forces acting on a small particle in an acoustical field in an ideal fluid. *Sov. Phys. Dokl.* **6**, 773–775.

Gould, R.K. and Coakley, W.T. (1974). The effects of acoustic force on small particles in suspension. *Proc. Symp. Finite Wave Effects in Fluids.* IPC Science and Tech. Press, Lyngby, Denmark.

Graham, E., Hedges, M., Leeman, S. and Vaughan, P. (1980). Cavitational bio-effects at 1.5 MHz. *Ultrasonics* **18**, 224–228.

Greenspan, M. and Tschiegg, C.E. (1967). Radiation-induced acoustic cavitation; apparatus and some results. *J. Res. NBS (C) Eng. Instrum.* **71C**, 299–312.

Griffing, V. and Sette, D. (1955). Luminescence produced as a result of intense ultrasonic waves. *J. Chem. Phys.* **23**, 503.

Gross, D.R., Miller, D.L. and Williams, A.R. (1985). A search for ultrasonic cavitation within the canine cardiovascular system. *Ultrasound Med. Biol.* **11**, 85–97.

ter Haar, G.R. (1977). The effect of ultrasonic standing wave fields on the flow of particles, with special reference to biological media. PhD thesis, University of London.

ter Haar, G.R. and Daniels, S. (1981). Evidence for ultrasonically induced cavitation *in vivo. Phys. Med. Biol.* **26**, 1145–1149.

ter Haar, G.R., Daniels, S., Eastaugh, K.C. and Hill, C.R. (1982). Ultrasonically induced cavitation *in vivo. Br. J. Cancer* **45** (Suppl. V), 151–155.

ter Haar, G.R., Duck, F.A., Starritt, H.C. and Daniels, S. (1989). Biophysical characterisation of diagnostic ultrasound equipment – preliminary results. *Phys. Med. Biol.* **34**, 1533–1542.

ter Haar, G.R., Dyson, M. and Smith, S.P. (1979). Ultrastructural changes in the mouse uterus brought about by ultrasonic irradiation at therapeutic intensities in standing wave fields. *Ultrasound Med. Biol.* **5**, 167–179.

ter Haar, G.R. and Hopewell, J.W. (1982). Ultrasonic heating of mammalian tissues in vivo. *Br. J. Cancer* **45** (Suppl. V), 65–67.

ter Haar, G.R., Stratford, I.J. and Hill, C.R. (1980). Ultrasonic irradiation of mammalian cells *in vitro* at hyperthermic temperatures. *Br. J. Radiol.* **53**, 784–789.

ter Haar, G.R. and Wyard, S.J. (1978). Blood cell banding in ultrasonic standing wave fields: a physical analysis. *Ultrasound Med. Biol.* **4**, 111–123.

Harvey, E.N. (1930). Biological aspects of ultrasonic waves: a general survey. *Biol. Bull.* **59**, 306–325.

Harvey, E.N. (1939). Sonoluminescence and sonic chemiluminescence. *J. Am. Chem. Soc.* **61**, 2392–2398.

Hedges, M.J., Leeman, S. and Vaughan, P. (1977). Acoustic cavitation. *Proc. Underwater Acoust. Group*, **5**, 19.

Herrick, J.F. (1953). Temperatures produced in tissues, by ultrasound:experimental study using various techniques. *J. Acoust. Soc. Am.* **25**, 12–16.

Hill, C.R. (1972). Ultrasonic exposure thresholds for changes in cells and tissues. *J. Acoust. Soc. Am.* **52**, 667–672.

Hill, C.R., Clarke, P.R., Crowe, M.R. and Hammick, J.W. (1969). Biophysical effects of cavitation in a 1 MHz ultrasonic beam. *Proc. Conf. Ultrasonics for Industry*, Illiffe, London, pp. 26–30.

Hill, C.R. and Joshi, G.P. (1970). The significance of cavitation in interpreting the biological effects of ultrasound. *Proc. Conf. on Ultrasonics in Biol. & Med. UBIOMED-70*, Polish Academy of Sciences, Warsaw.

Holland, C.K. and Apfel, R.E. (1990). Thresholds for transient cavitation produced by pulsed ultrasound in a controlled nuclei environment. *J. Acoust. Soc. Am.* **88**, 2059–2069.

Holland, C.K., Deng, C.X., Apfel, R.E., Alderman, J.L., Fernandez, L.A. and Taylor, K.J.W. (1996). Direct evidence of cavitation *in vivo* from diagnostic ultrasound. *Ultrason. Med. Biol.* **22**, 917–925.

Horder, M.M., Barnett, S.B., Vella, G.J., Edwards, M.J. and Wood, A.K.W. (1998). *In vivo* heating of the guinea pig fetal brain by pulsed ultrasound and estimates of thermal index. *Ultrasound Med. Biol.* **24**, 1467–1474.

Hsieh, D.-Y. and Plesset, M.S. (1961). Theory of rectified diffusion of mass into gas bubbles. *J. Acoust. Soc. Am.* **33**, 206–215.

Huber, P., Debus, J., Peschke, P., Hahn, E.W. and Lorenz, W.J. (1994). *In vivo* detection of ultrasonically induced cavitation by a fibre optic technique. *Ultrason. Med. Biol.* **20**, 811–825.

Hug, O. and Pape, R. (1954). Nachweis der Ultraschallkavitation in Gewebe. *Strahlentherapie* **94**, 79–99.

Hynynen, K. (1991). The threshold for thermally significant cavitation in dog's thigh muscle *in vivo*. *Ultrasound Med. Biol.* **17**, 157–169.

Hynynen, K., Watmough, D.J., and Mallard, J.R. (1981). The effects of some physical factors on the production of hyperthermia by ultrasound in neoplastic tissues. *Radiat. Environ. Biophys.* **19**, 215–226.

Jackson, F.J. and Nyborg, W.L. (1958). Small scale acoustic streaming near a locally excited membrane. *J. Acoust. Soc. Am.* **30**, 614–619.

Keller, J.B. and Miksis, M. (1980). Bubble oscillations of large amplitude. *J. Acoust. Soc. Am.* **68**, 628.

Kolios, M.C., Sherar, M.D. and Hunt, J.W. (1996). Blood flow cooling and ultrasound lesion formation. *Med. Phys.* **23**, 1287–1298.

Lamb, H. (1945). *Hydrodynamics*. Dover, New York.

Landau, L.D. and Lifshitz, E.M. (1966). *Fluid Mechanics*. Pergamon Press, Oxford.

Lauterborn, W. (1976). Numerical investigation of non-linear oscillations of gas bubbles in liquids, *J. Acoust. Soc. Am.* **59**, 283–293.

Lauterborn, W. (1986). Acoustic turbulence. In *Frontiers in Physical Acoustics*, D. Sette (ed.). North Holland, Amsterdam, pp. 123–124.

Lauterborn, W. and Bolle, H. (1975). Experimental investigations of cavitation-bubble collapse in the neighbourhood of a solid boundary. *J. Fluid Mech.* **72**, 391–399.

Lauterborn W. and Cramer E (1981). Subharmonic route to chaos observed in acoustics. *Phys. Rev. Lett.* **47**, 1445–1448.

Lauterborn, W., Hinsch, K., and Bader, F. (1972). Holography of bubbles in water as a method to study cavitation bubble dynamics. *Acustica* **26**, 170–171.

Lauterborn, W. and Parlitz, U. (1988). Methods of chaos physics and their applications to acoustics. *J. Acoust. Soc. Am.* **84**, 1975–1993.

Lauterborn, W. and Suchla, E. (1984). Bifurcation superstructure in a model of acoustic turbulence. *Phys. Rev. Lett.* **53**, 2304–2307.

Lehmann, J.F. and Herrick, J.F. (1953). Biologic reactions to cavitation, a consideration for ultrasonic therapy. *Arch. Phys. Med.* **3**, 86–98.

Lehmann, J.F., Delateur, B.J., Stonebridge, J.B. and Warren, C.G. (1967b). Therapeutic temperature distribution produced by ultrasound as modified by dosage and volume of tissue exposed. *Arch. Phys. Med. Rehab.* **48**, 662–666.

Lehmann, J.F., Delateur, B.J., Warren, C.G. and Stonebridge, J.B. (1967a). Heating produced by ultrasound in bone and soft tissue. *Arch. Phys. Med. Rehab.* **48**, 397–401.

Lehmann, J.F., McMillan, J.A., Brunner, G.D. and Blumberg, J.B. (1959). Comparative study of the efficiency of short wave, microwave and ultrasonic diathermy in heating the hip joint. *Arch. Phys. Med. Rehab.* **40**, 510–512.

Leighton T.G. (1994). *The Acoustic Bubble*. Academic Press, London.

Leighton, T.G., Lingard, R.J., Walton, A.J. and Field, J.E. (1992). Bubble sizing by the nonlinear scattering of two acoustic frequencies. In *Natural Physical Sources of Underwater Sound*, B.R. Kerman (ed.). Kluwer, Dordrecht, The Netherlands.

Leighton, T.G., Pickworth, M.J.W., Tudor, J. and Dendy, P.P. (1990). A search for sonoluminescence *in vivo* in the human cheek. *Ultrasonics* **28**, 181–184.

Leighton, T.G., White, P.R. and Marsden, M.A. (1995). Applications of one-dimensional bubbles to lithotripsy, and to diver response to low frequency sound. *Acta Acoust.* **3**, 517–529.

Leverett, L. B., Hellums, J. D., Alfrey, C. P. and Lynch, E. C. (1972). Red cell damage by shear stress. *Biophys. J.* **12**, 257–273.

Lizzi, F.L., Coleman, D.J., Driller, J., Franzen, L.A. and Leopold, M. (1981). Effects of pulsed ultrasound on ocular tissue. *Ultrasound Med. Biol.* **7**, 245–252.

Mackay, R.S. and Rubissow, G. (1978). Decompression studies using ultrasonic imaging of bubbles. *IEEE Trans. BME* **25**, 537–544.

Magee, T.R. and Davies, A.H. (1993). Auditory phenomena during trans-cranial Doppler insonation of the basilar artery. *J. Ultrasound Med.* **12**, 747–750.

Makino, K., Mossoba, M.M. and Riesz, P. (1983). Chemical effects of ultrasound on aqueous solutions. Formation of hydroxyl radicals and hydrogen atoms. *J. Phys. Chem.* **104**, 1369–1377.

Marinesco, N. and Trillat, J.J. (1933). Action des ultrasons sur les plaques photographiques. *C. R. Acad. Sci. (Paris)* **196**, 856–860.

Martin, C.J. and Gemmell, H.G. (1979). A study of ultrasonically induced pulsations of gas filled channels in Elodea. *Phys. Med. Biol.* **24**, 600–612.

Martin, C.J., Gregory, D.W. and Hodgkiss, M. (1981). The effects of ultrasound in vivo on mouse liver in contact with an aqueous coupling medium. *Ultrasound Med. Biol.* **7**, 253–265.

McLean, J.R. and Mortimer, A.J. (1988). A cavitation and free radical dosimeter for ultrasound. *Ultrasound Med. Biol.* **14**, 59–64.

Meaney, P.M., Clarke, R.L., ter Haar, G.R. and Rivens, I.H. (1998). A 3D finite element model for computation of temperature profiles and regions of thermal damage during focused ultrasound surgery exposures. *Ultrasound Med. Biol.* **24**, 1489–1499.

Miller, D.L. (1977). The effects of ultrasonic activation of gas bodies in Elodea leaves during continuous and pulsed irradiation at 1 MHz. *Ultrasound Med. Biol.* **3**, 221–240.

Miller, D.L. (1979a). A cylindrical-bubble model for the response of plant-tissue gas bodies to ultrasound. *J. Acoust. Soc. Am.* **65**, 1313–1321.

Miller, D.L. (1979b). Cell death thresholds in Elodea for 0.45–10 MHz ultrasound compared to gas-body resonance theory. *Ultrasound Med. Biol.* **5**, 351–357.

Miller, D.L. (1981). Ultrasonic detection of resonant cavitation bubbles in a flow tube by their second-harmonic emissions. *Ultrasonics* **19**, 217–224.

Miller, D.L., Nyborg, W.L. and Whitcomb, C.C. (1978). In vitro clumping of platelets exposed to low intensity ultrasound. In *Ultrasound in Medicine*, Vol. 4. Plenum Publishing, New York, pp. 545–553.

Miller, D.L., Nyborg, W.L. and Whitcomb, C.C. (1979). Platelet aggregation induced by ultrasound under specialized conditions *in vitro*. *Science* **205**, 505.

Miller, D.L. and Thomas, R.M. (1993a). A comparison of hemolytic and sonochemical activity of ultrasonic cavitation in a rotating tube. *Ultrasound Med. Biol.* **19**, 83–90.

Miller, D.L. and Thomas, R.M. (1993b). Ultrasonic gas body activation in *Elodea* leaves and the mechanical index. *Ultrasound Med. Biol.* **19**, 343–351.

Minnaert, M. (1933). On musical air-bubbles and the sounds of running water. *Philos. Mag.* **16**, 235–248.

Morris, J.V. and Coakley, W.T. (1978). Detection of ultrasonic cavitation emissions from insonated plant tissues. *Proc. Ultrasonics International* 1977. IPC Business Press, Lyngby, Denmark, pp. 206–211.

Morris, J.V. and Coakley, W.T. (1980). The non-thermal inhibition of growth and the detection of acoustic emissions from bean roots exposed to 1 MHz ultrasound. *Ultrasound Med. Biol.* **6**, 113–126.

Morton, K.I., ter Haar, G.R., Stratford, L.J. and Hill, C.R. (1982). The role of cavitation in the interaction of ultrasound with V79 Chinese hamster cells *in vitro*. *Br. J. Cancer* **45** (Suppl. V), 147–150.

Morton, K.I., ter Haar, G.R., Stratford, L.J. and Hill, C.R. (1983). Subharmonic emission as an indicator of ultrasonically induced biological damage. *Ultrasound Med. Biol.* **9**, 629–633.

Nassiri, D.K., Nicholas, D. and Hill, C.R. (1979). Attenuation of ultrasound in skeletal muscle. *Ultrasonics* **17**, 230–232.

NCRP (1992). Exposure criteria for medical diagnostic ultrasound: 1. Criteria based on thermal mechanisms. *Report No. 113*. National Council for Radiation Protection and Measurements, Bethesda, MD.

Negeshi, K. (1961). Experimental studies on sonoluminescence and ultrasonic cavitation. *J. Phys. Soc. Jpn.* **16**, 1450–1465.

Neppiras, E.A. (1968). Subharmonic and other low frequency emission from bubbles in sound-irradiated liquids. *J. Acoust. Soc. Am.* **46**, 587–601.

Neppiras, E.A. (1969a). Subharmonic and other low frequency signals from sound irradiated liquids. *J. Sound Vib.* **10**, 176–186.

Neppiras, E.A. (1969b). Subharmonic and other low frequency emission from bubbles in sound-irradiated liquids. *J. Acoust. Soc. Am.* **46**, 587–601.

Neppiras, E.A. (1980a). Acoustic cavitation. *Phys. Rep.* **61**, 159–251.

Neppiras, E.A. (1980b). Acoustic cavitation thresholds and cyclic processes. *Ultrasonics* **18**, 201–209.

Neppiras, E.A. and Coakley, W.T. (1976). Acoustic cavitation in a focused field in water at 1 MHz. *J. Sound Vib.* **45**, 341–373.

Neppiras, E.A. and Noltingk, B.E. (1951). Cavitation produced by ultrasonics: theoretical conditions for the onset of cavitation. *Proc. Phys. Soc. B* **64**, 1032–1038.

Nightingale, K.R., Kornguth, P.J., Walker, W.F., McDermott, B.A. and Trahey, G.E. (1995). A novel technique for differentiating cysts from solid lesions: preliminary results in the breast. *Ultrasound Med. Biol.* **21**, 745–751.

Noltingk, B.E. and Neppiras, E.A. (1950). Cavitation produced by ultrasonics. *Proc. Phys. Soc. B* **63**, 674–685.

Nyborg, W.L. (1965). Acoustic streaming. In *Physical Acoustics*, Vol. IIB, W. P. Mason (ed.). Academic Press, New York, Chapt. 11.

Nyborg, W.L. (1967). Radiation pressure on a small rigid sphere. *J. Acoust. Soc. Am.* **42**, 947–952.

Nyborg, W.L. (1975). Ultrasound. In *Intermediate Biophysical Mechanics*. Cummings Publishing, California, Chapt. 14, Section 9.

Nyborg, W.L. (1978a). Physical mechanisms for biological effects of ultrasound. *HEW Publication (FGDA)* 78–8062.

Nyborg, W.L. (1978b). Physical principles of ultrasound. In *Ultrasound: Its Applications in Medicine and Biology* (1st edn), F.J. Fry (ed.). Elsevier, New York, pp. 1–75.

Nyborg, W.L. and Dyer, H.J. (1960). Ultrasonically induced motions in single plant cells. *Conf. on Medical Electronics*, Paris, France, 24–27 June 1959. Iliffe & Sons, London, pp. 391–396.

Nyborg, W.L. and Steele, R.B. (1983). Temperature elevation in a beam of ultrasound. *Ultrasound Med. Biol.* **9**, 611–620.

Parke, A.V.M. and Taylor, D. (1956). The chemical action of ultrasonic waves. *J. Chem. Soc.* **4**, 4442–4450.

Parlitz, U., Englisch, V., Scheffczyk, C. and Lauterborn, W. (1990). Bifurcation structure of bubble oscillators. *J. Acoust. Soc. Am.* **88**, 1061–1077.

Patton, C.A., Harris G.R. and Phillips R.A. (1994). Output levels and bio-effects indices from diagnostic ultrasound exposure data reported to the FDA. *IEEE Trans. UFFC* **41**, 353–359.

Paul, W. D. and Imig, C. J. (1955). Temperature and blood flow studies after ultrasonic irradiation. *Am. J. Phys. Med.* **34**, 370–375.

Pennes, H.H. (1948). Analysis of tissue and arterial blood temperatures in the resting human forearm. *J. Appl. Physiol.* **1**, 93–122.

Penney, D.P., Schenk E.A., Maltby K., *et al.* (1993). Morphological effects of pulsed ultrasound in the lung. *Ultrasound Med. Biol.* **19**, 127–135.

Plesset, M.S. (1949). The dynamics of cavitation bubbles. *J. Appl. Mech.* **16**, 277–282.

Polotskii, I.G. (1949). *Z. Fizi. Khim.* **22**, 387.

Poritsky, H. (1952). The collapse or growth of a spherical bubble or cavity in a viscous fluid. In *Proceedings of the First US National Congress on Applied Mechanics*. E. Sternberg (ed.). New York, pp. 813–821.

Price, G.J. (1998). Sonochemistry and drug delivery. In *Ultrasound in Medicine*, F.A. Duck, A.C. Baker and H.C. Starritt (eds). Institute of Physics Publishing, Bristol, pp. 241–259.

Price, G.J. and Lenz, E.J. (1993). The use of dosimeters to measure radical production in aqueous sonochemical systems. *Ultrasonics* **31**, 451–456.

Pritchard, N. J., Hughes, D. E. and Peacocke, A. R. (1966). The ultrasonic degradation of biological macromolecules under conditions of stable cavitation. 1. Theory, methods and applications to deoxyribonucleic acid. *Biopolymers* **4**, 259–273.

Prosperetti, A., Crum, L.A. and Commander, K.W. (1988). Nonlinear bubble dynamics. *J. Acoust. Soc. Am.* **83**, 502–514.

Rayleigh, Lord (1917). On the pressure developed in a liquid during the collapse of a spherical cavity. *Philos. Mag.* **34**, 94–98.

Rooney, J.A. (1970). Haemolysis near an ultrasonically pulsating gas bubble. *Science* **169**, 869–871.

Rooney, J.A. (1972). Shear as a mechanism for sonically induced biological effects. *J. Acoust. Soc. Am.* **52**, 1718–1724.

Rosenberger, H. (1950). Über den Wirkungsmechanismus der Ultraschallbehandlung, ins besondere bei Ischias und Neuralgien. *Der Chirurg.* **21**, 404–406.

Roy, R.A., Atchley, A.A., Crum, L.A., Fowlkes, J.B. and Reidy, J.J. (1985). A precise technique for the measurement of acoustic cavitation thresholds and some preliminary results. *J. Acoust. Soc. Am.* **78**, 1799–1805.

Roy, R.A., Madanshetty, S. and Apfel, R.E. (1990). An acoustic backscatter technique for the detection of transient cavitation produced by microsecond pulses of ultrasound. *J. Acoust. Soc. Am.* **87**, 2451–2455.

Rozenberg, L.D. and Sirotyuk, M.G. (1961). Radiation of sound in a liquid with cavitation present. *Sov. Phys. Acoust.* **6**, 477–479.

Rubissow, G.J. and Mackay, R.S. (1971). Ultrasonic imaging of *in vivo* bubbles in decompression sickness. *Ultrasonics* **9**, 225–234.

Saksena, T.K. and Nyborg, W.L. (1970). Sonoluminescence from stable cavitation. *J. Chem. Phys.* **53**, 1722–1734.

de Santis, P., Sette, D. and Wanderlingh, F. (1967). Cavitation detection: the use of subharmonics. *J. Acoust. Soc. Am.* **42**, 514–516.

Schmitz, W. (1950). Ultraschall als biologisches Forschungsmittel. *Strahlentherapie* **83**, 654–662.

Schrope, B. and Newhouse, V.L. (1993). Second harmonic ultrasonic blood perfusion measurement. *Ultrasound Med. Biol.* **19**, 567–579.

Sette, D. and Wanderlingh, F. (1962). Nucleation by cosmic rays in ultrasonic cavitation. *Phys. Rev.* **125**, 409–417.

Starritt, H.C., Duck, F.A. and Humphrey, V.F. (1989). An experimental investigation of streaming in pulsed diagnostic ultrasound beams. *Ultrasound Med. Biol.* **15**, 363–373.

Staudenraus, J. and Eisenmenger, W. (1988). Optisches Sondenhydrophon. *Fortschritte der Akustik*. DAGA GmbH, pp. 476–479.

Staudenraus, J. and Eisenmenger, W. (1993). Fibre optic probe hydrophone for ultrasonic and shock wave measurements in water. *Ultrasonics* **4**, 267–273.

Strasberg, M. (1959). Onset of ultrasonic cavitation in tap water. *J. Acoust. Soc. Am.* **31**, 163–176.

Tarantal, A.F. and Canfield, D.R. (1994). Ultrasound induced lung haemorrhage in the monkey. *Ultrasound Med. Biol.* **20**, 65–72.

Tarantal A.F., Chu F., O'Brien W.D. and Hendrickx, A.G. (1993). Sonographic heat generation *in vivo* in the gravid long-tailed Macaque (*Macaca fascicularis*). *J. Ultrasound Med.* **5**, 285–295.

Thomenius, K.E. (1990). Thermal dosimetry models for diagnostic ultrasound. In *Proc. IEEE Ultrasonics Symposium*. IEEE, New York, pp. 1399–1408.

Todd, J.H. (1970). Measurement of chemical activity of ultrasonic cavitation in aqueous solutions. *Ultrasonics* **8**, 234–238.

Tucker, D.G. (1965). The exploitation of non-linearity in underwater acoustics. *J. Sound Vib.* **2**, 429–434.

Vaughan, P.W. (1968). Investigation of acoustic cavitation thresholds by observation of the first subharmonic. *J. Sound. Vib.* **7**, 236–246.

Wang, S-W., Feng, R., Xu, J.-Y. and Shi, Q. (1993). Effect of ultrasound pulse width on cavitation in a small size reverberation field. *Ultrasonics* **31**, 39–44.

Weissler, A. (1959). Formation of hydrogen peroxide by ultrasonic waves:free radicals. *J. Am. Chem. Soc.* **81**, 1077–1081.

Weissler, A., Cooper, H.W. and Snyder, S. (1950). Chemical effects of ultrasonic waves: oxidation of KI solution by CCl_4. *J. Am. Chem. Soc.* **72**, 1769.

Westervelt, P.J. (1957). Acoustic radiation pressure. *J. Acoust. Soc. Am.* **29**, 26–29.

WFUMB (1992). Issues and recommendations regarding thermal mechanisms for biological effects of ultrasound. *Ultrasound Med. Biol.* **18**, 731–814.

WFUMB (1998). Conclusions and recommendations regarding nonthermal mechanisms for biological effects of ultrasound. *Ultrasound Med. Biol.* **24** (Suppl. 1).

Willard, G.W. (1953). Ultrasonically induced cavitation in water – a step by-step process. *J. Acoust. Soc. Am.* **25**, 669–686.

Williams, A.R. (1971). Hydrodynamic disruption of human erythrocytes near a transversely oscillating wire. *Rheol. Acta* **10**, 67–70.

Williams, A.R. (1977). Intravascular mural thrombi produced by acoustic microstreaming. *Ultrasound Med. Biol.* **3**, 191–203.

Williams, A.R., Delius, M., Miller, D.L. and Schwarze, W. (1989). Investigation of cavitation in flowing media by lithotriptor shock waves both *in vitro* and *in vivo*. *Ultrasound Med. Biol.* **15**, 53–60.

Williams, A.R., Hughes, D.E. and Nyborg, W.L. (1970). Hemolysis near a transversely oscillating wire. *Science* **169**, 871–873.

Williams, A.R. and Miller, D.L. (1980). Photometric determination of ATP release from human erythrocytes exposed to ultrasonically activated gas-filled pores. *Ultrasound Med. Biol.* **6**, 251–256.

Wilson, W.L., Wiercinski, F.J., Nyborg, W.L., Schnitzler, R.M. and Sichel, F.J. (1966). Deformation and motion produced in isolated living cells by localized ultrasonic vibration. *J. Acoust. Soc. Am.* **40**, 1363–1370.

Wojcik, J., Filipczynski, F. and Kujawska, T. (1999). Temperature elevations computed for three-layer and four-layer obstetrical tissue models in nonlinear and linear ultrasonic propagation cases. *Ultrasound Med. Biol.* **25**, 259–267.

Wood, R.W. and Loomis, A.L. (1927). The physical and biological effects of high frequency sound waves of great intensity. *Philos. Mag.* **4** (7), 417–436.

Wu, J., Chase, J.D., Zhu, Z. and Holzapfel, T.P. (1992). Temperature rise in a tissue-mimicking material generated by unfocused and focused ultrasonic transducers. *Ultrasound Med. Biol.* **18**, 495–512.

Wu, J. and Nyborg, W.L. (1992). Temperature rise generated by a focussed Gaussian beam in a two-layer medium. *Ultrasound Med. Biol.* **18**, 293–302.

Yosioka, K. and Kawasima, Y. (1955). Acoustic radiation pressure on a compressible sphere. *Acustica* **5**, 167–173.

Zeman, R.K., Davros, W.J., Garra, B.S. and Horii, S.C. (1990a). Cavitation effects during lithotripsy. Part I: results of *in vitro* experiments. *Radiology* **177**, 157–161.

Zeman, R.K., Davros, W.J., Goldberg, J.A., *et al.* (1990b). Cavitation effects during lithotripsy. Part II: Clinical observations. *Radiology* **177**, 163–166.

13

Therapeutic and Surgical Applications

GAIL R. TER HAAR

Institute of Cancer Research, Royal Marsden Hospital, UK

13.1 INTRODUCTION

As we have seen from Chapter 12 (and *cf.* Harvey & Loomis 1928) it has been known for some time that ultrasound interacts with tissue to produce biological change. Although there has been natural concern about possible hazard associated with diagnostic ultrasonic imaging, most of the early effort was put into using ultrasonically induced changes in tissue for therapeutic benefit.

There is an extensive literature covering the subject of ultrasound therapy, although unfortunately most reports are anecdotal and contain little hard scientific information. It is intended in this chapter largely to confine the discussion to work that has a reasonably well-established scientific basis.

Therapeutic ultrasound can be divided broadly into two classes: at low intensities (0.125–3.0 W cm^{-2} SATA (spatial average, temporal average intensity) at frequencies of a few megahertz) the aim is to produce non-destructive heating or other, non-thermal effects, and to stimulate or accelerate normal physiological response to injury; at higher intensities (> 5 W cm^{-2}) the aim is rather to produce controlled selective destruction of tissues. The first category includes the majority of physiotherapeutic uses, whereas beam surgery falls into the second category.

13.2 PHYSIOLOGICAL BASIS FOR ULTRASOUND THERAPY

13.2.1 HEAT

The temperature distributions that may be obtained in mammalian tissues during ultrasonic heating have been discussed in some detail in Chapter 12, Section 12.1. The controlled delivery of heat to deep-seated tissues may give therapeutic benefit in a number of ways, some of which are outlined in this section.

In general, reports that the thermal effects of ultrasound are of therapeutic benefit have not been accompanied by accurately measured temperature distributions, nor by rigorous dosimetry, and so the effects described here are largely based on qualitative evidence.

The high absorption coefficients exhibited by large protein molecules mean that collagenous tissues may be heated preferentially using ultrasound. It is often these tissues that the physiotherapist would like to treat.

Physical Principles of Medical Ultrasonics, Second Edition. Edited by C. R. Hill, J. C. Bamber and G. R. ter Haar.
© 2004 John Wiley & Sons, Ltd: ISBN 0 471 97002 6

13.2.2 NON-THERMAL EFFECTS

The non-thermal mechanisms by which ultrasound may act on tissue have been outlined in Chapter 12. As far as consideration of physiological effects is concerned, these mechanisms may be divided into two classes: cyclic and non-cyclic.

Cyclic effects arise from the periodic nature of the sound pressure field and have been referred to as 'micro-massage' (Summer & Patrick 1964). This oscillatory motion may help in loosening adhesions present in soft tissue injuries.

The main non-cyclic effect thought to produce therapeutic benefit is acoustic streaming (see Chapter 12, Section 12.3.2). This may be due to stable, oscillating cavities or to radiation forces in intra- or extracellular fluids. Acoustic streaming can modify the local environment of membranes, altering concentration gradients and changing the diffusion of ions and molecules across them. Mihran *et al.* (1990) attributed the change in excitability of myelinated sciatic nerve in frogs to radiation pressure effects. It has been shown that the potassium content of some cells may be reduced following irradiation with ultrasound *in vitro* (Chapman *et al.* 1979), although cavitation bubbles may be involved in this type of experiment. Changes in the calcium content of smooth muscle cells may account for the increase in uterine contractions in mice induced by ultrasound (ter Haar *et al.* 1978), and Al Karmi *et al.* (1994) demonstrated that the increase in ionic conductance in frog skin induced by ultrasound was influenced by the presence of calcium ions. Mortimer and Dyson (1988) showed that exposure of cultured fibroblasts *in vitro* to intensities of $0.5–1.0\,\mathrm{W\,cm^{-2}}$ increased the amount of intracellular calcium but that $1.5\,\mathrm{W\,cm^{-2}}$ did not. It is extremely difficult to identify positively the different non-thermal effects that may arise in tissues, and indeed to isolate such effects from any tissue heating that must necessarily occur when sound is absorbed in tissue. It is probably easiest to identify effects due to cavitation by the criterion that application of increased ambient pressure will suppress them.

Some of the non-thermal effects of ultrasound may be detrimental if care is not exercised in its application. If a reflecting surface is contained within the irradiated volume, standing waves may be set up. If a blood vessel lies within this volume, red blood cell banding may occur, and if this is maintained for a significant length of time, tissues downstream may be deprived of oxygen.

Where cavitation bubbles are formed in tissue, a variety of effects may be observed. As mentioned earlier, streaming motions are set up around a stably oscillating bubble.

13.2.2.1 Increase in Extensibility and Strength of Collagenous Tissues

A major factor that often impedes the recovery of soft tissue to injury is contracture associated with the injury, which may lead to an inhibition of normal motion. Slight tissue heating may increase mobility. Lehmann *et al.* (1970), for example, have described how the application of heat during stretching exercises may increase the elastic properties of collagenous structures. Gersten (1955) has shown that ultrasonic heating can lead to an increase in tendon extensibility. Scar tissue may also be rendered more supple by the use of ultrasonic treatment. Specific applications in physiotherapy are discussed in Section 13.3.

Enwemeka *et al.* (1990) found that when $0.5\,\mathrm{W\,cm^{-2}}$ (1 MHz) ultrasound was used for 5 min daily for 9 days to treat severed rabbit tendons, the tensile strength and energy absorption capacity were significantly increased. This was in contrast to the earlier findings of the same group (Enwemeka 1989) in which $1\,\mathrm{W\,cm^{-2}}$ was not effective in increasing these properties. This finding – that effects of ultrasound may be more beneficial at low intensities than at higher ones – has been found in other model systems, such as calcium transport across membranes (Mortimer & Dyson 1988; see Section 13.2.2) and in wound healing (Byl *et al.* 1992, 1993). This may indicate that non-thermal mechanisms of action may also be playing a therapeutic role. Da Cunha *et al.* (2002) found similar results, showing that pulsed ultrasound (1 MHz; 0.5 W cm^{-2} SATA; pulsed 1:4) enhanced healing of the rat Achilles tendon, whereas continuous wave exposure at the same intensity retarded it. Takakura *et al.* (2002) exposed rat medial collateral ligaments to low-intensity pulsed ultrasound (1.5 MHz; r.f. 1 kHz; 200 μs pulses; 30 mW cm^{-2}). They found that 12 days following injury the exposed ligaments were stronger than the controls, but that this difference had disappeared by 21 days. The mean diameter of the collagen fibres was greater in the exposed ligaments than in the controls.

13.2.2.2 Decrease in Joint Stiffness

The range of motion of stiff joints may be increased when the contractures around them are heated (Backlund & Tiselius 1967). Ultrasound may be the heating modality of choice when the joint has significant soft tissue cover because its penetration into muscle is better than that of other forms of diathermic energy (Lehmann *et al.* 1959; Hand & ter Haar 1981).

13.2.2.3 Pain Relief

Many patients report pain relief following heat treatment of an affected area. This may be instantaneous and long lasting. Ultrasound appears to be particularly beneficial in producing pain relief in some patients. For example, Rubin and Kuitert (1955) found it useful in producing relief from pain arising from phantom limbs, scars and neuromas. Mechanisms for pain relief are poorly understood and, if this is a localised effect in the tissue, non-thermal effects may be involved.

13.2.2.4 Changes in Blood Flow

Vascular changes are often seen in response to localised tissue heating and may be observed at a distance from the heated volume. It has been shown that muscle blood flow may increase two- to threefold following ultrasonic heating to temperatures in the range 40–45°C (ter Haar & Hopewell 1983). Similar effects have been reported by Paul and Imig (1955). Imig *et al.* (1954) attributed blood flow changes to local vasodilation and found similar effects with ultrasound and electromagnetic heating. Abramson *et al.* (1960) have shown blood flow changes following pulsed irradiation. The changes persisted for about half an hour following treatment.

Local dilation increases the oxygen supply and thus improves the environment of cells. This may have therapeutic benefit. An increased inflammatory response also may be seen.

A study of the microvascular dynamics of rat cremaster muscle has shown that, for sufficiently high intensities (> 5 W cm^{-2} in the case quoted), there may be a decrease both in vessel lumen and volume flow in some vessels. This was, however, thought not to be a thermal effect but more likely to be due to cavitation or some other mechanical cause (Hogan *et al.* 1982).

13.2.2.5 Decrease in Muscle Spasm

Heat may induce a reduction in muscle spasm. This is thought to be a sedative effect of increased temperature on peripheral nerve endings (Fountain *et al.* 1960). Ultrasound may be used to produce this effect.

The extent of physiological response to heating may depend on a number of factors, including temperature achieved, time of heating, heated volume and rate of temperature rise. Ultrasound provides a method of rapidly heating a well-defined volume. The highly collagenous regions of superficial cortical bone, periosteum, menisci, synovium and capsules of joints, myofascial interfaces, intermuscular scars, fibrotic muscle, tendon sheaths and major nerve trunks are among the anatomical structures that are heated selectively by ultrasound.

In some conditions ultrasound can be the most effective form of thermotherapy (compared with short-wave diathermy, wax baths and infrared) and may be the treatment method of choice (Middlemast & Chatterjee 1978).

13.2.3 ULTRASONICALLY ENHANCED DRUG DELIVERY

13.2.3.1 Sonophoresis

Sonophoresis, or phonophoresis as it is sometimes called, is the term used to describe the ultrasonically induced increase in penetration of pharmocologically active agents through the skin or through other anatomical barriers or membranes (Skauen & Zenter 1984). The possible mechanisms responsible for sonophoresis are heating, cavitation and micro-streaming. It seems improbable that heating is responsible because similar effects are not achieved by other heating techniques (Meidan *et al.* 1995). Bommannan *et al.* (1992a, b) have suggested that cavitation may be involved, although this seems unlikely at the exposure levels generally used. The 'stirring' produced by acoustic streaming may perturb any barriers to perfusion at the skin, thus allowing enhanced perfusion (Ziskin & Michlovitch 1986). Griffin and Touchstone (1963, 1972) and Griffin *et al.* (1965) showed an increase in cortisol level intramuscularly and within the paravertebral nerve as a result of ultrasound exposure. As a result of these findings, small-scale clinical trials of the effects of the combination of ultrasound and either injected or topically applied hydrocortisone on pain relief and reduction of inflammation have been undertaken (Griffin *et al.* 1967; Kleinkort & Wood 1975; Davick *et al.* 1988; Muir *et al.* 1990), with variable results.

Attempts to increase anaesthetic effect transdermally with ultrasound have yielded inconsistent results (Novak 1964; Cameroy 1966; Moll 1977; Antich *et al.* 1986; Smith *et al.* 1986; Williams 1990; Singh & Vyas 1996). Anaesthetics studied include lignocaine, lidocaine and xylocaine.

In general, studies of sonophoresis lack the scientific rigour necessary to provide convincing proof that ultrasound can enhance transdermal drug delivery. An exception to this appears to be the work of Bommannan *et al.* (1992a, b). This group has studied the ability of ultrasound to enhance the transport of salicylic acid through the skin. They found that whereas a 20-min exposure of $0.2\,W\,cm^{-2}$ at $2\,MHz$ had no effect, the same exposure time and intensity at 10 and $16\,MHz$ increased transport by 4- and 2.5-fold, respectively (Bommannan *et al.* 1992b). A study of mechanisms involved (Bommannan *et al.* 1992a) led them to investigate the transport of the electron dense colloidal tracer lanthanum hydroxide across the skin. They found that lanthanum hydroxide penetrated the stratum corneum and underlying epidermal layers via an intercellular route under the influence of ultrasound. The cellular morphology of these layers was unaffected at $0.2\,W\,cm^{-2}$ when a $10\,MHz$ frequency was used for 5 or 20 min or $16\,MHz$ was used for 5 min. A frequency of $16\,MHz$ for 20 min at $0.2\,W\,cm^{-2}$ showed cellular damage typical of cavitation effects, although this seems surprising at this intensity level and high frequency. Some degree of local heating could not be ruled out.

The field of sonophoresis is tantalising. There appears to be anecdotal evidence that it may be a real and useful phenomenon, but proper scientific evidence for this is lacking. A comprehensive review of the literature has been carried out by Meidan *et al.* (1995). They concluded that there were no discernible trends between ultrasonic exposure conditions, molecular structure and degree of enhancement. The most convincing results have been observed when the enhanced absorption of molecules was obtained by exposing tissues to ultrasound prior to application of the drug (Murphy & Hadgraft 1990; Bommannan *et al.* 1992a; McElnay *et al.* 1993). This indicates that the effect is obtained by inducing perturbations to the stratum corneum such that it is permeabilised to drug delivery. Electron microscopy of the skin surface has revealed deep crater-like clefts where superficial capillaries are visible. This disruption may facilitate the absorption of drugs into the bloodstream (Tachibana & Tachibana 1999).

Weimann and Wu (2002) have reported an effect that they term sonomacroporation. This is the enhancement of transdermal delivery of high-molecular-weight drugs (such as poly-L-lysine (51 kDa), insulin (6 kDa) and erythropoietin (48 kDa)) by the transient generation of large pores (1–100 μm) in the stratum corneum. Weimann and Wu (2002) demonstrated the effect with poly-L-lysine using 20 kHz ultrasound at intensities in the range 2–50 W cm^{-2}. They saw a considerably higher flux of these large molecules than did Mitragotri and Blankschtein (1995), who used intensities of < 2 W cm^{-2}. Sonomacroporation provides the potential for using these pathways to facilitate the delivery of micron-sized liposomes loaded with drugs through the skin.

13.2.3.2 Thrombolysis

The potential for ultrasound to dissolve blood clots has been investigated fairly extensively for a number of years (Tachibana & Tachibana 1996). The thrombus resembles a fibrin net with spaces between the fibrin or red cells. The transport of fibrinolytic drugs into the thrombus determines the clot lysis rate. Ultrasound appears to enhance the transport of these drugs through the clot via a non-thermal mechanism. Acoustic streaming appears to be an important factor, presumably because it increases the availability of drug at the thrombus surface. It has been demonstrated that the effect is considerably enhanced when cavitation centres in the form of microbubbles are introduced (Tachibana & Tachibana 1995). Fibrinolysis with urokinase was increased in an artificial blood clot from 26.6% for the drug alone. 33% for drug plus ultrasound exposure (170 kHz; 0.5 W cm^{-2}; 2 ms on/4 ms off; 60 s) to 51.3% when exposed to drug and ultrasound in the presence of albumin-coated gas bubbles. Drugs that have been investigated for their efficacy in combination with ultrasound *in vitro* include rt-PA (recombinant tissue plasminogen activator), t-PA (tissue plasminogen activator), urokinase and streptokinase (Olsson *et al.* 1994).

Tachibana and Tachibana (1996) used an acoustic horn driven at 224 kHz (30 mW) to demonstrate enhanced fibrinolysis in combination with urokinase *in vitro*. They have also described a catheter with a ceramic source (0.7–2.0 MHz) mounted at the tip, for use intravascularly. Sobbe *et al.* (1974) used a 26 kHz catheter probe to dissolve blood clots in animals *in vivo*. Suction removed the dissolved clot material through the centre of the catheter. Similar success has been demonstrated by Rosenschein *et al.* (1990), Siegel *et al.* (1996b) and Atar *et al.* (1999). Behrens *et al.* (2001) compared the efficacy of 185 kHz ultrasound (2 W cm^{-2}) exposure to that from a 1 MHz diagnostic probe (524 mW cm^{-2}) in producing thrombolysis when clots placed in a post-mortem skull were exposed to rt-PA with and without ultrasound. They showed that under these conditions 185 kHz was more effective.

This is an interesting and evolving field. The reader is referred to extensive reviews by Siegel (1996) and Tachibana and Tachibana (1999) for more detail. Ultrasound is also used to recanalise vessels blocked by atherosclerotic plaque (see Section 13.5) and, conversely, to occlude patent vessels (Section 13.5.1.2.5).

13.2.3.3 Gene Therapy

There is considerable interest in developing systems that facilitate the transfer of genes into diseased tissues and organs. The main goal is to increase the efficiency of delivery of exogenous nucleic acid to the intended target. A perfect system would enhance gene expression in the target while having no effect in non-target tissues. Ultrasound might be able to provide this localisation. It has been shown that ultrasound can enhance gene transfer into cells *in vitro* (Kim *et al.* 1996; Bao *et al.* 1997; Lawrie *et al.* 1999; Tata *et al.* 1999). This enhancement has also been demonstrated *in vivo* (Bao *et al.* 1998; Bednarski *et al.* 1998). However, it is clear that transfection is significantly improved in the presence of cavitation (Bao *et al.* 1998; Greenleaf *et al.* 1998). There is therefore considerable interest in the effects of ultrasound on gene transfer in the presence of artificially introduced cavitation nuclei, namely gas-filled contrast agents (Price & Kaul 2002). It is known that diagnostic levels of ultrasound (with mechanical index (MI) levels around 1.6–2.0) can burst these microbubble contrast agents. If a drug or gene were contained within the bubble it would be released into the bloodstream in the vicinity of the ultrasound beam. In addition, the interaction between ultrasound and the bubble can increase the permeability of blood vessel walls. Extravasation of red blood cells has been seen following ultrasound exposure of contrast agents *in vivo*, but only in positions in which the bubbles were constrained (Price *et al.* 1998; Skyba *et al.* 1998). This permeabilisation allows transport of large molecules across the membrane. Ultrasound exposures of the gas bodies can lead to enhanced gene transfer either when the bubbles are in the vicinity of the genetic material or when the genes are encapsulated within or bound to the bubbles. Both strategies have been investigated *in vitro* (Huber & Pfisterer 2000; Lawrie *et al.* 2000; Frenkel *et al.* 2002) and *in vivo* (Miller *et al.* 1999; Tachibana *et al.* 1999; Anwer *et al.* 2000; Huber & Pfisterer 2000; Manome *et al.* 2000; Shohet *et al.* 2000; Taniyama *et al.* 2002a, b).

In principle there are two main vehicles for gene transfer – viral and non-viral vectors. Viral vectors (adeno- and retroviruses), which account for the majority of clinical trials to date, may produce unwanted side effects because they can provoke immunogenic responses. Non-viral vectors are easier to prepare. Pure plasmid DNA can be attached to microbubble walls. Lawrie *et al.* (2000) showed that ultrasound exposures that enhanced transgene expression after naked DNA transfection by up to a factor of 10 in the absence of bubbles gave an approximately 300-fold increase when contrast agents were present. Tachibana *et al.* (1999) have reported significant increases in reporter gene expression *in vivo* in mouse quadriceps following 1 MHz ultrasound exposure, and Manome *et al.* (2000) have demonstrated gene expression enhancement in solid tumours. Frenkel *et al.* (2002) showed that, when plasmid DNA was attached to albumin microbubbles, gene expression and transfection were enhanced more than if the two were not bound together. Shohet *et al.* (2000) injected perfluoropropane microbubbles to which were bound recombinant adenovirus containing the complementary DNA encoding the β-galactoside gene into rats. The rat hearts were exposed to pulsed 1.3 MHz ultrasound. Four days after exposure a 10-fold enhancement of β-galactosidase expression was found.

Ultrasound-enhanced gene therapy is a rapidly expanding field. It is intriguing because the exposure levels required to destroy microbubbles lie in the diagnostic range. In fact, if exposure levels are too high, unacceptable levels of cell killing may be seen (Huber *et al.* 1999) and extended exposure times may result in lower levels of DNA transfer (Wyber *et al.* 1997).

13.2.3.4 Sonodynamic Therapy

Photodynamic therapy has been used with some success in the treatment of a number of cancers, including those of the colon and bladder (Fromm *et al.* 1996; Dougherty *et al.* 1998; Nseyo *et al.*

1998). The principle of the technique is that photosensitive drugs (usually haematoporphyrin derivatives) delivered to tumours systemically or locally are excited by exposure to laser light of appropriate wavelength. However, photodynamic therapy is limited by the necessity to gain close access to the tumour for the laser light, and by the limited penetration of light into a solid tumour mass. It has been shown that acoustic cavitation can also activate photosensitive drugs such as haematoporphyrin and ATX-70 (Yumita *et al*. 1989; Umemura *et al*. 1990, 1993; Miyoshi *et al*. 1995; Kessel *et al*. 1994). This has been termed sonodynamic therapy. It has the clear advantage over photodynamic therapy that the activating ultrasound beam has better penetration and better localisation potential than laser light. Ogawa *et al*. (2001) have demonstrated that the combination of ultrasound (255 kHz; 0.4 W cm^{-2}; 30 s) and the photosensitising drug merocyanine 540 (MC 540) leads to an increase in membrane porosity. This may be useful if genes or drugs are to be delivered selectively. Tachibana *et al*. (1997) showed that ultrasound in combination with a photosensitive drug (porfimer sodium) reduced the survival of leukaemic cells exposed *in vitro* to 34% compared with 70% when exposed to ultrasound alone and 96.7% when exposed to drug alone. Normal cell survivals were 86.9% for ultrasound plus drug, 84.6% for ultrasound alone and 98.9% for drug alone.

In order to achieve tumour selectivity, photosensitisers have been conjugated with antibodies against tumour-associated antigens. Abe *et al*. (2002) have investigated the exposure of carcinoembryonic antigen (CEA)-expressing cells to ultrasound (1 MHz, 1 W cm^{-2}; 50% duty cycle; 60 s) and a photoimmunoconjugate between the sensitiser ATX-70 and a monoclonal antibody specific to CEA. They found in both *in vitro* and *in vivo* models that sonodynamic therapy with the conjugate was the most effective. Sonodynamic therapy is still in its infancy. It seems likely that it will find its niche in selected tumours such as those in the bladder. Ultrasound may prove to be preferable to laser light for these photosensitive drugs.

13.3 PHYSIOTHERAPY

Ultrasound is used in physical medicine. Originally it was thought of as one of several different techniques for diathermy treatment, competing with hot packs, microwave and radiofrequency methods. The main use of ultrasonic therapy has been in the treatment of soft tissue injuries, although it has been used also for wound healing and for the treatment of bone and joint injuries. As the basic understanding of interaction mechanisms improves, there is a move by some physiotherapists to alter their treatment regimes in an attempt to make use of any beneficial non-thermal mechanisms that may exist (by use of lower intensities and of pulsed beams). There is a dearth of scientifically designed controlled clinical trials, and so the ultrasonic treatment regime that is used is usually empirically determined, and often to each department's particular 'recipe'. It is true, however, that, as more education is given to physiotherapists on the subject of ultrasound, more treatment 'planning' occurs. It would be unfair, though, to be too critical of the physiotherapists' methods of choosing the ultrasound exposure because the necessary information is not readily available to them. It is not known which intensities are important in determining therapeutic benefit and whether, for example, the SATP or SATA intensity is of most importance (see Chapter 3, Section 3.8). Intuitively one might think that where a thermal effect is required the SATA intensity (i.e. 'total energy') would be important, whereas if a non-thermal effect is required it may be the peak intensity that dominates (SATP).

13.3.1 EQUIPMENT AND TECHNIQUES

There are a variety of ultrasound physiotherapy units available commercially. The majority are small and light enough to be readily portable. Most offer spatial average intensities up to

$3\,\mathrm{W\,cm^{-2}}$ (over the effective radiating area; but see below) and operate at frequencies in the range 0.75–5 MHz. The energy is delivered in either continuous or pulsed mode. Pulsed irradiations are mainly chosen when a predominantly non-thermal effect is required. Precise treatment regimes are usually determined empirically. The choice of carrier frequency is determined by the depth of lesion to be treated, higher frequencies being used for the more superficial injuries. These commercial generators usually offer the choice of two or three discrete frequencies (often with interchangeable transducers) and either discrete intensity settings or a continuously variable intensity control. Most machines have a pulsing facility, with one or two pulsing regimes offered. Commonly available pulsing regimes are 2 ms : 2 ms (mark : space) and 2 ms : 8 ms. (Pulsing regimes are expressed as either a mark : space ratio or as a duty factor [mark/(mark+space) %]; in either case, a pulse length must be given for the pulsing to be described fully.) A timer is usually included so that treatment times may be pre-set. Published surveys of ultrasound therapy generators in hospital use have revealed that the calibrations supplied by the machine manufacturers may be grossly inaccurate (for example, see Stewart *et al.* 1974; Repacholi & Benwell 1979). Repacholi and colleagues found that, for the 37 devices in use in the Ottawa area that were tested, the acoustic output varied from +200% to −250% of the meter reading, with 72% of the devices giving less than the set value in the continuous mode. Similar results were found by Hekkenberg *et al.* (1986), Pye and Milford (1994) and Pye (1996).

The timers were also checked and, although the majority were accurate to within 5%, 40% were in error by more than this and in some cases by as much as 20%. In the Stewart survey, and also in the author's experience, equipment has been found that gave no output despite a positive meter reading.

There are some easy tests to give a quick assessment of whether or not there is acoustic output from the therapy transducer. Some physiotherapists apply a layer of coupling medium to the transducer face and turn up the intensity until 'ripples' form on the surface of the coupling agent. Alternatively, the transducer may be held under water, pointing towards the surface. As the intensity is increased, a disturbance, often described as a 'fountain', may be seen on the water surface. Martin and Fernandez (1997) have described the use of thermochromic material sandwiched between layers that absorb ultrasound to visualise an ultrasonic field. If the absorbent layers are optically transparent, the thermal image obtained when the sandwich intercepts a physiotherapy beam shows the beam shape. Using this method, spatial peak intensities down to $0.2\,\mathrm{W\,cm^{-2}}$ may be detected with a spatial resolution of ca. 0.5 mm, in times of the order of 5 s.

Spatial average intensities at therapy levels can be measured using a simple radiation balance (Hill 1970; Shotton 1980; Davidson *et al.* 1991), and beam profiles may be obtained using small heat- or pressure-sensitive devices (Woolley *et al.* 1975). These methods are discussed in Chapter 3.

Standard methods for characterisation of the output and performance of physiotherapy equipment have been developed (Hekkenberg *et al.* 1994). Exposure levels for physiotherapy treatment are usually quoted as spatial averages. The International Electrotechnical Commission (IEC) standard method (IEC 1996) calculates an average over the 'effective radiating area'. This is the part of a plane at, or close to, the treatment head through which almost all the ultrasound passes. A beam non-uniformity ratio also has been defined. This parameter takes into account the existence of high local pressures (hot spots) and represents the ratio of the peak to spatial average intensity in the beam. In a survey of 37 treatment heads, the beam non-uniformity ratio was normally found to be in the range 3–7, but eight heads had values of $\geqslant 8$. Beam non-uniformity ratio values > 8 are thought to be characteristic of a 'hot spot'. This threshold value is twice the maximum value for an ideal piston transducer and represents a spatial peak/temporal peak intensity of $48\,\mathrm{W\,cm^{-2}}$ and a spatial peak/temporal average intensity of $24\,\mathrm{W\,cm^{-2}}$ At these levels, adverse biological effects might be anticipated.

Therapy transducers are usually made from discs of low-loss lead zirconate titanate (e.g. 'PZT4'). They are mounted in a waterproof housing, often of aluminium or stainless steel, at the end of a lightweight handle and are air-backed. A typical method of crystal mounting is shown in Figure 13.1. Examples of field profiles for a commercial therapy transducer are shown in Figure 13.2.

A variety of techniques may be used to introduce the ultrasonic energy into the treatment site. The most common method is a 'contact' application in which the transducer is applied directly to the skin and adequate transmission is obtained through a thin layer of coupling medium (with acoustic impedance matching that of the skin).

Water bath immersion may be used where awkward geometries are to be irradiated, such as the elbow or ankle. Alternatively, water bags may be used. The water is contained within a flexible bag of acoustically transparent material. The bag can be made to conform to the surface geometry of the region to be treated and is acoustically coupled to the skin by a thin layer of coupling medium.

Commonly used coupling media are easily sterilisable liquids with suitable acoustic impedance, such as mineral oil or liquid paraffin. Thixotropic substances are also used. These are easy to apply because they are quite viscous but they become more liquid under the action of ultrasound. A comparison of commonly used coupling agents has been published that shows that the amount of energy transmitted through the different media is very similar for the thin layers used, more difference being measured on changing the pressure exerted by the transducer on the film than on changing the coupling medium (Warren *et al.* 1976).

Open wounds may be treated through sterile wound dressings, provided that they have similar acoustic properties to soft tissues and that air can be excluded from the wound. An example of such a dressing is Geliperm (Geistlich Pharmaceuticals). This is a transparent polyacrylamide agar gel containing 96% water. This dressing, which has been shown to transmit 95% of ultrasound energy at 1 MHz, is used to dress skin graft donor sites, burns, pressure sores and varicose ulcers. Geliperm has been used successfully as an ultrasound contact medium for chronic varicose ulcers, unhealed amputation stumps and ligament injuries (Brueton & Campbell 1987). Sterile saline is first applied to the wound and then the dressing, moistened on both sides with sterile saline, is applied, taking care to exclude all air.

The transducer may be held still in one position during treatment ('stationary head technique') or may be moved continuously over the affected area ('moving head technique').

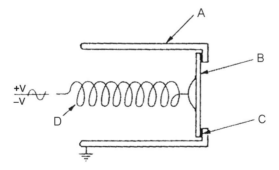

Figure 13.1. Schematic diagram to show typical method of crystal mounting for air-backed therapy transducers: (A) metal housing (earthed); (B) piezoelectric crystal silvered on both faces; (C) solder; (D) spring-loaded contact to back face

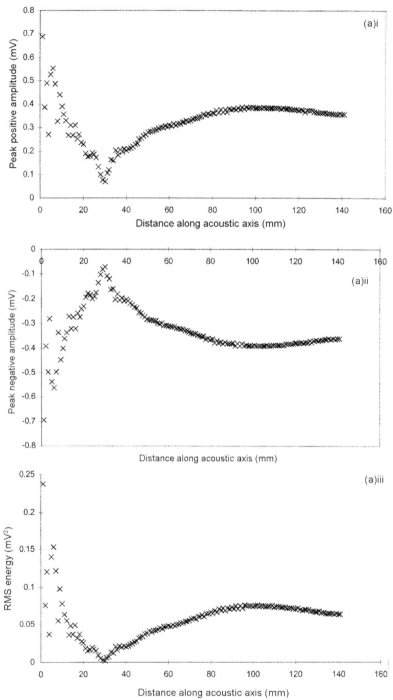

Figure 13.2a For caption see page 419

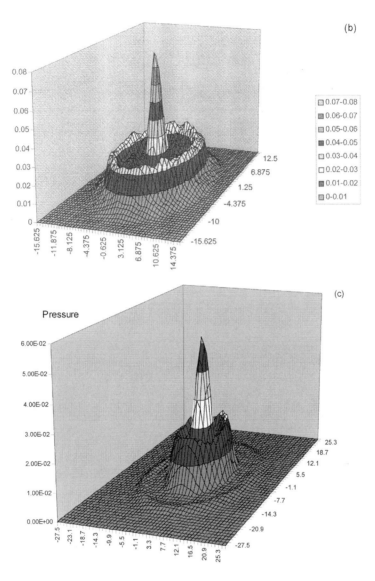

Figure 13.2b, c

The stationary head method should be avoided where possible because standing waves can be set up and 'hot spots' in the field can lead to local damage.

13.3.2 APPLICATIONS OF ULTRASOUND IN PHYSIOTHERAPY

Ultrasound is used mainly in the treatment of soft tissue injuries for the acceleration of wound healing, the resolution of oedema, softening of scar tissue and for many other conditions. It is also used, among other things, for bone injuries and circulatory disorders.

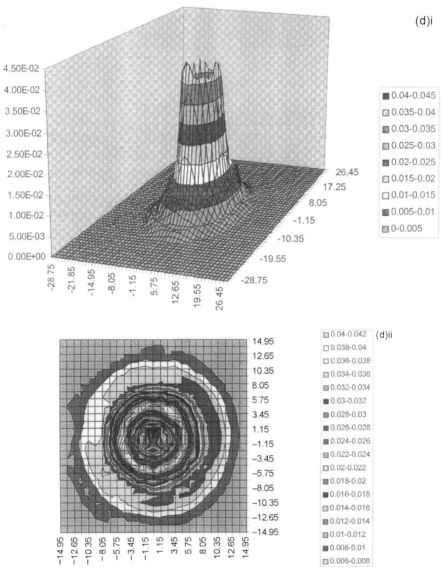

Figure 13.2d

13.3.2.1 Soft Tissue Injuries

One of the most common applications of ultrasound in physiotherapy is for the stimulation of tissue repair and wound healing. The evidence for the value of its use in this way is largely anecdotal, but a useful scientific study of the situation has been made using rabbits' ears (Dyson *et al.* 1968, 1970; Dyson & Pond, 1970). Tissue was excised from the pinnae of both ears; one side was irradiated with ultrasound while the other was treated as a control. Figure 13.3 shows the way in which the treated ear healed compared with the control. It can be seen

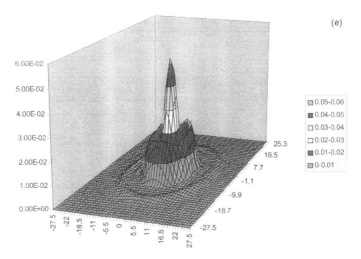

Figure 13.2. Typical field from a physiotherapy transducer. (a 1 cm diameter disc operating at 1.1 MHz): (a) axial plots of peak positive pressure, peak negative pressure and intensity; (b) transaxial profile of intensity measured 1 cm from transducer face; (c) transaxial profile of intensity measured 2 cm from transducer face; (d) two- and three-dimensional transaxial profiles of intensity measured 4 cm from transducer face; (e) transaxial profile of intensity measured 8 cm from transducer face. *Source*: Courtesy of Dr Zeqiri at the National Physical Laboratory, UK

that two waves of healing occurred. If the ultrasound was pulsed 2 ms on: 8 ms off at $0.5\,W\,cm^{-2}$ (SATP intensity), the best increase in healing was seen, although $0.1\,W\,cm^{-2}$ delivered in continuous mode gave a similar effect. With $8\,W\,cm^{-2}$ pulsed 1 ms on : 79 ms off there was an increase in lesion size. All three treatment regimes had the same time-averaged intensity. For pulsed ultrasound, $0.5\,W\,cm^{-2}$ (2 ms : 8 ms) gave more rapid healing than 0.25, 1.0, 1.5, 2.0 or $4.0\,W\,cm^{-2}$ pulsed in the same fashion.

Tissue repair can best be described in terms of three overlapping phases. During an 'inflammatory' phase, phagocytic activity of macrophages and polymorphonuclear leukocytes leads to the removal of cell debris and pathogens. The digestion of this material is largely carried out by lysosomal enzymes from the macrophages. It is known that ultrasound at therapy intensities may assist in accelerating this phase (Dyson 1990; Young & Dyson 1990; De Deyne & Kirsch-Volders 1995). It has been shown that ultrasound can stimulate the release of histamine by mast cell degranulation (Fyfe & Chahl 1982), possibly by an increase of calcium ion transport across their membranes (Mortimer & Dyson 1988). Although therapeutic ultrasound can accelerate this inflammatory phase of wound healing, it appears not to be an anti-inflammatory agent (Goddard *et al* 1983; Snow & Johnson 1988).

The second phase in wound healing, which starts about 3 days after injury, is 'proliferative'. Cells migrate to the injured region and start to divide. Granulation tissue is formed and fibroblasts begin to synthesise collagen. The strength of the wound begins to increase and specially adapted cells, myofibroblasts, cause the wound to contract. Ultrasound has been shown to have considerable effect on the synthesis of collagen by fibroblasts both *in vitro* and *in vivo* (Dyson & Smalley 1983).

Harvey *et al*. (1975) have demonstrated that, when primary diploid human fibroblasts were irradiated with 3 MHz ultrasound at an intensity of $0.5\,W\,cm^{-2}$ *in vitro*, the amount of protein synthesised was increased. Electron microscopic examination of irradiated cells revealed that,

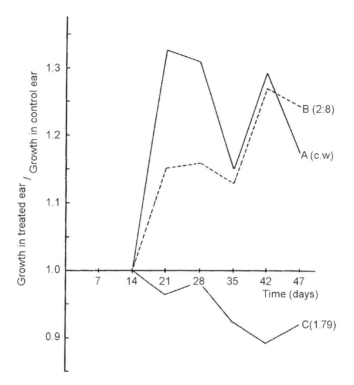

Figure 13.3. Effect on regeneration of rabbits' ears of different ultrasonic treatments with equivalent thermal dose: (A) 0.1 W cm^{-2} continuous wave, ΔT=1.3°C; (B) 0.5 W cm^{-2}, 2 ms : 8 ms, ΔT=1.6°C; (C) 8.0 W cm^{-2}, 1 ms : 79 ms, ΔT=1.6°C. *Source*: Adapted from Dyson *et al.* (1970)

in comparison with control cells, there were more free ribosomes, more dilatation of rough endoplasmic reticulum, more cytoplasmic vacuolation, more autophagic vacuoles and more damage to lysosomal membranes and mitochondria. Subsequent work from the same group (Webster *et al.* 1978, 1980) has shown that cavitation may be involved in producing this stimulation of collagen synthesis. Increased collagen synthesis also has been shown as a result of ultrasonic irradiation of fibroblasts *in vivo* (Webster *et al.* 1979). Ultrasound has been shown to stimulate the formation of granulation tissue (Pospisilova *et al.* 1974; Pospisilova 1976).

The third phase is that of remodelling. Normal connective tissue derives its elasticity from the way in which the network of collagen is arranged, allowing the tissue to tense and relax without undue strain. In scar tissue, the fibres are often laid down in an irregular, matted fashion that does not allow stretch without tearing the tissue. This leads to a reduction in the strength and elasticity of the scar compared with that of the normal tissue surrounding it. There is evidence that scar tissue treated with ultrasound is stronger and more elastic than 'normal' scar tissue, indicating that ultrasound may influence the fashion in which new collagen is deposited, and therefore aid the remodelling process.

Drastichova *et al.* (1973) have studied the effect of ultrasound (0.85 W cm^{-2}) on the strength of scars in guinea pigs. Incisions on the back were irradiated 3 and 4 days after cutting. The breaking strength of the scars was 189% of that in controls in one series, and 271% in another.

Dyson *et al.* (1979) have studied the effect of ultrasound (3 MHz, $0.5\,W\,cm^{-2}$) on the healing of cryosurgical lesions in rats. The lesions were irradiated on days 0, 1, 3, 5 and 7. The ultrasonically treated scar tissue was found to have a breaking strength of 109% of mock-irradiated scars at one month and 126% of untreated scars after 2 months. After 2 months the breaking strength of the treated scars was 42% of that of normal skin at the same site.

Byl *et al.* (1992, 1993) studied the wound breaking strength and collagen deposition of incisions in pig skin subjected to two intensity levels of therapeutic ultrasound ($1.5\,W\,cm^{-2}$, continuous wave, 1 MHz, 5 min; and $0.5\,W\,cm^{-2}$, pulsed 20%, 1 MHz, 5 min). They found that during the first week following injury either intensity could be used and an enhanced breaking strength was measured. However, after this time it was necessary to use the lower intensity in order to retain a beneficial effect.

It is disappointing that, despite the widespread use of therapy ultrasound, very few large-scale clinical trials have taken place. One condition, however, for which a trial has been carried out is that of chronic varicose ulcers on the leg (Dyson *et al.* 1976). Treated ulcers were irradiated with pulsed 3 MHz ultrasound (2 ms : 8 ms) at a SATP intensity of $1.0\,W\,cm^{-2}$. After 12 treatments (three times weekly for 4 weeks) insonated ulcers had an average surface area of 66.4±8.8% of their area at the beginning of treatment, whereas control ulcers had an area 99.6±8.9% of the initial area. Temperature rises in the treated area were measured and found to be less than 1°C. Such a temperature rise, if obtained by other means, would be insufficient to account for the observed stimulation of healing, and the mechanism is thus believed to be non-thermal. Callam *et al.* (1987) found similar results, although their treatment regime was slightly different, being once a week for 12 weeks (1 MHz, $0.5\,W\,cm^{-2}$, pulsed). In a separate study, it has been shown that ultrasound may increase the 'take' of skin grafts at trophic ulcer sites (Galitsky & Lavina 1964). McDiarmid *et al.* (1985) were able to demonstrate an improvement in the healing rate of infected pressure sores, but not of clean ones (3 MHz, SATA $0.2\,W\,cm^{-2}$, 2 ms : 8 ms, three treatments a week). A possible explanation for this finding may be that infected sores may contain more macrophages than clean ones, and thus ultrasonic stimulation of these cells into the production of wound factors will have more effect here than in the clean wounds, which may already be healing at an 'optimum' rate.

Ultrasound is used with some success to soften and increase the elasticity of scar tissue and contractures (Bierman 1954; Markham & Wood 1980; Pospisilova *et al.* 1980). The evidence for this is again anecdotal but it seems a fairly universal finding. The mechanism by which this may occur is unclear, but may relate to the combination of mild heating and exercise as described earlier in this chapter.

It is thought that ultrasound can be used to some benefit in reducing oedema associated with soft tissue injuries. Fyfe and Chahl (1980) have investigated this oft-heard claim (see, for example, Patrick 1973). They treated experimentally induced oedema in rats with $0.5\,W\,cm^{-2}$ pulsed ultrasound at a range of frequencies (0.75 MHz, 1.5 MHz and 3.0 MHz). A frequency-dependent effect was reported, 0.75 MHz being the only effective frequency. The pulsing regime (2 ms : 8 ms or 2 ms : 2 ms) was not important. The mechanism producing this resolution of oedema is not known. It may be due to increased blood flow or to localised tissue changes due to acoustic streaming.

Until more rigorous scientific studies of these and other reported effects are undertaken, the mechanism by which therapeutic benefit, if any, is obtained will be the subject of speculation and it will not be possible to optimise treatments using an understanding of interaction mechanisms. Robertson (2002) undertook a survey of randomised clinical trials of physiotherapy ultrasound. She was unable to find a relationship between 'dose' and therapeutic outcome, although the majority of effective treatments were pulsed, with spatial average temporal average intensities lying between 0.16 and $0.5\,W\,cm^{-2}$.

13.3.2.2 Bone Injuries

The repair of soft tissue injuries and bone injuries shows some similarities. Both processes have inflammatory, proliferative and remodelling phases. It is this similarity, and the fact that the cells involved initially are of the same type, that have prompted the investigation of the potential of ultrasound in bone healing, although little has been published on this topic.

It has been found in experimental studies of fracture in rat fibulae that ultrasonic irradiation during the inflammatory and early proliferative phases accelerates and enhances healing. Direct ossification, with little cartilage production, is seen. Treatment in the late proliferative phase, however, was found to be disadvantageous: cartilage growth is stimulated, with delay to bony union (Dyson & Brookes 1983). In their study, it was found that 1.5 MHz was more effective than 3.0 MHz (SATP 0.5 W cm^{-2}, 2 ms : 8 ms, 5 min) and so a non-thermal effect is suggested, although the precise mechanism still needs elucidation. This finding has been repeated by a number of authors. Pilla et al. (1990) showed that the strength of intact bone was reached in ultrasonically treated rabbit fibulae 17 days after osteotomy, compared with 28 days for control animals (1.5 MHz, SATA 0.03 W cm^{-2}, 200 μs : 800 μs, 20 min daily). Heckman et al. (1994) demonstrated similar acceleration of healing in a human clinical trial. They treated open fractures of the tibial shaft and found a significant reduction in the time needed to achieve clinical and radiographic healing: 96±4.9 days for the ultrasonically treated group and 154±13.7 days for the control group (1.5 MHz, SATA 0.03 W cm^{-2}, 200 μs : 800 μs, daily, starting within 7 days of fracture).

There appears to be evidence that it is not only the time at which treatment is started that is important, but also the dose level. Too high an intensity can lead to inhibition of protein synthesis or, at worst, to deleterious effects. Tsai et al. (1992) found that whereas 0.5 W cm^{-2} (SATA) significantly accelerated bone repair, 1.0 W cm^{-2} (SATA) suppressed the repair process (1.5 MHz, 200 μs, 5–20 min daily). Reher et al. (1997), in an in vitro study of the effect of ultrasound exposure on mouse calveria bone, found that whereas 0.1 W cm^{-2} (3 MHz, 2 ms : 8 ms, 5 min) stimulated collagen and non-collagenous protein synthesis, intensities of 0.5–2 W cm^{-2} inhibited these. The observed protein synthesis stimulation was attributed to osteoblastic activity. Yang et al. (1996) found a statistically significant increase in mechanical strength in fractured rat femurs at 0.05 W cm^{-2} (SATA, 0.5 MHz) but not at 0.1 W cm^{-2}. They noted a shift in the expression of genes associated with cartilage formation in the treated bones. Aggrecan gene expression was higher than control values on day 7 but lower than control on day 21. There are a number of other reports supporting the finding that very low intensities are effective in promoting bone repair (Kristiansen et al. 1997; Mayr et al. 2000, 2001; Shimazaki et al. 2000; Nolte et al. 2001; Rubin et al. 2001; Takikawa et al. 2001; Heybeli et al. 2002). Heybeli et al. (2002), for example, have reported stimulation of fracture repair in rats following five exposures to diagnostic levels of ultrasound (7.5 MHz; 11.8 mW cm^{-2}; 1 ms pulses; r.f. 1 Hz; 10 min; 5-day intervals).

Wang et al. (1994) found ultrasonically accelerated fracture repair at 21 days in a rat femoral model, but only at 1.5 MHz (SATA 0.03 W cm^{-2}, 200 μs : 800 μs) and not at 0.5 MHz.

It seems clear that, at the correct exposure levels, ultrasound may have a role to play in the acceleration of the rate of bone fracture repair, but the evidence from human clinical trials is sparse.

13.4 ULTRASOUND IN TUMOUR CONTROL

In this section, the use of ultrasound at intensity levels (SPTA) less than about 5 W cm^{-2} is discussed. The aim at these levels is generally to achieve cellular reproductive death. This is distinct from the 'high'-intensity focused beam applications for tumour ablation discussed in Section 13.5 for which the aim is instantaneous cell killing induced by temperatures in excess of 55°C.

The first mention of the possibility of using ultrasound for the treatment of cancer was in a report published in *Nature* in 1933, which stated that it had no specific effect on Ehrlich's carcinoma (Szent-Györgi 1933). From this time, enthusiasm for the potential of ultrasound as an antitumour agent has come in waves, reflecting, by and large, the popularity of hyperthermia.

In the years up to 1949 a number of groups studied the possibility of using ultrasound either on its own or in conjunction with X-rays. In 1944, the first report of the successful application of ultrasound to human tumours (skin metastases) appeared (Horvath 1944). In 1949 a conference in Erlangen, Germany, concluded that the excessive enthusiasm for the potential of ultrasound was not backed up by clinical results, and that 'its use should be discontinued' (Kremkau 1979). Following this, the research effort was considerably reduced for a while.

A revival in interest in the use of heat for cancer therapy either alone or with X-rays or chemotherapy (Field & Bleehen 1979) led to renewed interest in the ultrasonic treatment of tumours.

Three lines of study have evolved, namely the use of ultrasound on its own, the possibility of synergy with x- or γ-irradiation and the possibility of synergy with cytotoxic agents.

Ultrasound of sufficient intensity can undoubtedly heat localised regions of tissue to required hyperthermic temperatures ($> 42°C$; see Chapter 12, Section 12.1.2). Techniques for achieving specific temperature distributions have been discussed in Chapter 2 and in several review articles (see, for example, ter Haar & Hand 1981; Hunt, 1982). These include the use of lens systems, curved transducers, mirror systems, crossed beams and phased arrays. The temperature distribution required depends on the size and shape of the tumour to be treated and its position in the body. In general, the aim is to heat the tumour mass to a uniform temperature while maintaining the 'normal' tissue at a physiologically acceptable level. In practice, the tumour is generally heated to give an acceptable minimum tumour temperature and some normal tissue is heated to a comparable degree because it is important that the tumour periphery reaches hyperthermic levels. The wide range of distributions required means that the heating technique must be extremely flexible. Temperatures must be measured accurately and this is usually done invasively using thermocouple probes.

There are indications that ultrasound may have some cytotoxic effect over and above that due to the temperature rise. This has been shown by the *in vitro* irradiation of cells maintained at hyperthermic temperatures (Li *et al.* 1977; ter Haar *et al.* 1980). The loss of reproductive integrity (as shown by clonogenic assay) is found to be greater in the heated and ultrasonically irradiated samples than in the samples that had only been heated (Figure 13.4a). The mechanism of killing is not known but has been shown to be non-thermal and non-cavitational in origin (Morton *et al.* 1983). A similar effect has been seen in multicellular spheroids (Figure 13.4b). This is an effect of ultrasound on cells maintained at hyperthermic temperatures; irradiation at 37°C under similar conditions does not alter cell survival.

Evidence for a synergistic effect between ultrasound and X-rays is somewhat equivocal. The earliest reports from Woeber (1957, 1965) indicated that, if ultrasound was used in conjunction with X-rays for both rat Walker carcinoma and some human tumours (mainly basal cell cancer and squamous cell carcinoma), the radiotherapy dose could be reduced by 30–40% to give the same tumour response as obtained with radiotherapy alone. Ultrasound alone had no effect on the tumour.

Other investigators have found that the effectiveness of ultrasound added to x-irradiation may be tumour type dependent (Witcofski & Kremkau 1978) and in some cases may be

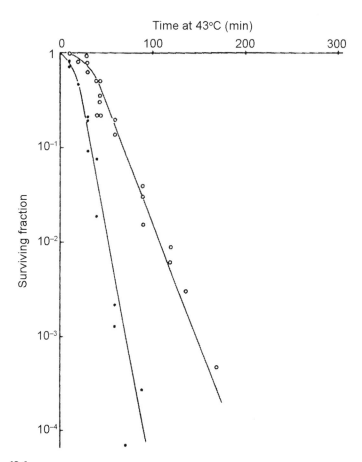

Figure 13.4a

non-existent (Clarke *et al.* 1970). It is likely that the effect is dependent on the radiosensitivity of the tumour and the temperature distribution achieved within the tumour itself. If the tumour is not heated uniformly it is likely that the minimum temperature achieved determines the success of the treatment (Hahn & Pounds 1976).

Study of the combination of ultrasound with chemotherapeutic agents has produced equally confusing results. The first suggestion that ultrasound might be used in conjunction with nitrogen mustard (mechlorethamine) came in 1967 (Hill 1967), but no synergistic effect was found at this time. However, nine years later, Kremkau *et al.* (1976) found that if mice were challenged with tumour cells (L1210 leukaemia) that had been treated with ultrasound and nitrogen mustard *in vitro* prior to injection, the mice survived longer than if they were challenged with cells that had been treated with either agent alone. In similar experiments with other drugs, five out of ten produced a similar enhancement but no mechanistic pattern emerged. It has been postulated that the presence of these cytotoxic agents prevents the cells from repairing ultrasonically induced damage, or vice versa (Kremkau 1979). The mechanism of action may be partially thermal in origin.

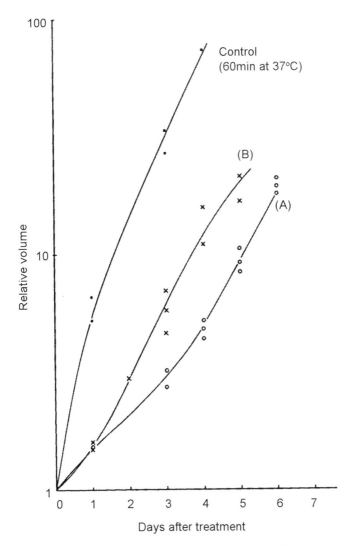

Figure 13.4. (a) Survival curve for cells irradiated with 3 MHz, 3 W cm^{-2} ultrasound *in vitro* while being held at 43°C. (b) Growth curves for multicellular spheroids that have been maintained at 43°C for 60 min with (A) or without (B) simultaneous irradiation with ultrasound

If ultrasound is to be used as a means of inducing hyperthermia in conjunction with chemotherapeutic agents, several factors should be taken into account in selecting potentially suitable drugs. The drug should be more cytotoxic at hyperthermic temperatures than at 37°C, and should be activated at the tumour site so that selective heating of the tumour can give therapeutic benefit. This requirement rules out cyclophosphamide, for example, which is activated in the liver (Lele 1979).

Umemura *et al.* (1996, 1997) have investigated the use of acoustic cavitation in conjunction with some of the porphyrins (haematoporphyrin, protoporphyrin and a

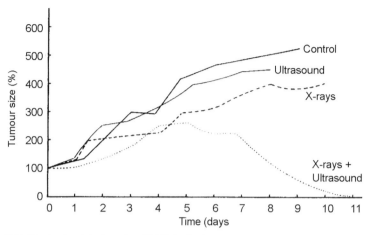

Figure 13.5. Woeber's original results (1965) indicating that ultrasound and X-rays given to rat tumours together give more effective tumour control than either agent on its own

gallium-deuteroporphyrin ATX-70) to produce cytotoxic effects on tumour cells. They found that a considerable enhancement of porphyrin toxicity could be obtained if the tumour is simultaneously exposed to the fundamental and second harmonic – a method known as second harmonic superposition. This technique halves the intensity needed to produce a given effect, such as a specified level of 'cavitation intensity' as measured using a potassium iodide test.

It is difficult to draw general conclusions as to the efficacy of this type of ultrasound exposure in cancer therapy. Woeber's original (1965) results (shown in Figure 13.5) showed a substantial increase in effectiveness of x-irradiation when combined with ultrasound. In a series of treatments of superficial human neoplasms (Hahn *et al.* 1980), 12% showed complete response, 42% showed partial response and 46% showed no response. Squamous cell carcinomas of the head and neck responded best. Figure 13.6 summarises results presented in the literature up until 1979 on tumour growth. It seems reasonable enough to expect that heat-sensitive tumours may be treated successfully with ultrasound, and the possibility exists that other tumours also may be affected because the non-thermal effects of ultrasound may be effective in producing tumour regression.

Evidently ultrasound may have an important role to play in hyperthermic therapy for tumours. Although it seems that the technology for heating superficial tumours (< 3–4 cm deep) exists (Anhalt *et al.* 1995) and is in routine clinical use in some centres, further improvements in understanding and a good deal of engineering will be required to produce reliable, reproducible methods for heating deep-seated tumours. In general, it should be true that, if it is possible to produce an ultrasound scan of a tumour, it should be possible to heat it.

The introduction of thermal therapies into the treatment of cancer has necessitated the formulation of a dose parameter so that different regimes may be compared. Early protocols described treatments in terms of the time for which a given temperature is held. However, because it is not always possible to reach predetermined temperature levels (for reasons related to technology, patient physiology or patient comfort), a more meaningful description has been sought. One chosen solution (Sapareto & Dewey 1984) records the times for which temperatures are held and, from this, estimates an equivalent time at one reference temperature (usually taken to be 43°C). It is now generally accepted that there is an

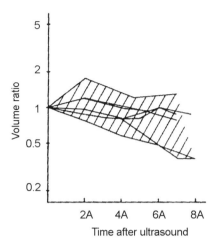

Figure 13.6. Graph showing response of a variety of tumours to ultrasound therapy (A indicates either 1 or 3 days, depending on the tumour type). This demonstrates the spread of responses that has been reported. *Source*: Adapted from Kremkau (1979)

exponential relationship between temperature and exposure time for a given biological effect. In most biological systems, a 1°C temperature rise requires a halving of the exposure time to achieve the same level of effect for temperatures above 43°C, whereas below this temperature the time must be reduced by a factor of 3–4. Mathematically this may be expressed as:

$$t_1 = t_2 R^{(T_1 - T_2)}$$

where t is the heating time, T is the temperature and R is 0.5 for temperatures above 43°C and 0.25 for temperatures below 43°C.

In order to compare the thermal 'dose' accumulated by tissues exposed to a complex heating regime with that experienced if the temperature had been held at 43°C, an equivalent time t_{43} is calculated, for which:

$$t_{43} = \int_{t=0}^{final} R^{(43-T)} dt$$

Thermal doses are therefore often quoted in terms of t_{43}. It has been shown by a number of authors that the required temperature–time combination at the boundary of a high-intensity focused ultrasound lesion (see Section 13.5.1) is 56°C for 1–2 s. Using the above formulation, a temperature of 56°C held for 1.75 s gives an equivalent time at 43°C of 240 min.

The biophysics of ultrasonic killing of cells at elevated temperatures is poorly understood. It seems likely that non-thermal interactions will occur that are secondary to the heating effect. If this is the case, then extracellular membranes seem the most likely target for damage in the cell. This may be especially important where synergism between heating and other cytotoxic agents is sought. The subject requires more effort to pinpoint mechanisms for action. Once mechanisms are established, then it should be possible to plan the ultrasound exposure conditions to maximise cytotoxicity.

When ultrasound is used at low power levels, such as those used in physiotherapy, caution should be exercised when malignant tumours are exposed. Sicard-Rosenbaum *et al.* (1995) found that when implanted tumours in mice were treated with 3 MHz ultrasound for 5 min at 1 W cm^{-2} ten times in a 2-week period, they grew faster than the control group of sham-irradiated tumours. The maximum temperature measured during treatment was 41°C. It was postulated that although this temperature was not cytotoxic, it was sufficient to increase blood flow and stimulate tumour growth. There was no measurable change in metastatic rate.

A concern that arises with any new procedure for cancer management is its potential for promoting metastatic spread. It is difficult to investigate this rigorously, but some early reports with ultrasound suggested that there might be some enhancement of metastatic disease (Fry & Johnson 1978). However, the evidence does not generally support this suggestion (Kremkau 1979; Smachlo *et al.* 1979; Goss & Fry 1984), and one group has reported that rates of lung metastases were lower in high-intensity focused ultrasound-treated animals than in controls (Yang *et al.* 1991). This is an area of research that requires careful investigation.

13.5 SURGERY

There are two main ways in which ultrasound finds application in surgery. The first makes use of the potential of a highly focused beam to produce local tissue destruction, and the second uses mechanical vibrations at ultrasonic frequencies to drive a blade, saw, metal tip or other instrument.

13.5.1 FOCUSED BEAM SURGERY

13.5.1.1 Principles and Techniques

A technique that is to replace a conventional surgical knife should be reproducible and controllable in its ability to destroy tissue, it should be able to affect a sharply defined region only and preferably should be quick and associated with the minimum of blood loss. High-intensity focused ultrasonic beams have most of these qualities. Focal spots about 1–2 mm in diameter and 3–4 mm in length may typically be achieved. The tissue ablation technique based on these high-intensity focused beams has come to be known interchangeably as HIFU (high-intensity focused ultrasound) or FUS (focused ultrasound surgery). The principle of this technique is shown in Figure 13.7.

The use of sharply focused beams to produce lesions in organs at depth within the body without damage to intervening tissue was initially investigated in the brain because interest was expressed in the use of these lesions for experimental neuroanatomy. Other organs that have been studied since include the liver, prostate, spinal cord, kidney and eye.

As described in Chapter 2, focusing may be achieved by a variety of methods (see also ter Haar & Hand 1981). The simplest way is to use a spherical, curved shell of piezoelectric material as the transducer. The focus of such a shell lies on the central axis, near the centre of curvature of the bowl. Field distributions for such transducers can be calculated (see Chapter 2; O'Neil 1949; Kossoff 1979). Focal lesions have been produced in the brain tissue of rats and cats using these focused bowl transducers (Warwick & Pond 1968; Robinson & Lele 1972) and in the prostate, liver, breast and kidney in humans (ter Haar 1995).

Although sharply defined heated volumes can be achieved in this fashion, there is no flexibility as to focal distance. Different focal depths may be achieved using a plane transducer in conjunction with a variety of acoustic lenses. These are usually made from materials in which the velocity of sound is greater than that in water, and so concave lenses are needed to

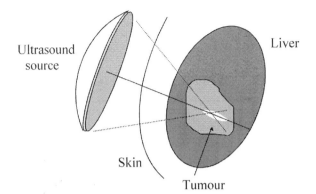

Figure 13.7. Schematic diagram of the principle of focused ultrasound surgery. The focus is placed within the target volume. Tissue overlying and surrounding the target is undamaged

obtain a converging beam (Chapter 2). The main limitation of such a lens system is absorption in the lens material. Maximum power transmission is obtained when the transducer and lens are separated by a quarter of a wavelength of impedance-matched material. Such transducer/ lens combinations have been used to produce sharply defined lesions in rat and rabbit livers, and in experimental tissues *in vitro* and *in vivo* (Linke *et al.* 1973; Lee *et al.* 1979; ter Haar *et al.* 1989).

Fry (1958) described the use of four plane transducers, each fronted by a planoconcave spherical lens. The four beams were brought to a coincident focus and the intensity maximised by suitable phasing of the individual beams.

Emerging phased array technology for high-power ultrasound applications has led to the design of transducers that allow electronic beam steering to facilitate the 'painting out' of tissue volumes larger than that of the focal region (Ebbini & Cain 1991; Goss *et al.* 1996; Daum & Hynynen 1999; Lizzi *et al.* 1999).

Two types of transducers have been developed for clinical use: trans-rectal devices (for urological applications) and those designed for extracorporeal use. The trans-rectal devices have both an imaging and a therapy transducer incorporated into one unit that can be inserted *per rectum* for treatment of the prostate. In one device (Foster *et al.* 1993) the same 4 MHz transducer is used alternately for imaging and therapy, whereas in another (Gelet *et al.* 1993), imaging is achieved by a retractable 7.5 MHz transducer and therapy undertaken with a 2.25 MHz source.

Vallancien *et al.* (1993) modified a commercial lithotripter to make an extracorporeal focused surgery device. In this clinical unit, the 1 MHz source consisted of multiple confocal transducer elements and had a focal length of 320 mm. A 3.5 MHz imaging transducer was placed at the centre of the therapy elements. The ultrasound source was placed below the bed in a large water bath and the beam coupled to the target via a waterproof membrane on which the patient lay. A similar coupling geometry has been used by Cline *et al.* (1992) in which the single-element ultrasound source is designed to be an integral part of a magnetic resonance scanner. In this device the 1.5 MHz spherical bowl source (10.3 cm focal length) lies in the water bath below the scanner couch. A third device (ter Haar *et al.* 1998) also uses a 1.7 MHz single-element spherical bowl transducer with a focal length of 140 mm. The treatment geometry for this device is such that a small water bag is placed over the patient in good acoustic contact with the skin, and the therapy source is placed into this bag. Imaging is achieved in this prototype by reproducible interchange of the therapy and diagnostic transducers.

Köhrmann *et al.* (2002b) have described a handheld device for FUS ablation. In this probe, the ultrasound energy from a 1 MHz cylindrical source is focused using a parabolic reflector. A 3.5 MHz diagnostic probe is positioned in the centre of the cylinder. The handheld probe used to produce haemostasis, developed in Seattle, comprised a spherically concave piezoelectric disc bonded to a solid coupling aluminium cone using a thin layer of epoxy (Vaezy *et al.* 1997; Brentnall *et al.* 2001).

Focused ultrasound surgery applicators are also under construction for endoscopic use. Lafon *et al.* (1998, 2001) have described a device that has been used clinically for the treatment of bile duct carcinoma (Prat *et al.* 2001). The applicator is constructed around a 2 m long flexible metal shaft of diameter 3.8 mm. The active transducer was a plane piezo-ceramic, gilded element (8×2.8 mm) embedded in a brass head 1 cm long, backed by an air cavity, operating at 10 MHz. A 12 μm thick polyethylene envelope encases the transducer. When 14 W cm^{-2} is used for 20 s, a lesion 8 mm long and 3 mm wide can be produced at a depth of 10 mm. A cylindrical phased array for trans-oesophageal use also has been described (Melodelima *et al.* 2002).

In general, the focal region used in beam surgery is cigar shaped: an ellipsoid of revolution about the central axis of the field. The distribution of pressure at the focus has the form $[2J_1(x)/x]$, the width W_A of the focal spot being given by (*cf.* equation (2.5)):

$$W_A = (1.22t_0\lambda)/a \tag{13.1}$$

where t_0 is the focal length, a is the transducer radius and λ is the wavelength in the tissue.

For a non-attenuating medium, diffraction theory predicts that 84% of the energy at the surface of a circular radiator passes through the focal region (Chapter 2; Hueter *et al.* 1956). However, in tissue where absorption takes place, and/or with other shapes of radiator, this proportion will be reduced.

The precise shape of any lesion produced will depend on the tissue being irradiated. In homogeneous tissue the lesion may be approximately ellipsoidal. If, however, two tissue types are present, one being less absorptive of ultrasound than the other, the lesion shape is less predictable. This would be the case, for example, in the brain where white matter may be damaged selectively, with grey matter and vascular structures being less sensitive (Fry *et al.* 1955). The vascularity of the tissue also affects the lesion size. Part of the appeal of this technique is that, if sufficient energy is delivered very rapidly, tissue effects are effectively perfusion independent (Billard *et al.* 1990; Chen *et al.* 1993a; Hill *et al.* 1994). Chen *et al.* (1993a) have suggested that, in order to achieve this, exposures of <3 s should be used. This agrees with the theoretical predictions of Hill *et al.* (1994).

Geometrically, the ratio of the length to the width of the ellipsoid depends on the solid angle of irradiation. It can be seen from equation (13.1) that, as the frequency is increased, the width of the focal region decreases for a given amount of absorbed energy. For a brief, intense exposure the lesion volume is approximately linearly dependent on the amount of energy absorbed by the tissue (Johnston & Dunn 1976). The optimum frequency for a specific application becomes a compromise between the need to keep the attenuation low in order to allow sufficient energy to reach the target, and the necessity to have sufficient absorption in the target to ensure an adequate temperature rise. Hill (1994) has shown that the optimum frequency in this regard is one that leads to a total attenuation in tissue of the order of 10 dB. Assuming, for illustration, a representative tissue attenuation of 0.7 dB cm^{-1} MHz^{-1}, then this would imply an optimum frequency of 2.6 MHz for a target depth of 5 cm and of 1.4 MHz for a depth of 10 cm. An extra consideration is that, in general, a smaller focal region is obtained at higher frequencies if all other source geometries remain the same.

There have been various attempts to collate available data pertaining to threshold intensities for lesion production (see, for example, Fry et al. 1970; Lerner et al. 1973; Frizzell et al. 1977; Johnston & Dunn 1981). It has been suggested empirically (and apparently without rigorous assessment of degree of conformity) that, on a log-log plot of intensity as a function of exposure time three collinear regions can be identified. For intensities of $>2\times10^3\,\mathrm{W\,cm^{-2}}$ and exposure times of $<4\times10^{-2}\,\mathrm{s}$, cavitation mechanisms are thought to be involved (Fry et al. 1970); for exposure times of $>1\,\mathrm{s}$ (Lerner et al. 1973) and intensities of $<200\,\mathrm{W\,cm^{-2}}$ (Frizzel et al. 1977), thermal mechanisms may be responsible. In the region between (shown on Figure 13.8), the mechanism for lesion production is unclear. Cavitation thresholds (as determined by subharmonic emissions) in brain appear to agree with this classification (Gavrilov 1974). A threshold intensity in the region of 30–40 $\mathrm{W\,cm^{-2}}$ seems to exist for exposure times of 10^2–$10^3\,\mathrm{s}$ (Johnston & Dunn 1981). It has been proposed that the relationship between intensity and exposure time to produce a lesion is:

$$It^{1/2} = c(f,T) \tag{13.2}$$

where c is a weak function of frequency and possibly of the base temperature of the tissue (Dunn et al. 1975). In an attempt to determine the mechanism for lesion development, it has been shown that the threshold curves can be predicted if it is assumed that the relationship between stress and strain in tissue is non-linear and exhibits hysteresis (Johnston & Dunn 1981) and that the sound travels as plane waves in tissue.

Hill et al. (1994) have proposed a general thermal model for lesion development. The basis for this model is the assumption that, for the short, high-intensity exposures used in FUS only those cells whose temperature is raised above a certain hypothetical threshold temperature are killed. This assumption has been the starting point for a number of models (Lizzi & Ostromogilsky 1987) that have given good agreement with measured temperature distributions for specific transducer configurations. The model of Hill et al. (1994) has more general application because it assumes that the focal beam profiles, both axially and laterally, are Gaussian.

It is known from the 'conventional' hyperthermia field that, for the temperature range 42–46°C, the probability of cell death is a function both of exposure temperature and exposure time, given quantitatively by the empirical relationship:

$$\ln(S/S_0) = -kt$$

where k is given by the Arrhenius equation

$$k = A\exp(E/R_g T)$$

Here, A is a constant, E is the activation energy of the process, R_g is the gas constant and T is the absolute temperature.

Although this relationship has only been tested experimentally for temperatures up to about 50°C, there is reasonable evidence that it will hold good for exposure times down to 1 s (ter Haar 1986). For shorter time scales than this, it is necessary to extrapolate from longer exposures. The relationship suggests that only a fraction of 10^{-6} of cells would survive an exposure of 60°C for 0.1 s. At this temperature, lesioned tissue takes on a 'cooked' appearance (Clarke & ter Haar 1997). Experimental and theoretical evidence have led to a general consensus that the temperature at the edge of the FUS lesion lies between 55°C and 60°C (Robinson & Lele 1972; Hill & ter Haar 1995).

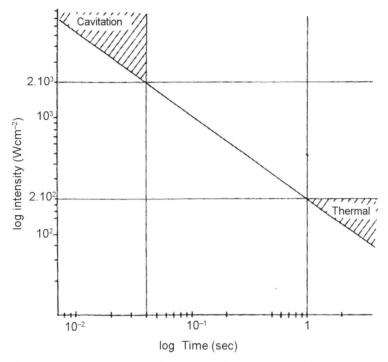

Figure 13.8. Plot of log(Intensity) against log(Time) to show the threshold for lesion production using focused beams. The line has the form $It^{1/2}=c(f,T)$ (see text). The domains for thermal and cavitational mechanisms of damage are shown

The Arrhenius relationship and the assumption of Gaussian beam profiles are used by Hill *et al.* (1994) to derive a 'lesioning rate parameter', R, which is the reciprocal of the time required to achieve a lesion threshold in the absence of thermal redistribution. Theory and experiment have been shown to be in good agreement at low-intensity exposures (see Figure 13.9). The deviation of experimental measurement from theoretical prediction at the higher intensities is probably a result of non-linear and cavitation effects.

Figure 13.10 shows two lesions. The one on the left is a clinically 'useful' lesion, ellipsoidal in shape and falling symmetrically across the focal plane. It is made using an exposure close to the threshold. The lesion on the right is misshapen and is the result of either too high an intensity or too long an exposure time. In a detailed study of the effect of increasing intensity and exposure time, Watkin *et al.* (1996a) showed that, at intensity/time combinations above the threshold for lesion production, the lesion moves forward through the focus towards the source and forms a 'bulbous'-shaped head. Meaney *et al.* (1998, 2000) have modelled this phenomenon theoretically and have shown that it can, in part, be explained by the increase in acoustic absorption coefficient due to the raised ambient temperature in the beam path. These effects must be taken into consideration when attempting to 'paint out' large tissue volumes by placing single lesions side by side in arrays (Malcolm & ter Haar 1996). In order to avoid effects due to a gradual rise in ambient tissue temperature, it is necessary to wait up to 60 s between successive exposures. An alternative method of delivering the required energy is to move the transducer while it is excited, thus forming scanned 'tracks' as shown in Figure 13.13b. Typical scan rates are $1-4\,\mathrm{mm\,s^{-1}}$.

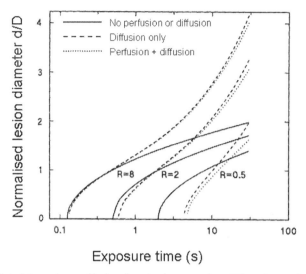

Figure 13.9. Predicted dependence of lesion diameter (expressed as *d/D*) on three values of lesioning rate parameter, *R*, which is defined as the reciprocal of the time required to achieve a lesion threshold in the absence of thermal redistribution. The distribution is shown for three different conditions of thermal redistribution: none (solid line), diffusion only (dashed line) and diffusion plus perfusion (dotted line). *Source*: Adapted from Hill *et al.* (1994)

The field of FUS lacks a consistent way of describing the incident acoustic field and the absorbed energy at the target site. Exposures are usually given in terms of the focal peak intensity, and this may be quoted as a free field value or 'de-rated' to give an *in situ* value. In an attempt to identify a single quantity that would be usefully predictive of tissue ablation, Hill *et al.* (1994) proposed the use of the parameter I_{SAL}, the acoustic intensity Spatially Averaged over the area enclosed by the half-pressure maximum contour as determined under Linear conditions (see also Chapter 2). It has been shown that following an initial rapid growth of lesion diameter, and before thermal diffusion, tissue water boiling or cavitation effects come into play, this lesion diameter is close to or just less than the full width at half-pressure maximum contour. The area over which I_{SAL} is calculated is therefore appropriate for an ablative lesion.

It can be shown readily (O'Neil 1949; see also Chapter 2) that I_{SAL} is $0.557I_{SP}$ (the spatial pressure maximum of the linear beam profile). Estimation of I_{SAL} requires a good estimate of the total acoustic power (measured, for example, using a radiation force balance; Davidson 1991), and beam pressures profiles that can be determined under low-power, linear conditions. A hydrophone used for this does not require calibration.

Microscopy of these ultrasonically produced lesions reveals 'island and moat' structures, the boundary between normal and affected tissue being sharp (Warwick & Pond 1968). Similar lesions have been observed to result from heating by a fine wire embedded in the tissue (Pond 1970). In brain tissue, the 'island' is a coagulated core and the 'moat' shows liquefaction of the nerve cells, although intact blood vessels may be found. Electron microscopy of the tissue reveals that mitochondria are among the first structures to be damaged; they may be swollen and of low electron density, but in brain the synapses may be more sensitive and exhibit damage earlier (Fallon *et al.* 1973; Borrelli *et al.* 1981).

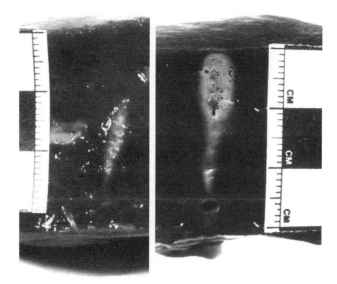

Figure 13.10. Photograph showing two focused ultrasound lesions in liver. In both cases, the sound entered the liver through the capsule at the top of the picture. The focal plane was set approximately 1.7 cm from the capsule. The lesion on the left is 'clinically useful' because it is of predictable shape and position. The one on the right, showing more unpredictable damage, is the result of overexposure

This 'island' and 'moat' structure has also been seen in the prostate and liver (Linke *et al.* 1973; ter Haar & Robertson 1993; ter Haar 1995). In the liver, 2 h after formation, the boundary of the lesion contained a rim of glycogen-free cells that otherwise appear to be histologically normal. This rim is no more than 10 cells thick (see Figure 13.11) and the cells within it are found to be dead 48 h later (ter Haar & Robertson 1993).

If the ultrasound exposure conditions used are well above the threshold for a purely thermal lesion, then light microscopy reveals not only the coagulative necrosis characteristic of thermal injury but also the 'holes' and tissue tearing that are characteristic of tissue water boiling or acoustic cavitation (Chen *et al.* 1993b). In general, it is felt that cavitation should be avoided because it renders the extent and position of damage unpredictable (Lele 1986; Watkin *et al.* 1996a), although Holt and Roy (2001) have shown that cavitation bubble activity enhances heating at the focus.

There is little doubt that a highly focused ultrasound beam can produce a well-demarcated volume of ablated tissue. So that this potential of achieving a very high degree of spatial localisation may be fully used clinically, it is important not only that the target tissue volume is properly identified prior to treatment but also that it can be monitored both during and after the procedure. The initial hope was that ultrasound could be used not only for treatment planning but also for real-time monitoring and follow-up of tissue response. This would allow the use of a single treatment head that could incorporate both the diagnostic and therapeutic transducers. This has been realised in trans-rectal probes designed for the treatment of benign prostate disease (Foster *et al.* 1993; Gelet *et al.* 1993) and in sources intended for ophthalmological use (Coleman *et al* 1985a, b).

Bush *et al.* (1993) showed that in *ex vivo* liver, although the attenuation coefficient of lesioned tissue was significantly greater than that of 'normal' tissue (see Figure 13.12), both the

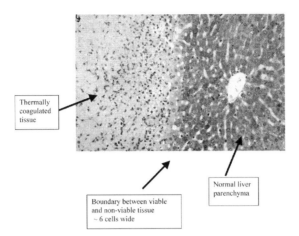

Figure 13.11. Transaxial histological section of a lesion in rat liver produced by focused ultrasound surgery. The sharp boundary between live and dead cells is clearly seen

speed of sound and the backscatter were unchanged. This was true for purely 'thermal' lesions in which there was no visible evidence of bubble activity. If bubbles were present within the lesioned volume, then there was a considerable increase in backscatter, as seen in Figure 13.13. This therefore leads to the conclusion that only 'bubbly' lesions are visible on a conventional diagnostic ultrasound B-scan. Thermally induced damage appears only because there is an acoustic shadow created behind the target volume. Thermal ablation therefore requires an imaging method that is sensitive to attenuation changes in order to become visible. One such method that has been proposed is reflex transmission imaging (Chapter 9). Another method that may prove successful is elastography (Chapter 9) because the ablated tissue is palpably harder than its surroundings.

An alternative method of monitoring focused ultrasound treatments is provided by magnetic resonance imaging (MRI). If the ultrasound therapy transducer is constructed of MR-compatible materials, then the focused ultrasound treatment can be conducted within the bore of an MR scanner. The heated tissue volume can be visualised using conventional T1-weighted, SE or spoiled gradient refocused echo (SPGR) pulse sequences (Cline *et al.* 1992, 1994). The necrosed volume can be demonstrated with T2-weighted fast spin-echo images (Hynynen *et al.* 1993, 1996a). Hardy *et al.* (1994) demonstrated that a temperature sensitivity of ca. 2°C with a time resolution of 300 ms could be obtained along a line through the ultrasonic focus. This temperature sensitivity is sufficient to allow an initial low-power pulse to be used to indicate the location of the focal volume prior to full power treatment. Such a technique needs to be used with care because the ablated volume may move forward with increasing incident intensity (Watkin *et al.* 1996a).

Magnetic resonance imaging can also be a useful tool for monitoring the response of tissue to FUS treatment, especially when used in conjunction with contrast agents such as gadolinium (Gd)-DTPA (Rowland *et al.* 1997).

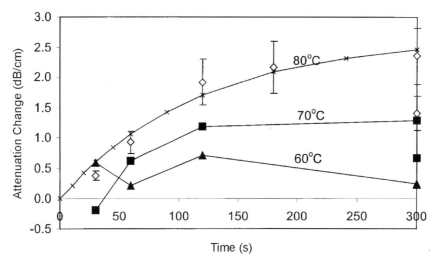

Figure 13.12. Graph showing the change in attenuation coefficient for ox liver held at 60°C, 70°C or 80°C for different times. Tissue 'lesioning' occurs at temperatures above 56°C held for 1–2 s. Attenuation coefficients are measured with tissue held at room temperature following heating

13.5.1.2 Clinical Applications

Although the first description of the use of high-intensity focused ultrasound beams was published in 1942 (Lynn *et al.* 1942) and the first report of application of FUS to humans was in 1960 (Ballantine *et al.* 1960; Fry & Fry 1960), this technique did not really gain much clinical acceptance until the 1990s, despite successful ophthalmological treatments. There are probably two main reasons for this. Early equipment was heavy and cumbersome and the original applications proposed were in the brain, which involved surgical intervention to lift a skull flap. Just as FUS was being developed, the drug L-dopa was brought out. This proved to be a more acceptable treatment for Parkinson's disease, from the patient's perspective. The second factor restricting the growth of FUS in its early days was the lack of good and precise imaging. In order to capitalise on the precision of the cell killing proffered by FUS, it is necessary to be able to place 'lesions' accurately within the target volume. This requires precise targeting and treatment follow-up, which is only now available with diagnostic ultrasound scanning and MRI techniques.

The clinical applications that have been widely explored lie in neurosurgery, ophthalmology, urology and oncology. In addition to these, a number of other applications, including synovectomy (Foldes *et al.* 1999) and as an alternative to vasectomy (Roberts *et al.* 2002), have been proposed.

13.5.1.2.1 Neurosurgery

First attempts at placing ultrasound lesions in the brain were unsuccessful, probably because the skull bone was left intact (Lynn *et al.* 1942; Lynn & Putnam 1944). Although small lesions were found in the brain, there was profound damage to the scalp. Mode conversion and the high acoustic absorption of bone lead to a high degree of attenuation in the skull bone. Once a

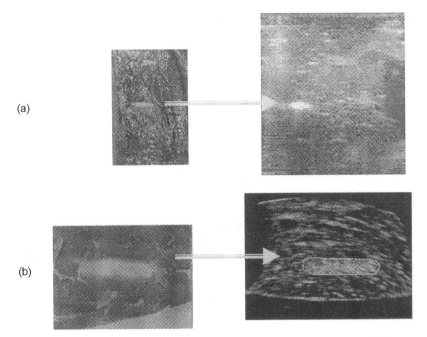

Figure 13.13. The B-mode images of (a) a single lesion and (b) a scanned track. The bright appearance of the thermally coagulated tissue on the image (arrowed) implies the existence of gas bubbles

window had been made in the skull, discrete lesions could be placed deep within the brain (Wall *et al.* 1951; Fry *et al.* 1955; Bakay *et al.* 1957). Fry *et al.* (1955, 1970) demonstrated that white matter was more susceptible to damage than grey matter.

Fry *et al.* (1960) reported the results of treating Parkinson's disease in 50 patients. Following craniotomy, the substantia negra and ansa lenticularis were exposed through the dura under local anaesthetic. The total procedure took 14 hours. Despite the claim that symptoms of Parkinsonism were eliminated, this treatment does not appear to have been taken further, probably because of the development of L-dopa at this time.

Ballantine *et al.* (1960) reported complete pain relief in seven patients with painful subcutaneous neuromata who were treated with 2.7 MHz (1700 W cm^{-2}, 0.14 s pulses) ultrasound. This does not appear to have been followed up.

The requirement to remove a skull flap, combined with targeting complexity, limited the progress of this research. However, phase correction techniques may allow the focus to be reconstructed following transmission through bone (Hynynen & Jolesz 1998). The feasibility of this has been demonstrated using large-area hemispherical phased arrays (Sun & Hynynen 1999; Clement *et al.* 2000).

13.5.1.2.2 Ophthalmology

The first suggestion that FUS could be used to destroy specific targets within the eye came from Lavine *et al.* (1952), who demonstrated cataract formation when the lens of the eye was targeted. Laboratory studies have demonstrated that FUS can decrease intra-ocular pressure (Rosenberg & Purnell 1967) and produce lesions in the vitreous, lens, retina and choroid (Purnell *et al.* 1964; Coleman *et al.* 1971).

Focused ultrasound surgery has been used successfully in the treatment of glaucoma. This was first established in experimental models (Coleman *et al.* 1985a, b) using intensities up to 2000 W cm^{-2} at 4.6 MHz. Histology showed focal thinning of the sclera and focal disruption of the ciliary body. The conjunctiva remained intact. The first human treatments were undertaken in 1982 and produced encouraging results. Of the 880 patients treated, 79.3% had a sustained lowering of intra-ocular pressure after 1 year (Silverman *et al.* 1991).

Focused ultrasound surgery has also been used with success in experiments to seal traumatic capsular tears (Coleman *et al.* 1985c) and in the laboratory treatment of intra-ocular tumours (Lizzi *et al.* 1984; Burgess *et al.* 1985), retinal detachment (Rosecan *et al.* 1985) and vitreous haemorrhage (Coleman *et al.* 1980).

Although FUS has shown considerable promise for ophthalmological applications, laser surgery has enjoyed wider success and application, presumably because of its apparently simpler technology.

13.5.1.2.3 Urology – Benign Prostate Disease

Urological sites of interest are readily available to focused ultrasound treatment by either a trans-rectal route or trans-abdominally through a full bladder.

A problem area in urology is the successful treatment of benign prostate hyperplasia (BPH). The 'gold standard' method of trans-urethral resection (TURP) has a significant morbidity rate associated with it and requires general anaesthetic. Focused ultrasound surgery has been investigated as a non-invasive technique that could be conducted on an outpatient basis. Coagulative necrosis has been induced in canine prostates (Foster *et al.* 1993; Gelet *et al.* 1993). Temperatures of 55–60°C have been recorded (Foster *et al.* 1993). Four weeks after exposure cystic cavities lined with urothelium are observed. In humans the ultrasound damage is seen 1 week after exposure as haemorrhagic necrosis, which is replaced by granulation tissue within 10 weeks (Susani *et al.* 1993). Initial results from clinical trials (Gelet *et al.* 1993; Madersbacher *et al.* 1994, 1995; Sanghvi *et al.* 1996; Mulligan *et al.* 1997; Sullivan *et al.* 1997) showed encouraging results with increase in flow rate and decreases in post-void residual volume, with treatments that included the bladder neck being the most successful (Sanghvi *et al.* 1996; Sullivan *et al.* 1997). However, the long-term results of Madersbacher *et al.* (2000) were disappointing, with 43.8% of patients requiring a salvage TURP within 4 years. An acceptable alternative to TURP would require a re-intervention rate of less than 16% at 8 years (Schatzl *et al.* 2000). Treatment times for FUS ablation of BPH were restricted to be comparable to those required for TURP. This meant that smaller volumes were treated. In addition, whereas tissue is removed in TURP, ablated tissue must be phagocytosed. This may be the reason for the disappointing results.

13.5.1.2.4 Malignant Tumour Ablation

As discussed above, hyperthermia (in which the tissue temperature is maintained at 43–45°C for times of the order of 1 h) has been used extensively for the treatment of malignant tumours on its own or in conjunction with radio- or chemotherapy (Watmough & Ross 1986). Focused ultrasound surgery, which relies on temperatures in excess of 55°C held for times of the order of 1 s, has the advantage that, if the energy is deposited sufficiently rapidly, temperatures achieved are independent of vascular perfusion. This means that, provided the temperature achieved exceeds the threshold required for instantaneous cell killing for the exposure times used, the absolute temperature within the target volume is unimportant. Temperatures drop rapidly at the edge of the lesion volume (Hill *et al.* 1994; Clarke & ter Haar 1997). Tumours in rat, mouse and hamster have been treated successfully with FUS (Fry & Johnson 1978; ter

Haar *et al.* 1991a,b). The success of a treatment depends to a large extent on good treatment planning and targeting. However, it has been shown that, when comprehensive coverage of a tumour is achieved, complete tumour kill can be obtained (Chen *et al.* 1993b, 1999). The appeal of FUS for tumour therapy arises from its non-invasive nature and, more importantly, it appears to be without side effects. This means that re-treatment, which is usually not an option for radiotherapy, is possible.

Liver tumours. Kopecky *et al.* (1993) have reviewed much of the early experimental work on the treatment of liver tumours with high-intensity ultrasound. Visioli *et al.* (1999) have published the preliminary results of a phase I clinical trial for the treatment of soft tissue tumours, including the liver. They demonstrated that FUS can be used as an outpatient procedure without the use of anaesthetic or other form of sedation. It was well tolerated by patients and, when the correct exposure level was used, tissue changes corresponding to the ablated volumes could be seen on diagnostic ultrasound and MR scans after 1 week. An *in situ* ablative intensity of $1500\,W\,cm^{-2}$ (spatial peak intensity 1.7 MHz) has been defined. A phase II study was undertaken for the treatment of liver metastases using this technique. Early results are promising (Allen *et al.* 2003). Wu *et al.* (2002) have reported the treatment of 68 patients with liver cancer. Where treated tissue was subsequently excised, total ablation of the tumour was seen in all cases. These treatments are continuing in China with more than 700 patients having been treated for both primary and secondary masses. Contrast-enhanced MRI 1–2 weeks following treatment has proved to be the best imaging modality for assessment of the treated volume.

Urological cancers. Selected regions of the bladder wall have been ablated *in situ* through the intact skin in experimental models (Watkin *et al.* 1996b), and this has led to the treatment of superficial bladder tumours in humans (Vallancien *et al.* 1993, 1996).

Experience in treating kidneys is not extensive. *In vivo* animal studies have demonstrated the potential of the technique (Linke *et al.* 1973; Frizzell *et al.* 1977; Chapelon *et al.* 1992; Watkin *et al.* 1995, 1997; Adams *et al.* 1996; Daum *et al.* 1999; Tu *et al.* 1999) but this has not been fully exploited clinically, although renal tumours have been targeted successfully (Susani *et al.* 1993; ter Haar *et al.* 1998; Visioli *et al.* 1999; Köhrmann *et al.* 2000, 2002a).

Prostate cancer has also been treated with some early success in a number of patients (Bihrle *et al.* 1994; Madersbacher *et al.* 1994; Gelet *et al.* 1996; Chapelon *et al.* 1998). Treatment of cancer in the prostate presents different problems from treatment of BPH. For prostate cancer there is no 'gold standard' treatment. It is a multi-focal disease, the foci of which are difficult to detect with diagnostic ultrasound. It is important in the control of prostate cancer that all these foci are destroyed. The most successful FUS treatments have been those that have ablated the whole gland (Beerlage *et al.* 1999a, b; Chaussy *et al.* 1999; Vallancien *et al.* 1999). Madersbacher *et al.* (1995) were the first to report successful treatment of whole tumours. With experience, local control rates have risen from 50% at 8 months in the early days to 90% more recently (Gelet *et al.* 1996; Chaussy *et al.* 2003). Focused ultrasound surgery is currently finding a role in the treatment of prostate cancer for patients who would not otherwise be offered surgery or who have local recurrence (following failed surgery, radiotherapy or brachytherapy). If the long-term clinical results continue to be good, it may find favour as a primary therapy.

Gynaecological tumours. A number of teams have been investigating the potential of FUS in the treatment of uterine fibroids. Vaezy *et al.* (2000) demonstrated the feasibility in a nude mouse model. Köhrmann *et al.* (2000) have published preliminary results of a clinical trial (15 patients in a phase I trial; 3 in a phase II trial). They used a handheld extracorporeal transducer. Chan *et al.* (2002) have described a vaginal FUS device designed specifically for the treatment of uterine fibroids under diagnostic ultrasound guidance. Keshavarzi *et al.* (2002) have demonstrated in a mouse model that uterine leiomyosarcomas can also be treated with FUS.

Breast cancer. The trans-cutaneous non-invasive ablation of breast cancer would have the potential to be a breast-conserving treatment with good cosmetic effect. Hynynen *et al*. (2001) have reported the successful treatment of eight out of eleven benign breast masses (fibroadenomas) under MR guidance. Gianfelice *et al*. (2000) have used a similar device to treat 20 patients with localised malignant breast disease. At 6 months, 53% had negative core biopsies, and of the remaining patients 66% became tumour-free following retreatment.

13.5.1.2.5 Vascular Occlusion

An intriguing use of FUS is for the interruption of blood flow. This has been demonstrated in a number of biological models (Delon-Martin *et al*. 1995; Hynynen *et al*. 1996b,c; Rowland *et al*. 1997; Vaezy *et al*. 1997, 1999a, b; Rivens *et al*. 1999). The mechanisms by which flow is stopped are not clear, but thermal effects are clearly important. Fallon *et al*. (1972) were able to demonstrate focal lesions in exposed rabbit arterial wall, but did not describe occlusion of flow. A possible explanation for this was that they only reached 'lesioning' temperatures ($\geqslant 60°C$) (see Section 13.5.1.1) when $100\,W\,cm^{-2}$ was used for 40 s or $400\,W\,cm^{-2}$ was used for 1.5 s. It is not clear from this paper where the thermocouple was placed in relation to the blood vessel. It is possible that these temperatures were not achieved in the vessels.

Hynynen *et al*. (1996b, c) achieved occlusion in rabbit renal arteries (with diameter about 0.6 mm) by using a combination of high and low intensities. Using a 1.5 MHz transducer mounted within an MR scanner, exposures of $6500\,W\,cm^{-2}$ for 1 s were used with the intention of inducing transient cavitation and, once flow was seen to have stopped on an MR angiogram, thermal coagulation was achieved by placing a close-packed array of 10-s $2800\,W\,cm^{-2}$ lesions around the artery. The authors postulate that the first, high-intensity exposure causes a transient constriction (spasm) in the vessel. This eliminates the cooling effect of blood and allows subsequent thermal coagulation of the vessel wall. Fujiwara *et al*. (2002) were also able to occlude the femoral arteries in the rat when using 3 MHz ultrasound (free field spatial peak intensity $10\,kW\,cm^{-2}$; 5–10 s exposures), but not at 1 MHz free field spatial peak intensity ($0.8\,kW\,cm^{-2}$; 5–10 s exposures). They postulated a thermal mechanism and presented histological evidence to support this. Focused ultrasound surgery can also be used to seal punctures in blood vessels (Vaezy *et al*. 1998).

Rivens *et al*. (1998) used a lower intensity ($960\,W\,cm^{-2}$, 1.7 MHz) to place an array of lesions across rat femoral vessels (diameter 0.5–1.5 mm). In this study, aimed at investigating the role of FUS in fetal medicine for the occlusion of blood vessels for the treatment of feto-fetal transfusion syndrome and in oncology for the destruction of tumour vessels, complete occlusion was demonstrated using MRA angiography and Gd-DTPA contrast agents (Figure 13.14). Wu *et al*. (2002) have shown tumour vessel occlusion following treatment of malignant human solid tumours.

Delon-Martin *et al*. (1995) were able to induce thrombosis in the rat femoral vein using a 7.31 MHz transducer to create an array of 3-s $167\,W\,cm^{-2}$ exposures in a study of the potential role of FUS as a physical sclerosing agent for varicose veins. This treatment produced thermal damage but not disruption of the vessel wall.

Vaezy *et al*. (1997) have described a potential application of FUS in the treatment of hepatic trauma. They demonstrated that it is possible to stop bleeding from the cut liver by sweeping a 3.3 MHz, $3000\,W\,cm^{-2}$ (spatial peak) focused beam over incisions in rat livers. Profuse bleeding was slowed to an 'ooze' in < 2 min, and complete haemostasis could be achieved in < 3 min in 80% of cases. Temperatures up to 86°C were reported. The same group have sought to induce haemostasis following splenic injury (Vaezy *et al*. 1999b; Noble *et al*. 2002). They used a handheld device operating at 9.6 MHz ($\sim 3\,kW\,cm^{-2}$ focal intensity). It took, on

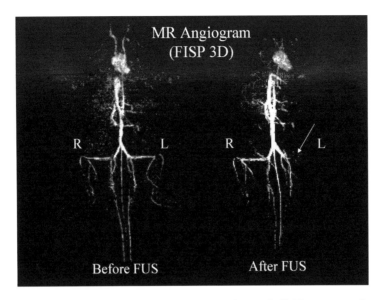

Figure 13.14. Magnetic resonance angiograms of rat vasculature. (Left) The pattern prior to focused ultrasound treatment of the left femoral vessels. (Right) Vascular occlusion due to ultrasound exposure (arrowed)

average, 96 s to seal an incision 8–10 mm long and 4–5 mm deep. The authors postulated that the ultrasound raised the temperature to ca. 100°C, leading to tissue coagulation. In addition, they suggested that the boiling of tissue fluids may create microbubbles that can enhance cavitation effects. Cavitation causes platelet activation and aggregation, and tissue homogenisation (Poliachik *et al.* 2001). It was proposed that the ensuing blood clot and hardened tissue homogenate act as a plug that occludes blood vessels in the region.

13.5.2 MENIÈRE'S DISEASE

Ultrasound may be used in the place of more conventional surgery to treat the symptoms of Menière's disease, a disorder of the inner ear that leads to attacks of vertigo. The aim of the treatment is to relieve the vertigo while preserving the existing level of hearing. A fine ultrasonic beam is directed to the lateral semicircular canal of the ear and a high intensity is used to destroy the sensory neuro-epithelium of the cristae and maculae in the labyrinth. Accurate dosimetry is essential for this technique (Wells *et al.* 1963; Angell James 1967) because the facial nerve lies close to the semicircular canal, and damage to this nerve may result in facial paralysis. Although the use of ultrasound for this purpose was first proposed in 1948 (Sjoberg *et al.* 1963), the first full report of its use to destroy vestibular function was not published until 1952 when Krejci used an intensity of 4 W cm^{-2} for 15 min. Eleven months later this patient was free from tinnitus and vertigo but hearing was somewhat impaired.

The irradiation method frequently used is that described by Arslan (1953). A groove is made by removal of mastoid cells, and the transducer is inserted into this groove. This allows irradiation of the labyrinth. Nystagmus is induced (the patient feels unbalanced and the eyes drift towards the direction in which he/she feels he/she is falling). When the nerve endings in the labyrinth are destroyed, the nystagmus changes direction. This is used as an indicator of the operation's success, because the patient is usually treated under local anaesthetic.

Sorensen and Andersen (1979) found, using a modified Arslan technique, that 72% of patients got lasting relief from attacks of vertigo, the hearing of the majority of patients being unchanged. In a review of the results of ultrasonic treatment in Menière's disease, Sjoberg *et al.* (1963) showed that relief from vertigo had good success, the rate varying from 67% to 95%, while the results on hearing mainly showed either no change or slight improvement. In the majority of cases, tinnitus was unaffected.

One risk of the technique developed by Arslan lies in irradiation of the facial nerve, leading to paralysis. The round window technique has been developed to reduce this risk (Kossoff & Khan 1966; Kossoff *et al.* 1967). In a series of 59 patients, none developed facial paralysis and 80% had their vertigo attacks abolished by one or two irradiations.

13.5.3 TOOL SURGERY

Ultrasonically driven surgical tools generally comprise a half-wavelength rod of magneto-strictive or piezoceramic transducer, coupled to a waveguide and terminated in a working end that has a shape relevant for specific jobs. The amplitude of vibration of the tip may be in the range 15–350 µm and the working frequency is up to 0–30 kHz.

Ultrasonic tools require less force than conventional knives to achieve a cut because the friction between two surfaces is reduced if one surface is vibrating (Goliamina 1974). The high temperatures that may be reached at the tip of an ultrasonic scalpel can cauterise vessels of < 2 mm in diameter (Derderian *et al.* 1982). This reduces bleeding in the area and thus facilitates surgery.

The advantage of ultrasound over cryosurgical techniques is that the tip does not stick to tissue and the cut surfaces do not exhibit late damage. An advantage that the ultrasonic scalpel has over laser surgery is that the surgeon has tactile feedback and the tissue destruction is less indiscriminate (Hodgson 1979).

Clinically, ultrasonically driven tools have found a number of applications. Two main types of use can be identified, the first of which is in tissue aspiration. Perhaps the most common use here is the removal of cataracts from the eye (phaco-emulsification). The instrument tip is in the form of a hollow tube (Kelman 1967). A similar technique may be used for debulking solid tumours, such as rectal tumours (Hodgson 1979).

The second type of use for these instruments is tissue cutting. As mentioned above, this has some advantages in being relatively bloodless. The technique has been used successfully on highly vascular organs such as the liver and spleen. It has also been used for tracheotomies, tonsillectomies, and in the lungs, bronchial tubes, thoracic walls and eye (Goliamina 1974; Hodgson 1979; Derderian *et al.* 1982). An ultrasonic saw may also be used to cut bone. In one comparative study the cut surface was found to be rougher when produced by an ultrasonic saw than when made by a conventional saw but did not have the microfractures seen with those instruments (Aro *et al.* 1981). The ultrasonic saw was thought to be smooth and easy to use, and better for performing accurate osteotomies. Bone healing appeared to be slower initially following ultrasonic cutting, but after 6 weeks healing appeared to be the same with both types of cutting.

The field of ultrasonic surgical tools is one that has been little explored. It appears from the various poorly quantified reports that exist that it may be of some considerable use. It awaits some careful science and engineering to maximise its full potential.

13.5.4 ULTRASOUND ANGIOPLASTY

The use of intravascular, ultrasonically driven wire tips has been investigated both for the ablation of atherosclerotic plaque and for accelerating the dissolution of blood clots by thrombolytic drugs.

Siegel *et al.* (1996a) demonstrated, using a flexible 2.6 Fr solid wire probe ensheathed in a 7 Fr catheter driven by an ultrasonic lithotripsy generator at 20 kHz, that they could recanalise sections of human atherosclerotic arteries 0.5–5 cm in length in < 60 s. The amplitude of vibration of the probe tip was 50±25 µm and the acoustic power was 20–50 W. The speed of recanalisation depended on the speed with which the probe was moved through the vessel. The probe was cooled by irrigation, and there was no evidence of thermal injury or perforation of the vessels. Ninety per cent of the particles produced by the procedure were < 10 µm in diameter.

Similar results have been obtained in animal experiments *in vivo*. Sections of guide-wire-resistant obstructed atherosclerotic vessels were surgically implanted into dogs prior to treatment (Siegel *et al.* 1996a). Using a mean acoustic power of 40±13 W these vessels were recanalised in 15 s–4 min. In 10/12 cases ultrasonic treatment was followed by balloon angioplasty.

Human clinical trials combined of ultrasound and balloon angioplasty for the 'unblocking' of blood vessels have yielded promising results. In one trial, 96% of 163 patients treated had < 50% residual stenosis following treatment (Siegel 1996b).

13.5.5 DENTISTRY

It was first suggested that ultrasound could be used in periodontics in 1955, by Zinner, who proposed its use for calculus removal.

The instrument used for dentistry consists of a rod of transducer material terminated in a tip shaped for the job in hand (Ewen & Glickstein 1968). The tip undergoes longitudinal vibrations at a frequency in the range 25–42 kHz with an amplitude in the range 6–100 µm (Suppipat 1974).

Ultrasonic scaling dislodges and cleanses adherent accumulations from tooth and root surfaces. The tip can scale, plane, rub and abrade teeth to rid them of calculus, plaque, food debris, stain and softened cementum. Ultrasound is an important technique in the treatment of ulcerative gingivitis, marginal gingivitus and pericoronitis. Ultrasonic tools can be used for curretage. In this case, the tip is placed against soft tissue to produce a small, controlled burn.

A comparison of a number of reports on the efficiency of ultrasound for scaling indicates that it may require less operator effort, reduce patient discomfort and decrease scaling time relative to hand scaling, although the final result is much the same. Ultrasound was thought to be more efficient for stain removal (Suppipat 1974). Photomicrographic studies have shown that the tooth surface is smoother following ultrasonic scaling than after hand scaling (Ewen 1966). The field of ultrasound in dentistry has been reviewed by Walmsley (1988).

REFERENCES

Abe, H., Kuroki, M., Tachibana, K., Li, T., Awasthi, A., Ueno, A., Matsumoto, H., Imakiire, T., Yamauchi, Y., Yamada, H., Ariyoshi, A. and Kuroki, M. (2002). Targeted sonodynamic therapy of cancer using a photosensitizer conjugated with antibody against carcinoembryonic antigen. *Anticancer Research* **22**, 1575–1580.

Abramson, D.I., Burnett, C., Bell, Y., Tuck, S., Rejal, H. and Fleischer, C.J. (1960). Changes in blood flow, oxygen uptake and tissue temperatures produced by therapeutic physical agents. 1. Effect of ultrasound. *Am. J. Phys. Med.* **39**, 51–62.

Adams, J.B., Moore, R.G., Anderson, J.H., Strandberg, J.D., Marshall, F.F. and Davoussi, L.R. (1996). High-intensity focused ultrasound ablation of rabbit kidney tumours. *J. Endourol.* **10**, 71–75.

Al Karmi, A.M., Dinno, M.A., Stolz, D.A., Crum, L.A. and Matthews, J.C. (1994). Calcium and the effects of ultrasound on frog skin. *Ultrasound Med. Biol.* **20**, 73–81.

Allen, M., Rivens, I., Visioli, A. and ter Haar, G. (2003). Focused Ultrasound Surgery (FUS): a non-invasive technique for the thermal ablation of liver metastases. *Proc. 2nd International Symposium on Therapeutic Ultrasound* 2003, pp. 17–25. University of Washington, USA.

Angell James, J. (1967). Clinical aspects of the surgical treatment of Menière's disease with ultrasound. *Ultrasonics* **5**, 102–104.

Anhalt, D.P., Hynynen, K. and Roemer, R.B. (1995). Patterns of change sof tumour temperatures during clinical hyperthermia: implications for treatment planning, evaluation and control. *Int. J. Hypertherm.* **11**, 425–436.

Antich, T.J., Randall, C.C., Westbrook, R.A., Morrissey, M.C. and Brewster, C.E. (1986). Physical therapy treatment of knee extensor disorders: comparison of four treatment modalities. *J. Orthopt. Sports. Phys. Ther.* **8**, 255–259.

Anwer, K., Kao, G., Proctor, B., Anscombe, I., Florack, V., Earls, R., Wilson, E., McCreery, T., Unger, E., Rolland, A. and Sullivan, S.M. (2000). Ultrasound enhancement of cationic lipid-mediated gene transfer to primary tumours following systemic administration. *Gene Ther.* **7**, 1833–1839.

Aro, H., Kallioniemi, H., Aho, A.J. and Kellokumpu-Lehtinen, P. (1981). Ultrasonic device for bone cutting. *Acta Orthopt. Scand.* **52**, 5–10.

Arslan, M. (1953). Treatment of Menière's syndrome by direct application of ultrasound waves to the vestibular system. *Proc. 5th Int. Cong. Otorhinolaryngol.*, Amsterdam, pp. 429–436.

Atar, S., Luo, H., Nagai, T. and Siegel, R. (1999). Ultrasonic thrombolysis: catheter delivered and transcutaneous applications. *Eur. J. Ultrasound* **9**, 39–54.

Backlund, L. and Tisellius, P. (1967). Objective measurement of joint stiffness in rheumatoid arthritis. *Acta Rheum. Scand.* **13**, 275.

Bakay, L., Hueter, T.F., Ballantine, H.T. and Sosa, D. (1957). Ultrasonically produced changes in the blood-brain barrier. *A.M.A. Arch. Neurol. Psychol.* **76**, 457–467.

Ballantine, H.T., Bell, E. and Manlapaz, J. (1960). Progress and problems in the neurological application of focused ultrasound. *J. Neurosurg.* **17**, 858–876.

Bao, S., Thrall, B.D., Gies, R.A. and Miller, D.L. (1998). *In vivo* transfection of melanoma cells by lithotripter shock waves. *Cancer Res.* **58**, 219–221.

Bao, S., Thrall, B.D. and Miller, D.L. (1997). Transfection of reporter plasmid into cultured cells by sonoporation *in vitro*. *Ultrasound Med. Biol.* **23**, 953–959.

Bednarski, M.D., Lee, J.W., Callstrom, M.R. and Li, K. (1997). *In vivo* target specific delivery of macromolecular agents with MR guided focused ultrasound. *Radiology* **204**, 263–268.

Beerlage, H.P., van Leenders, J.L.H., Oosterhof, G.O.N., Witjes, J.A., van de Kaa, C.A., Debruyne, F.M.J. and de la Rosette, J.J.M.C.H. (1999a). High-intensity focused ultrasound followed after one to two weeks by radical retropubic prostatectomy: Results of a prospective study. *Prostate* **39**, 41–46.

Beerlage, H.P., Thuroff, S., Debruyne, F.M.J., Chaussy, C. and de la Rosette, J.J.M.C.H. (1999b). Transrectal high-intensity focused ultrasound using the Ablatherm device in the treatment of localised prostate carcinoma. *Urology* **54**, 273–277.

Behrens, S., Spengos, K., Daffertshofer, M., Schroeck, H., Dempfle, C.E. and Hennerici, M. (2001). Transcranial ultrasound-improved thrombolysis: diagnostic vs therapeutic ultrasound. *Ultrasound Med. Biol* **27**, 1683–1689.

Bierman, W. (1954). Ultrasound in the treatment of scars. *Arch. Phys. Med. Rehab.* **35**, 209–214.

Bihrle, R., Foster, R.S., Sanghvi, N.T., Donohue, J.P. and Hood, P.J. (1994). High intensity focused ultrasound for the treatment of benign prostatic hyperplasia: early United States clinical experience. *J. Urol.* **151**, 1271–1275.

Billard, B.E., Hynynen, K. and Roemer, R.B. (1990). Effects of physical parameters on high temperature ultrasound hyperthermia. *Ultrasound Med. Biol.* **16**, 409–420.

Bommannan, D., Menon, G.K., Okuyama, H., Elias, P.M. and Guy, R.H. (1992a). Sonophoresis. II. Examination of the mechanism(s) of ultrasound enhanced transdermal drug delivery. *Pharm. Res.* **9**, 1043–1047.

Bommannan, D., Okuyama, H., Stauffer, P. and Guy, R.H. (1992b). Sonophoresis. I. The use of high frequency ultrasound to enhance trans-dermal drug delivery. *Pharm. Res.* **9**, 559–564.

Borrelli, M.J., Bailey, K.I. and Dunn, F. (1981). Early ultrasonic effects upon mammalian CNS structures (chemical synapses). *J. Acoust. Soc. Am.* **69**, 1514–1516.

Brentnall, M.D., Martin, R.W., Vaezy, S., Kaczkowski, P.J., Forster, F. and Crum, L.A. (2001). A new high intensity focused ultrasound applicator for surgical applications. *IEEE Trans. Ultrason. Ferroelectr. Freq. Control* **48**, 53–63.

Brueton, R.H. and Campbell, B. (1987). The use of Geliperm as a sterile coupling agent for therapeutic ultrasound. *Physiotherapy* **73**, 653.

Burgess, S.E.P., Chang, S., Svitra, P., Driller, J., Lizzi, F.L. and Coleman, D.J. (1985). Effect of hyperthermia on experimental choroidal melanoma. *Br. J. Ophthalmol.* **69**, 854–860.

Bush, N.L., Rivens, I., ter Haar, G.R. and Bamber, J. (1993). Acoustic properties of lesions generated with an ultrasound therapy system. *Ultrasound Med. Biol.* **19**, 789–801.

Byl, N.N., McKenzie, A.L., West, J.M., Whitney, J.D., Hunt, T.K. and Scheuenstuhl, B.S. (1992). Low dose ultrasound effects on wound healing: a controlled study with Yucatan pigs. *Arch. Phys. Med. Rehab.* **73**, 656–664.

Byl, N.N., McKenzie, A., Wong, T., West, J. and Hunt, T.K. (1993). Incisional wound healing: A controlled study of low and high dose ultrasound. *J. Orthopt. Sports Phys. Ther.* **18**, 619–628.

Callam, M.J., Harper, D.R., Dale, J.J., Ruckley, C.V. and Prescott, R.J. (1987). A controlled trial of weekly ultrasound therapy in chronic leg ulceration. *Lancet ii*, 204–206.

Cameroy, B.M. (1966). Ultrasound enhanced local anaesthesia. *Am. J. Orthopt.* **8**, 47.

Chan, A.H., Fujimoto, V.Y., Moore, D.E., Martin, R.W. and Vaezy, S. (2002). An image guided high intensity focused ultrasound device for uterine fibroid treatment. *Med. Phys.* **29**, 2611–2620.

Chapelon, J.Y., Gelet, A., Souchon, R., Pangaud, C., Blanc, E. (1998). Therapy using ultrasound: application to localised prostate cancer. *Journal d'Echografie et de Medicine par Ultrasons* **19**, 260–264.

Chapelon, J.Y., Margonari, J., Theillère, Y., Gorry, F., Vernier, F., Blanc, E. and Gelet, A. (1992). Effects of high energy focused ultrasound on kidney tissue in the rat and the dog. *Eur. Urol.* **22**, 147–152.

Chapman, I.V., Macnally, N.A. and Tucker, S. (1979). Ultrasound induced changes in rates of influx and efflux of potassium ions in rat thymocytes *in vitro*. *Ultrasound Med. Biol.* **6**, 47–58.

Chaussy, C., Thuroff, S. and Zimmermann, R. (1999). Localized prostate cancer treated by transrectal high-intensity focused ultrasound (HIFU): Outcome of 150 patients after 3 years. *J. Urol.* **161**, 331.

Chaussy, C., Thuroff, S., Lacoste, F. and Gelet, A. (2003). HIFU and prostate cancer: the European experience. *Proc. 2nd International Symposium on Therapeutic Ultrasound*, pp. 1–7. University of Washington, USA.

Chen, L., ter Haar, G.R., Hill, C.R., Dworkin, M., Carnochan, P., Young, H. and Bensted, J.P.M. (1993a). Effect of blood perfusion on the ablation of liver parenchyma with high intensity focused ultrasound. *Phys. Med. Biol.* **38**, 1661–1673.

Chen L., ter Haar, G.R., Hill, C.R., Eccles, S.A. and Box, G. (1999). Treatment of implanted liver tumours with focused ultrasound. *Ultrasound Med. Biol.* **25**, 847–856.

Chen, L., Rivens, I., Riddler, S., Hill, C.R. and Bensted, J.P.M. (1993b). Histological changes in rat liver tumours treated with high intensity focused ultrasound. *Ultrasound Med. Biol.* **19**, 67–74.

Clarke, R.L. and ter Haar, G.R. (1997). Temperature rise recorded during lesion formation by high intensity focused ultrasound. *Ultrasound Med. Biol.* **23**, 299–306.

Clarke, P.R., Hill, C.R. and Adams, K. (1970). Synergism between ultrasound and X-rays in tumour therapy. *Br. J. Radiol.* **43**, 97–99.

Clement, G.T., White, J. and Hynynen, K. (2000). Investigation of a large-area phased array for focused ultrasound surgery through the skull. *Phys. Med. Biol.* **45**, 1071–1083.

Cline, H.E., Hynynen, K., Hardy, C.J., Watkins, R.D., Schenck, J.F. and Jolesz, F.A. (1994). MR temperature mapping of focused ultrasound surgery. *Magnetic Resonance in Medicine* **31**, 628–636.

Cline, H.E., Schenck, J.F., Hynynen, K., Watkins, R.D., Souza, J.P. and Jolesz, F.A. (1992). MR-guided focused ultrasound surgery. *J. Comput. Assist. Tomogr.* **16**, 956–965.

Coleman, D.J., Lizzi, F.L., Burt, W. and Wen, H. (1971). Properties observed in cataracts produced experimentally with ultrasound. *Am. J. Ophthalmol.* **71**, 1284–1288.

Coleman, D.J., Lizzi, F.L., Driller, J., Rosado, A.L., Chang, S., Iwamoto, T. and Rosenthal, D. (1985a). Therapeutic ultrasound in the treatment of glaucoma. I. Experimental model. *Ophthalmology* **92**, 339–346.

Coleman, D.J., Lizzi, F.L., Driller, J., Rosado, A.L., Burgess, S.E.P., Torpey, J.H., Smith, M.E., Silverman, R.H., Yablonski, M.E., Chang, S. and Rondeau, M.J. (1985b). Therapeutic ultrasound in the treatment of glaucoma. II. Clinical applications. *Ophthalmology* **92**, 347–353.

Coleman, D.J., Lizzi, F.L., El-Mofty, A.A.M., Driller, J. and Franzen, L.A. (1980). Ultrasonically accelerated resorption of vitreous membranes. *Am. J. Ophthalmol.* **89**, 490–499.

Coleman, D.J., Lizzi, F.L., Torpey, J.H., Burgess, S.E.P., Driller, J., Rosado, A.L. and Nguyen, H.T. (1985c). Treatment of experimental lens capsular tears with intense focused ultrasound. *Br. J. Ophthalmol.* **69**, 645–649.

da Cunha, A., Parizotto, N.A. and Vidal, B. de C. (2001). The effect of therapeutic ultrasound on repair of the Achilles tendon (*Tendon calcaneus*) of the rat. *Ultrasound Med. Biol.* **27**, 1691–1696.

Daum, D.R. and Hynynen, K. (1999). Theoretical design of a spherically sectioned phased array for ultrasound surgery of the liver. *Eur. J. Ultrasound* **9**, 61–69.

Daum, D.R., Smith, N.B., King, R. and Hynynen, K. (1999). *In vivo* demonstration of non-invasive thermal surgery of the liver and kidney using an ultrasonic phased array. *Ultrasound Med. Biol.* **25**, 1087–1098.

Davick, J.P., Martin, R.K. and Albright, J.P. (1988). Distribution and deposition of tritiated cortisol using phonophoresis. *Phys. Ther.* **68**, 1672–1675.

Davidson, F. (1991). Ultrasonic power balances. In *Output measurements for medical ultrasound* R.C. Preston (ed.). Springer, London, pp. 75–90.

De Deyne, P.G. and Kirsch-Volders, M. (1995). *In vitro* effects of therapeutic ultrasound on the nucleus of human fibroblasts. *Phys. Ther.* **75**, 629–634.

Delon-Martin, C., Vogt, C., Chignier, E., Guers, C., Chapelon, J.Y. and Cathignol, D. (1995). Venous thrombosis generation by means of high intensity focused ultrasound. *Ultrasound Med. Biol.* **21**, 113–119.

Derderian, G. P., Walshaw, R. and McGehee, J. (1982). Ultrasonic surgical dissection in the dog spleen. *Am. J. Surg.* **143**, 269–273.

Dougherty, T.J., Gomer, C.J., Henderson, B.W., Jori, G., Kessel, D., Korbelik, M., Moan, J. and Peng, Q. (1998). Photodynamic therapy. *J. Natl. Cancer Inst.* **90**, 889–905.

Drastichova, V., Samohyl, J. and Slavetinska, A. (1973). Strengthening of sutured skin wound with ultrasound in experiments on animals. *Acta Chir. Plast. (Praha)* **15**, 114–119.

Dunn, F., Lohnes, J.E. and Fry, F.J. (1975). Frequency dependence of threshold ultrasonic dosages for irreversible structural changes in mammalian brain. *J. Acoust. Soc. Am.* **58**, 512–514.

Dyson, M. (1990). Role of ultrasound in wound healing. In *Wound Healing: Alternatives in Management*, L.C. Kloth, J.M. McCulloch and J.A. Feedar (eds). FA Davis, Philadelphia, pp. 259–285.

Dyson, M. and Brookes, M. (1983). Stimulation of bone repair by ultrasound. In *Ultrasound '82* R.A. Lerski and P. Morley (eds). Pergamon Press, Oxford, pp. 61–66.

Dyson, M., Franks, C. and Suckling, J. (1976). Stimulation of healing of varicose ulcers by ultrasound. *Ultrasonics* **14**, 232–236.

Dyson, M. and Pond, J.B. (1970). The effect of pulsed ultrasound on tissue regeneration. *Physiotherapy* **56**, 136–142.

Dyson, M., Pond, J.B., Joseph, J. and Warwick, R. (1968). The stimulation of tissue regeneration by means of ultrasound. *Clin. Sci.* **35**, 273–285.

Dyson, M., Pond, J.B., Joseph, J. and Warwick, R. (1970). Stimulation of tissue regeneration by pulsed plane wave ultrasound. *IEEE Trans. Son. Ultrason.* **SU-17**, 133–144.

Dyson, M. and Smalley, D. (1983). Effects of ultrasound on wound contraction. In *Ultrasound Interactions in Biology and Medicine*, R. Millner and U. Corbet (eds). Plenum Press, New York, p. 151.

Dyson, M., Webster, D.F., Pell, R. and Crowder, M. (1979). Improvement in the mechanical properties of scar tissue following treatment with therapeutic levels of ultrasound in vivo. *Proc. 4th Eur. Symp. Ultrasound Biol. Med.* **1**, 129–134.

Ebbini, E.S. and Cain, C.A. (1991). A spherical-section ultrasound phased array applicator for deep localized hyperthermia. *IEEE Trans. Biomed. Eng.* **38**, 634–643.

Enwemeka, C.S. (1989). The effect of therapeutic ultrasound on tendon healing – a bio-mechanical study. *Am. J. Phys. Med. Rehab.* **68**, 383–387.

Enwemeka, C.S., Rodriguez, O. and Mendosa, S. (1990). The biomechanical effects of low intensity ultrasound on healing tendons. *Ultrasound Med. Biol.* **16**, 801–807.

Ewen, S.J. (1966). A photomicrographic study of root scaling. *Periodontics* **4**, 273–277.

Ewen, S.J. and Glickstein, C. (1968). Ultrasonic instrumentation for dentistry. In *Ultrasonic Therapy in Periodontics*. C. C. Thomas, Springfield, IL, Chapt. 2.

Fallon, J.T., Stehbens, W.E. and Eggleton, R.C. (1972). Effect of ultrasound on arteries. *Arch. Pathol.* **94**, 380–388.

Fallon, J.T., Stehbens, W.E. and Eggleton, R.C. (1973). An ultrastructural study of the effect of ultrasound on arterial tissue. *J. Pathol.* **111**, 275–284.

Field, S.B. and Bleehen, N.M. (1979). Hyperthermia in the treatment of cancer. *Cancer Treat. Rev.* **6**, 63–94.

Foldes, K., Hynynen, K., Shortkroff, S., Winalski, C.S., Collucci, V., Koskinen, S.K., McDannold, N. and Jolesz, F. (1999). Magnetic resonance imaging-guided focused ultrasound synovectomy. *Scand. J. Rheumatol.* **28**, 233–237.

Foster, R.S., Bihrle, R., Sanghvi, N.T., Fry, F.J. and Donohue, J.P. (1993). High intensity focused ultrasound in the treatment of prostate disease. *Eur. Urol.* **23**(Suppl. 1), 29–33.

Fountain, F.P., Gersten, J.W. and Sengir, O. (1960). Decrease in muscle spasm produced by ultrasound, hot packs and infrared radiation. *Arch. Phys. Med.* **41**, 293–298.

Frenkel, P.A., Chen, S., Thai, T., Shohet, R.V. and Grayburn, P.A. (2002). DNA-loaded albumin microbubbles enhance ultrasound mediated transfection *in vitro*. *Ultrasound Med. Biol.* **28**, 817–822.

Frizzell, L.A., Linke, C.A., Carstensen, E.L. and Fridd, C.W. (1977). Thresholds for focal ultrasonic lesions in rabbit kidney, liver and testicle. *IEEE Trans. Biomed. Eng.* **BME-24**, 393–396.

Fromm, D., Kessel, D. and Webber, J. (1996). Feasability of photodynamic therapy using endogenous photosensitisation for colon cancer. *Arch. Surg.* **131**, 667–669.

Fry, F.J. (1958). Precision high intensity focusing ultrasound machines for surgery. *Am. J. Phys. Med.* **37**, 152–156.

Fry, F.J. (1978). Intense focused ultrasound: its production, effects and utilization. In *Ultrasound: Its Applications in Medicine and Biology*, F.J. Fry (ed.), Part 11, Vol. III. Elsevier Scientific, New York, pp. 689–736.

Fry, W.J., Barnard, J.W., Fry, F.J., Krumins, R.F. and Brennan, J.F. (1955). Ultrasonic lesions in the mammalian central nervous system. *Science* **122**, 517–518.

Fry, W.J. and Fry, F.J. (1960). Fundamental neurological research and human neurosurgery using intense ultrasound. *IRE Trans. Med. Electron.* **ME-7**, 166–181.

Fry, F.J. and Johnson, L.K. (1978). Tumour irradiation with intense ultrasound. *Ultrasound Med. Biol.* **6**, 33–38.

Fry, F.J., Kossoff, G., Eggleton, R.C. and Dunn, F. (1970). Threshold ultrasonic dosages for structural changes in the mammalian brain. *J. Acoust. Soc. Am.* **48**, 1413–1417.

Fujiwara, R., Sasaki, K., Ishikawa, T., Susuki, M., Umemura, S., Kushima. M. and Okai, T. (2002). Arterial blood flow occlusion by high intensity focused ultrasound and histological evaluation of its effect on arteries and surrounding tissues. *J. Med. Ultrasonics* **29**, 85–90.

Fyfe, M. and Chahl, L.A. (1980). The effect of ultrasound on experimental oedema in rats. *Ultrasound Med. Biol.* **6**, 107–111.

Fyfe, M. and Chahl, L.A. (1982). Mast cell degranulation: a possible mechanism of action of therapeutic ultrasound. *Ultrasound Med. Biol.* **8** (Suppl. 1), 62.

Galitsky, A.B. and Levina, S.I. (1964). Vascular origin of trophic ulcers and application of ultrasound as pre-operative treatment to plastic surgery. *Acta Chir. Plast. (Praha)* **6**, 271–278.

Gavrilov, L.R. (1974). Physical mechanism of the lesion of biological tissue by focused ultrasound. *Sov. Phys. Acoust.* **20**, 16–18.

Gelet, A., Chapelon, J.Y., Bouvier, R., Souchon, R., Pangaud, C., Abdelrahim, A.F., Cathignol, D. and Dubernard, J.M. (1996). Treatment of prostate cancer with trans-rectal focused ultrasound: early clinical experience. *Eur. Urol.* **29**, 174–183.

Gelet, A., Chapelon, J.Y., Margonari, J., Theillere, Y., Gorry, F., Souchon, R. and Bouvier, R. (1993). High intensity focused ultrasound experimentation on human benign prostatic hypertrophy. *Eur. Urol.* **23** (Suppl.1), 44–47.

Gersten, J.W. (1955). Effect of ultrasound on tendon extensibility. *Am. J. Phys. Med.* **34**, 362–369.

Gianfelice, D.C., Hail, M. and Lepanto, L. (2000). Initial treatment protocol for breast neoplasms with MR-guided focused ultrasound ablation (MR-FUS) apparatus: works in progress. *86th Meeting of Radiol. Soc. North Am.* **Abstract C04–273**.

Goddard, D.H., Revell, P.A., Cason, J., Gallagher, S. and Currey, H.L.F. (1983). Ultrasound has no anti-inflammatory effect. *Ann. Rheum. Dis.* **42**, 582–584.

Goliamina, I.P. (1974). Ultrasonic surgery. In *Acoustics. Proc. 8th Int. Congress on Acoustics*, London. pp. 63–69.

Goss, S.A., Frizzell, L.A., Kouzmanoff, J.T., Barich, J.M. and Yang, J.M. (1996). Sparse random ultrasound phased array for focal surgery. *IEEE Trans. Ultrason. Ferroelect. Freq. Control* **43**, 1111–1121.

Goss, S.A. and Fry, F.J. (1984). The effect of high intensity ultrasonic irradiation on tumour growth. *IEEE Trans. Son. Ultrason.* **SU-28**, 21–26.

Greenleaf, W.J., Bolander, M.E., Sarkar, G., Goldring, M.B. and Greenleaf, J.F. (1998). Artificial cavitation nuclei significantly enhance acoustically induced cell transfection. *Ultrasound Med. Biol.* **24**, 587–595.

Griffin, J.E., Echternach, E.L., Price, R.M., *et al.* (1967). Patients treated with ultrasonically driven hydrocortisone and with ultrasound alone. *Phys. Ther.* **47**, 595–601.

Griffin, J.E. and Touchstone, J.C. (1963). Ultrasonic movement of cortisol into pig tissue. I. Movement into skeletal muscle. *Am. J. Phys. Med.* **42**, 77–85.

Griffin, J.E. and Touchstone, J.C. (1972). Effects of ultrasonic frequency on phonophoresis of cortisol into some tissues. *Am. J. Phys. Med.* **51**, 62–78.

Griffin, J.E., Touchstone, J.C. and Liu, A.C.-Y. (1965). Ultrasonic movement of cortisol into pig tissue. II. Movement into paravertebral nerve. *Am. J. Phys. Med.* **44**, 20–25.

ter Haar, G.R. (1986). Effects of increased temperature on cells, on membranes and on tissues. In *Hyperthermia*, D.J. Watmough and W.M. Ros (eds). Blackie, Glasgow, pp. 14–41.

ter Haar, G.R. (1995). Ultrasound focal beam surgery. *Ultrasound Med. Biol.* **21**, 1089–1100.

ter Haar, G.R., Clarke, R.L., Vaughan, M.G. and Hill, C.R. (1991a). Trackless surgery using focused ultrasound technique and case report. *Min. Invas. Ther.* **1**, 13–19.

ter Haar, G.R., Dyson, M. and Talbert, D. (1978). Ultrasonically induced contractions in mouse uterine smooth muscle *in vivo*. *Ultrasonics* **16**, 275–276.

ter Haar, G.R. and Hand, J.W. (1981). Heating techniques in Hyperthermia. III. Ultrasound. *Br. J. Radiol.* **54**, 459–466.

ter Haar, G.R. and Hopewell, J.W. (1983). The induction of hyperthermia by ultrasound: its value and associated problems. 1. Single, static, plane transducer. *Phys. Med. Biol.* **28**, 889–896.

ter Haar, G.R., Rivens, I., Chen, L. and Riddler, S. (1991b). High intensity focused ultrasound for the treatment of rat tumours. *Phys. Med. Biol.* **36**, 495–501.

ter Haar, G.R., Rivens, I.H., Moskovic, E., Huddart, R. and Visioli, A.G. (1998). Phase I clinical trial of the use of focused ultrasound surgery for the treatment of soft tissue tumours. *SPIE* **3249**, 270–276.

ter Haar, G.R. and Robertson, D. (1993). Tissue destruction with focused ultrasound *in vivo*. *Eur. Urol.* **23** (Suppl. 1), 8–11.

ter Haar, G.R., Sinnett, D. and Rivens, I. (1989). High intensity focused ultrasound – a surgical technique for the treatment of discrete liver tumours. *Phys. Med. Biol.* **34**, 1743–1750.

ter Haar, G.R., Stratford, I.J. and Hill, C.R. (1980). Ultrasonic irradiation of mammalian cells *in vitro* at hyperthermic temperatures. *Br. J. Radiol.* **53**, 784–789.

Hahn, G.M., Li, G.C., Marmor, J.B. and Pounds, D.W. (1980). Thermal and nonthermal effects of ultrasound. In *Radiation Biology in Cancer Research*, R.E. Meyn and H.R. Wither (eds). Raven Press, New York, pp. 623–636.

Hahn, G.M. and Pounds, D. (1976). Heat treatment of solid tumours: why and how. *Appl. Radiol.* **5**, 131–144.

Hand, J.W. and ter Haar, G.R. (1981). Heating techniques in hyperthermia. *Br. J. Radiol.* **54**, 443–466.

Hardy, C.J., Cline, H.E. and Watkins, R.D. (1994). One dimensional NMR thermal mapping of focused ultrasound surgery. *J. Comput. Assist. Tomogr.* **18**, 476–483.

Harvey, E.N. and Loomis, A.L. (1928). High frequency sound waves of small intensity and their biological effects. *Nature* **121**, 622.

Harvey, W., Dyson, M., Pond, J.B. and Grahame, R. (1975). The *in vitro* stimulation of protein synthesis in human fibroblasts by therapeutic levels of ultrasound. In *Ultrasonics in Medicine*, E. Kazner *et al.* (eds), International Congress Series No. 363. Excerpta Medica, Amsterdam, pp. 10–21.

Heckman, J.D., Ryaby, J.P., McCabe, J., Frey, J.F. and Kilcoyne, R.F. (1994). Acceleration of tibial fracture healing by non-invasive, low intensity pulsed ultrasound. *J. Bone Joint Surg.* **76**, 26–34.

Hekkenberg, R.T., Oosterbaan, W.A. and van Beekum, W.T. (1986). Evaluation of ultrasound therapy devices. *Physiotherapy* **72**, 390–395.

Hekkenberg, R.T., Reibold, R. and Zeqiri, B. (1994). Development of standard measurement methods for essential properties of ultrasound therapy equipment. *Ultrasound Med. Biol.* **20**, 83–98.

Heybeli, N., Yeşildağ, Oyar, O., Gülsoy, U.K., Tekinsoy, M.A. and Mumcu, E.F. (2002). Diagnostic ultrasound treatment increases the bone fracture healing rate in an internally fixed rat femoral osteotomy model. *J. Ultrasound Med.* **21**, 357–363.

Hill, C.R. (1967). Changes in tissue permeability produced by ultrasound. *Br. J. Radiol.* **40**, 317.

Hill, C.R. (1970). Calibration of ultrasonic beams for biomedical applications. *Phys. Med. Biol.* **15**, 241–248.

Hill, C.R. (1994). Optimum acoustic frequency for focused ultrasound surgery. *Ultrasound Med. Biol.* **20**, 259–269.

Hill, C.R. and ter Haar, G.R. (1995). Review article: high intensity focused ultrasound – potential for cancer treatment. *Br. J. Radiol.* **68**, 1296–1303.

Hill, C.R., Rivens, I., Vaughan, M.G. and ter Haar, G.R. (1994). Lesion development in focused ultrasound surgery: a general model. *Ultrasound Med. Biol.* **20**, 259–269.

Hodgson, W.J.B. (1979). The ultrasonic scalpel. *Bull. NY Acad. Med.* **55**, 908–915.

Hogan, R.D., Franklin, T.D., Fry, F.J., Avery, K.A. and Burke, K.M. (1982). The effect of ultrasound on microvascular hemodynamics in skeletal muscle: effect on arterioles. *Ultrasound Med. Biol.* **8**, 45–55.

Holt, R.G. and Roy, R. (2001). Measurements of bubble-enhanced heating from focused MHz frequency ultrasound in tissue mimicking material. *Ultrasound Med. Biol.* **27**, 1399–1412.

Horvath, J. (1944). Ultraschallwirkung beim menschlichen Sarkom. *Strahlentherapie* **75**, 119–125.

Huber, P.E., Jenne, J., Debus, J., Wannenmacher, M.F. and Pfisterer, P. (1999). A comparison of shock wave and sinusoidal-focused ultrasound induced localised transfection of HeLa cells. *Ultrasound Med. Biol.* **25**, 1451–1457.

Huber, P.E. and Pfisterer, P. (2000). *In vitro* and *in vivo* transfection of plasmid DNA in the Dunning prostate tumour R3327-AT1 is enhanced by focused ultrasound. *Gene Ther.* **7**, 1516–1525.

Hueter, T.F., Ballantinme, H.T. and Cotter, W.C. (1956). Production of lesions in the central nervous system with focused ultrasound: a study of dosage factors. *J. Acoust. Soc. Am.* **28**, 192–201.

Hunt, J.W. (1982). Applications of microwave, ultrasound and radiofrequency heating. In *Third International Symposium: Cancer Therapy by Hyperthermia, Drugs and Radiation*. National Cancer Institute Monograph 61, NIH Publication 82-2437. National Cancer Institute, pp. 447–456. USA.

Hynynen, K., Chung, A., Calucci, V. and Jolesz, F.A. (1996b). Potential adverse effects of high intensity focused ultrasound exposure. *Ultrasound Med. Biol.* **22**, 193–201.

Hynynen, K., Colucci, V., Chung, A. and Jolesz, F. (1996c). Noninvasive arterial occlusion using MRI-guided focused ultrasound. *Ultrasound Med. Biol.* **22**, 1071–1077.

Hynynen, K., Darkazanli, A., Unger, E. and Schenck, J.F. (1993). MRI-guided noninvasive ultrasound surgery. *Med. Phys.* **20**, 107–115.

Hynynen, K., Freund, W.R., Cline, H.E., Chung, A.H., Watkins, R.D., Vetro, J.P. and Jolesz, F.A. (1996a). A clinical, noninvasive, MR imaging-monitored ultrasound surgery method. *Radiographics* **16**, 185–195.

Hynynen, K. and Jolesz, F.A. (1998). Demonstration of potential non-invasive ultrasound brain therapy through an intact skull. *Ultrasound Med. Biol.* **24**, 275–283.

Hynynen, K., Pomeroy, O., Smith, D.N., Huber, P.E., McDannold, N.J., Kettenbach, J., Baum, J., Singer, S. and Jolesz, F.A. (2001). MR imaging-guided focused ultrasound surgery of fibroadenomas in the breast: a feasibility study. *Radiology* **219**, 176–185.

IEC (1996). *International Electrotechnical Commission European Standard EN 61689. Ultrasonics – Physiotherapy systems – Performance requirements and methods of measurement in the frequency range 0.5 MHz–5 MHz*. IEC.

Imig, C.J., Randall, B.F. and Hines, H.M. (1954). Effect of ultrasonic energy on blood flow. *Am. J. Phys. Med.* **33**, 100–102.

Johnston, R.L. and Dunn, F. (1976). Ultrasonic absorbed dose, dose rate, and produced lesion volume. *Ultrasonics* **14**, 153–155.

Johnston, R.L. and Dunn, F. (1981). Ultrasonic hysteresis in biological media. *Environ./Biophys.* **19**, 137–148.

Kelman, C.D. (1967). Phaco-emulsification and aspiration: a new technique of cataract removal. *Am. J. Ophthalmol.* **64**, 23–35.

Kesharvarzi, A., Vaezy, S., Noble, M.L., Chi, E.Y., Walke, C., Martin, R.W. and Fujimoto, V.Y. (2002). Treatment of uterine leiomyosarcoma in a xenograft nude mouse model using high intensity focused ultrasound: a potential treatment modality for recurrent pelvic disease. *Gynecol. Oncol.* **86**, 344–350.

Kessel, D., Jeffers, R., Fowlkes, J. and Cain, C. (1994). Porphyrin induced enhancement of ultrasound cytotoxicity. *Int. J. Radiat. Biol.* **66**, 221–228.

Kim, H.J., Greenleaf, J.F., Kinnick, R.R. and Bronk, J.T. (1996). Ultrasound mediated transfection of mammalian cells. *Hum. Gene Ther.* **7**, 1339–1346.

Kleinkort, J.A. and Wood, F. (1975). Phonophoresis with 1 percent *versus* 10 percent hydrocortisone. *Phys. Ther.* **55**, 1320–1324.

Köhrmann, K.U., Michel, M.S., Fruhauf, J., Volz, J., Back, W., Gaa, J., *et al.* (2000). High intensity focused ultrasound for non-invasive tissue ablation in the kidney, prostate and uterus. *J. Urol.* **163** (Suppl. 4), 156.

Köhrmann, K.U., Michel, M.S., Gaa, J., Marlinghaus, E. and Alken, P. (2002a). High intensity focused ultrasound as non-invasive therapy for multifocal renal cell carcinoma: case study and review of the literature. *J. Urol.* **167**, 2397–2403.

Köhrmann, K.U., Michel, M.S., Steidler, A., Marlinghaus, E., Kraut, O. and Alken, P. (2002b). Technical characterization of an ultrasound source for non-invasive thermoablation by high-intensity focused ultrasound. *BJU Int.* **90**, 248–252.

Kopecky, K.K., Yang, R., Sanghvi, N.T. and Rescolla, F.J. (1993). Liver tumour ablation with high-intensity focused ultrasound. *Semin. Intervent. Radiol.* **10**, 125–131.

Kossoff, G. (1979). Analysis of focusing action of spherically curved transducers. *Ultrasound Med. Biol.* **5**, 359–365.

Kossoff, G. and Khan, A.E. (1966). Treatment of vertigo using the ultrasonic generator. *Arch. Otol.* **84**, 181–188.

Kossoff, G., Wadsworth, J.R. and Dudley, P.F. (1967). The round window ultrasonic technique for the treatment of Menière's disease. *Arch. Otolaryngol.* **86**, 534.

Kremkau, F.W. (1979). Cancer therapy with ultrasound: an historical review. *J. Clin. Ultrasound* **7**, 287–300.

Kremkau, F.W., Kaufmann, J.S., Walker, M.M., Burch, P.G. and Spurr, C.L. (1976). Ultrasonic enhancement of nitrogen mustard cytotoxicity in mouse leukaemia. *Cancer* **37**, 1643–1647.

Kristiansen, T.K., Ryaby, J.P., McCabe, J., Frey, J.J. and Roe, L.R. (1997). Accelerated healing of distal radial fractures with the use of specific low intensity ultrasound: a multi-centre, prospective, randomised, double blind, placebo controlled study. *J. Bone Joint Surg. Am.* **79**, 961–973.

Lafon, C., Chapelon, J.Y., Prat, F., Gorry, F., Margonari, J., Theillére, Y. and Cathignol, D. (1998). Design and preliminary results of an ultrasound applicator for interstitial thermal coagulation. *Ultrasound Med. Biol.* **24**, 113–122.

Lafon, C., Theillére, Y., Prat, F., Arefiev, A., Chapelon, J.Y. and Cathignol, D. (2001). Development of an interstitial ultrasound applicator for endoscopic procedures: animal experimentation. *Ultrasound Med. Biol.* **26**, 669–675.

Lavine, O., Langenstrass, K., Bowyer, C., Fox, F., Griffing, V. and Thaler, W. (1952). Effect of ultrasonic waves on the refractive media of the eye. *Arch. Ophthalmol.* **47**, 204–219.

Lawrie, A., Brisken, A.F., Francis, S.E., Cumberland, D.C., Crossman, D.C. and Newman, C.M. (2000). Microbubble enhanced ultrasound for vascular gene therapy. *Gene Ther.* **7**, 2023–2027.

Lawrie, A., Brisken, A.F., Francis, S.E., Tayler, D.I., Chamberlain, D.C. and Newman, C.M. (1999). Ultrasound enhances reporter gene expression after transfection of vascular cells *in vitro*. *Circulation* **99**, 2617–2620.

Lee, A.J., Taberner, P.V. and Halliwell, M. (1979). Severing the corpus callosum in rats using ultrasound: theoretical and experimental correlations. *J. Acoust. Soc. Am.* **66**, 1292–1298.

Lehmann, J.F., McMillan, J.A., Brunner, G.D. and Blumberg, J.B. (1959). Comparative study of the efficiency of short wave, microwave and ultrasonic diathermy in heating the hip joint. *Arch Phys. Med. Rehab.* **40**, 510–512.

Lehmann, J.F., Masock, A.J., Warren, C.G. and Kobtanski, J.N. (1970). Effect of therapeutic temperatures on tendon extensibility. *Arch Phys. Med. Rehab.* **51**, 481–487.

Lele, P.P. (1979). A strategy for localized chemotherapy of tumours using ultrasonic hyperthermia. *Ultrasound Med. Biol.* **5**, 95–97.

Lele, P.P. (1986). Effects of ultrasound on 'solid' mammalian tissues and tumours *in vivo*. In *Ultrasound: Medical Applications, Biological Effects and Hazard Potential*, M. Repacholi, M. Grandolfo and A. Rindi (eds). Plenum, New York, pp. 275–306.

Lerner, R.M., Carstensen, E.L. and Dunn, F. (1973). Frequency dependence of thresholds for ultrasonic production of thermal lesions in tissue. *J. Acoust. Soc. Am.* **54**, 504–506.

Li, G.C., Hahn, G.M. and Tolmach, L.J. (1977). Cellular inactivation by ultrasound. *Nature* **267**, 163–165.

Linke, C.A., Carstensen, E.L., Frizzell, L.A., Elbadawi, A. and Fridd, C.W. (1973). Localised tissue destruction by high intensity focused ultrasound. *Arch. Surg.* **107**, 887–891.

Lizzi, F.L., Coleman, D.J., Driller, J. and Franzen, L.A. (1978). Experimental ultrasonically induced lesions in the retina, choroid and sclera. *Invest. Ophthalmol.* **17**, 350.

Lizzi, F.L., Coleman, D.J., Driller, J., Ostromogilsky, M., Chang, S. and Greenall, P. (1984). Ultrasonic hyperthermia for ophthalmic surgery. *IEEE Trans. Son. Ultrason.* **SU-31**, 473–480.

Lizzi, F.L., Deng, C.X., Lee, P., Rosado, A., Silverman, R.H. and Coleman, D.J. (1999). A comparison of ultrasonic beams for thermal treatment of ocular tumours. *Eur. J. Ultrasound* **9**, 71–78.

Lizzi, F.L. and Ostromogilsky, M. (1987). Analytical modelling of ultrasonically induced tissue heating. *Ultrasound Med. Biol.* **13**, 607–618.

Lynn, J.G. and Putnam, T.J. (1944). Histological and cerebral lesions produced by focused ultrasound. *Am. J. Pathol.* **20**, 637–649.

Lynn, J.G., Zwemmer, R.L., Chick, A.J. and Miller, A.F. (1942). A new method for the generation and use of focused ultrasound in experimental biology. *J. Gen. Physiol.* **26**, 179–193.

Madersbacher, S., Kratzik, C., Susani, M. and Marberger, M. (1994). Tissue ablation in benign prostatic hyperplasia with high intensity focused ultrasound. *J. Urol.* **152**, 1956–1961.

Madersbacher, S., Pedevilla, M., Vingers, L., Susani, M. and Marberger, M. (1995). Effect of high intensity focused ultrasound on human prostate cancer *in vivo*. *Cancer Res.* **55**, 3346–3351.

Madersbacher, S., Schatzl, G., Djavan, R., Stuling, T. and Marberger, M. (2000). Long-term outcome of transrectal high-intensity focused ultrasound therapy for benign prostatic hyperplasia. *Eur Urol.* **37**, 687–694.

Malcolm, A.L. and ter Haar, G.R. (1996). Ablation of tissue volumes using high intensity focused ultrasound. *Ultrasound Med. Biol.* **22**, 659–669.

Manome, Y., Nakamura, M., Ohno, T. and Furuhata, H. (2000). Ultrasound facilitates transduction of naked plasmid DNA into colon carcinoma cells *in vitro* and *in vivo*. *Hum. Gene Ther.* **11**, 1521–1528.

Markham, D.E. and Wood, M.R. (1980). Ultrasound for Dupuytren's contracture. *Physiotherapy* **66**, 55–58.

Martin, K. and Fernandez, R. (1997). A thermal beam shape phantom for ultrasound therapy transducers. *Ultrasound Med. Biol.* **23**, 1267–1274.

Mayr, E., Frankel, V. and Ruter, A. (2000). Ultrasound: an alternative healing method for nonunions? *Arch. Orthopt. Trauma Surg.* **120**, 1–8.

Mayr, E., Laule, A., Suger, G., Ruter, A. and Claes, L. (2001). Radiographic results of callus distraction aided by pulsed low intensity ultrasound. *J. Orthopt. Trauma* **15**, 407–414.

McDiarmid, T., Burns, P.N., Lewith, G.T. and Machin, D. (1985). Ultrasound and the treatment of pressure sores. *Physiotherapy* **71**, 66–70.

McElnay, J.C., Benson, H.A.E., Harland, R. and Hadgraft, J. (1993). Phonophoresis of methyl nicotinate: a preliminary study to elucidate the mechanism of action. *Pharm. Res.* **10**, 1726–1731.

Meaney, P.M., Cahill, M.D. and ter Haar, G.R. (2000). The intensity dependence of lesion position shift during focused ultrasound surgery. *Ultrasound Med. Biol.* **26**, 441–450.

Meaney, P.M., Clarke, R.L., ter Haar, G.R. and Rivens, I.H. (1998). A 3D finite element model for computation of temperature profiles and regions of thermal damage during focused ultrasound surgery exposures. *Ultrasound Med. Biol.* **24**, 1489–1499.

Meidan, V.M., Walmsley, A.D. and Irwin, W.J. (1995). Phonophoresis – is it a reality? *Int. J. Pharm.* **118**, 129–149.

Melodelima, D., Lafon, C., Prat, F., Birer, A. and Cathignol, D. (2002). Ultrasound cylindrical phased array for transoesophageal thermal therapy: initial studies. *Phys. Med. Biol.* **47**, 1–13.

Middlemast, S. and Chatterjee, D.S. (1978). Comparison of ultrasound and thermotherapy for soft tissue injuries. *Physiotherapy* **64**, 331–332.

Mihran, R.T., Barnes, F.S. and Wachtel, H. (1990). Temporally specific modification of myelinated axon excitability *in vitro* following a single ultrasound pulse. *Ultrasound Med. Biol.* **16**, 297–309.

Miller, D.L., Bao, S., Gies, R.A. and Thrall, B.D. (1999). Ultrasonic enhancement of gene transfection in murine melanoma tumours. *Ultrasound Med. Biol.* **25**, 1425–1430.

Mitragotri, S. and Blankschtein, D. (1995). Ultrasound mediated transdermal protein delivery. *Science* **269**, 850–853.

Miyoshi, N., Misik, V., Fukuda, M. and Riesz, P. (1995). Effect of gallium-porphyrin analogue ATX-70 on nitroxide formation from a cyclic secondary amine by ultrasound on the mechanism of sonodynamic activation. *Radiat. Res.* **143**, 194–202.

Moll, M.J. (1977). A new approach to pain: lidocaine and decadron with ultrasound. *USAF Med. Serv. Dig.* **30**, 8–11.

Mortimer, A.J. and Dyson, M. (1988). The effect of therapeutic ultrasound on calcium uptake in fibroblasts. *Ultrasound Med. Biol.* **14**, 499–506.

Morton, K.I., ter Haar, G.R., Stratford, I.J. and Hill, C.R. (1983). Subharmonic emission as an indicator of ultrasonically induced biological damage. *Ultrasound Med. Biol.* **9**, 629–633.

Muir, W.S., Magee, F.P., Longo, J.A., Karpman, R.R. and Finlay, P.R. (1990). Comparison of ultrasonically applied vs intra-articular injected hydrocotisone levels in canine knees. *Orthopaed. Rev.* **19**, 351–356.

Mulligan, E.D., Lynch, T.H., Mulvin, D., Greene, D., Smith, J.M. and Fitzpatrick, J.M. (1997). High intensity focused ultrasound in the treatment of benign prostatic hyperplasia. *Br. J. Urol.* **79**, 177–180.

Murphy, T.M. and Hadgraft, J. (1990). A physico-chemical interpretation of phonophoresis in skin penetration enhancement. In *Prediction of Percutaneous Penetration: Methods, Measurements and Modelling*, R.C. Scott, R.H. Guy and J. Hadgraft (eds). IBC, London, pp. 333–336.

Noble, M.L., Vaezy, S., Keshavarzi, A., Paun, M., Prokop, A.F., Chi, E.Y., Cornejo, C., Sharar, S.R., Jurkovich, G.J., Martin, R.W. and Crum, L.A. (2002). Spleen haemostasis using high intensity ultrasound: survival and healing. *J. Trauma* **53**, 1115–1120.

Nolte, P.A., van der Krans, A., Patka, P., *et al.* (2001). Low intensity pulsed ultrasound in the treatment of nonunions. *J. Trauma* **51**, 693–702.

Novak, E.J. (1964). Experimental transmission through intact skin by ultrasound. *Arch. Phys. Med. Rehabil.* **64**, 231–232.

Nseyo, U.O., Shumaker, B., Klein, E.A. and Sutherland, K. (1998). Photodynamic therapy using porfimer sodium as an alternative to cystectomy in patients with refractory transitional cell carcinoma *in situ* of the bladder. *J. Urol.* **160**, 39–44.

Ogawa, K., Tachibana, K., Uchida, T., Tai, T., Yamashita, N., Tsujita, N. and Miyauchi, R. (2001). High resolution scanning electron microscopic evaluation of cell-membrane porosity by ultrasound. *Med. Electron. Microsc.* **34**, 249–253.

Olsson, S.B., Johansson, B., Nilsson, A.M., Olsson, Ch. and Roijer, A. (1994). Enhancement of thrombolysis by ultrasound. *Ultrasound Med. Biol.* **20**, 375–382.

O'Neil, H.T. (1949). Theory of focusing radiators. *J. Acoust. Soc. Am.* **21**, 516–526.

Patrick, M.K. (1973). Ultrasonic therapy – has it a place in the 70's? *Physiotherapy* **59**, 282–283.

Paul, W.D. and Imig, C.J. (1955). Temperature and blood flow studies after ultrasonic irradiation. *Am. J. Phys. Med.* **34**, 370–375.

Pilla, A.A., Mont, M.A., Nasser, P.R., Khan, S.A., Figueiredo, M., Kaufman, J.J. and Siffert, R.S. (1990). Non-invasive low intensity pulsed ultrasound accelerates bone healing in the rabbit. *J. Orthopaed. Trauma* **4**, 246–253.

Poliachik, S.L., Chandler, W.L., Mourad, P.D., Ollas, R.J. and Crum, L.A. (2001). Activation, aggregation and adhesion of platelets exposed to high intensity focused ultrasound. *Ultrasound Med. Biol.* **27**, 1567–1576.

Pond, J.B. (1970). The role of heat in the production of ultrasonic focal lesions. *J. Acoust. Soc. Am.* **47**, 1607–1611.

Pospisilova, J. (1976). Effect of ultrasound on collagen synthesis and deposition in experimental granuloma tissue. *Acta Chir. Plast. (Praha)* **18**, 176–183.

Pospisilova, J., Brazdova, K. and Velecky, R. (1974). Effect of ultrasound multiplied by non-pathogenic infection on collagen tissue formation. *Experientia* **30**, 755–757.

Pospisilova, J., Samohyl, J., Koprivova, M. and Jelinkova, A. (1980). Our experience with the use of ultrasound in rehabilitation of hand. *Acta Chir. Plast. (Praha)* **22**, 191–199.

Prat, F., Lafon, C., Theilliére, J.Y., Fritsch, J., Choury, A.D., Lorand, I. and Cathignol, D. (2001). Destruction of a bile duct carcinoma by intraductal high intensity ultrasound during ERCP. *Gastrointest. Endosc.* **53**, 797–800.

Price, R.J. and Kaul, S.J. (2002). Contrast ultrasound targeted drug and gene delivery: an update on a new therapeutic modality. *J. Cardiovasc. Pharmacol. Ther.* **7**, 171–180.

Price, R.J., Skyba, D.M., Kaul, S.J. and Skalak, T.C. (1998). Delivery of colloidal particles and red blood cells to tissue through microvessel ruptures created by targeted microbubble destruction with ultrasound. *Circulation* **98**, 1264–1267.

Purnell, E.W., Sokollu, A., Torchia, R. and Taner, N. (1964). Focal chorioretinitis produced by ultrasound. *Invest. Ophthalmol.* **3**, 657–664.

Pye, S. (1996). Ultrasound therapy equipment – does it perform? *Physiotherapy* **82**, 39–44.

Pye, S. and Milford, C. (1994). The performance of ultrasound therapy machines in Lothian region, 1992. *Ultrasound Med. Biol.* **20**, 347–359.

Reher, P., Elbeshir, E.-N.I., Harvey, W., Meghji, S. and Harris, M. (1997). The stimulation of bone formation *in vitro* by therapeutic ultrasound. *Ultrasound Med. Biol.* **23**, 1251–1258.

Repacholi, M.H. and Benwell, D.A. (1979). Using surveys of ultrasound therapy devices to draft performance standards. *Health Phys.* **36**, 679–686.

Rivens, I., Rowland, I., Denbow, M., Fisk, N., Leach, M. and ter Haar, G. (1998). Focused surgery induced vascular occlusion in fetal medicine. *SPIE* **3249**, 260–265.

Rivens, I.H., Rowland, I.J., Denbow, M., Fisk, N.M., ter Haar, G.R. and Leach, M.O. (1999). Vascular occlusion using focused ultrasound surgery for use in fetal medicine. *Eur. J. Ultrasound* **9**, 89–97.

Roberts, W.W., Wright, E.J., Fried, N.M., Nicol, T., Jarrett, T.W., Kavoussi, L.R. and Solomon, S.B. (2002). High intensity focused ultrasound ablation of the epididymis in a canine model: a potential alternative to vasectomy. *J. Endourol.* **16**, 621–625.

Robertson, V. (2002). Dosage and treatment response in randomised clinical trials of therapeutic ultrasound. *Phys. Ther. Sport* **3**, 124–133.

Robinson, T.C. and Lele, P.P. (1972). An analysis of lesion development in the brain and in plastics by high intensity focused ultrasound at low megahertz frequencies. *J. Acoust. Soc. Am.* **51**, 1333–1351.

Rosecan, L.R., Iwamoto, T., Rosado, A., Lizzi, F. and Coleman, D.J. (1985). Therapeutic ultrasound in the treatment of retinal detachment: clinical observation and light and electron microscopy. *Retina* **5**, 115–122.

Rosenberg, R.S. and Purnell, E.W. (1967). Effects of ultrasonic radiation on the ciliary body. *Am. J. Ophthalmol.* **63**, 403–409.

Rosenschein, U., Bernstein, J., Di Segni, E., Kaplinsky, E., Bernheim, J. and Rozenszain, L.A. (1990). Ultrasonic angioplasty: disruption of atherosclerotic plaques and thrombi *in vitro* and arterial recanalization *in vivo*. *J. Am. Coll. Cardiol.* **15**, 711–717.

Rowland, I.J., Rivens, I., Chen, L., Lebozer, C.H., Collins, D.J., ter Haar, G.R. and Leach, M.O. (1997). MRI study of hepatic tumours following high intensity focused ultrasound surgery. *Br. J. Radiol.* **70**, 144–153.

Rubin, C., Bolander, M., Ryaby, J.P. and Hadjiargyrou, M. (2001). Current concepts review. The use of low intensity ultrasound to accelerate the healing of fractures. *J. Bone Joint Surg.* **83**, 258–270.

Rubin, D. and Kuitert, J.H. (1955). Use of ultrasonic vibration in the treatment of pain arising from phantom limbs, scars and neuromas: a preliminary report. *Arch. Phys. Med. Rehab.* **35**, 445–452.

Sanghvi, N.T., Fry, F.J., Bihrle, R., Foster, R.S., Phillips, M.H., Syrus, J., Zaitsev, A.V. and Hennige, C.W. (1996). Non-invasive surgery of prostate tissue by high-intensity focused ultrasound. *IEEE Trans. Ultrason. Ferroelectr. Freq. Control* **43**, 1099–1110.

Sapareto, S.A. and Dewey, W.C. (1984). Thermal dose determination in cancer therapy *Int. J. Radiat. Oncol. Biol. Phys.* **10**, 787–800.

Schatzl, G., Madersbacher, S., Djavan, B., Lang, T. and Marberger, M. (2000). Two-year results of transurethral resection of the prostate versus four 'less invasive' treatment options. *Eur. Urol.* **37**, 695–701.

Shimazaki, A., Inui, K., Azuma, Y., Nishimura, N. and Yamano, Y. (2000). Low intensity pulsed ultrasound accelerates bone maturation in distraction osteogenesis in rabbits. *J. Bone Joint Surg. Br.* **82**, 1077–1082.

Shohet, R.V., Chen, S., Zhou, Y.T., Wang, Z., Meidell, R.S., Unger, R.H. and Grayburn, P.A. (2000). Echocardiographic destruction of albumin microbubbles directs gene delivery to the myocardium. *Circulation* **101**, 2554–2556.

Shotton, K.C. (1980). A tethered float radiometer for measuring the power from ultrasonic therapy equipment. *Ultrasound Med. Biol.* **6**, 131–133.

Sicard-Rosenbaum, L., Lord, D., Danoff, J.V., Thom, A.K. and Eckhaus, M.A. (1995). Effects of continuous therapeutic ultrasound on growth and metastasis of subcutaneous murine tumours. *Phys. Ther.* **75**, 3–13.

Siegel, R.J. (1996). *Ultrasound Angioplasty.* Kluwer Academic, Dordrecht.

Siegel, R.J., Fischell, T.A., Cumberland, D.C. and Fishbein, M.C. (1996a). Ultrasound angioplasty: experimental studies. In *Ultrasound Angioplasty*, R.J. Siegel (ed.). Kluwer Academic, Dordrecht, pp. 69–91.

Siegel, R.J., Steffan, W., Luo, H., Marzelle, J. and Fishbein, M.C. (1996b). High intensity, low frequency catheter delivered ultrasound for thrombus dissolution. In *Ultrasound Angioplasty*. R.J. Siegel (ed.). Kluwer Academic, Dordrecht, pp. 135–150.

Silverman, R.H., Vogelsang, B., Rondeau, M.J. and Coleman, D.J. (1991). Therapeutic ultrasound for the treatment of glaucoma. *Am. J. Ophthalmol.* **111**, 327–337.

Singh, R. and Vyas, S.P. (1996). Topical liposomal system for localized and controlled drug delivery. *J. Dermatol. Sci.* **13**, 107–111.

Sjoberg, A., Stable, J., Johnson, S. and Sahl, R. (1963). Treatment of Menière's disease by ultrasonic irradiation. *Acta Otolaryngol. Suppl.* **178**, 171–175.

Skauen, D.M. and Zenter, G.M. (1984). Phonophoresis. *Int. J. Pharm.* **20**, 235–245.

Skyba, D.M., Price, R.J., Linka, A.Z., Skalak, T.C. and Kaul, S. (1998). Direct *in vivo* visualization of intravascular destruction of microbubbles by ultrasound and its local effects on tissue. *Circulation* **98**, 290–293.

Smachlo, K., Field, C.W., Child, S.J., Hare, J.D., Linke, C.A. and Carstensen, E.L. (1979). Ultrasonic treatment of tumors: I. Absence of metastases following treatment of a hamster fibrosarcoma. *Ultrasound Med. Biol.* **5**, 45–49.

Smith, W., Win, F. and Parette, R. (1986). Comparative study using four modalities in shin splint treatments. *J. Orthopt. Sports Phys. Ther.* **8**, 77–80.

Snow, C.J. and Johnson, K.A. (1988). Effect of therapeutic ultrasound on acute inflammation. *Physiother. Can.* **40**, 162–167.

Sobbe, A., Stumpff, U., Trubestein, G., Figge, H. and Kozuschek, W. (1974). Die Ultraschall Auflösung von Thromben. *Klin. Wochenschr.* **52**, 1117–1121.

Sorensen, H. and Andersen, M.S. (1979). Long term results of ultrasonic irradiation in Menière's disease. *Clin. Otolaryngol.* **4**, 125–129.

Stewart, H.F., Harris, G. Herman, B.A., Robinson, R.A., Haran, M.E., McGall, G.R., Carless, G. and Rees, D. (1974). Survey of use and performance of ultrasonic equipment in Pinellas county, Florida. *Phys. Ther.* **54**, 707–715.

Sullivan, L.D., McLoughlin, M.G., Goldenberg, L.G., Gleave, M.E. and Marich, K.W. (1997). Early experience with high-intensity focused ultrasound for the treatment of benign prostatic hyperplasia. *Br. J. Urol.* **79**, 172–176.

Summer, W. and Patrick, M.K. (1964). *Ultrasonic Therapy: A Textbook for Physiotherapists.* Elsevier, London.

Sun, J. and Hynynen, K. (1999). The potential of transskull ultrasound therapy and surgery using the maximum available skull surface area. *J. Acoust. Soc. Am.* **105**, 2519–2527.

Suppipat, N. (1974). Ultrasonics in periodontics. *J. Clin. Periodont.* **1**, 206–213.

Susani, M., Madersbacher, S., Kratzik, C., Vingers, L. and Marberger, M. (1993). Morphology of tissue destruction induced by focused ultrasound. *Eur. Urol.* **23**(Suppl. 1), 34–38.

Szent-Györgi, A. (1933). Chemical and biological effects of ultrasonic radiation. *Nature* **131**, 278.

Tachibana, K. and Tachibana, S. (1995). Albumin microbubble echo-contrast material as an enhancer for ultrasound accelerated thrombolysis. *Circulation* **92**, 1148–1150.

Tachibana, K. and Tachibana, S. (1996). Ultrasound energy for enhancement of fibrinolysis and drug delivery: special emphasis on the use of transducer tipped ultrasound system. In *Ultrasound Angioplasty*, R.J. Siegel (ed.). Kluwer Academic, Dordrecht, pp. 121–133.

Tachibana, K. and Tachibana, S. (1999). Application of ultrasound energy as a new drug delivery system. *Jpn. J. Appl. Phys.* **38**, 3014–3019.

Tachibana, K., Uchida, T., Hisano, S. and Morioka, E. (1997). Eliminating adult T-cell leukaemia cells with ultrasound. *Lancet* **349**, 325.

Takakura, Y., Matsui, N., Yoshiya, S., Fujioka, H., Muratsu, H., Tsunoda, M. and Kurosaka, M. (2002). Low intensity pulsed ultrasound enhances early healing of medial collateral ligament injuries in rats. *J. Ultrasound Med.* **21**, 283–288.

Takikawa, S., Matsui, N., Kokubu, T., *et al.* (2001). Low intensity pulsed ultrasound initiates bone healing in rat non-union fracture model *J. Ultrasound Med.* **20**, 197–205.

Taniyama, Y., Tachibana, K., Hiraoka, K., Aoki, M., Yamamoto, S., Matsumoto, K., Nakamura, T., Ogihara, T., Kaneda, Y. and Morishita, R. (2002a). Development of safe and efficient novel nonviral gene transfer using ultrasound: enhancement of transfection efficiency of naked plasmid DNA in skeletal muscle. *Gene Ther.* **9**, 372–380.

Taniyama, Y., Tachibana, K., Hiraoka, K., Namba, T., Yamasaki, K., Hashiya, N., Aoki, M., Ogihara, T., Yasufumi, K. and Morishita, R. (2002b). Local delivery of plasmid DNA into rat carotid artery using ultrasound. *Circulation* **105**, 1233–1239.

Tata, D.B., Dunn, F. and Tindall, D.J. (1999). Selective clinical ultrasound signals mediate differential gene transfer and expression in two human prostate cancer cell lines: LnCap and PC-3. *Biochim Biophys. Res. Commun.* **234**, 64–67.

Tsai, C.-L., Chang, W.H. and Liu, T.-K. (1992). Preliminary studies of duration and intensity of ultrasonic treatments on fracture repair. *Chin. J. Physiol.* **35**, 21–26.

Tu, G., Qiao, T., He, S., *et al.* (1999). An experimental study on high-intensity focused ultrasound in the treatment of VX2 rabbit kidney tumours. *Chin. J. Urol.* **20**, 456–458.

Umemura, S., Kawabata, K., Sasaki, K. (1997). *In vitro* and *in vivo* enhancement of sonodynamically active cavitation by second harmonic superimposition. *J. Acoust. Soc. Am.* **101**, 569–577.

Umemura, S., Kawabata, K. and Sasaki, K., Yumita, N., Umemura, K. and Nishigaki, R. (1996). Recent advances in sonodynamic approach to cancer therapy. *Ultrason. Sonochem.* **3**, S187–S191.

Umemura, S., Yumita, N. and Nishigaki, R. (1993). Enhancement of ultrasonically induced cell damage by a gallium-porphyrin complex ATX-70. *Jpn J. Cancer Res.* **84**, 582–588.

Umemura, S., Yumita, N., Nishigaki, R. and Umemura, K. (1990). Mechanism of cell damage by ultrasound in combination with haematoporphyrin. *Jpn J. Cancer Res.* **81**, 962–966.

Vaezy, S., Fujimoto, V.Y., Walker, C., Martin, R.W., Chi, E.Y. and Crum, L.A. (2000). Treatment of uterine fibroid tumour in a nude mouse model using high-intensity focused ultrasound. *Am. J. Obstet. Gynecol.* **183**, 6–11.

Vaezy, S., Martin, R., Keilman, G., Kaczkowski, P., Chi, E., Yazaji, E., Caps, M., Poliachik, S., Carter, S., Sharar, S., Cornejo, C. and Crum, L.A. (1999a). Control of splenic bleeding by using high intensity ultrasound. *J. Trauma Injury, Infection and Critical Care.* **47**, 521–524.

Vaezy, S., Martin, R., Mourad, P. and Crum, L. (1999b). Hemostasis using high intensity focused ultrasound. *Eur. J. Ultrasound* **9**, 79–87.

Vaezy, S., Martin, R., Schmiedl, U., *et al.* (1997). Liver haemostasis using high intensity focused ultrasound. *Ultrasound Med. Biol.* **23**, 1413–1420.

Vaezy, S., Martin, R.W., Yaziji, H., *et al.* (1998). Hemostasis of punctured blood vessels during high intensity focused ultrasound. *Ultrasound Med. Biol.* **24**, 903–910.

Vallancien, G., Chartier-Kastler, E., Bataille, N., Chopin, D., Harouni, M. and Bougaran, J. (1993). Focused extra-corporeal pyrotherapy. *Eur. Urol.* **23** (Suppl. 1), 48–52.

Vallancien, G., Guillonneau, B., Desgrandchamps, F., Leduc, A., Thuroff, S., Chaussy, C., Kiel, H.J., Wieland, W. and Gelet, A. (1999). Local control of prostate cancer by transrectal high-intensity focused ultrasound therapy (HIFU): preliminary results of European study. *J. Urol.* **161** (Suppl. 4), 330.

Vallancien, G., Harouni, M., Guillonneau, B., Veillon, B. and Bougaran, J. (1996). Ablation of superficial bladder tumors with focused extracorporeal pyrotherapy. *Urology* **47**, 204–207.

Visioli, A.G., Rivens, I.H., ter Haar, G.R., Horwich, A., Huddart, R.A., Moskovic, E., Padhani, A. and Glees, J. (1999). Preliminary results of a phase I dose escalation clinical trial using focused ultrasound in the treatment of localised tumours. *Eur. J. Ultrasound* **9**, 11–18.

Wall, P.D., Fry, W.J., Stephens, R., Tucker, D. and Lettvin, J.Y. (1951). Changes produced in the central nervous system by ultrasound. *Science* **114**, 686–687.

Walmsley, A.D. (1988). Applications of ultrasound in dentistry. *Ultrasound Med. Biol.* **14**, 7–14.

Wang, S.J., Lewallen, D.G., Bolander, M.E., *et al.* (1994). Low intensity ultrasound treatment increases strength in a rat femoral fracture model. *J. Orthopt. Res.* **12**, 40–47.

Warren, C.G., Koblanski, J.N. and Sigelmann, R.A. (1976). Ultrasound coupling media: their relative transmissivity. *Arch Phys. Med. Rehab.* **57**, 218–222.

Warwick, R. and Pond, J.B. (1968). Trackless lesions in nervous tissues produced by high intensity focused ultrasound (high frequency mechanical waves). *J. Anat.* **102**, 387–405.

Watkin, N.A., ter Haar, G.R., Morris, S.B. and Woodhouse, C.R.J. (1995). The urological applications of focused ultrasound surgery. *Br. J. Urol.* **75** (Suppl. 1), 1–8.

Watkin, N.A., ter Haar, G.R. and Rivens, I. (1996a). The intensity dependence of the site of maximal energy deposition in focused ultrasound surgery. *Ultrasound Med. Biol.* **22**, 483–491.

Watkin, N.A., Morris, S.B., Rivens, I. and ter Haar, G.R. (1997). High intensity focused ultrasound ablation of the kidney in a large animal model. *J. Endourol.* **11**, 191–196.

Watkin, N.A., Morris, S.B., Rivens, I.H., Woodhouse, C.R.J. and ter Haar, G.R. (1996b). A feasibility study for the non-invasive treatment of superficial bladder tumours with focused ultrasound. *Br. J. Urol.* **78**, 715–721.

Watmough, D.J. and Ross, W.M. (1986). *Hyperthermia.* Blackie, Glasgow.

Webster, D.F., Dyson, M. and Harvey, W. (1979). Ultrasonically induced stimulation of collagen synthesis *in vivo. Proc. 4th Eur. Symp. Ultrasound Biol. Med.* **1**, 135–140.

Webster, D.F., Harvey, W., Dyson, M. and Pond, J.B. (1980). The role of ultrasound-induced cavitation in the *in vitro* stimulation of collagen synthesis in human fibroblasts. *Ultrasonics* **18**, 33–37.

Webster, D.F., Pond, J.B., Dyson, M. and Harvey, W. (1978). The role of cavitation in the *in vitro* stimulation of protein synthesis in human fibroblasts by ultrasound. *Ultrasound Med. Biol.* **4**, 343–351.

Weimann, L.J. and Wu, J. (2002). Transdermal delivery of poly-L-lysine by sonomacroporation. *Ultrasound Med. Biol.* **28**, 1173–1180.

Wells, P.N.T., Bullen, M.A., Follett, D.M., Freundlich, H.F. and James, J.A. (1963). The dosimetry of small ultrasonic beams. *Ultrasonics* **1**, 106–110.

Williams, A.R. (1990). Phonophoresis: an *in vivo* evaluation using three topical anaesthetic preparations. *Ultrasonics* **28**, 137–141.

Witcofski, R.L. and Kremkau, F.W. (1978). Ultrasonic enhancement of cancer radiotherapy. *Radiology* **127**, 793–797.

Woeber, K. (1957). Diminution of X-ray dosage in cancer by simultaneous X-ray and ultrasound treatment (Biological basis and clinical results). *Acta Dermatol. Venereol.* **2**, 434–436.

Woeber, K. (1965). The effect of ultrasound in the treatment of cancer. In *Ultrasonic Energy*, E. Kelly (ed.). University of Illinois Press, Urbana, pp. 137–149.

Woolley, P.E., Barnett, R.J. and Pond, J.B. (1975). The use of probes to measure megahertz ultrasonic fields in liquids. *Ultrasonics* **13**, 68–72.

Wu, F., Chen, W.Z., Bai, J., Zou, J.Z., Wang, J.L., Zhu, H. and Wang, Z. (2002). Tumor vessel destruction resulting from high intensity focused ultrasound in patients with solid malignancies. *Ultrasound Med. Biol.* **28**, 535–542.

Wyber, J.A., Andrews, J. and D'Emanuele, A. (1997). The use of sonication for the efficient delivery of plasmid DNA into cells. *Pharma. Res.* **14**, 750–756.

Yang, K.-H., Parvizi, J., Wang, S.J., Lewallen, D.G., Kinnick, R.R., Greenleaf, J.F. and Bolander, M.E. (1996). Exposure to low intensity ultrasound increases aggrecan gene expression in a rat femur fracture model. *J. Orthopt. Res.* **14**, 802–809.

Yang, R., Reilly, C.R., Rescorla, F.J., *et al.* (1991). High intensity focused ultrasound in the treatment of experimental liver cancer. *Arch. Surg.* **126**, 1002–1009.

Young, S.R. and Dyson, M. (1990). Effect of therapeutic ultrasound on the healing of full-thickness excised skin lesions. *Ultrasonics* **28**, 175–180.

Yumita, N., Nishigaki, R., Umemura, K. and Umemura, S. (1989). Hematoporphyrin as a sensitiser of cell damaging effect of ultrasound. *Jpn J. Cancer Res.* **80**, 219–222.

Zinner, D.D. (1955). Recent ultrasonic dental studies, including periodentia, without the use of an abrasive. *J. Dent. Res.* **34**, 748–749.

Ziskin, M.C. and Michlovitch, S.L. (1986). Therapeutic ultrasound. In *Contemporary Perspectives in Rehabilitation.* Vol. 1, S.L. Michlovitch (ed.). F.A. Davis, Philadelphia, pp. 141–176.

14

Assessment of Possible Hazard in Use

GAIL R. TER HAAR

Institute of Cancer Research, Royal Marsden Hospital, UK

14.1 INTRODUCTION

As must be the case for any physical agent capable of depositing energy in the human body, it is not only scientifically interesting but professionally imperative to enquire whether the medical use of ultrasound may be hazardous in any way to either patient or operator. Such enquiry dates from the earliest days of both therapeutic and diagnostic ultrasound and, in view of the logical impossibility of absolute proof of safety for any given agent, is likely to continue indefinitely as a matter for discussion and controversy.

The purpose of this chapter is to consider the various lines of evidence that can be brought to bear on this question, and in doing so it will be necessary to discuss definitions not only of relevant biological endpoints but also of the concepts of 'safety' and 'hazard' in the context of either therapeutic or diagnostic practice. We shall also review some of the guidelines and recommendations in the field that have evolved from the deliberations of various international and other expert groups.

In what follows we shall first somewhat extend previous discussion (Chapter 3, Section 3.8) of the measurement of ultrasonic exposure in medical practice. Then, in subsequent sections, we shall consider the biological evidence and, here, if only for didactic convenience, we shall consider in turn the systems of successively increasing levels of organisational complexity.

14.2 EXPOSURE PRACTICE AND LEVELS

Assessment of the exposure of human tissues that arises from medical ultrasound equipment is a complex task. Output is normally characterised by measurements made under free field conditions in a water bath. A full description of an ultrasonic field entails a number of quantities. These may include the frequency, source dimensions, duty factor in a pulsed field, peak positive and negative pulse pressure amplitudes, temporal average power and temporal and spatial peak intensities. These quantities, and their determination, have been discussed in Chapter 3, Section 3.8.

Representative values of exposure quantities for different classes of medical ultrasound units are shown in Table 14.1. This is not a complete list.

During ultrasonic exposure, acoustic energy is transmitted into tissue through some form of coupling medium. For the majority of diagnostic investigations, coupling is obtained by an

---

Physical Principles of Medical Ultrasonics, Second Edition. Edited by C. R. Hill, J. C. Bamber and G. R. ter Haar.
© 2004 John Wiley & Sons, Ltd: ISBN 0 471 97002 6

Table 14.1. Output characteristics of ultrasound devices

Equipment type	Frequency range (MHz)	Typical source area (mm²)	Typical duty factor	Power (mW)	External probes Spatial peak, temporal average intensity I_{SPTA} (mW cm⁻²)	Peak negative acoustic pressure p^- (MPa)	Intra-cavitary probes Spatial peak, temporal average intensity I_{SPTA} (mW cm⁻²)	Peak negative acoustic pressure p^- (MPa)
Diagnostic								
Pulse–echo								
B-mode	1–20	100–3000	0.001	4–256 (64)	1–1330 (175)	0.45–5.54 (2.09)	0.8–284 (64.60)	0.66–3.5 (2.32)
M-mode	1–20	100–3000	0.001	0.5–213 (46)	4.2–604 (127)	0.45–5.54 (2.09)	2.0–210 (62.7)	0.66–3.5 (2.32)
Doppler								
Fetal heart detector	2–4	100	1	5–30		0.01		
Pulsed Doppler	5–10	100	0.01	11–324 (144)	36–9080 (1570)	0.67–5.32 (2.18)	97.1–1440 (747)	0.97–3.53 (2.26)
Colour flow	5–10	100	0.01	35–295 (138)	21–2150 (429)	0.46–4.25 (2.41)	0.97–3.53 (2.26)	1.14–3.04 (2.47)
Therapeutic								
Physiotherapy								
Continuous wave	0.75–3	300	1	0–15 000	500			
Pulsed	0.75–3	300	0.2	0–3000		0.5		
Surgery	0.5–10	5000	1	200 000		5		

Source: From Henderson *et al.* (1995) and Whittingham (2000).

aqueous gel applied directly to the skin surface. For more awkward geometries either the area to be exposed is immersed in a bath of degassed water or a water-filled bag that conforms to the surface geometry is placed on the skin.

Contact scanning inevitably results in irradiation of tissues in the near-field region of the transducer. Sharp peaks of intensity occur in this region, particularly in a continuous wave beam, and high cumulative doses may be delivered if the beam is not moved continually and/ or pulsed. In order to avoid near-field effects, a stand-off tube containing coupling medium is sometimes fitted to the transducer face.

It has become good practice in literature reports to quote ultrasonic exposure levels for bio-effect studies in terms either of the spatial, temporal average intensities measured under free field conditions at the position of the biological sample (and, where possible, to give details of the beam profile at this position and the value of the spatial, temporal peak intensity) or in terms of the pressure field at the sample, with the peak positive and negative pressure amplitudes being given. Although this does not provide a complete description of the field, it enables a reasonable assessment to be made. It has been pointed out previously (Chapter 3, Section 3.8) that it has not yet been possible to identify any quantitative predictors of biological effect of ultrasound, in the sense that absorbed dose serves this function in ionising radiation biology and the use of ultrasonic 'intensity' in any form is in this sense arbitrary and usually not directly relevant biologically. In particular it will be evident from the discussion of Chapter 12 that acoustic pressure may be more relevant in some instances, especially where cavitation is involved. Pressures are usually measured using hydrophone probes and intensity can be derived from the pressure values obtained. The relationship $I = P_0^2/2\rho c$, although only strictly valid for plane progressive wave conditions (Chapter 1), can be considered to be a useful approximation in many situations.

Although the best bio-effect reports contain a rigorous description of the ultrasonic exposure conditions, the fact remains that the absorbed dose cannot be quantified adequately. Furthermore, because of the effects of absorption, scattering, reflection and non-linear propogation, the free field exposure condition may not be exactly the same as the exposure conditions within the biological sample *in situ*, even in a laboratory experiment.

14.3 STUDIES OF ISOLATED CELLS

The study of isolated cells in culture can provide useful information at a fundamental level about ultrasonically induced changes produced under closely defined exposure conditions. Under optimum conditions the cells should be contained in sample holders that perturb the ultrasonic field as little as possible.

It is impossible in a chapter of this kind to cite all the evidence that exists for ultrasonically induced changes in cells. Instead, representative examples will be given that are drawn from work with mammalian cells.

There are a number of endpoints that have been used to study the effect of external agents on cells. It is convenient here to distinguish between 'gross' effects, such as lysis, destruction of reproductive ability and damage to cellular ultrastructure, and more subtle effects, such as chromosomal changes, functional changes and altered growth patterns.

14.3.1 CELL LYSIS

The evidence that ultrasound exposure of cells in suspension can lead to cell lysis is extensive and unquestionable. Cavitation has been shown to be a major mechanism in producing complete cellular disruption of this sort, and a number of studies have been published on this subject (e.g. Kaufman *et al.* 1977; Morton *et al.* 1982). It is not clear, however, that ultrasound can produce lysis in the absence of cavitation effects. Several authors (including Elwart *et al.* 1988) have demonstrated that the amount of lysis obtained depends on the concentration of cells in suspension, with higher cell concentrations exhibiting proportionally less lysis than low ones. It is postulated that this is because high cell densities interfere with bubble activity in the suspension. Brayman *et al.* (1992) investigated this further and suggested that this 'cell density effect' was, in part, due to respiratory consumption of dissolved oxygen and concomitant release of CO_2 into the suspension medium, thus reducing the probability of lysis-inducing effects (Carstensen *et al.* 1993). In a later publication, Brayman *et al.* (1996b) studied existing data and concluded that, although the proportion of cells that are lysed decreases with increasing cell density, the total number of cells lysed actually increases. These authors hypothesise that cell size is an important determinant of the extent of cell lysis because of its effect on cell–cell and cell–bubble spacings in suspensions of a given concentration. Cell size is also important in the formation of cell aggregates around pulsating bubbles (Nyborg & Miller 1982; Brayman & Miller 1993). Lysis, where it occurs, appears to be an immediate consequence of ultrasound exposure rather than a delayed effect, and may affect cells in mitosis more than those in other stages of the cell cycle (Clarke & Hill 1969).

14.3.2 REPRODUCTIVE ABILITY

A common measure of biological effect in conventional radiobiology is the clonogenic assay. This assesses the ability of a cell to divide and produce viable progeny following a specific treatment.

In general, cells that survive ultrasonic exposure as intact cells go on to produce progeny in the same way as their untreated counterparts (Bleaney *et al.* 1972; Morton *et al.* 1982). The exception to this appears to be cells that are exposed to ultrasound while being maintained at an elevated temperature (Li *et al.* 1977; ter Haar *et al.* 1980). It has been found that there is a loss of reproductive ability in the heated, irradiated cells over and above that of cells subjected to heat alone. The mechanism for this effect is not understood, but is thought to be non-thermal and non-cavitational in origin (Morton *et al.* 1983). (See section 13.4).

14.3.3 ULTRASTRUCTURAL CHANGES

Most aspects of cellular ultrastructure have been studied following ultrasonic irradiation. A variety of changes have been seen, many of which may not necessarily be lethal.

Changes to the extracellular membrane following ultrasonic irradiation are usually manifested as changes in permeability to ion transport. Examples of this are the sublethal alteration in the thymocyte plasma membrane that leads to a decrease in potassium content following $1\,\mathrm{W\,cm^{-2}}$ irradiation *in vitro* at $1.8\,\mathrm{MHz}$ (Chapman 1974), and the reversible increase in calcium ion uptake in fibroblasts demonstrated by Mortimer and Dyson (1988) ($1\,\mathrm{MHz}$, $0.5–1.0\,\mathrm{W\,cm^{-2}}$ SPPA).

Electron microscopy of cells following ultrasonic treatment at therapy intensities has revealed damage to a variety of organelles, primarily to mitochondria. When intact tissues have been studied using this technique, damage to lysosomes has been seen, with consequent release of lysosomal enzymes. It is not clear whether lysosomal damage is a direct, or indirect, result of ultrasonic exposure (Dvorak & Hrazdira 1966; Hrazdira 1970; Taylor & Pond 1972).

Damage to the plasma membrane of the luminal aspect of endothelial cells of blood vessels irradiated in standing wave fields has also been reported both in chick embryos and mouse uterine vessels (Dyson *et al.* 1974; ter Haar *et al.* 1979).

Where cavitation is implicated in causing damage, not only has membrane and mitochondrial damage been seen but dilated rough endoplasmic reticulum and some irregular lesions have been observed (Harvey *et al.* 1975).

In general, it seems that the cell nucleus is relatively unaffected by ultrasonic irradiation, the only lesions being slit-like vacuoles at the nuclear membrane (ter Haar *et al.* 1979). Watmough *et al.* (1977) have suggested that cavitation microbubbles may be produced within cells and that nuclear, mitochondrial and granular endoplasmic reticulum membranes could act as nucleation sites. These organelles would be specifically affected and damage might manifest itself as lesions next to the membrane. There is, however, no direct evidence for this hypothesis.

14.3.4 *CHROMOSOMAL AND CYTOGENETIC EFFECTS*

Ultrasound of sufficiently high intensity may lead to degradation of DNA in solution. It appears that cavitation is a prerequisite for this and that the damage is due to hydrodynamic shear stresses, free radical formation or excessive heating (Thacker 1973; Miller & Thomas 1995, 1996). Such conditions are unlikely to pertain for diagnostic ultrasound exposures.

There has been considerable effort exerted in looking for ultrasonically induced chromosomal alterations and sister chromatid exchanges. The vast majority of evidence is that ultrasound up to quite high intensities ($100 \, \mathrm{W \, cm^{-2}}$ SPTP) does not produce chromosomal damage (for a comprehensive review see: Rott 1981; EFSUMB 1994). There is, however, some indication that there may be some synergistic interaction producing chromosomal aberrations when $3 \, \mathrm{W \, cm^{-2}}$ ultrasound (810 kHz) follows x-irradiation to 1 Gy (100 rad) but not when it precedes it (Kunze-Muhl 1981).

Sister chromatid exchange analysis has been applied frequently as an assay for the effect of potentially mutagenic agents on mammalian cells, although the implications for the cell or whole organism are poorly understood (Latt & Schreck 1980; Gebhart 1981). A report that diagnostic ultrasound may be able to produce sister chromatid exchanges *in vitro* (Liebeskind *et al.* 1979a) stimulated a flurry of publications on this topic, some of which are summarised in Table 14.2, with a majority showing negative results even for intensities up to $3.0 \, \mathrm{W \, cm^{-2}}$ (3.15 MHz, continuous wave).

Although there has been the occasional report that ultrasound may produce chromosomal damage, no such report has ever been substantiated by investigators in laboratories other than those of the original authors, and the majority of the most carefully documented literature on the subject have yielded negative reports (EFSUMB 1994). In addition, the majority of these studies have been carried out *in vitro* – where interaction mechanisms need not necessarily be the same as those that will pertain in intact tissues *in vivo*.

14.3.5 *FUNCTIONAL CHANGES*

Ultrasound may stimulate or inhibit cellular function. An example of its stimulatory action – the increase in protein synthesis following irradiation of human fibroblasts *in vitro* – has already been discussed (see Chapter 13, Section 13.3.2.1).

Most other functional changes involve interactions at the level of the extracellular membrane. For example, it has been reported that the electrophoretic mobility of cells may be affected by ultrasound (Taylor & Newman 1972). This reflects a change in cell surface charge density, probably due to volume changes (Mummery 1978), but appears only to occur under *in vitro* conditions in association with cavitationally induced cell lysis (Joshi *et al.* 1973).

Table 14.2. Sister chromatid exchange induction by ultrasound

Reference	Cell type	Ultrasound	Result
Morris *et al.* (1978)	Human leucocytes *in vitro*	Continuous wave 15.3–36 W cm^{-2} SP	Negative
Liebeskind *et al.* (1979b)	HeLa *in vitro*	Pulsed 35.4 W cm^{-2} SPTP 6.6 W cm^{-2} SATA	Negative
Liebeskind *et al.* (1979a)	Human lymphocytes *in vitro*	Pulsed 2.7 W cm^{-2} SATA	Positive
Wegner *et al.* (1980)	CHO (G$_2$) *in vitro*	Pulsed 10 mW cm^{-2} SPTA	Negative
Haupt *et al.* (1981)	Human lymphocytes *in vitro*	Pulsed 1.3 W cm^{-2} SPTP 0.02 mW cm^{-2} SPTA	Negative
Zheng *et al.* (1981)	Amniotic cells *in vivo*	Pulsed	Negative
Ehlinger *et al.* (1991)	Human lymphocytes *in vivo*	Pulsed	Positive
Barrass *et al.* (1982)	Fibroblasts *in vitro*	Continuous wave 3 W cm^{-2} SP	Negative
Wegner & Meyenburg (1982)	CHO (G$_1$, S) *in vitro*	Pulsed 0.01 W cm^{-2} SPTP	Negative
Lundberg *et al.* (1982)	Amniotic cells *in vivo*	Pulsed 5 mW cm^{-2} SATP	Negative
Au *et al.* (1982)	Bone marrow *in vivo*	Continuous wave 0.3–0.6 W cm^{-2} SP	Negative
Stella *et al.* (1984)	Human lymphocytes *in vivo*		Positive
Ciaravino *et al.* (1986)	Human lymphocytes *in vitro*		Negative
Barnett *et al.* (1988)	CHO *in vitro*	Pulsed 2500 W cm^{-2} I_m	Positive
Miller *et al.* (1985)	CHO *in vitro*	Pulsed 1400 W cm^{-2} I_m 2 W cm^{-2} TA	Negative
Miller *et al.* (1991)	Human lymphocytes *in vivo*	1 1.2 W cm^{-2} SA	Negative

Time lapse photomicrography studies of cellular movements have revealed ultrasonically induced changes that may last for several generations (Liebeskind *et al.* 1982). The implication of this finding for *in vivo* irradiation with ultrasound is far from clear.

14.4   STUDIES ON MULTICELLULAR ORGANISMS

The search for biological effect produced by ultrasound has been carried out on a wide range of multicellular structures. These include plants, insects, small animals and humans. However, it is only practicable here to discuss work that has been carried out in mammalian systems.

14.4.1 BONE AND SOFT TISSUE EFFECTS

The question of hazard arising from irradiation of adult bone and tissue is a difficult one because, in many cases, as for example in physiotherapy, controlled biological change is the objective of the exposure. As has been stressed before, change does not necessarily constitute a hazard.

When one considers thermal effects it is necessary to realise that different tissues have different sensitivities to heating. Figure 14.1 demonstrates this for a range of adult tissues. Here, the threshold for damage is presented in terms of the time of exposure required at a temperature of 43°C.

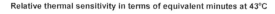

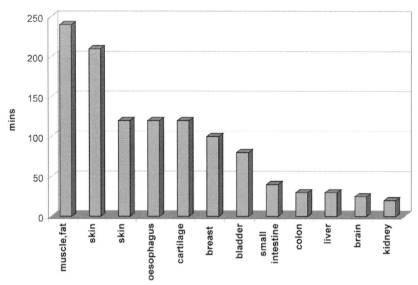

Figure 14.1. Relative thermal sensitivities of a number of different adult tissues expressed as time required at 43°C to produce damage. Data taken from Dewey (1991), Fajardo (1984) and Lyng *et al.* (1991a, b)

14.4.1.1 Bone Effects

The influence of bone lying within soft tissue on the absorption of an ultrasonic field has been discussed in Chapter 12. The main effect that is likely to occur in the bone itself is heating at the periosteum, because the absorption of ultrasonic energy by bone is too high to allow significant penetration at medical frequencies. Herman and Harris (2002) have calculated that, during millisecond pulses or pulsed bursts of ultrasound at intensities near the 1993 Food and Drug Administration limits (FDA 1993), transient temperature rises in bone at or near the focus may reach biologically significant levels and thus is an important consideration for safety.

Surprisingly little has been done to study the effects of ultrasonic exposure to bone (Goldblat 1969; Dyson & Brookes 1983). Dyson and Brookes have shown that ultrasonic irradiation at a fracture site is only beneficial if carried out during the inflammatory or early proliferative phase of healing, and is disadvantageous (stimulating cartilaginous growth) if undertaken in the late proliferative phase. Goldblat (1969) reported that the fracture healed more rapidly shortly after treatment but thereafter began to weaken, being no stronger than the control 6–7 weeks later. Bone fracture repair has been discussed in more detail in Chapter 13, Section 13.3.2.2.

Barth and Wachsmann (1949) have looked at the effect of irradiation of bone in dogs of different ages using either a stationary or a moving transducer head. They found a thickening in young bones, followed by loss of periosteum. The intensity threshold for a stationary transducer lay in the region 0.5–1 W cm^{-2}. Similar effects were seen in old bone but they took longer to develop. These changes were presumably due to heating of the periosteum.

Generally, the problem most likely to arise when irradiating over bone – periosteal heating – is likely to be a limiting factor in physiotherapy or hyperthermic treatments over superficial bone. It may also prove to be a problem with pulsed Doppler examinations performed at the maximum available output level of the device. In the aware human with normal temperature sensitivity, excessive periosteal heating from this cause is likely to lead to pain (e.g. Lehmann *et al.* 1967) and if treatment is stopped when pain is felt then damage is likely to be avoided. Particular care needs to be taken, however, with patients who have reduced pain sensitivity and who may not have this 'early warning system'.

Obstetric applications of pulsed Doppler ultrasound are of particular concern from the thermal hazard viewpoint. This is particularly so because proliferating tissue has been shown to be especially susceptible to thermal injury (Edwards 1986, 1993; Miller & Ziskin 1989) and abnormal brain development has been reported in rodents following temperature elevations of 4°C for 5 min *in utero* (Barnett *et al.* 1994; WFUMB 1992). Bosward *et al.* (1993) measured temperature rises of 4.7°C in brain tissue adjacent to the occipital bone of 60-day gestation guinea pigs and 5.2°C in the vicinity of the parietal bone (120 s exposure; 2.9 W cm^{-2} I_{SPTA}; 260 mW power). Carstensen *et al.* (1990) reported a 5.6°C temperature rise in the cranial bone of young mice *in vivo* (I_{SPTA}=1.5 W cm^{-2}; 45 s). These intensities are similar to the maxima found in pulsed Doppler equipment (see Table 14.1). Similar studies have been undertaken in fetal sheep *in vivo* by Duggan *et al.* (1995). They reported temperature rises of 1.7°C after 120 s in response to an ultrasonic power of 0.6 W (0.26 W cm^{-2} SATA); this rose to 8.8°C for a power level of 2.0 W. For unperfused tissue, 0.6 W led to a temperature increase of 3.0°C after 120 s.

14.4.1.2 Soft Tissue Effects

Ultrastructural changes following ultrasonic irradiation of intact tissue *in vivo* have been discussed previously (Section 14.3.3). In summary, extracellular membranes, lysosomes and mitochondria are the cellular components most often affected.

Soft tissue effects have principally been investigated because of the widespread interest in the use of ultrasound for physiotherapy. Observations of accelerated wound healing (Dyson *et al.* 1968) have been discussed in Chapter 13, Section 13.3.2.1.

When mammalian smooth muscle has been irradiated with ultrasound a variety of effects have been seen. These range from alteration of contractile activity (Talbert 1975; ter Haar *et al.* 1978) to inhibition of action potentials (Hu *et al.* 1978). These effects have been seen at intensities above 1 W cm^{-2} and are thought to be due to changes in ion transport across cell membranes, produced by acoustic streaming.

14.4.2 EFFECTS ON BLOOD COMPONENTS AND VASCULATURE

Erythrocytes form the component of the blood that is least sensitive to ultrasonic damage. Haemolysis is usually mediated by cavitation and/or high hydrodynamic shear stresses (Rooney 1970; Williams *et al.* 1970). There has, however, been some indication that haemolysis may occur at therapeutic intensities in the presence of collapse cavitation and in regions of turbulent flow (Wong & Watmough 1980), and ATP may be released at low spatial average intensities (20–30 W cm^{-2}) when erythrocytes are irradiated *in vitro* in the presence of stable gas bodies (Williams & Miller 1980).

The most fragile component of whole blood is the population of platelets. Where localised haemolysis will generally not be important, damage to platelets with the associated possibility of thrombus formation may be a significant hazard.

Williams (1974) has shown *in vitro* that platelet damage can result from shear stresses within the suspending fluid that are very low relative to those required to damage erythrocytes and other blood constituents. Thus, when stable bubbles are introduced into a platelet suspension, damage may be seen at spatial average intensities as low as 0.8 W cm^{-2} (Miller *et al.* 1979).

Cavitation appears to be difficult to induce in whole blood, possibly because it is continuously filtered of impurities by the body and so is not rich in cavitation nuclei. However, if the acoustic pressure is high enough (e.g. 17 MPa (=100 atm.) at 1 MHz) it has been demonstrated that cavitation can be induced (Brayman *et al.* 1996b). It has also been demonstrated that the addition of contrast agents to whole or diluted blood can lead to detectable haemolysis at ultrasonic exposure levels that produce no such effect in the absence of these agents (Brayman *et al.* 1995; Miller & Thomas 1995, 1996). In one study, not only did the presence of contrast agent increase the amount of haemolysis induced, but it also lowered the threshold pressure for its induction by a factor of 1.78 (Miller & Thomas 1996). For example, using burst mode (0.1 ms:10 ms; 1.28 MHz), the pressure amplitude needed to induce haemolysis changed from in excess of 17.8 MPa without contrast agent to 10 MPa in its presence. Other investigators have established thresholds in the range 11–24 MPa (Brayman *et al.* 1995; Ivey *et al.* 1995). These levels are significantly higher than those found in commercial diagnostic units (see Table 14.1). Brayman *et al* (1996a) have studied the frequency dependence of haemolysis production for cells in suspension. They showed that, for a fixed pressure amplitude, the amount of haemolysis decreased with increasing frequency, showing an inverse third or fourth power dependency. Brayman and Miller (1999) also showed that the haemolytic yield for different pulse lengths and pulse numbers was approximately constant for a given 'on-time'. Miller and Gies (1998a) have shown that perfluorocarbon-filled bubbles yield more haemolysis than air-filled agents, presumably because of their longer persistence.

However, most *in vivo* attempts to detect damage to blood components following ultrasonic irradiation of humans have proved negative so far (Williams *et al.* 1977). It seems unlikely that such damage would be detected easily *in vivo*, because a small population of damaged cells could be diluted rapidly by normal cells flowing through the area. Dalecki *et al.* (1997) have demonstrated haemolysis in mouse blood following ultrasonic exposure through the chest wall: 10 μs pulses (100 kHz p.r.f; 1.15 MHz) were used in 5 min exposures and a threshold of $p^+=3.5\pm0.9$ MPa, $p^-=2$ MPa was found. However, the amount of haemolysis observed was clinically insignificant ($<4\%$). At a frequency of 2.35 MHz only 0.46% haemolysis was seen at a pressure amplitude of 10 MPa.

Irradiation of blood vessels in standing wave fields has been shown to cause damage to the luminal aspect of the plasma membrane both in the *area vasculosa* of the chick embryos (Dyson *et al.* 1974) and in uterine vessels in the mouse (ter Haar *et al.* 1979). From the appearance and site of this damage it was thought to be caused by shear stresses set up by acoustic streaming. Where the damage was most severe, extravasation of erythrocytes into surrounding tissue could be seen. The damage mechanism associated with standing wave formation appears to require a finite time in which to become effective and its consequences thus can be avoided by using a moving sound head.

Child *et al.* (1990) were the first to report the induction of haemorrhage in mouse lung tissue by ultrasonic exposures (1.2 MHz, 10 μs pulse, $I_{SPTA}=1$ mW cm^{-2} for 3 min, $p^+ =0.7$ MPa). This has since been reported by a number of authors and has been observed in rodents, swine and monkeys (Penney *et al.* 1993; Frizzell *et al.* 1994; Tarantal & Canfield 1994; Zachary & O'Brien 1995; Holland *et al.* 1996). The damage manifests itself as localised lesions located on the lung surface. Peri-alveolar capillaries are ruptured, thus allowing plasma proteins and erythrocytes to spill out into alveolar spaces. A similar phenomenon has been observed in the gas-containing intestine (Dalecki *et al.* 1995) but has never been seen in the absence of gas, and so does not present a hazard in, for example, the fetal lung. The biological significance of this observation is not known. It is certainly true that surface haemorrhages can be induced by coughing and that premature babies often have observable lung haemorrhages that are not considered adverse. The mechanism of action by which this effect is produced is not fully understood. One possible explanation is that the gas interface serves as a pressure release boundary that causes a reversal of the incident pressure pulse, leading to high local negative pressures.

The introduction of gas-filled contrast agents (see Chapter 9) might be expected to alter the threshold for induction of haemorrhage. However, Raeman et al. (1997) have demonstrated that the presence of Albunex did not significantly increase the amount of haemorrhage observed in the mouse lung. Animals were exposed to 10 μs pulses of 1.15 MHz ultrasound for 5 min at a peak positive pressure of 2 MPa. The experiments indicated also that the threshold pressure for induction of the effect was not altered by the presence of Albunex.

Dalecki et al. (1997) used 5-min exposures of 10 μs pulses (100 Hz p.r.f.) at 1.15 MHz (peak pressures 0–10 MPa) and at 2.35 MHz (10 MPa). They studied the extent of haemolysis in mouse blood following ultrasonic exposure of the heart through the chest wall. The experimental group of animals were given four 0.05-ml boluses of commercial concentration Albunex at 1-min intervals during this exposure. It was found that, although the threshold for inducing haemolysis ($p^+ \sim 3.5 \pm 0.9$ MPa, $p^- = 2$ MPa) was not changed by the introduction of the contrast agent, significantly more haemolysis was measured in its presence. Nevertheless, at the highest pressures used the amount of haemolysis seen ($\sim 4\%$) is not considered to be clinically significant. At 2.35 MHz, only 0.46% haemolysis was seen at 10 MPa.

Miller and Gies (1998b) showed that the induction of petechiae was proportional to the dose of contrast agent. The activation of these gas bodies leads to capillary leakage, with 100 ms pulses being more damaging than shorter ones (10–100 μs). Skyba et al. (1998) observed microvessel rupture in rat cremaster muscle following exposure to 2.3 MHz ultrasound in harmonic imaging mode with MI values (see Section 14.6) between 0.4 and 1.0. Similar results have been reported for an MI of 0.4 by Miller and Quddus (2000). Kobayashi et al. (2002) demonstrated similar effects using lower, more clinically relevant, microbubble concentrations. Miller and Gies (1999) investigated the incidence of haemorrhage and petechiae in mouse intestine in the presence of contrast agent. They showed a frequency dependence of $f^{0.7}$ for haemorrhage and $f^{0.94}$ for petechiae, but found that the threshold for haemorrhage was not altered by the presence of gas-filled microbubble contrast agents.

Van der Wouw (2000) reported premature ventricular contractions during second harmonic imaging of a contrast agent for myocardial perfusion in humans. Zachary et al. (2002) have shown that pulsed ultrasound (3.1 MHz, 1.3 μs pulses, 1.7 kHz p.r.f., $p^- = 15.9$ MPa, MI = 5.8) could trigger arrhythmias (atrial premature contractions, ventricular premature contractions, ventricular tachycardia) in 10 out of 20 rats hearts exposed when contrast agents in concentrations at least 14 times those used clinically in echocardiography are present. Clearly more work is required to establish thresholds for these effects.

A new observation with acoustic contrast agents is the phenomenon of so-called 'acoustically stimulated acoustic emission' (Uhlendorf & Scholle 1996). This occurs during exposure of some agents to B-mode or colour Doppler ultrasound and is thought to be a transient response arising from the breakdown of these hollow microbubbles. This effect has been seen at p^+ values of about 1 MPa at frequencies above 2 MHz and manifests itself as the emission of a broadband acoustic signal. Where this phenomenon is seen following the transmission of one pulse, it is not seen for subsequent pulses. Although at first sight, this bubble disintegration appears to be similar to that resulting from inertial cavitation, there is no published evidence of biological damage arising from acoustically stimulated acoustic emission. This is clearly an area that requires careful study.

14.4.3 CONSEQUENCES OF ULTRASONIC EXPOSURE OF EMBRYOS IN UTERO

There has naturally been a lot of interest in the biological consequences of irradiation of embryos *in utero*, primarily because of the widespread usage of diagnostic ultrasound in obstetrics. The search has been for gross teratogenic effects, for developmental changes and for genetic effects.

Miller *et al*. (2002) have analysed the available thermal teratology data in terms of 'thermal dose' (see Chapter 13, Section 13.4). They converted the temperature–time information for the induction of known embryological defects into an 'equivalent time' that would be required to get the same effect if the temperature rise were $4°C$ (t_4). They showed that when the percentage of embryos with defects is plotted against t_4 the best-fit line passes through zero. This would suggest that no temperature rise is without biological hazard. However, there is sufficient scatter on the data for a more probable interpretation to be that there is a threshold at $t_4 \sim 5$ min. (This threshold can also be interpreted as 2.5 min for a temperature rise of $4.5°C$ or 10 min for $3.5°C$.)

Inevitably, the bulk of mammalian safety studies have been carried out in rats and mice. Such experiments have a number of limitations. In particular, it is difficult to quantify the field in these small mammals and is generally impracticable to scale down the exposure field to avoid exposing a large fraction of the animal with consequent whole-body heating.

It is impossible to detail all the studies that have been carried out on embryonic development but some are listed in Table 14.3. It appears that, in most of the cases for which fetal abnormalities have been seen, a rise in temperature to above $41.5°C$ was induced in the uterus (Shoji *et al*. 1975; Hara *et al*. 1977; Hara 1980). In general, where no such rise has been seen, the fetuses have appeared normal. Lele (1979) and Edwards (1986, 1993) have shown that uterine hyperthermia can lead to a number of teratological effects, fetal resorption and growth retardation.

Curto (1976) found an increased mortality rate in mouse offspring following ultrasonic irradiation using $125–500$ W cm^{-2} (SATA), 1 MHz (continuous wave). Edmonds *et al*. (1979) could not repeat this finding at 2 MHz (440 mW cm^{-2}) at a different gestational age.

There are a number of literature reports dealing with a reduction in mean fetal weight following ultrasonic irradiation *in utero* (O'Brien 1976; Tachibana *et al*. 1977; Stolzenberg *et al*. 1980). Barnett and Williams (1990) concluded that the adverse fetal effects seen were caused by changes in maternal physiology, largely due to the high temperatures that can be achieved in maternal tissues such as the bladder and spine.

Many of these studies have been carried out at the stage of organogenesis for the fetus (about 8 days for the mouse and 9 days for the rat). Despite this, no adverse effects have been seen at intensities used diagnostically (see Tables 14.1 and 14.3). The evidence would therefore indicate that it is unlikely that current practice in obstetric diagnostic ultrasound will give rise to teratogenic or developmental changes. This conclusion is reinforced when one notes that the exposure conditions for experimental rats and mice are significantly different from those pertaining to human exposures. In rodent experiments the ultrasound beam is wide in relation to the fetal size, whereas this is not the case for the human fetus at the stage of most diagnostic scans. A significant temperature rise is unlikely to occur during human exposures of soft tissues to B-mode ultrasound. Prior to 1991 all diagnostic ultrasound devices were required to have maximum derated I_{SPTA} values below 720 mW cm^{-2} for peripheral vascular applications, 430 mW cm^{-2} for cardiac use, 94 mW cm^{-2} for fetal and 17 mW cm^{-2} for ophthalmic applications. After this date regulations were changed to permit an upper limit of 720 mW cm^{-2} for all applications, except those in ophthalmology, provided that the thermal and mechanical indices (MI and TI; see Section 14.6) are displayed. This change has led to considerable increase in I_{SPTA} for both B-mode and Doppler mode (Whittingham 2000).

Table 14.3. Biological effects resulting from ultrasonic exposures *in utero*

Biological system exposed	Exposure conditions	Biological endpoint assayed	Finding	Reference
(a)				
Pregnant mice (8 days GA)	1–3 MHz, 5 min SPTP 200–490 W cm^{-2} SPTA 0.75–27 W cm^{-2} Pulsed 10 μs–10 ms	Litter size Resorption rate Abnormalities	No significant effect	Warwick *et al.* (1970)
Pregnant mice, 2 strains (8 days GA)	2.25 MHz 5 h c.w. TA c.w. 40 mW cm^{-2}	Fetal weight Fetal death Malformation	Significant effect on fetal death rate in one strain	Shoji *et al.* (1975)
Pregnant rats	1.9 MHz 10 min SATP 100 W cm^{-2} SATA 1 W cm^{-2} Pulsed 0.6–10 ms	Fetal viability Resorption	No significant effect	Garrison *et al.* (1973)
Pregnant mice (14 days GA)	1 MHz, 3 min c.w. SA 0.5 W cm^{-2}	21 days survival of offspring	Significant decrease in survival at 0.125 W cm^{-2}	Curto (1976)
(b)				
Pregnant mice (8 days GA)	1 MHz SA 0.5–0.7 W cm^{-2}, 300 s 2–3 W cm^{-2}, 20 s 3–5.5 W cm^{-2}, 10 s	Fetal weight	Significant decrease in average weight	O'Brien (1976)
Pregnant mice (8 days GA)	2.3 MHz, 5–60 min c.w. 0.16–10 W cm^{-2}	Structural changes Congenital malformations Chromosome aberrations	No significant effect	Mannor *et al.* (1972)
Pregnant mice (8 days GA)	2 MHz, 5 min SATA 50 mW cm^{-2} Pulsed TP 22 W cm^{-2}	Maternal weight Fetal malformation	Reduced maternal weight Fetal abnormalities	Hara *et al.* (1977)
Pregnant mice (8 days GA)	2 MHz, 5 min 2 W cm^{-2}	Fetal malformation	Abnormalities seen	Hara *et al.* (1977)

(c)

Subject	Conditions	Parameter	Effect	Reference
Pregnant mice (1, 2, 4, 7, 13 days GA)	2 MHz c.w. 0.5 W cm^{-2}, 140 s 1 W cm^{-2} 60 s	Fetal weight	Significant decrease	Stolzenburg et al. (1980)
Pregnant mice	2.3 MHz c.w. SATA 80–100 mW cm^{-2}	Fetal weight	Significant decrease	Tachibana et al. (1977)
Pregnant mice (8 days GA)	2 MHz c.w. SATA 0.44 W cm^{-2}	Neonatal mortality	No significant effect	Edmonds et al. (1979)
Pregnant mice (8 days GA)	2 MHz 0.1, 0.6 W cm^{-2} 10 μs pulse, 5 min 200, 1000 Hz p.r.f.	Teratogenic effects	None found	Child et al. (1988)
Pregnant mice (8 days GA)	1 MHz 5.5 W cm^{-2} (10–20 s) SP 55 W cm^{-2} (10 ms) SP	Birthweight	No effect found	Child et al. (1989)
Pregnant rats (9 days GA)	3.2 MHz c.w. 0.32, 4 W cm^{-2} SA 15 mins	Fetal size and abnormalities	No significant effect for intensities <3 W cm^{-2}	Sikov & Hildebrand (1976)

(d)

Subject	Conditions	Parameter	Effect	Reference
Pregnant rats (8, 9, 10, 11, 12, 13 days GA)	2.5 MHz c.w. 10 mW cm^{-2} SA 1.5–2 h	Litter size Resorption rate Fetal weight	No significant effect	McClain et al. (1972)
Pregnant rats (8, 9, 10, 11, 12, 13 days GA)	2.5 MHz c.w. 10 mW cm^{-2} SA 1.5–2 h	Litter size Resorption rate Fetal weight	No significant effect	McClain et al. (1972)
Pregnant rats (15–20 days GA)	1 MHz c.w. 2.6–4.2 W cm^{-2} SATA 0–600 s	Fetal, intra-abdominal temperature measurement	Temp. rise 0°C (1.3 W cm^{-2}) 6–8°C (2.6 W cm^{-2}) 11–12.8°C (4.2 W cm^{-2})	Abraham et al. (1989)

(continued)

Table 14.3. (*continued*)

Biological system exposed	Exposure conditions	Biological endpoint assayed	Finding	Reference
(d) (*continued*)				
Pregnant rats (9.5 days GA)	3.14 MHz 1.2 W cm^{-2} SPTA 3.1 µs 2 kHz p.r.f. 0–30 min 38°C, 40°C	Morphological and biochemical damage	No gross effects Decrease in somite number	Angles *et al.* (1990)
(e)				
Pregnant rats (4–9 days GA)	3 MHz 0–30 W cm^{-2} SPTA	Teratogenic effects (birthweight, malformations)	No effect	Vorhees *et al.* (1991)
Pregnant *Macaques* (33 exposures throughout gestation)	7.5 MHz 0.28 mW cm^{-2} SPTA 2.34 W cm^{-2} SPPA 10–20 min	Birthweight Blood counts Behavioural studies	Reduced birthweight Transient reduction in neutrophil and monocyte count Increase in 'quiet activities'	Tarantal *et al.* (1989 a, b)
Pregnant *Macaques* (21–153 days GA)	5.6 MHz 146–556 mW cm^{-2} SPTA (de-rated) (MI 0.9–1.5)	Birthweight Blood counts	Transient reduction in birthweight and neutrophil counts	Tarantal *et al.* (1995)

GA, gestational age; c.w., continuous wave.

While the increase has been greatest for B-mode, the thermal hazard is greatest in pulsed Doppler exposures where the highest I_{SPTA} intensities are found.

14.4.4 ULTRASOUND IN CANCER TREATMENT

The potential of ultrasound in cancer treatment has been discussed in Chapter 13, Sections 13.4 and 13.5. The general aim has been to raise the tumour tissue to hyperthermic or ablative temperatures while maintaining normal tissue temperatures at non-toxic levels. Any hazard arising from such treatment lies in damaging healthy normal tissue around the tumour or in disseminating malignant cells around the body, thus increasing metastasis.

Careful localisation of the acoustic beam should minimise the hazard to normal tissues. In addition, a normal response to elevated temperatures in muscle is an increased blood flow, which can lead to tissue cooling (see ter Haar & Hopewell 1983). It is not clear whether such a cooling mechanism exists in tumours.

The question as to whether or not hyperthermia may increase the rate of metastasis of a tumour is still largely unresolved. It appears that, in mice, whole-body hyperthermia may increase metastatic spread but there is no evidence to suggest that localised heating has any effect on metastasis (Hahn 1982). Smachlo *et al.* (1979) carried out a study on a hamster fibrosarcoma line using 5 MHz ultrasound (3 W cm^{-2} SATA) and found no increase in metastasis. This is discussed in more detail in Chapter 13, Section 13.4.

Thus it appears that careful use of ultrasound for the treatment of cancer is unlikely to be hazardous, except perhaps where tumours overlie bone. In such cases it may be that intensities high enough to produce adequate tumour heating may give rise to sufficient periosteal heating to cause pain. Experience has shown that this can be a limiting factor in the treatment of some patients.

14.5   HUMAN FETAL STUDIES

In view of the long-established and widespread use of ultrasound in obstetrics, it is extremely likely that any non-stochastically determined effects on the fetus that might have occurred would have been detected and reported by now. In order, however, to detect any possible rare stochastic effects on the fetus arising from ultrasonic exposure (as opposed to those occurring either spontaneously or from other factors), large-scale epidemiological studies are necessary. These are necessarily time-consuming and costly, but a number of such studies now exist in the literature. These have employed a range of study designs, including retrospective case control and prospective randomised control trials. Descriptive studies are used to generate hypotheses, whereas analytical studies are used to test such hypotheses. Published surveys that deal with human exposures to diagnostic ultrasound *in utero* are summarised in Table 14.4. They fall roughly into four categories – investigation of the incidence of childhood malignancies, studies of neurological development, studies of speech development and investigation of birthweight of children exposed *in utero* to ultrasound. Salvesen (2000) has written an excellent review of this field.

14.5.1 CHILDHOOD CANCER

An understandable concern (stemming from experience with ionising radiation) that arises from the use of any form of radiation is the induction of malignancies. Although it has always been felt improbable that ultrasound can induce cancer, given its inability to induce genetic effects *in vitro* in the absence of cavitation (see Chapter 13, Section 13.4), two surveys on this topic have been conducted. The correct design for studying outcomes that are likely to be rare

Table 14.4. Epidemiological studies of human exposure to diagnostic ultrasound during pregnancy

Type of study	Publication	Effect	Population studied
Observational studies			
Descriptive			
Longitudinal design	Scheidt *et al.* (1978)	123 variables, including neurological effects, hearing, birthweight	1907
Analytical			
Case–control design	Kinnier-Wilson & Waterhouse (1984)	Childhood malignancies	3462
	Cartwright *et al.* (1984)	Childhood malignancies	1665
	Shu *et al.* (1994)	Childhood malignancies	642
	Soharan *et al.* (1995)	Childhood malignancies	520
	Campbell *et al.* (1993)	Speech delay	216
Cohort design	Stark *et al.* (1984)	17 variables, including dyslexia, neurological effects, hearing	806
	Moore *et al.* (1988)	Birthweight	2129
	Lyons *et al.* (1988)	Birthweight and growth to 6 years	298
	Kieler *et al.* (2001)	Handedness	179 395
Experimental studies			
Randomised trial	Salvesen *et al.* (1990, 1992, 1993a, b)	Six hypotheses (age 8–9 years): vision, dyslexia, handedness, growth, neurology, hearing	2161
	Kieler *et al.* (1997)	Hypothesis: association of ultrasound exposure *in utero* with handedness	3265
	Kieler *et al.* (1998)	Hypothesis: delayed speech development	3265
	Newnham *et al.* (1993)	Hypothesis: benefit of routine use of ultra-sound – effect found on birthweight	2834
	Waldenstrom *et al.* (1988)	Hypothesis: benefit of routine use of B-mode imaging ultrasound – effect reported on birthweight	4997

is that of case–control. The two studies, which are well conducted and cover an adequately sized population, used this method and could find no association between ultrasonic exposure *in utero* and childhood malignancy (Cartwright *et al.* 1984; Kinnier-Wilson & Waterhouse 1984; Shu *et al.* 1994; Sorahan *et al.* 1995). Uniquely among epidemiological studies, this appears to be a clearcut result.

14.5.2 NEUROLOGICAL DEVELOPMENT

A total of 123 variables were chosen for investigation in the longitudinal study of Scheidt *et al.* (1978). They found that a significantly higher proportion of children exposed to ultrasound *in utero* had an abnormal grasp, or tonic reflex, than those not exposed to ultrasound. There was no difference between the exposed and control groups for any of the other variables. The biological importance of abnormal reflexes is unknown and there is also a question mark over this study because the multiple hypothesis testing involved increases the possibility of chance findings.

Stark *et al.* (1984) designed a cohort study for 425 ultrasonically exposed children and 381 unexposed children between the ages of 7 and 12 years. The outcomes studied included hearing measurements, visual acuity and colour vision assessment, studies of cognitive function and behaviour and detailed neurological examinations. None of these outcomes showed an association with ultrasonic exposure *in utero*, with the exception of dyslexia. A significantly greater number of ultrasonically exposed children were found to be dyslexic. This finding could not be repeated in two subsequent published Norwegian studies. The incidence of dyslexia was the main objective of two long-term prospective randomised controlled trials (Salvesen *et al.* 1990, 1992, 1993a, b). In addition to dyslexia, visual acuity, hearing and impaired neurological development were studied. None of these outcomes showed any association with *in utero* ultrasound exposure. In this study design, the dyslexia results are less susceptible to being a chance finding than in the original study. A sixth outcome – handedness, was also studied and a weak association between ultrasonic exposure and incidence of non-right-handedness was found (19% of exposed children, and 15% of control children were left-handed). A randomised controlled trial to test the association between ultrasound and non-right-handedness has been carried out in Sweden (Kieler *et al.* 1997). They found that there was no statistically significant difference between ultrasonically screened and control groups. However, a gender-specific analysis according to exposure showed that slightly more boys were found to be non-right-handed (odds ratio 1.30; 95% confidence interval 1.01–1.69). Meta-analysis of the two Scandinavian trials (Salvesen & Eik-Nes 1999) has revealed no statistically significant difference between the ultrasound screened groups and the controls, but there was a statistically significant difference in subgroup analysis among the boys. Analysis by 'intention to treat' indicated no association between ultrasound exposure *in utero* and subsequent non-right-handedness. A follow-up paper by Kieler *et al.* (2001) reported a cohort study of men born between 1973 and 1978 who had enrolled for military service. There were 6858 men in the 'exposed' group and 172 537 in the 'unexposed' group. Assignment to left-handedness was done on the basis of the way in which the subject handled a rifle. No difference in handedness was found between groups for men born between 1973 and 1975 when ultrasound scanning was relatively unusual, but for those born between 1976 and 1978 (when ultrasound was more widely offered) the risk of left-handedness was higher in the 'exposed' group. Because allocation to study group was on the basis of the hospital in which birth occurred, there is a high chance of mis-classification. In itself, non-righthanded-ness does not constitute a public health problem, but if it is an indication that diagnostic ultrasound exposures can affect the central nervous system then this must be clarified. It seems clear that this is a topic for which a properly designed prospective randomised trial is needed so that the question may be resolved.

14.5.3 SPEECH DEVELOPMENT

As yet, no definitive answer can be given to the question of whether ultrasonic exposure *in utero* can lead to a delay in speech development because the two published surveys (Campbell *et al.* 1993; Salvesen *et al.* 1994) both have statistical limitations.

Campbell *et al.* (1993) compared 72 children having delayed speech with 144 matched controls. They reported that the odds of suffering delayed speech were 2.8 times higher among children exposed to ultrasound *in utero* than for those who were not. The information about the ultrasonic exposures received by the children was not assessed in a blind fashion and so the results could be subject to bias. In contrast, in the Norwegian study on this topic (Salvesen *et al.* 1994), it was found that ultrasonically exposed children were not referred to a speech therapist as often as those who had not been scanned *in utero*. However, although this is the better designed of the two surveys, speech delay was not a prior hypothesis of this study and so this finding might also be due to chance.

14.5.4 BIRTHWEIGHT

The first report that diagnostic ultrasound might be able to affect birthweight was that by Moore et al. (1988). In a cohort study examining 198 ultrasonically exposed and 198 control babies, the group of children who had been subject to ultrasound in utero had a lower average birthweight. The authors' conclusion was that maternal and fetal risk factors, rather than the ultrasound exposure, might explain their finding.

Newnham et al. (1993) performed a randomised controlled trial on 2834 pregnant women. Half of the group received only one diagnostic imaging scan at 18 weeks but otherwise had standard antenatal care. The other half were offered Doppler ultrasound examinations five times in the third trimester. Although they concluded that the frequent Doppler examinations conferred no benefit on pregnancy outcome, they reported a statistically significant increased number of babies with a birthweight below the tenth centile in this group. The difference in mean birthweight between the two groups was 25 g (not statistically significant). The birthweight analysis was not a prior hypothesis of this study and so this result is not conclusive (but could be the basis for a new study). These results are not consistent with other published studies. In fact, several other studies have reported higher birthweights in ultrasonically screened babies than in unexposed groups (Waldenstrom et al. 1988; Neilson 1993).

Lyons et al. (1988) compared growth during childhood for ultrasonically exposed and non-exposed children. They could find no difference in height or body weight at birth or at 6 months and 1, 2, 3, 4, 5 and 6 years of age. Salvesen et al. (1993b) found a similar result in their Norwegian study. Interestingly, in this study the only statistically significant difference in child growth curves was between the screened children of mothers who were smokers at the first antenatal visit and the unscreened children of smoking mothers. The former group of children were heavier at birth and showed better growth during childhood. Similar results were shown by Waldenstrom et al (1988). Neither study provides an explanation for this finding and it is not clear that the reason is due to maternal cessation of smoking.

Another published survey is a retrospective (not case controlled) study of 1114 'normal' pregnant women at different stages of pregnancy (Hellman et al. 1970). For the group of women receiving ultrasound there was a 2.7% incidence of congenital fetal abnormalities, the incidence being 4.8% in the control group.

In summary, existing epidemiological studies have indicated that there is no association between diagnostic ultrasound exposure in utero and childhood malignancies. Possible associations between diagnostic ultrasound exposure in utero and dyslexia, delayed speech development and handedness have not been confirmed. There are conflicting data about a possible association between ultrasound and birthweight. On the one hand, B-mode ultrasound imaging may lead to a slight increase in birthweight, whereas Doppler ultrasound may lead to reduced birthweights. This is difficult to understand from a mechanistic viewpoint and the possibility of chance findings cannot be ruled out.

14.6 SUMMARY OF RECOMMENDATIONS AND GUIDELINES FOR EXPOSURE

From the evidence that has been presented in this chapter and in Chapters 12 and 13 it will be clear that a number of ultrasonically induced biological changes may occur in experimental and clinical situations. Although any biological change in the wrong place may constitute a hazard, it is practically useful to concentrate attention on any potential effects that may lead to serious possibility of disease, e.g. cancer or genetic malformations, and particularly where these may arise in a stochastically determined manner, possibly with an appreciable latent period. The following statements can, however, be made:

1. Therapeutic ultrasound should be administered by experts (e.g. trained physiotherapists) and with care. Standing wave formation should be avoided near blood vessels and care should be taken, when irradiating over gas or bone, that excessive heating does not occur.
2. There is no evidence that ultrasound, as currently used in clinical diagnosis, causes damage to human embryos *in utero*. No chromosomal aberrations have been detected either in maternal or fetal lymphocytes following exposure.
3. No hazard should arise from the careful use of ultrasound to produce localised heating for cancer treatment. There is no evidence that the rate of metastasis might increase. Care should, however, be exercised in this respect when local heating is administered simultaneously with whole-body hyperthermia.

A number of official national and international bodies have published statements pertinent to the safety of medical ultrasound (Barnett & ter Haar 2000, www.efsumb.org, www.aium.org, www.bmus.org). Generally these statements deal with the risks associated with diagnostic ultrasound examinations, and particularly with obstetric applications.

The Australian Ultrasound Society (ASUM) has issued a number of statements on safety issues (Barnett & ter Haar 1999). Its statement on 'Thermal biological effects' contains the following recommendations:

(a) A diagnostic exposure that produces a maximum temperature rise of 1.5°C above normal physiological levels (37°C) may be used without reservation in clinical examinations.
(b) A diagnostic exposure that elevates embryonic or fetal temperature above 41°C (i.e. 4°C above normal body temperature) for 5 minutes or more should be considered potentially hazardous.
(c) The effects of heating should be reduced by minimising the duration of exposure.
(d) Owing to the possible influence of potentiating factors, duplex/Doppler ultrasound in the febrile patient might present an additional embryonic and fetal risk.
(e) Care should be taken to use the minimum output consistent with obtaining the required diagnostic information and to minimise the duration of pulsed Doppler examinations in pregnancy.

The American Institute of Ultrasound in Medicine (AIUM) has an official statement regarding heating (1993) that is slightly more specific. It specifies that 'For exposure durations up to 50 hours, there have been no significant biological effects observed due to temperature increases less than or equal to 2°C above normal'. In addition they state that 'For temperature increases greater than 2°C above normal, there have been no significant biological effects observed due to temperature increases less than or equal to

$$\frac{6 - \log_{10}t}{0.6}$$

where t is the exposure duration in minutes ranging from 1 to 250. For example, for temperature increases of 4°C and 6°C, the corresponding limits for the exposure duration t are 16 minutes and 1 minute, respectively.'

It is, in practice, impossible for the user to know the temperature rise that is induced by a specific application of an ultrasound beam *in vivo* in every circumstance or, for that matter, for the user to assess the probability of a specific exposure inducing cavitation. Two biophysical indices – the thermal index (TI) and the mechanical index (MI) – have therefore been developed to provide the user with information with which to make safety judgements (EFSUMB 1996; Abbott 1999). The equations used for calculating these indices are contained in the AIUM/NEMA Output Display Standard (ODS) (AIUM/NEMA 1992).

The thermal index is a number that provides an estimate of the tissue temperature rise (in °C) that might be possible under 'reasonable worst case conditions'. Three thermal indices are defined – a soft tissue index (TIS) and two bone indices (TIB, TIC). The thermal index is defined as the ratio of the acoustic power emitted to the power required to heat the target tissue by 1°C. The calculation of TI assumes a tissue model that consists of a homogeneous attenuating medium with attenuation coefficient $0.3\,\mathrm{dB\,cm^{-1}\,MHz^{-1}}$. Bone is included as a strongly absorbing surface perpendicular to the ultrasonic beam. The TIB is designed for use when the bone lies near the beam focus and is appropriate, according to the ODS, for second and third trimesters of pregnancy and for neonatal cephalic studies. The TIC (cranial TI) is designed for heating of bone close to the transducer and is for paediatric and adult transcranial applications. For precise formulation of these indices, the reader is referred to the ODS (AIUM/NEMA 1992). The formulae differ for scanned and unscanned beams and for wide and narrow beams.

The European Federation of Societies for Ultrasound in Medicine and Biology (EFSUMB 1996) shows that the form of TI for soft tissue heating is $\mathrm{TIS} = (Wf\kappa_1)$, where W is the acoustic power, f is the frequency and κ_1 is a factor determined by the relationship assumed between power and intensity and on the rates of energy absorbed and lost. If power is in mW and f is in MHz, $\kappa_1 = 0.00476$. For bone heating, the formulae are $\mathrm{TIB} = W\kappa_2$ and $\mathrm{TIC} = W\kappa_3$, where κ_2 and κ_3 are always greater than κ_1 and depend on the chosen tissue model.

For all soft tissue imaging, including M-mode and pulsed Doppler operation using small transducers, the maximum heating occurs in the tissue next to the transducer. For M-mode and pulsed Doppler, heating is predicted to be greatest when bone lies near the focus. For transcranial studies, the greatest heating is in the bone next to the transducer.

The mechanical index is calculated from the expression

$$\mathrm{MI} = p^- / \sqrt{f}$$

where f is the frequency (in MHz) and p^- is the peak negative pressure (in MPa) measured in water and 'de-rated' to give the *in situ* value using an attenuation coefficient of $0.3\,\mathrm{dB\,cm^{-1}\,MHz^{-1}}$. This index is designed to give some indication of the probability that cavitation will occur in the target tissues, and relies on the fact that there is a frequency-dependent threshold acoustic pressure above which cavitation may occur.

The ODS requires manufacturers to display one of these indices, depending on the mode of operation, the clinical application and the maximum value that the indices may achieve. For B-mode the MI is usually displayed, whereas for Doppler and M-mode the TI is more usually shown. An index is required to be displayed if it may reach a value of 1.0 for any machine setting. If it can reach this level then it is shown whenever it is 0.4 or more, so that the user has some prior warning as the index climbs towards 1.0. The choice of TI to be displayed is decided by the manufacturer and should be appropriate to the mode of application. The TIC is displayed for transcranial applications and the TIB is clearly always greater than TIS because the potential for bone heating is always greater than that for soft tissue heating. The user needs to be careful, however, when bone is likely to be exposed incidentally simply because it lies in the beam, albeit not being the target tissue of interest. It is likely that the TIS is displayed under these circumstances. Jago *et al.* (1999) have demonstrated that when bone is exposed to ultrasound through an overlying low-attenuation liquid layer, such as may occur in the third trimester of pregnancy, the TI may substantially underestimate the maximum temperature rise that could occur.

The British Medical Ultrasound Society (www.bmus.org) has issued guidelines for the safe use of diagnostic ultrasound equipment. These give guidance for scanning practice when the MI and TI reach different values:

(a) Since for MI > 0.3 there is a possibility of minor damage to neonatal lung or intestine, neonatal exposure times at these levels should be kept to a minimum.
(b) When MI > 0.7 there is the risk of cavitation if gas bubble contrast agents are used. There is also a theoretical risk of cavitation in the absence of these agents.
(c) When TI > 0.7, scan times of the fetus or embryo should be restricted as follows: for TI = 0.7, 60 min; for TI = 1.0, 30 min; for TI = 0.5, 15 min; for TI = 2.0, 4 min; for TI = 2.5, 1 min.
(d) When TI > 1.0 ophthalmic scanning is not recommended.
(e) When TI ⩾ 3.0 fetal and embryonic scanning is not recommended.

The increasing use of gas bubble contrast agents introduces new concern for ultrasound safety because cavitation effects become more likely. The American Institute for Ultrasound in Medicine and Biology issued a statement about the 'Bioeffects of diagnostic ultrasound with gas body contrast agents' in 2002 (www.aium.org):

> Induction of petechiae and extravasation from capillaries in mammalian tissue *in vivo* have been reported and independently confirmed for diagnostic ultrasound exposure with a mechanical index above about 0.4 and gas-body contrast agent present in the circulation. The clinical significance of these findings is presently uncertain. Only apparently minor side effects have been reported in clinical testing and use of ultrasound contrast agents. However, on the basis of these reports and a large body of data from laboratory studies *in vitro* and *in vivo* it should be noted that the potential for any diagnostic ultrasound-induced adverse effects will depend not only on the composition, dosage and administration of the agent but also on operator-controlled settings of ultrasound machines, such as timing, mode, frequency and power, as well as the anatomy scanned. Therefore, physicians and sonographers should be cognisant of the possible enhancement of non-thermal bioeffects during contrast-enhanced diagnostic ultrasound and factor this potential into risk–benefit considerations.'

The EFSUMB publishes an annual Clinical Safety Statement for Diagnostic Ultrasound. The full EFSUMB 2003 Clinical Safety Statement for Diagnostic Ultrasound is:

> 'Diagnostic ultrasound has been widely used in clinical medicine for many years with no proven deleterious effects. However, as the use of ultrasound increases, with the introduction of new techniques, with a broadening of the medical indications for ultrasound examinations and with increased exposure, continuous vigilance is essential to ensure its continued safe use.

A broad range of ultrasound exposure is used in the different diagnostic modalities currently available. Doppler imaging and measurement techniques may use higher exposures than those used in B- and M-modes, with pulsed Doppler techniques having the potential for the highest levels.

The recommendations contained in this statement assume that commercial ultrasound equipment conforming to international safety standards is being used and that it is used prudently by competent personnel who are trained in safety matters.

B- AND M-MODES

Based on scientific evidence of ultrasonically induced biological effects to date, there is no reason to withhold B- or M-mode scanning for any clinical application, including the routine clinical scanning of every woman during pregnancy. Some techniques, such as tissue harmonic imaging and coded excitation, may use higher exposures than conventional imaging. The user is advised to make use of any exposure information provided by the manufacturer, e.g. in the form of displayed safety indices. Scanning for three-dimensional imaging does not introduce any additional safety considerations.

DOPPLER MODES (COLOUR FLOW AND POWER DOPPLER IMAGING AND SPECTRAL PULSED DOPPLER)

Exposures used in these Doppler modes are commonly higher than for B- and M-modes. The highest powers, and therefore the greatest potential for thermal effects, occur in spectral pulsed Doppler mode at maximum machine output setting and in Doppler imaging modes when using narrow colour boxes.

The informed use of Doppler ultrasound is not contraindicated. However, at maximum machine output settings significant thermal effects at bone surfaces cannot be excluded. The user is advised to make use of any exposure information provided by the manufacturer (e.g. in the form of displayed safety indices) to gain awareness of the output conditions and to act prudently to limit exposure of critical structures, including bone and regions including gas. Particular care should be taken to minimise exposure times.

DOPPLER FOR FETAL HEART MONITORING

The power levels used for fetal heart monitoring are sufficiently low that the use of this modality is not contraindicated, on safety grounds, even when it is to be used for extended periods.

GAS-FILLED CONTRAST AGENTS

Particular safety considerations are associated with the use of gas-filled contrast agents. High values of the MI should be used only when required for a particular clinical study and with limited exposure times.

ULTRASOUND EXPOSURE DURING PREGNANCY

The embryonic period is known to be particularly sensitive to any external influences. Until further scientific information is available, investigations should be carried out with careful control of output levels and exposure times. With increasing mineralisation of the fetal bone as the fetus develops, the possibility of heating fetal bone increases. The user should prudently limit exposure of critical structures such as the fetal skull or spine during Doppler studies.

SAFETY CONSIDERATIONS FOR OTHER ORGANS

Particular care should be taken to reduce the risk of heating during investigations of the eye. Extra care is also appropriate when carrying out neonatal cardiac and cranial investigations.'

Practical quantification of ultrasonic exposures is often difficult and may be complex. There is no international consensus as to the important quantities that should be measured to give a meaningful indicator of emission or exposure as far as biological effects are concerned. One suggested useful set of quantities may be:

1. For the case of pulse–echo devices, the spatial peak pressure amplitude (the sum of the peak positive and negative pressure amplitudes), where this is at its maximum value in the beam (generally near the focus). There may be cases for which this cannot be measured, in these cases then the maximum value in the beam of the spatial peak, temporal peak intensity may be a satisfactory alternative.
2. In addition, for the case of therapeutic, surgical and diagnostic Doppler (continuous wave and pulsed) devices, the total acoustic (time averaged) power.

If the quantification is for biological effects experimentation, these values should be measured at the position of the sample of interest.

Specific protection of the user against solid- or liquid-borne ultrasound should seldom be necessary. Care should, however, be taken where the operator's hands may be immersed in the coupling medium, as in the case of immersion physical therapy.

14.7 CONCLUSION

The subject of medical ultrasonic safety has a long history and is assured of a long future. Definitive answers to many important questions may be impossible to find, and new and potentially controversial evidence is likely to arise from time to time.

The subject is one where the quantitative approach of physics will always be important. This is particularly so in the matter of measurement and reporting of exposure and, although hydrophone and allied technology can now provide a good basis for measurement, the logic of the approach to metrology is seriously flawed at present through our inability to identify one or even a small set of physical quantities that will serve as adequately quantitative predictors of ultimate biological effect.

The biology of the subject is complex and can sometimes seem bafflingly so. However, considerable resolution of the complexity will come about if it is borne in mind: first, that reports of new biological phenomena generally need clear documentation, and preferably independent confirmation, before they can be taken seriously into account; and second, that one needs in this field to distinguish between an effect (something observable) and a hazard (a major deleterious consequence for a human individual). In this context it will probably be appropriate to concentrate attention on evidence concerning mutagenesis, carcinogenesis and teratogenesis. As already discussed in detail, there is increasingly good evidence in these areas (derived from a number of different biological systems and with a wide variety of ultrasonic exposure conditions) against the induction of such changes. Such evidence will need to be taken into account in assessing the significance of any new and apparently conflicting reports. In the absence of adequate information on which to base maximum allowable levels of medical ultrasound exposures, it may be more useful to put forward some criteria for *appropriate* use for each application. One set of such criteria may be summarised as follows:

1. The operator should be aware of exposure levels and use minimum exposure of a patient consistent with effective achievement of the desired clinical benefit. The on-screen display of thermal and mechanical indices is designed to increase this awareness. The quantification of exposure level has been discussed in Section 14.6.
2. Staff and other personnel should not be deliberately exposed in any unnecessary manner or degree.

3. All procedures should be carried out only by (or under supervision of) well and appropriately trained staff.

If such guidelines are followed, medical ultrasound may be used effectively and with a high degree of confidence in its safety.

REFERENCES

Abbott, J.G. (1999). Rationale and derivation of MI and TI – a review. *Ultrasound Med. Biol.* **25**, 431–441.

Abraham, V., Ziskin, M.C. and Heyner, S. (1989). Temperature elevation in the rat fetus due to ultrasound exposure. *Ultrasound Med. Biol.* **15**, 443–449.

AIUM/NEMA (American Institute of Ultrasound in Medicine/National Electrical Manufacturers Association) (1992). *Standard for the Real-Time Display of Thermal and Mechanical Acoustic Output Indices on Diagnostic Ultrasound Equipment.* AIUM, Rockville, Maryland.

Angles, J.M., Walsh, D.A., Li, K., Barnett, S.B. and Edwards, M.J. (1990). Effects of pulsed ultrasound on the development of rat embryos in culture. *Teratology* **42**, 285–293.

Au, W.W., Obergoenner, N., Goldenthal, K.L., Corry, P. and Willingham, V. (1982). Sister chromatid exchanges in mouse embryos after exposure to ultrasound *in vitro. Mutat. Res.* **103**, 315.

Barnett, S.B. and ter Haar, G.R. (2000). Guidelines and recommendations for the safe use of diagnostic ultrasound: the users' responsibilities. In *The Safe Use of Ultrasound in Medical Diagnosis*, G.R. ter Haar and F.A. Duck (eds). British Institute of Radiology, London, pp. 102–112.

Barnett, S.B., ter Haar, G.R., Ziskin, M.C., Nyborg, W.L. and Maeda, K. (1994). Current status of research on biophysical effects of ultrasound. *Ultrasound Med. Biol.* **20**, 205–218.

Barnett, S.B., Miller, M.W., Cox, C. and Carstensen, E.L. (1988). Increased sister chromatid exchanges in Chinese hamster ovary cells exposed to high intensity pulsed ultrasound. *Ultrasound Med. Biol.* **14**, 397–403.

Barnett, S.B. and Williams, A.R. (1990). Identification of possible mechanisms responsible for fetal weight reduction in mice following exposure. *Ultrasonics* **28**, 159–165.

Barrass, N., ter Haar, G.R. and Casey, G. (1982). The effect of ultrasound and hyperthermia on sister chromatid exchange and division kinetics of BHK21 C13/A3 cells. *Br. J. Cancer* **45**, (Suppl. V), 187.

Barth, G. and Wachsmann, F. (1949). Biological effects of ultrasound therapy. *Kongress Bericht*, Erlanger Ultraschall Tagung, pp. 162–205.

Bleaney, B.I., Blackbourne, P. and Kirkley, J. (1972). Resistance of CHLF hamster cells to ultrasonic radiation of 1.5 MHz frequency. *Br. J. Radiol.* **45**, 354–357.

Borrelli, M., Thompson, L.L., Cain, C.A. and Dewey, W.C. (1990). Time–temperature analysis of cell killing of BHK cells heated at temperatures in the range of 43.5°–57°C. *Int. J. Radiat. Oncol. Biol. Phys.* **19**, 389–399.

Bosward, K., Barnett, S.B., Wood, A.F.K., Edwards, M.J. and Kossoff, G. (1993). Heating of guinea pig fetal brain during exposure to pulsed ultrasound. *Ultrasound Med. Biol.* **19**, 415–424.

Brayman, A.A., Azadniv, M., Cox, C. and Miller, M.W. (1996a). Haemolysis of Albunex-supplemented, 40% haematocrit human erythrocytes *in vitro* by 1 MHz pulsed ultrasound: acoustic pressure and pulse length dependence. *Ultrasound Med. Biol.* **22**, 927–938.

Brayman, A.A., Azadniv, M., Makin, I.R.S., *et al.* (1995). Effect of a stabilised microbubble contrast agent on haemolysis of human erythrocytes exposed to high intensity pulsed ultrasound. *Echocardiography* **12**, 13–21.

Brayman, A.A., Church, C.C. and Miller, M.W. (1996b). Re-evaluation of the concept that high cell concentrations 'protect' cells *in vitro* from ultrasonically induced lysis. *Ultrasound Med. Biol.* **22**, 497–514.

Brayman, A.A., Doida, Y. and Miller, M.W. (1992). Apparent contribution of respiratory gas exchange to the *in vitro* 'cell density effect' in ultrasonic cell lysis. *Ultrasound Med. Biol.* **18**, 701–714.

Brayman, A.A. and Miller, M.W. (1993). Cell density dependence of the ultrasonic degassing of fixed erythrocyte suspensions. *Ultrasound Med. Biol.* **19**, 243–252.

Brayman, A.A. and Miller, M.W. (1997). Acoustic cavitation nuclei survive the apparent ultrasonic destruction of Albunex microspheres. *Ultrasound Med. Biol.* **23**, 793–796.

Brayman, A.A. and Miller, M.W. (1999). Sonolysis of Albunex supplemented, 40% hematocrit human erythrocytes by pulsed 1 MHz ultrasound: pulse number, pulse duration and exposure vessel rotation dependence. *Ultrasound Med. Biol.* **25**, 307–314.

Campbell, J.D., Elford, R.W. and Brant, R.F. (1993). Case control study of prenatal ultrasonography exposure in children with delayed speech. *Can. Med. Assoc. J.* **149**, 1435–1440.

Carstensen, E.L., Child, S.Z., Norton, S. and Nyborg, W.L. (1990). Ultrasonic heating of the skull. *J. Acoust. Soc. Am.* **87**, 1310–1317, *Ultrasound Med. Biol.* **20**, 205–218.

Carstensen, E.L., Kelly, P., Church, C.C., Brayman, A.A., Child, S.Z., Raeman, C.H. and Schery, L. (1993). Lysis of erythrocytes by exposure to CW ultrasound. *Ultrasound Med. Biol.* **19**, 147–165.

Cartwright, R.A., McKinney, P.A., Hopton, P.A., Birch, J.M., Hartley, A.L. Mann, J.R., Waterhouse, J.A.H., Johnston, H.E., Draper, G.J. and Stiller, C. (1984). Ultrasound examinations in pregnancy and childhood cancer. *Lancet* **2**, 999–1000.

Chapman, I.V. (1974). The effect of ultrasound on the potassium contents of rat thymocytes *in vitro*. *Br. J. Radiol.* **47**, 411–415.

Child, S.Z., Carstensen, E.L., Gates, A.H. and Hall W.J. (1988). Testing for the teratogenicity of pulsed ultrasound in mice. *Ultrasound Med. Biol.* **14**, 493–498.

Child, S.Z., Hartman, C.L., Schery, L.A. and Carstensen, E.L. (1990). Lung damage from exposure to pulsed ultrasound. *Ultrasound Med. Biol.* **16**, 817–825.

Child, S.Z., Hoffman, D., Strassner, D., Carstensen, E.L., Gates, A.H., Cox, C. and Miller, M.W. (1989). A test of I^2t as a dose parameter for fetal weight reduction from exposure to ultrasound. *Ultrasound Med. Biol.* **15**, 39–44.

Ciaravino, V., Miller, M.W. and Carstensen, E.L. (1986). Sister chromatid exchanges in human lymphocytes exposed to *in vitro* therapeutic ultrasound. *Mutat. Res.* **172**, 185–186.

Clarke, P.R. and Hill, C.R. (1969). Biological action of ultrasound in relation to the cell cycle. *Exp. Cell. Res.* **58**, 443.

Curto, K.A. (1976). Early postpartum mortality following ultrasound radiation. In *Ultrasound in Medicine*, Vol. 2, D.N. White and R. Barnes (eds). Plenum Press, New York, pp. 535–536.

Dalecki, D., Raeman, C.H., Child, S.Z. and Carstensen, E.L. (1995). Intestinal haemorrhage from exposure to pulsed ultrasound. *Ultrasound Med. Biol.* **21**, 1067–1072.

Dalecki, D., Raeman, C.H., Child, S.Z., Cox, C., Francis, C.W., Meltzer, R.S. and Carstensen, E.L. (1997). Haemolysis *in vivo* from exposure to pulsed ultrasound. *Ultrasound Med. Biol.* **23**, 307–313.

Dewey, W.C. (1991). Arrhenius relationships from the molecule and cell to the clinic. *Int. J. Hypertherm.* **10**, 457–483.

Duggan, P.M., Liggins, G.C. and Barnett, S.B. (1995). Ultrasonic heating of the brain of the fetal sheep *in utero*. *Ultrasound Med. Biol.* **21**, 553–560.

Dvorak, M. and Hrazdira, I. (1966). Changes in the ultrastructure of bone marrow cells in rats following exposure to ultrasound. *Z. Mikrosk. Anat. Forsch.* **4**, 451–460.

Dyson, M. and Brookes, M. (1983). Stimulation of bone repair by ultrasound. In *Ultrasound 82*, R.A. Lerski and P. Morley (eds). Pergamon Press, pp. 61–66.

Dyson, M., Pond, J.B., Joseph, J. and Warwick, R. (1968). The stimulation of tissue regeneration by means of ultrasound. *Clin. Sci.* **35**, 273–295.

Dyson, M., Pond, J.B., Woodward, B. and Broadbent, J. (1974). The production of blood cell stasis and endothelial damage in the blood vessels of chick embryos treated with ultrasound in a stationary wave field. *Ultrasound Med. Biol.* **1**, 133–148.

Edmonds, P.D., Stolzenberg, S.J., Torbit, C.A., Madan, S.M. and Pratt, D. (1979). Postpartum survival of mice exposed *in utero* to ultrasound. *J. Acoust. Soc. Am.* **66**, 590–593.

Edwards, M.J. (1986). Hyperthermia as a teratogen: a review of experimental studies and their clinical significance. *Teratogen. Carcinogen. Mutagen.* **6**, 563–582.

Edwards, M.J. (1993). Hyperthermia and birth defects. *Cornell Vet.* **83**, 1–7.

EFSUMB (European Federation of Societies for Ultrasound in Medicine & Biology) (1994). Tutorial paper: genetic effects. *Eur. J. Ultrasound* **1**, 91–92.

EFSUMB (European Federation of Societies for Ultrasound in Medicine & Biology) (1996). Tutorial paper: thermal and mechanical indices. *Eur. J. Ultrasound* **4**, 145–150.

Ehlinger, C.A., Katayama, K.P., Reeler, N.R. and Mattingly, R.F. (1991). Diagnostic ultrasound increases sister chromatid exchange; preliminary report. *Wisconsin Med. J.* **80**, 21.

Elwart, J.W., Brettel, H. and Kober, L.O. (1988). Cell membrane damage by ultrasound at different cell concentrations. *Ultrasound Med. Biol.* **14**, 43–50.

Fajardo, L.F. (1984). Pathological effects of hyperthermia of normal tissues. *Cancer Res. Suppl.* **44**, 4826s–4833s.

FDA (Food and Drug Administration, Center for Devices and Radiological Health) (1993). *Revised (510k) Diagnostic Ultrasound Guidance for 1993*. FDA, Rockville, MD.

Frizzell, L.A., Chen E. and Lee, C. (1994). Effects of pulsed ultrasound on the mouse neonate: hind limb paralysis and lung haemorrhage. *Ultrasound Med. Biol.* **20**, 53–63.

Garrison, B.M., Walter, J., Krueger, W.A., Kremkau, F.W. and McKinney, W.M. (1973). The influence of ovarian sonication on fetal development in the rat. *J. Clin. Ultrasound* **1**, 316–319.

Gebhart, E. (1981). Sister chromatid exchange (SCE) and structural chromosome aberration in mutagenicity testing. *Hum. Genet.* **58**, 235–254.

Goldblat, V.I. (1969). Processes of bone tissue regeneration under the effect of ultrasound (in Russian). *Ortop. Travmato. Protez.* **30**, 57–61.

ter Haar, G.R., Dyson, M. and Talbert, D. (1978). Ultrasonically induced contractions in mouse uterine smooth muscle *in vivo*. *Ultrasonics*, **16**, 275–276.

ter Haar, G.R., Dyson, M. and Smith, S.P. (1979). Ultrastructure changes in the mouse uterus brought about by ultrasonic irradiation at therapeutic intensities in standing wave fields. *Ultrasound Med. Biol.* **5**, 167–179.

ter Haar, G.R. and Hopewell, J.W. (1983). The induction of hyperthermia by ultrasound: its value and associated problems. 1. Single, static, plane transducer. *Phys. Med. Biol.* **28**, 889–896.

ter Haar, G.R., Stratford, L.J. and Hill, C.R. (1980). Ultrasonic irradiation of mammalian cells *in vitro* at hyperthermic temperatures. *Br. J. Radiol.* **53**, 784–789.

Hahn, G.M. (1982). *Hyperthermia and Cancer*. Plenum Press, New York.

Hara, K. (1980). Effect of ultrasonic irradiation on chromosomes, cell division and developing embryos. *Acta Obstet. Gynaecol. Jpn.* **32**, 6148.

Hara, K., Minoura, S., Okai, T. and Sakamoto, S. (1977). Symposium on recent studies in the safety of diagnostic ultrasound, safety of ultrasonics on organism. *Jpn. J. Med. Ultrason.* **4**, 256–258.

Harvey, W., Dyson, M., Pond, J.B. and Grahame, R. (1975). The *in vitro* stimulation of protein synthesis in human fibroblasts by therapeutic levels of ultrasound. In *Ultrasonics in Medicine*. E. Kazner, *et al.* (eds). Excerpta Medica, Amsterdam, pp. 10–21.

Haupt, M., Martin, A.O., Simpson, J.L., lqbal, M.A., Elias, S., Dyer, A. and Sabbagha, R.E. (1981). Ultrasonic induction of sister chromatid exchanges in human lymphocytes. *Hum. Genet.* **59**, 221.

Hellman, L.M., Duffus, G.M., Donald, L. and Sunden, B. (1970). Safety of diagnostic ultrasound in obstetrics. *Lancet* **i**, 1133.

Henderson, J., Willson, K., Jago, J.R. and Whittingham, T.A. (1995). A survey of the acoustic outputs of diagnostic ultrasound equipment in current clinical use. *Ultrasound Med. Biol.* **21**, 699–705.

Herman, B.A. and Harris, G.R. (2002). Models and regulatory considerations for transient temperature rise during diagnostic ultrasound pulses. *Ultrasound Med. Biol.* **28**, 1217–1224.

Holland, C.K., Deng, C.X., Apfel, R.E., Alderman, J.L., Fernandez, L.A. and Taylor, K.J.W. (1996). Direct evidence of cavitation *in vivo* from diagnostic ultrasound. *Ultrasound Med. Biol.* **22**, 917–925.

Hrazdira, L. (1970). Changes in cell ultrastructure under direct and indirect action of ultrasound. In *Ultrasonographia Medica*, J. Bock and K. Ossoinig (eds). Vienna Academy of Medicine, Vienna, pp. 457–463.

Hu, J.H., Taylor, J.D., Press, H.C. and White, J.E. (1978). Ultrasonic effects on mammalian interstitial muscle membrane. *Aviat. Space Environ. Med.* **49**, 607–609.

Ivey, J.A., Gardner, E.A., Fowlkes, J.B., Rubin, J.M. and Carson, P.L. (1995). Acoustic generation of intra-arterial contrast boluses. *Ultrasound Med. Biol.* **21**, 757–767.

Jago, J.R., Henderson, J., Whittingham, T.A. and Mitchell, G. (1999). A comparison of AIUM/NEMA thermal indices with calculated temperature rises for a simple third trimester pregnancy model. *Ultrason. Med. Biol.* **25**, 623–628.

Joshi, G.P., Hill, C.R. and Forrester, J.A. (1973). Mode of action of ultrasound on the surface charge of mammalian cells. *Ultrasound Med. Biol.* **1**, 45–48.

Kaufman, G.E., Miller, M.W., Griffiths, T.D. and Ciaravino, V. (1977). Lysis and viability of cultured mammalian cells exposed to 1 MHz ultrasound. *Ultrasound Med. Biol.* **3**, 21–25.

Kieler, H., Ahlsten, G., Haglund, B., Salvesen, K. and Axelsson, O. (1998). Routine ultrasound screening in pregnancy and aspects of the children's subsequent neurological development. *Obstet. Gynecol.* **91**, 750–756.

Kieler, H., Axelsson, O., Haglund, B., Nilsson, S and Salvesen, K. (1997). Routine ultrasound screening in pregnancy and the children's subsequent handedness. *Early Hum. Dev.* **50**, 233–245.

Kieler, H., Cnattingius, S., Haglund, B., Palmgren, J. and Axelsson, O. (2001). Sinistrality – a side-effect of prenatal sonography: a comparative study of young men. *Epidemiology* **12**, 618–623.

Kinnier-Wilson, L.M. and Waterhouse, J.A.H. (1984). Obstetric ultrasound and childhood malignancies. *Lancet* **2**, 997–998.

Kobayashi, N., Yasu, T., Yamada, S., Kudo, N., Kuroki, M., Kawakami, M., Miyatake K. and Saito, M. (2002). Endothelial cell injury in venule and capillary induced by contrast ultrasonography. *Ultrasound Med. Biol.* **28**, 949–956.

Kunze-Muhl, E. (1981). Observations on the effect of X-ray alone and in combination with ultrasound on human chromosomes. *Hum. Genet.* **57**, 257–260.

Latt, S.A. and Schreck, R.R. (1980). Sister chromatid exchange analysis. *Am. J. Hum. Genet.* **32**, 297.

Lehmann, J.F., DeLateur, B.J., Stonebridge, J.B. and Warren, C.G. (1967). The therapeutic temperature distribution produced by ultrasound as modified by dosage and volume of tissue exposed. *Arch. Phys. Med. Rehab.* **48**, 662–666.

Lele, P.P. (1979). Safety and potential hazards in the current applications of ultrasound in obstetrics and gynaecology. *Ultrasound Med. Biol.* **5**, 307–320.

Li, G.C., Hahn, G.M. and Tolmach, L.J. (1977). Cellular inactivation by ultrasound. *Nature* **267**, 163–165.

Liebeskind, D., Bases, R., Eliequin, F., Neubort, S., Leifer, R., Goldberg, R. and Koenigsberg, M. (1979a). Diagnostic ultrasound: effects on DNA and growth patterns of animal cells. *Radiology* **131**, 177–184.

Liebeskind, D., Bases, R., Mendez, F., Elequin, F. and Koenigsberg, M. (1979b). Sister chromatid exchanges in human lymphocytes after exposure to diagnostic ultrasound. *Science* **205**, 1274–1275.

Liebeskind, D., Padawer, J., Wolley, R. and Bases, R. (1982). Diagnostic ultrasound: time lapse and transmission electron microscopic studies of cells insonated *in vitro*. *Br. J. Cancer* **45** (Suppl. V), 176–186.

Lyng, H., Monge, O.R., Bohler, P.J. and Rofstad, E.K. (1991a). Relationships between thermal dose and heat-induced tissue and vascular damage after thermoradiotherapy of locally advanced breast carcinoma *Int. J. Hypertherm.* **7**, 403–415.

Lyng, H., Monge, O.R., Bohler, P.J. and Rofstad, E.K. (1991b). Changes in temperatures and thermal doses with fraction number during hyperthermic treatment of locally advanced breast carcinoma. *Int. J. Hypertherm.* **7**, 815–825.

Lyons, E.A., Dyke, C., Toms, M. and Cheang, M. (1988). *In utero* exposure to diagnostic ultrasound: a 6-year follow-up. *Radiology* **166**, 687–690.

Lundberg, M., Jerominski, L., Livingston, G., Kochenour, N., Lee, T. and Fineman, R. (1982). Failure to demonstrate an effect of *in vivo* diagnostic ultrasound on sister chromatid exchange frequency in anniotic fluid cells. *Am. J. Med. Genet.* **11**, 31.

Mannor, S.M., Serr, D.M., Tamari, I., Meshorer, A. and Frei, E.H. (1972). The safety of ultrasound in fetal monitoring. *Am. J. Obstet. Gynaecol.* **113**, 653–661.

McClain, R.M., Hoar, R.M. and Saltzman, M.B. (1972). Teratological study of rats exposed to ultrasound. *Am. J. Obstet. Gynaecol.* **114**, 39–42.

Miller, D.L. and Gies, R.A. (1998a). Enhancement of ultrasonically induced haemolysis by perfluorocarbon-based compared to air-based echo-contrast agents. *Ultrasound Med. Biol.* **24**, 285–292.

Miller, D.L. and Gies, R.A. (1998b). Gas-body-based contrast agent enhances vascular damage to mouse intestine. *Ultrasound Med. Biol.* **24**, 1201–1208.

Miller, D.L. and Gies, R.A. (1999). Ultrasonically induced vascular damage to the mouse intestine. *J. Acoust. Am.* **105**, 1324–1325.

Miller, D.L., Nyborg, W.L., Dewey, W.C., Edwards, M.J., Abramowicz, J.S. and Brayman, A.A. (2002). Hyperthermic teratogenicity, thermal dose and diagnostic ultrasound during pregnancy: implications of new standards on tissue heating. *Int. J. Hypertherm.* **18**, 361–384.

Miller, D.L., Nyborg, W.L. and Whitcomb, C.C. (1979). Platelet aggregation induced by ultrasound under specialized conditions *in vitro*. *Science* **205**, 505–507.

Miller, D.L. and Quddus, J. (2000). Diagnostic ultrasound activation of contrast agent gas bodies induces capillary rupture in mice. *Proc. Nat. Acad. Sci.* **20**, 10179–10184.

Miller, D.L. and Thomas, R.M. (1995). Ultrasound contrast agents nucleate inertial cavitation *in vitro*. *Ultrasound Med. Biol.* **21**, 1059–1065.

Miller, D.L. and Thomas, R.M. (1996). Contrast agent gas bodies enhance haemolysis induced by lithotriptor shock waves and high intensity focused ultrasound in whole blood. *Ultrasound Med. Biol.* **22**, 1089–1095.

Miller, D.L., Thomas, R.M. and Frazier M.E. (1991). Single strand breaks in CHO cell DNA induced by ultrasonic cavitation in vitro. *Ultrasound Med. Biol.* **17**, 401–406.

Miller, M.W. (1985). Does ultrasound induce sister chromatid exchanges? *Ultrasound Med. Biol.* **11**, 561–570.

Miller, M.W. and Ziskin, M.C. (1989). Biological consequences of hyperthermia. *Ultrasound Med. Biol.* **15**, 707–722.

Moore, R.M., Diamond, E.L. and Cavalieri, R.L. (1988). The relationship of birthweight and intrauterine diagnostic ultraound exposure. *Obstet. Gynecol.* **71**, 513–517.

Mortimer, A.J. and Dyson, M. (1988). The effect of therapeutic ultrasound on calcium uptake in fibroblasts. *Ultrasound Med. Biol.* **14**, 499–506.

Morton, K.I., ter Haar, G.R., Stratford, L.J. and Hill, C.R. (1982). The role of cavitation in the interaction of ultrasound with V79 Chinese Hamster cells *in vitro*. *Br. J. Cancer* **45**, 147–150.

Morton, K.I., ter Haar, G.R., Stratford, L.J. and Hill, C.R. (1983). Subharmonic emission as an indicator of ultrasonically induced biological damage. *Ultrasound Med. Biol.* **9**, 629–633.

Morris, S.M., Palmer, C.C., Fry, F.J. and Johnson, L.K. (1978). Effect of ultrasound on human leucocytes in sister chromatid exchange analysis. *Ultrasound Med. Biol.* **4**, 253.

Mummery, C.L. (1978). Effect of ultrasound on fibroblasts *in vitro*. PhD thesis, University of London.

Neilson, J.P. (1993). Routine ultrasound in early pregnancy. In *Cochrane Database of Systematic Reviews*, Review no. 03872, M.W. Enkin, M.J.N.C. Keirse, M.J. Renfrew and J.P. Meilson (eds). Oxford Update Software, Oxford.

Newnham, J.P., Evans, S.F., Michael, C.A., Stanley, F.J. and Landau, L.I. (1993). Effects of frequent ultrasound during pregnancy: a randomised controlled trial. *Lancet* **342**, 887–892.

Nyborg, W.L. and Miller, D.L. (1982). Biophysical implications of bubble mechanics. *Appl. Sci. Res.* **38**, 17–24.

O'Brien, W.D. (1976). Ultrasonically induced fetal weight reduction in mice. In *Ultrasound in Medicine*, D.N. White (ed.). Plenum Press, New York, pp. 531–532.

Penney, D.P., Schenk, E.A., Maltby, K., Harman-Raeman, C., Child, S.Z. and Carstensen, E.L. (1993). Morphological effects of pulsed ultrasound in the lung. *Ultrasound Med. Biol.* **19**, 127–135.

Raeman, C.H., Dalecki, D., Child, S.Z., Meltzer R.S. and Carstensen, E.L. (1997). Albunex does not increase the sensitivity of the lung to pulsed ultrasound. *Echocardiography* **14**, 553–557.

Rooney, J.A. (1970). Hemolysis near an ultrasonically pulsating gas bubble. *Science* **169**, 869–871.

Rott, H.-D. (1981). Zur Frage der Schadigungsmöglichkeit durch diagnostischen Ultraschall. *Ultraschall* **2**, 56.

Salvesen, K. (2000). Epidemiological studies of diagnostic ultrasound. In *The Safe Use of Ultrasound in Medical Diagnosis*, G.R. ter Haar and F.A. Duck (eds). British Institute of Radiology, London, pp. 86–93.

Salvesen, K.A., Bakketeig, L.S., Eik-Nes, S.H., Undheim, L.O. and Okland, O. (1990). Routine ultrasonography *in utero* and school performance at age 8–9 years. *Lancet* **339**, 85–89.

Salvesen, K.A. and Eik-Nes, S. (1999). Ultrasound during pregnancy and subsequent childhood non-right handedness – a meta-analysis. *Ultrasound Obstet. Gynecol.* **13**, 241–246.

Salvesen, K.A., Jacobsen, G., Vatten, L.J., Eik-Nes, S.H. and Bakketeig, L.S. (1993b). Routine ultrasonography *in utero* and subsequent growth during childhood. *Ultrasound Obstet. Gynecol.* **3**, 6–10.

Salvesen, K.A., Vatten, L.J., Bakketeig, L.S. and Eik-Nes, S.H. (1994). Routine ultrasonography *in utero* and speech development. *Ultrasound Obstet. Gynecol.* **4**, 101–103.

Salvesen, K.A., Vatten, L.J., Eik-Nes, S.H., Hugdahl, K. and Bakketeig, L.S. (1993a). Routine ultrasonography *in utero* and subsequent handedness and neurological development. *Br. Med. J.* **307**, 159–164.

Salvesen, K.A., Vatten, L.J., Jacobsen, G., Eik-Nes, S.H., Okland, O., Molne, K. and Bakketeig, L.S. (1992). Routine ultrasonography *in utero* and subsequent vision and hearing at primary school age. *Ultrasound Obstet. Gynecol.* **2**, 243–247.

Sapareto, S.A. and Dewey, W.C. (1984). Thermal dose determination in cancer therapy. *Int. J. Radiat. Oncol. Biol. Phys.* **10**, 787–800.

Scheidt, P.C., Stanley, F. and Bryla, D.A. (1978). One year follow-up of infants exposed to ultrasound *in utero*. *Am. J. Obstet. Gynecol.* **131**, 743–748.

Shoji, R., Murackami, U. and Shimizu, T. (1975). Influence of low intensity ultrasonic irradiation on prenatal development of two inbred mouse strains. *Teratology* **12**, 227–232.

Shu, X.O., Jin, F., Linet, M.S., Zheng, W., Clemens, J., Mills, J. and Gao, Y.T. (1994). Diagnostic X-ray and ultrasound exposure and risk of childhood cancer. *Br. J. Cancer* **70**, 531–536.

Sikov, M. and Hildebrand, B.P. (1976). Effects of ultrasound on the prenatal development of the rat. Part 1: 3.2 MHz continuous wave at nine days gestation. *Ultrasound* **4**, 357–363.

Skyba, D.M., Price, R.J., Linka, A.Z., Skalak, T.C. and Kaul, S. (1998). Direct *in vivo* visualization of intravascular destruction of microbubbles by ultrasound and its local effects on tissue. *Circulation* **98**, 290–293.

Smachlo, K., Fridd, C.W., Child, S.Z., Hare, J.D., Linke, C.A. and Carstensen, E.L. (1979). Ultrasonic treatment of tumors: 1. Absence of metastases following treatment of a hamster fibrosarcoma. *Ultrasound Med. Biol.* **5**, 45–49.

Sorahan, T., Lancashire, R., Stewart, A. and Peck, I. (1995). Pregnancy, ultrasound and childhood cancer: a second report from the Oxford survey of childhood cancers. *Br. J. Obstet. Gynaecol.* **102**, 831–832.

Stark, C.R., Orleans, M., Havercamp, A.D. and Murphy, J. (1984). Short and long term risks after exposure to diagnostic ultrasound *in utero*. *Obstet. Gynecol.* **63**, 194–200.

Stella, M., Trevison, L., Montaldi, A., Zaccaria, G., Rossi, G., Bianchi, V. and Levis, A.G. (1984). Induction of sister-chromatid exchanges in human lymphocytes exposed to *in vitro* and *in vivo* therapeutic ultrasound. *Mutat. Res.* **138**, 75–85.

Stolzenberg, S.J., Torbit, C.A., Pryor, G.T. and Edmonds, P.D. (1980). Toxicity of ultrasound in mice: neonatal studies. *Radiat. Environ. Biophys.* **18**, 37–44.

Tachibana, M., Tachibana, Y. and Suzuki, M. (1977). The present status of the safety of ultrasonic diagnosis in the area of obstetrics – the effect of ultrasound irradiation on pregnant mice as indicated in their fetuses. *Jpn. J. Med. Ultrason.* **4**, 279–283.

Talbert, D.G. (1975). Spontaneous smooth muscle activity as a means of detecting biological effects of ultrasound. In *Proceedings of Ultrasonics International 1975*. IPC Science & Technology Press, Guildford, pp. 279–284.

Tarantal, A.F. and Canfield, D.R. (1994). Ultrasound induced lung haemorrhage in the monkey. *Ultrasound Med. Biol.* **20**, 65–72.

Tarantal, A.F., Gargosky, S.E., Ellis, D.S., O'Brien, W.D. and Hendrickx, A.G. (1995). Hematologic and growth-related effects of frequent prenatal ultrasound exposure in the long-tailed Macaque (*Macaca Fascicularis*). *Ultrasound Med. Biol.* **21**, 1073–1081.

Tarantal, A.F. and Hendrickx, A.G. (1989a). Evaluation of the bio-effects of pre-natal ultrasound exposure in the Cynomolgus Macaque (*Macaca Fascicularis*): I. Neonatal/infant observations. *Teratology* **39**, 137–147.

Tarantal, A.F. and Hendrickx, A.G. (1989b). Evaluation of the bio-effects of pre-natal ultrasound exposure in the Cynomolgus Macaque (*Macaca Fascicularis*): II. Growth and behaviour during the first year. *Teratology* **39**, 149–162.

Taylor, K.J.W. and Newman, D.L. (1972). Electrophoretic mobility of Ehrlich suspensions exposed to ultrasound of varying parameters. *Phys. Med. Biol.* **17**, 270–276.

Taylor, K.J.W. and Pond, J.B. (1972). Primary sites of ultrasonic damage on cell systems. In *Interaction of Ultrasound and Biological Tissues*, Vol. 3, M. Reid and M.R. Sikov (eds). DHEW Publication No. (FDA)73-8008. DHEW, Washington, DC.

Thacker, J. (1973). The possibility of genetic hazard from ultrasonic radiation. *Curr. Top. in Radiat. Res. Q.* **8**, 235–258.

Uhlendorf, V. and Scholle, F.-D. (1996). Imaging of spatial distribution and flow of microbubbles using non-linear acoustic properties. *Acoust. Imag.* **22**, 233–238.

Van der Wouw, P.A., Brauns, A.C., Bailey, S.E., Powers, J.E. and Wilde, A.A.A. (2000). Premature ventricular contractions during triggered imaging with ultrasound contrast. *J. Am. Soc. Echocardiogr* **13**, 288–294.

Vorhees, C.V., Acuff-Smith, K.D., Weisenburger, W.P., Meyer, R.A., Smith, N.B. and O'Brien, W.D. (1991). A teratological evaluation of continuous wave, daily ultrasound exposure in unanaesthetised pregnant rats. *Teratology* **44**, 667–674.

Waldenstrom, U., Axelsson, O., Nilsson, S., Eklund, G., Fall, O., Lindeberg, S. and Sjodin, Y. (1988). Effects of routine ultrasound screening in pregnancy: a randomised controlled trial. *Lancet* **ii**, 585–588.

Warwick, R., Pond, J.B., Woodward, B. and Connolly, C.C. (1970). Hazards of diagnostic ultrasonography – study with mice. *IEEE Trans. Son. Ultrason.* **SU-17**, 158–164.

Watmough, D.J., Dendy, P.P., Eastwood, L.H., Gregory, D.W., Gordon, F.C.A. and Wheatley, D.N. (1977). The biophysical effects of therapeutic ultrasound in HeLa cells. *Ultrasound Med. Biol.* **3**, 205–219.

Wegner, R.-D. and Meyenburg, M. (1982). The effects of diagnostic ultrasonography on the frequencies of sister chromatid exchanges in Chinese hamster cells and human lymphocytes. *J. Ultrasound Med.* **1**, 355.

Wegner, R.-D., Obe, G. and Meyenburg, M. (1980). Has diagnostic ultrasound mutagenic effects? *Hum. Genet.* **56**, 95–98.

WFUMB (World Federation of Ultrasound in Medicine and Biology) (1992). WFUMB Symposium on Safety and Standardisation in Medical Ultrasound: issues and recommendations regarding thermal mechanisms for biological effects of ultrasound. *Ultrasound Med. Biol.* **18**, 731–814.

Whittingham, T.A. (2000). The output of diagnostic machines. In *The Safe Use of Ultrasound in Medical Diagnosis*, G.R. ter Haar and F.A. Duck (eds). British Institute of Radiology, London, pp. 16–31.

Williams, A.R. (1974). Release of serotonin from human platelets by acoustic microstreaming. *J. Acoust. Soc. Am.* **56**, 1640–1643.

Williams, A.R., Chatei, B.V., Sanderson, J.H., Taberner, D.A., May, S.J., Allen, K.A. and Sherwood, M.R. (1977). Beta-thromboglobulin release from human platelets after *in vivo* ultrasound irradiation. *Lancet* **2**, 931–932.

Williams, A.R., Hughes, D.E. and Nyberg, W.L. (1970). Hemolysis near a transversely oscillating wire. *Science* **169**, 871–873.

Williams, A.R. and Miller, D.L. (1980). Photometric detection of ATP release from human erythrocytes exposed to ultrasonically activated gas-filled pores. *Ultrasound Med. Biol.* **6**, 251–256.

Wong, Y.S. and Watmough, D.J. (1980). Hemolysis of red blood cells *in vitro* and *in vivo* caused by therapeutic ultrasound at 0.75 MHz. *Proc. Ultrasound Interaction in Biology and Medicine Symposium*, Paper C-14. Reinhardsbrunn, Germany, 10–14 November 1980.

Zachary, J.F., Hartleben, S.A., Frizzell, L.A. and O'Brien, W.D. (2002). Arrhythmias in rat hearts exposed to pulsed ultrasound after intravenous injection of a contrast agent. *J. Ultrasound Med.* **21**, 1347–1356.

Zachary, J.F. and O'Brien (1995). Lung haemorrhage induced by continuous and pulsed wave (diagnostic) ultrasound in mice, rabbits and pigs. *Vet. Pathol.* **32**, 43–54.

Zheng, H.Z., Mitter, N.S. and Chudley, A.C. (1981). *In vivo* exposure to diagnostic ultrasound and *in vitro* assay of sister chromatid exchange in cultured amniotic fluid cells. *IRCS Med. Sci.* **9**, 491.

15

Epilogue: Historical Perspectives

C. R. HILL

Institute of Cancer Research, Royal Marsden Hospital, UK

A systematic basis for the modern science of acoustics was laid in the late nineteenth century with the publication of the classical *Theory of Sound*, by Rayleigh (1877). It was by a seemingly strange chance that this was followed only three years later by the discovery, due to the brothers J. and P. Curie (1880), of the phenomenon of piezoelectricity, which was to make possible the effective extension of acoustics way beyond the audible region, and eventually to gigahertz frequencies. By the end of that century, however, acoustics had been overshadowed in the imagination of the physics community by the astonishing twin discoveries of X-rays and radioactivity, with their implications for the development of atomic and nuclear physics. It is thus only in recent years that the ultrasonic branch of acoustics has experienced a considerable revival of interest and has come to be seen as both a challenging and practically important branch of science.

The phenomenon of acoustic echoes has intrigued people throughout the ages – an example from the novelist Thomas Hardy, a contemporary of Rayleigh, has already been given on our title page. The modern, practical use of this phenomenon, in medicine and elsewhere, seems to have been stimulated by the disastrous collision with an iceberg suffered by the ocean liner *Titanic* on 15 April 1912. Within the following week a young British physicist, L. F. Richardson, then working for the Sunbeam Lamp Company and subsequently to become an outstanding meteorologist, had prepared a provisional patent for an 'Apparatus for warning a ship at sea of its nearness to large objects wholly or partly under water' (Richardson 1912; Ashford 1985). The idea of echo-sounding was not original at that time but Richardson's contribution was to emphasise the importance of using high frequencies in order to achieve good directivity. Whilst experimenting on the subject Richardson was to be seen in a rowing boat, using a tram horn as a sound source and an open umbrella as a 'parabolic' reflector, trying to record echoes from a nearby cliff. Ironically, his Quaker pacifist principles diverted him from following up this idea on the grounds of its likely military value.

Richardson's ideas were based on the use of airborne sound and a vital next step to the use of underwater propagation was taken by the French physicist P. Langevin, a former pupil of P. Curie. His work was stimulated by just the sort of objective that had inhibited Richardson: detection of wartime submarines. By 1917 he was able to achieve for the first time, for this purpose, the generation of high-frequency ultrasonic power. His achievement was all the greater because it was carried out prior to the invention of the thermionic valve and an intriguing account of the work, following its post-war declassification, was given by Wood

Physical Principles of Medical Ultrasonics, Second Edition. Edited by C. R. Hill, J. C. Bamber and G. R. ter Haar.
© 2004 John Wiley & Sons, Ltd: ISBN 0 471 97002 6

and Loomis (1927). They state that 'In Langevin's original apparatus the vibrations of the piezo-electric quartz plate were excited by a Poulsen arc, in connection with suitable condensers and coils. Voltages as high as 30 or 40,000 were applied to the plates and the amplitude of the waves raised to such a degree that small fish were killed by the radiation, and pain of considerable severity was experienced when the hand was thrust into the water in the tank.' The work thus represents a first record not only of the underwater echo technique on which medical diagnostic procedures are based but also of ultrasonic bioeffects.

It was the same Wood and Loomis, in the USA, who carried out the first systematic investigation of these bioeffects: the forerunner of what was to become a large but disappointingly qualitative and uncritical literature in the interwar years, much of which was reviewed by Bergmann (1954) in his *magnum opus*. Indeed, even by 1968, when the present author came to review the literature on possible biological hazards of ultrasound, there existed no systematic analytical framework for discussion of the various biophysical mechanisms of action that might be postulated (Hill 1968).

Although Langevin's work, in principle, laid the groundwork for the modern pulse–echo diagnostic technique, development of the necessary fast pulse electronic technology had to wait for a further 25 years. Meanwhile, although Röntgen's invention of X-ray shadow imaging had proved immensely powerful for many applications, it was found to have limitations, particularly for one very important organ – the brain – that possesses little in the way of naturally X-ray contrasting structures and is thus essentially invisible by this means. It was thus in the late 1930s that the brothers Dussik (1947) started their attempts at ultrasound transmission imaging of the brain, which they partially immersed in water and scanned using a transmitter/receiver pair of quartz crystals (and, of course, no time-gated electronics). What has only become clear with hindsight is that the brain, surrounded as it is by the mechanically very complex structure of the skull, is extremely difficult to work with, even using modern techniques, and that the images that they eventually published – pioneering achievements though they were – seem to have been entirely artefactual.

It was again the drive to satisfy military needs, this time in the development of radar, that provided the missing element – fast pulse techniques – required for the implementation of ultrasonic pulse–echo imaging on the scale of human anatomy. This opportunity was followed up, in a largely empirical manner, by several individuals independently, and notably by Howry in Denver, Colorado, and Wild in Minneapolis. These two had interestingly different conceptual approaches. Howry optimised his equipment to detect and map relatively large, what he conceived of as 'specular', echoes arising from organ interfaces; whereas Wild, a surgeon particularly interested in cancer, set out to record all the echoes that were backscattered from tissue parenchyma (Wild 1978). Initially, Howry's approach seems to have appealed to radiologists and engineers, and most of the early commercial equipment that came out in the 1960s was built on that principle. This eventually proved to have become something of a blind alley and by the mid-1970s, influenced by the work of Donald in Glasgow, the group of Kossoff in Australia and our own Royal Marsden group in London, Wild's 'grey-scale' imaging approach had become the accepted technique.

Prior to about 1970, medical ultrasonics had attracted only very scant interest as a significant branch of applied physics. In illustration of this point, even though it was becoming clear to any thoughtful physicist that the information retrieval mechanism underlying pulse–echo imaging was based on acoustic scattering, a search conducted at that time for literature on acoustic scattering from biological tissues found only two published papers, one of which was concerned with frozen fish (Chivers 1973; Hill *et al.* 1978). A number of physically- but predominantly engineering-oriented groups had indeed been working during the 1950s and 1960s on related issues – and outstandingly the group under W. J. Fry at the University of

Illinois – but their applied interest had generally been in potential surgical and therapeutic applications: a good picture of the state of the related science and technology in that period is given in a chapter by Fry and Dunn (1962).

Thus, in conclusion, although much of the theoretical basis underlying medical ultrasonic physics and biophysics is quite mature, most of the laboratory studies that have made it possible to start establishing a coherent intellectual framework for the subject are of relatively recent origin and often, indeed, ongoing. This book constitutes an attempt to record and clarify that framework.

REFERENCES

Ashford, O.M. (1985). *Prophet or Professor? The Life and Work of Lewis Fry Richardson*. Adam Hilger, Bristol/Boston.

Bergmann, L. (1954). *Der Ultraschall*. Hirzel Verlag, Stuttgart.

Chivers, R.C. (1973). The scattering of ultrasound by human tissues. PhD thesis. University of London.

Curie, J. and Curie, P. (1880). Sur l'électricité polaire dans cristaux hémièdres à face inclinées. *C. R. Acad. Sci.* **91**, 383–389.

Dussik, K.T., Dussik, F. and Wyt, L. (1947). Auf dem Wege zur Hypophonographie des Gehirnes. *Wien. Med. Ochenschr.* **97**, 425–429.

Fry, W.J. and Dunn, F. (1962). Ultrasound: analysis and experimental methods in biological research. In *Physical Techniques in Biological Research*, Vol. IV, W.L. Nastuk (ed.). Academic Press, New York.

Hill, C.R. (1968). The possibility of hazard in medical and industrial applications of ultrasound. *Br. J. Radiol.* **41**, 561–569.

Hill, C.R., Chivers R.C., Huggins R.W. and Nicholas, D. (1978). Scattering of ultrasound by human tissue. In *Ultrasound: Its Applications in Medicine and Biology*, W.J. Fry (ed.). Elsevier, Amsterdam, pp. 441–493.

Rayleigh, Lord (1877). *Theory of Sound*. Macmillan, London.

Richardson, M.L.F. (1912). *UK Patent 1125/1912*.

Wild, J.J. (1978). The use of pulse–echo ultrasound for early tumour detection: history and prospects. In *Ultrasound in Tumour Diagnosis*, C.R. Hill, *et al.* (eds). Pitman Medical, Tunbridge Wells.

Wood, R.W. and Loomis, A. (1927). The physical and biological effects of sound waves of great intensity. *Philos. Mag.* **4** (Suppl. 7), 417–436.

List of Symbols

The following list includes symbols that are widely used in several chapters or sections of the book, or may otherwise be of importance. It is not, however, exhaustive and generally does not include symbols that have been defined and introduced purely for use within a limited section of text.

Symbol		Section where symbol is first introduced or defined
$\mathbf{a}$	Particle acceleration	1.3
a	Radius of a circular radiator	2.3
$\hat{a}$	Average scale parameter (e.g. correlation length)	6.1.2
a_n	Component of emitter acceleration normal to vibrating surface	1.5
A	Wave amplitude	1.4.1
	Radius of a sphere/spherical radiator	2.5
	Particle acceleration amplitude	Table 2.3
A_C	Complex wave amplitude	1.6.1
$A(\dots)$	Angular spectrum	1.6.3
A_F	Array factor	1.6.6
A_I	Amplitude of incident wave	1.7.3
A_T	Amplitude of transmitted wave	1.7.3
A	First-order constant in expansion of p in powers of s	1.8
B	Wave amplitude	1.4.3
$B(\dots)$	Beam cross-section	1.6.5
B	Second-order constant in expansion of p in powers of s	1.8
B/A	Ratio of 1st and 2nd order constants in expansion of p	1.8
$C(c)$	$\bar{C}$ in constant medium: speed of sound for homogeneous equation	1.2.4
C	Specific heat	12.2.1
	(Gas) concentration	12.3.3.1
$\bar{C}$	$(\bar{\varrho}\bar{\beta})^{-1/2}$	
C_0	$(\varrho_0\beta_0)^{-1/2}$ in inhomogeneous medium	1.2.4
C_N	$[\partial p/\partial \varrho]_{ad}$	1.8.3
C_P	Heat capacity (at constant pressure)	4.3.1
D	Location of discontinuity or reflector	1.7.1
	Particle displacement amplitude	Table 2.3
D/Dt	Material (convective) derivative	1.2.1
$D(\dots)$	Directivity spectrum	1.6.4
D_n	Directivity spectrum of nth element in array	1.6.6
$D_{n,eff}$	Effective directivity spectrum of nth element in array	1.6.6
D_{array}	Directivity spectrum of multielement array	1.6.6

Physical Principles of Medical Ultrasonics, Second Edition. Edited by C. R. Hill, J. C. Bamber and G. R. ter Haar.
© 2004 John Wiley & Sons, Ltd: ISBN 0 471 97002 6

Symbol		Section where symbol is first introduced or defined
$(\dots)^E$	Denotes Eulerian description	1.2
E	Energy density per unit volume	1.3
F	Denotes general function	1.2.3
	Radiation force	3.4
f	Frequency	1.2.5
$f(\dots)$	Arbitrary function	1.6.3
F_f	Fourier transform of function f	1.6.3
f_Z	Echo from continuously varying impedance profile	1.7.2
f_R	Observed frequency of wave reflected from moving reflector	1.7.5
f_D	Doppler shift	1.7.5
$g(\dots)$	Arbitrary function	1.4.1
G	Green's function	1.5
	Shear elastic modulus	4.3.2
G_S	Free space Green's function	1.5
h	Transverse distance coordinate in cylindrical coordinate system	1.4.3
H	Pressure field impulse response/transfer function	1.6.2
H'	Time derivative of impulse response	1.6.2
H_S	Heaviside step function	1.6.2
$\mathbf{I}$	Intensity vector	1.3
I	Scalar intensity	1.3
I_{SPTA}	Spatial peak, temporal average intensity	3.8; 14.2
I_{SAL}	Spatial average intensity measured under linear conditions	3.8; 13.5.1.1
$\mathbf{i}$	Unit vector along x-axis	1.4.1
$\mathbf{j}$	Unit vector along y-axis	1.4.1
J	A Bessel function	2.5.1
k	Wave number	1.4.1
	Thermal conductivity	12.2.1
$\mathbf{k}$	Unit vector along z-axis	1.4.1
k_x	Spatial frequency conjugate to x	1.6.3
k_y	Spatial frequency conjugate to y	1.6.3
$(\dots)^L$	Denotes Lagrangian description	1.2
L	Barrier thickness	1.7.3
	Optical luminance	8.3.3
$\mathbf{M}$	Composite elastic modulus	4.3.2
$\mathbf{n}$	Unit vector in field propagation direction	1.3
N	Integer	1.6.1
n	Integer	1.6.6
	Standard deviation of refractive index	6.1.2
$\mathbf{n}_I$	Unit vector in direction of incident wave	1.7.4
$\mathbf{n}_R$	Unit vector in direction of reflected wave	1.7.4
$\mathbf{n}_T$	Unit vector in direction of transmitted wave	1.7.4
P	Acoustic pressure amplitude	Table 2.3
	General measure of a physical property	9.3.1
p_0	Undistorted density of medium	1.2
p_T	Total pressure	1.2
p	Acoustic pressure	1.2

Symbol		Section where symbol is first introduced or defined
p_ω	Amplitude of harmonic wave of (angular) frequency ω	1.2.5
p_x	Plane wave pressure	1.4.1
p_{Hx}	Harmonic plane wave pressure	1.4.1
p_{SWx}	Standing plane wave pressure	1.4.1
p_r	Spherical wave pressure	1.4.2
p_{Hr}	Harmonic spherical wave pressure	1.4.2
p_h	Cylindrical wave pressure	1.4.3
p_{Hh}	Harmonic cylindrical wave pressure	1.4.3
p_{A,ω_0}	On-axis pressure radiated by planar disc transducer, excited at frequency $\omega 0$	1.6.1
p_A	Axial pulse	1.6.5
p_I	Pressure of incident wave	1.7.4
p_R	Pressure of reflected wave	1.7.4
p_T	Pressure of transmitted wave	1.7.4
p_1	First-order term in expansion (in ε) of pressure	1.8.2
p_2	Second-order term in expansion (in ε) of pressure	1.8.2
q	Denotes arbitrary acoustic variable	1.2
$q(\dots)$	Arbitrary function	1.4.1
Q	Energy density flux vector	1.3
$\mathbf{r}$	Location vector	1.2
$\mathbf{r}_n$	Location of vector of nth element in array	1.6.6
r	Magnitude of location vector	1.4.2
R	Distance between two points	1.5
	Amplitude reflection coefficient	1.7.1
	Radiation pressure	1.8.1
	Gas constant	4.3.5
R_T	Radius of planar circular transducer	1.6
R_E	Intensity reflection coefficient	1.7.1
R_θ	Amplitude reflectivity for oblique incidence	1.7.4
R_I	Riemann invariant	1.8.3
s	Condensation	1.3
S	Denotes surface	1.5
	Geometrical aperture (a/A)	2.5
	Condensation amplitude	Table 2.3
	General measure of a signal value	9.3.1
S	Scattering distribution	1.7.2
$(.\bar{\,}.)$	Denotes time averaging	Table 1.1
t	Time	1.2
t_n	Excitation instant of nth element in array	1.6.6
T	Amplitude transmission coefficient	1.7.1
	Period	1.7.5
	Temperature	4.4.2.4
	Tissue impulse response	6.2.3
T_E	Intensity transmission coefficient	1.7.1
T_W	Pulse duration	1.7.2
T_θ	Amplitude transmissivity for oblique incidence	1.7.4
T_D	Duration of echo from moving reflector	1.7.5
T_S	Surface tension	4.3.3

Symbol		Section where symbol is first introduced or defined
u	Scalar particle velocity	1.2
$\mathbf{u}$	Particle velocity vector	1.3
u_1	First-order term in expansion (in ε) of particle velocity	1.8.2
u_2	Second-order term in expansion (in ε) of particle velocity	1.8.2
U	Particle velocity amplitude	Table 2.3
V	Volume	1.2.3
	Signal voltage amplitude	4.4.2.1
v_n	Normal component of transducer face velocity	1.6.1
V	Speed of moving interface	1.7.5
W	Acoustic power	4.2
x	Cartesian component of location vector	1.2
x_0	Value of x at time zero	1.2
x_s	Shock formation distance	1.8.2
y	Cartesian component of location vector	1.2
z	Cartesian component of location vector	1.2
Z	Specific acoustic impedance	1.3
	Frèsnel distance	4.4.2.2
$Z(\dots)$	Effective impedance	1.7.2
z	Axial distance component in cylindrical coordinate system	1.4.3
$Z_{\max,N}$	Nth axial maximum of pressure field	1.6.1
$Z_{\min,N}$	Nth axial minimum of pressure field	1.6.1
α	Acoustic amplitude attenuation coefficient	4.2
α_a	Acoustic amplitude absorption coefficient	4.2
α_s	Acoustic amplitude scattering coefficient	4.2
β_0	(Adiabatic) compressibility	1.2.3
$\bar{\beta}$	Mean value of compressibility	1.2.4
$\tilde{\beta}$	Compressibility fluctuation	1.2.4
β_N	Parameter of non-linearity	1.8.2
Γ	Impedance step	1.7.2
	Focusing strength (of a projector)	9.2.3.1
	Figure of merit of an interrogation procedure	9.3.1
γ	Parameter of non-linearity	1.8.2
	Ratio of specific heats	4.3.3
$\Delta(\dots)$	Denotes small increment	1.2.1
δ	Dirac delta function	1.5
Δ	Distance between two interfaces	1.7.1
ε	Denotes infinitesimal amount	1.5
η	Ratio of sound speeds	2.5.3
	Coefficient of viscosity	4.3.1
θ	Angle variable in spherical coordinate system	1.4.2
θ	Angle variable	1.6.2
θ_I	Angle of incidence	1.7.4
θ_R	Angle of reflection	1.7.4
$\hat{\theta}$	Angle for zero reflectivity at oblique incidence	1.7.4
θ_C	Critical angle	1.7.4

Symbol		Section where symbol is first introduced or defined
λ	Wavelength	1.4.1
μ	Total interaction (extinction) cross-section per unit volume	4.2
μ_a	Absorption cross-section per unit volume	4.2
μ_s	Scattering cross-section per unit volume	4.2
ν	Spatial frequency	9.2.3.1
∇	Gradient operator	1.2.4
∇^2	Laplacian operator	1.2.4
ξ	Particle displacement	1.2
Π	Rayleigh probability function	6.5.1
ϱ_0	Undisturbed density of medium	1.2
ϱ	Total density	1.2
ϱ_T	Density perturbation caused by wave	1.2
$\bar{\varrho}$	Mean value of density	1.2.4
$\tilde{\varrho}$	Density fluctuation	1.2.4
ϱ_1	First-order term in expansion (in ε) of acoustic density	1.8.2
ϱ_2	Second-order term in expansion (in ε) of acoustic density	1.8.2
σ	Coherent scattering/attenuation cross-section	6.2.6
	Surface tension	12.3.2
τ	Time interval	1.3
τ	Travel time variable	1.7.2
	Relaxation time	4.3.2
ϕ	Velocity potential	1.3
φ	Angle variable in spherical coordinate system	1.4.2
φ	Angle variable in cylindrical coordinate system	1.4.3
ψ	Phase angle	Table 1.1
	Scattering angle variable	6.2.2
χ	Thermal conductivity	4.3.1
ω	Angular frequency	1.2.5

Index

Note: page numbers in *italics* refer to figures and tables

A-scan image 199, 258
  multiple 258–9
absorption 93–4
  cavitation 118–19
  collagen fibrils 148–9
  cross-section 202
    per unit volume 94
  excess per molecule 96
  frequency dependencies 99
  gas bubbles 106–8
  homogeneous liquid-like media 97–100
  inhomogeneities 94
  inhomogeneous media 105–8
  intermolecular 145–6
  intramolecular 144–5
  microbubbles 118–19
  muscle 148–9
  non-linear propagation 113–16, *117*, 118
  pressure dependence 111
  related phenomena 112–13
  semi-solid media 100–5
  single relaxation process *98*
  solids 108–9
  temperature coefficient 110
  temperature dependence 109–11, 149–50
  theory of mechanisms 96–116, *117*, 118–19
  viscoelasticity 100–5
absorption coefficient 96, 106
  biopolymers 144
  classical 97, 99
  glycogen 153
  measurement 99
    direct 120, 147
    in tissue 119–41, 142, *143*
    phase-sensitive/-insensitive methods 146
    structural inhomogeneities 148–9
    temperature rise 135
    tissue methods 146
  proteins 144, 407
  published data 143–55
  scattering 203
  tissues 146–55
    composition 152–3
acoustic beam
  attenuation of incident 62
  deformation 249
  focusing 57–8
  formation 46–7, 279
    adaptive 279
    receive process 282
  profile/axial pulse description 24–5
  propagation and human body effects 56
  shaping 59
  size 269
  steering 57–8
  swinging 26
acoustic Bragg peak *62*
acoustic centre frequency, effective 282
acoustic emission, acoustically stimulated 466–7
acoustic field 41–2
  attenuation in overlying tissue 62
  detection 69–70
  focused 48–51, *52*, 53–6
  generation 42
    therapeutic 59–63
  interrogation 42
  magnitude of variables 63–4
  measurement 69–70
    acousto-electric effect 86
    biologically effective exposure/dose 86–8
    calorimetry 83–4
    hydrophones 71–3, *74–5*, 76–7
    optical diffraction methods 84–5
    particle displacement detectors 77–8
    piezoelectric devices 70–1
    radiation force 78–9, *80*, 81–3
  non-uniform sources 47
  particle displacement detectors 77–8
  particle velocity 349
  projected 42
  propagation 53
  pulsed 48
  receptive 42
  refraction in overlying tissue 62
  shape visualisation 85
  short-pulse 73
  standing wave 382, 387
  subharmonic emissions 365
  temperature distribution 60–2
  Toronto hybrid system 59
  travelling 35
  uniform sources 46–7
acoustic frequency
  broadband techniques 125
  spectrum 100
acoustic impedance 389
  cavitation 368–9
  media 213
  soft tissues 228, 234
  specific 9

acoustic impedance (*Contd*)
  tissues 234
  values 279
acoustic microscopy 192, 341
  far field 341, 342–4
  high-frequency 291
  near field 341
  techniques 341–4, *345*, 346
acoustic microstreaming 384–5
acoustic output of devices 36
acoustic pressure 2, 459
  bubble growth 361
acoustic streaming 382–3
  biological significance 388
  egg cells of marine vertebrates 389
  fluid motion 383
  mammalian tissues 396
  non-cavitational sources of shear stress 389
  regimes *387*
  sonophoresis 410
  velocity gradients 383, 384
acoustic transmission micrographs 343, *345*
acoustic vibrations, subharmonic *see* subharmonic
      signal emissions
acoustic waves
  amplitude 47
  cylindrical 12–13
  energy
    coupling to photo-excited charge carrier 86
    transport 8
  form focusing 59
  frequencies 1
  fronts *260*
  oscillatory action 118–19
  plane waves 9, 11, 48
    progressive 63, *64*
    reflection coefficient 213
    single-frequency 191
  propagation 101
    collagen fibres 177, 179
    finite amplitude 183–5
    medium 268–9
    non-linear 113–16, *117*, 118, 268–9, 291
  reflected 27
  shape change 114
  spherical 12
  standing 11
    mammalian tissues 396
  tissue interactions 94–6
  variables 7–9, *10*, 11–13
  wave quantities *10*
  see also absorption; attenuation; wave equation
acoustical holography 338, 340–1
acoustical inhomogeneity 135–7
acousto-electric effect 86
aerosomes 153–5
aggrecan gene expression 422
alanine, pressure/temperature dependency *231*, 232
American Institute of Ultrasound in Medicine
      (AIUM) 475–6, 477
amino acids *230*, 232
amplitude
  dependence 331–2
  distribution 41
  quantitation of displayed 238
anaesthetics, transdermal 410
angioplasty, ultrasound 442–3

angular dependence 194–6
angular distribution, scattering 200, *201*
angular spectrum approach 20–1, *22*
antinodes 11
apodisation 19, 47, 48
  deliberate amplitude 51
  edge wave suppression 48
  phase 53
  Toronto hybrid system 59
array factor 25–6
arterial wall
  muscle elasticity 218
  scattering frequency dependence 206–7
arteries, recanalisation of atherosclerotic 443
attenuation 83, 93–4, 288–9, *290*
  acoustic 268
  blood 148
  bone 179–80
  collagen level in tissues 152
  components 207
  cross-section per unit volume 94
  dispersion relationship 179
  energy 207
  frequency-dependent 116, 149, 331
  inhomogeneous media 105
  liver 148
  maximum measurable 129
  Maxwell model 104
  measurement
    in fluids 169
    by non-linear propagation 118
    techniques 119–27
  radiation damping 106
  Rayleigh law 109
  related phenomena 112–13
  scattering
    contribution 146–8
    relationship 207–9
  soft tissue temperature dependence 150
  solids 108–9
  spatial mapping 125
  temperature
    coefficient 152
    dependence 150
    rise 350
  thermal pulse decay 121
  tissue components 152
  variation 112–13
  Voigt model 104
attenuation coefficient 95, 96
  biologically relevant simple media 144–6
  bone 355
  fat 153
  frequency dependence 126, 292
  gas bubbles 107
  heat-induced tissue coagulation 150–2
  homogenised tissue 224
  image reconstruction 125
  intensity 350
  liver focused beam surgery *436*
  measurement
    accuracy improvement 131
    bone 148
    broadband techniques 124–5, 138
    buffered insertion techniques 132
    conditions 139–41, 142, *143*
    displaced coupling medium 131

equation 127–9
errors 127–41, *142*, 143
errors due to invalid assumptions 130–5
errors in homogeneous specimens 129–35
forward scattering 131
frequency specification 130
frozen tissues 140–1
gas bubbles 121, 140, 148
inherent biological variability 141
inhomogeneity effects 135–7
insertion technique 127, 132–4
interference exclusion 129–30
microscopic 125–6
narrow band techniques 121–4
non-linearity 130–6
path length 136
phase-sensitive/-insensitive methods 146
pressure 141
primary errors 129–30
pseudo-CW system 131
reflection at tissue boundaries 131
sound speed of tissue 131–5
spatial averaging of echo spectra 126–7
specimen ageing 139–40
speed 136
temperature 135, 141
tests on standard materials 137–8
tissue 119–41, 142, *143*
tissue changes in death 141, *143*
tissue fixation 141
tissue methods 146
tissue storage/measurement conditions 140
in vivo 126–7
microbubbles 154–5
muscle 353
non-linear propagation 118
published data 142–55
scattering 203
spatial distribution 127
speed of sound 177
tissues 146–55, 288, 289
viscosity of suspending fluid 111
Australian Ultrasound Society (ASUM) 475
autocorrelation 314
processing technique 327
theorem 314
autocorrelator technique 315–17
autoregression techniques 314, 315
autoregressive instantaneous estimator, low-order 318
axial beam translation 134
axial tomography 338
axicon fields 55–6

B-mode image 191, 199, 259
elastography 217–19
mechanical index 476
models 215–17
point spread function 265, *266*
properties 217
real-time two-dimensional 303
safety 478
signal-to-noise ratio of speckle 217
tissue movement 217–19
B-scanners, compounding mode 268
backscatter/backscattering 192
coefficient 138, 203, 209, *210*

frequency dependences 292
cross-section 202, 208
digital reconstruction 338
echoes 320
frequency dependence 202
measurement 196, 204
microbubbles 154–5, 280
orientation dependence 202
power intensity 212
pressure 197
pulse–echo systems 291
reconstruction 127
signal expression 291–2
substitution methods 204
temperature imaging 329
tissue ageing 140
tone-burst signals 204
see also B-mode image
ball and rod device 78
barrier, transmission through 30
beam-forming electronics, parallel-receive 261
beam-line 271
see also acoustic beam
benign prostate hyperplasia 438
Bessel functions 13
bio-effect studies 459
clonogenic assay 460
biopolymers
absorption coefficient 144
frequency dependence of ultrasonic absorption 145
molecular conformation 144
birthweight 474
bladder wall cancer 439
Blake threshold 362, 363
blood
attenuation 148
backscatter 209, *210*, 211
contrast media 330
echoes 320
cavitation 465
clots 411
contrast media 279, 465
envelope fluctuation methods 320
parametric colour flow imaging 321
perfusion 352
phase tracking methods 322
scattering 208–9, *210*, 211
ultrasonic damage 464–7
blood cells
extravasation into lung 395–6, 465–6
stasis 382
blood flow
interruption 440–1
measurement 329
microbubbles in visualisation 155
ultrasound therapy 409
blood vessels
endothelial damage 384, 460, 465
erythrocytes 382
hazards 464–7
radiation stress-induced compression 388
bone
attenuation 179–80
attenuation coefficient 355
measurement 148
hazards 462–4

Bone (*Contd*)
  healing 442
  heating 355, 463
  injuries 413
    dose level 422
    healing 422
  speed of sound 177, *178*, 179–80
    dispersion 169
  thermal index 398, 476
  transverse waves 180
Born approximation 30
  scattering 192, 194, *201*, 203
  spherical scatter 199
Bragg peak, acoustic *62*
brain
  focused beam surgery 436–7
  heating 356–8
  imaging 283–4
  speed of ultrasound and temperature 180, *181*
  synapse damage 433
breast, female
  acoustic shadowing 289
  attenuation coefficient 288
  benign mass treatment 440
  lump detection 251
  speed of sound 182
    measurement 171
  tomographic images *340*
  water bath imaging 281
breast cancer
  focused beam surgery 440
  malignant spicules 263
  screening 251
brightness 238
  contrast 241–3
British Medical Ultrasound Society 477
bubbles
  motion 363–4
  see also gas bubbles; microbubbles
bulk modulus, tissue 234
buoyant force 359

C-scan 262–3, 275
cadmium sulphide 86
  acoustoelectric receiver 124
calcium ions 408
calorimetry 83–4
cancer therapy 422–8
  childhood 472
  endoscopic focused beam surgery 430
  hazards 471–2
  metastasis risk 472
  see also tumour control
capacitance microphone 77
capillary leakage 466
carcinoembryonic antigen (CEA) 413
Cartesian diver radiometer 79, *80*
castor oil 137, 138
cataracts, removal 442
causality principle 28, 29
cavitation 118–19, 280, 358–78
  acoustic 359
    experimentally measured thresholds 374, 376–8
  acoustic emission 365–8, *370–1*
  acoustic pressure 362
  active detection 368
  activity monitoring 369

activity variation
  with intensity *367*, *370–1*, 376
  with pulsing conditions 377, *378*
blood 465
blood vessels 441
bubbles *360*
cell damage 461
cell lysis 459–60
collagen synthesis 420
definition 359
direct imaging 373
fibre optic methods 373–4
focused beam surgery 431, 434
haemolysis 464
harmonics 367
impedance change 368–9
inertial 359, 369
  thresholds 362
intensity threshold variation
  with ambient pressure 377, *379*
  with ambient temperature 378, *381*
  with frequency 376, *377*
  with gas content of medium 377, *380*
  with medium viscosity 378, *381*
liver 392
mammalian tissues 391–2, *393–4*, 395–6
monitoring 365–9, *370*, 371–4
  sensitivity of methods *375*
motes 361
non-inertial 359, 365, 367
nuclei 412
photosensitive drug activation 413
processes in free liquid 363, *364*
safety 477
second harmonic 367
stable 119
subharmonic emissions 365–7
thresholds 361–3
  non-inertial 361–2, *364*
tumour therapy with porphyrins 425–6
white noise 367–8
cavities, formation 359–61
cells
  chromosomal ultrasound effects 461
  cytogenetic effects 461
  damage 460–1
  death and temperature range 431
  functional changes 461–2
  ion transport permeability changes 460
  isolated 459–62
  lysis 459–60
  reproductive ability 460
  ultrastructural changes 460–1
central nervous system (CNS), heating 356
chemiluminescence 372
chemotherapeutic agents *see* cytotoxic agents
children
  handedness 473
  malignancy risk 472
  neurological development 472–3
  speech development 473–4
chloroplasts 391
chromosomal ultrasound effects 461
clonogenic assay 460
collagen 144, 233
  absorption 148–9
  arrangement 420

deposition 421
extensibility 408–9
selective heating 409
strength 408–9
synthesis 419, 420
tissue component 152
collagen fibres, acoustic wave propagation 177, 179
colloidal particle suspension 279
colour angiography 327
colour differentiation 247
colour Doppler imaging 293, 294
   energy 327
colour flow imaging 303, 304, 326
   clutter rejection filter 326
   parametric 321
   post-processing 326
   safety 478
   two-dimensional 326
   velocity estimation 326
compounding, spatial/temporal 276–7
compressibility 229
   determination in soft tissues 228
   fluctuations 196
   modulus 338
compression, ultrasonic longitudinal wave 100
connective tissue elasticity 420
constitutive equation 4–5
continuity equation 4
continuous wave techniques 305, 306–8
   coherent demodulation 311
   single scatterer *309*
contrast, visual 247
contrast agents, gas-filled 412, 466
   safety 477, 478
contrast media 330–2
   backscatter from blood 330
   blood 465
   instability effects 332
   microbubbles 118, 153–5
   performance enhancement 330
   pulse–echo systems 279–80
   signature recognition 330–2
   speed of sound 185
contrast resolution 241–3, 282, 285–6
   biological variance 285
   contrast-to-noise ratio 286
   differential signal 286
   noise level 286
   property values 285, 286
   spatial resolution 293
   technical precision 285–6
contrast transfer efficiency 295
cooling 352
cotton seed oil 138
coupling gel 30, 415, 457, 459
coupling medium
   displaced 131
   sound speed 131–2
cranial thermal index 398, 476
cross-correlation process 322, 323, 324
   one-bit 325
cross-section per unit volume 95
crossed beam method 171
crystals/crystalline materials
   natural 43
   photosensitive semiconductor 86
cylindrical waves 12–13

cytotoxic agents
   combination with ultrasound 424
   synergy with ultrasound 423–6

damping
   radiation 106
   thermal 105–6, 113
   viscous 105–6
dashpots 102
data acquisition, three-dimensional 261
deflection, refractive 249
demand modulation 242
demodulation
   coherent 310
   phase quadrature 311–13
density
   fluctuations 196
   modulus 338
dentistry 443
detection
   image interpretation 250
   of object 248
detective quantum efficiency 244
dextran 144
diagnostic probes, temperature rise in tissues 354
diaphragm, thoracic, specular reflection 268
diffraction
   corrections 93, 173–4
      computed 133
      experimental 134
   gain 134
   loss 134
   theory 200, 202, 430
diffraction error *133*
   corrections 132–3
diffraction tomography 196, 338
diffusion, rectified 118, 361
digital memory, looped 259
direct wave 19
directivity spectrum approach 22–3, *24*
discontinuity distance 115
disintegration 224
disk transducer element 44, *45*
dispersion 104
   attenuation relationship 179
   related phenomena 112–13
   single relaxation process *98*
   speed 110
dissipation parameter
   radiation 107, 108
   thermal 107, 108
   total 107
   viscous 107, 108
distributed aberrators 271
distributed scatterers 309
DNA
   aqueous suspension 144, *230*
   degradation 389, 461
   gene transfection 412
Doppler frequency-shift estimation strategies 313–18
   spectral estimation techniques 313–15
Doppler processing 303, 304, 305
Doppler shift 34, 304, 310
   detection 305–6
   equation 34
   frequency 322, *323*
      motion-induced 311

Doppler shift (*Contd*)
  measurement 308
  signal
    demodulation of returned 310–13
    power 327, *328*
    power spectrum 316
    sampling 318
    spectrum estimation 318
    spectrum 327, *328*
Doppler technique 305–20
  safety 478
  thermal index 476
  tissue imaging 320
dosimetry 71
drug delivery
  transdermal 410
  ultrasonically enhanced 410–13
dyslexia 473

echo 27, 487
  clutter 269, 321
  leading edge 33
  reflected sequence 28
  signal reception/manipulation 269, 271, *272*, 273–5
  signal-to-nose ratio 324
  strain imaging 328–9
  trailing edge 33
  see also speckle
echo-enhancement, gas bubbles 107
echo-sounding 487
echography 237, 238
  development 284
  noise in 243–6
edge wave 19, 55–6
  suppression 48
elastic moduli 101
elasticity
  estimation in soft tissues 227
  images 328
  modulus for soft tissue 226, 227
  ultrasonic imaging 234
elastography 217–19, 293, 328
  contrast transfer efficiency 295
  strain measurement 329
  tissue strain 294
electrolytes 229, *230*
electronic noise 245
embryo
  in utero exposure 467, *468–70*, 471
  see also fetus
endoscopy, focused beam surgery 430
energy
  absorption 97
  activation for relaxation process 109
  attenuation 207
  bimodal delivery 61
  conservation 32–3
  density 9
  flow 9
  Gibbs free energy 228
  instantaneous spatial distribution of deposition 60
  loss 93, 350
  transfer in harmonics 116
  transmission
    into tissue 457
    transducer to tissues 30
  transport 32–3, 35
enthalpy 228
entropy 228–9
envelope fluctuation methods 320–1
envelope tracking techniques 325–6
erythrocytes 382, 464, 465
  haemolysis 389
  inter-particle forces 386
ethyl alcohol 176
Euler formalism 2, 3, 4
Euler's equation 4
European Federation of Societies for Ultrasound in Medicine and Biology (EFSUMB) 476, 477–8
excitation
  amplitude shading 19
  continuous wave 46–7
  pulsed 45
  short pulse 53–4
  of source 46–7
exploso-scanning 261
exposimetry 71, 87
exposure
  expression 87–8
  guidelines 474–9
  levels 457, *458*, 459
  practice 457, *458*, 459
  recommendations 474–9
  safety 475
eye, human
  cataract removal 442
  dark adapted 371
  dynamic range of accommodation 240–1
  focused beam surgery 437–8
  safety in ultrasound investigations 479
  visual perception 239–48

facial nerve paralysis 442
fast pulse techniques 488
fat, body
  attenuation coefficient 153
  scattering coefficients 153
  speed of ultrasound 182
    temperature 180, *181*, 182
feature separation, noise-limited 252
Fermat's principle 192
ferroelectric ceramics 44–5
ferroelectrics 43
ferrous sulphate oxidation 372
fetal Doppler
  heart monitoring 478
  temperature rise 355
fetus
  heating 357–8
  human studies 472–4
  neurological development 472–3
  obstetric ultrasound risk 464
  in utero exposure 467, *468–70*, 471, 472
    birthweight 474
    safety 478
    speech development 473–4
fibrinolytic drugs 411
fibroblasts 419
ficoll 144
finite amplitude waves 34–9
  harmonic pumping 36–8
  measurement 183–4
  pressure-dependent velocity 38–9

radiation pressure 35–6
fixatives, histological 146
flash-echo technique 280
flicker sensitivity 246, *247*
flow imaging 303
fluctuation techniques 305
focused ultrasound surgery (FUS) 428
focusing strength 265
focusing systems 48–51, *52*, 53–6
  axicon fields 55–6
  edge waves 55–6
  limited diffraction fields 55–6
  shape 49
fogging, photographic plates 369
Fourier periodogram 313–14
Fourier slice theorem 23
Fourier transform 20, 21, 23
  analysis 315
  autocorrelation 314, 316
  bubble motion 364
  phase difference spectra 174
  scattering 196
  spectral estimation 313
fovea 240
fracture healing 463
Fraunhoffer diffraction zone 46, 282
frequency detectors, instantaneous 315–18
frequency spectrum analysis 292
Frèsnel distance 46, 50
Fricke ionising radiation dosimetry 372

gall bladder stone 269
gas bubbles 106–8
  acoustic microstreaming 384–5
  activity at megahertz frequencies 389–90
  adiabatic collapse 371–2
  attenuation coefficient 140
    measurement 148
  attenuation measurement 121
  attractive forces 389
  buoyancy 359, 360
  cavitation 359, *360*
    acoustic emission 365–8, *370–1*
    active detection 368
  compression 361
  diagnostic ultrasound imaging 392–3
  direct imaging 373
  fibre optic imaging 373–4
  growth 361, 362
    sonoluminescence 371
  harmonic signals 367
  impedance change 368–9
  mammalian tissues 391, 392, *393, 394,* 395
  optical detection 373
  organic molecule skin 360
  oscillations 384, 386
    chaotic 365–6
    forced 362
    non-linear 363
    vibrating wire model 389
  platelet aggregation 387
  pressure 359–60
  pulmonary capillaries 396
  radiation force 386–8
  scattering 205
  stabilisation 360–1
  stabilised 107

subharmonic emissions 365–7
surface tension 361
surface velocity 387
white noise 367–8
Gaussian function
  auto-correlation *206*
  B-mode image 216
gelatin 144
Geliperm 415
gene therapy 412
gene transfer vectors 412
Gibbs free energy 228
gingivitis 443
glaucoma 438
glycine, pressure/temperature dependency *231*, 232
glycogen, absorption coefficient 153
granulation 419
Green's function 13–14, 198
  impediography 214
grey-scale imaging 488

haematoporphyrin 412–13
haemolysis 464, 465
  critical stress 384, *386*
  red blood cells 389
  threshold stress 389
haemostasis, focused beam surgical 440–1
handedness studies 473
harmonic fields, angular spectrum approach 20–1
harmonic pressure amplitude distribution 21
harmonic pumping 36–8, 39, 343
harmonics/harmonic waves 6–7
  beam aberration alleviation 271
  cylindrical 13
  energy transfer 116
  frequency and beam size 269
  generation 331–2
  image derivation 268–9, *270*
  narrowband 331
  plane 11, *39*
  reflected 33–4
  second 280
    cavitation 367
    Oseen force 385
    pressure amplitude 291
    superposition 426
  spherical 12
  travelling 22
  wideband 280
  see also subharmonic signal emissions
heart, fetal monitoring 478
  see also temperature
heat
  physiological basis for therapy 407
  physiological responses 409
  safety 475–6
Heaviside step function 18, 29
Helmholtz equation 7, 20
high-intensity focused ultrasound (HIFU) 428
Hilbert transform 313
hip joint, heating 355
histamine release 419
hydration state 229
hydrophones 71–3, *74–5*, 76–7
  calibration 73, 76–7, 81
  fibre optic 373–4
  large aperture 23

hydrophones (*Contd*)
  measurements at a point 77
  membrane device 72–3, *74–5*
  needle 72
  point 24, 25
  preamplifier 72
  probes 459
  pulse–echo system performance assessment 282–3
  scattering error 204–5
  short-pulse fields 73
  small-aperture device 77
  wetting 73
hydrostatic pressure 359, 360
hyperthermia, localised *290*

I-beam configuration 264
identification of object 248
images
  classification 250
  data coherence 275–6
  high-quality rapid sequential 249
  interpretation 249–52
  noise content 241–2
  parameterisation 249
imaging 237
  human visual perception 239–48
  medical 248–9
  observer performance 248
  performance criteria 284–7, 329
  quantitative measures 238–9
  spatial characteristics 238–9
  system dynamic range 245
  time-dependent phenomena 293–5
  see also parametric imaging
impedance
  constant 29
  continuously varying 28–30
  effective 28, 214
impediography 213–14
impulse response technique 17–19, 20
incandescence 372
insertion techniques, buffered 127, 132–4
intensity 50
  acoustic 63, 82
  coefficient 95
  exposure 87
  gain 51, 93
  instantaneous 9
  linear-equivalent spatial average 88
  loss 93
  normalised 51
  plane wave 95
  transmission 28
    coefficient 30
inter-particle forces 385–8
interferometers, ultrasonic 123
  continuous wave 168
intra-ocular pressure decrease 437–8
ion transport, cell permeability changes 460

joints
  contractures 409, 421
  injuries 413
  stiffness 409

Kasai autocorrelator, instantaneous 318
kidney tumour treatment 439

Kupffer cells, contrast media 279

Lagrange formalism 3, 4
Laplacian operator 6
laser speckle 215, 217
  see also speckle
lattice dislocations 108
lead zirconate-titanates 44, 415
lens focusing 53, 54–5
line spread function 239
linear acoustics *see* wave equation, canonical inhomogeneous of linear acoustics
linear scanner, real-time 171
linearisation 4
lipids, acoustic propagation properties 145
liposomes, drug-loaded 411
liquid tissue
  speed of sound 177, *178*
  see also blood
lithotripsy
  extracorporeal 63, 77
    displacement detector 78
    measurement devices 88
  shock waves 395–6
  ultrasonic generator 443
liver
  adenocarcinoma acoustic micrograph *345*
  attenuation 148
    coefficient 224
  cavitation effects 392
  cirrhosis 183
  contrast medium 148
  focused beam surgery 434–5, *436*
  heating 356
  scattering 203–4, 205, 209, *210*
  speed of sound 183
    measurement 171
    non-linearity parameter 184
  trauma 440–1
  tumour treatment 439
localisation, image interpretation 250
loss of correlation imaging 280
luminance 238
lung
  haemorrhage 395–6, 465–6
  speed of sound 177, *178*

M (movement) scan
  cardiac application 259
  safety 478
  thermal index 476
macromolecular interactions 145–6
macroscope, ultrasound 125
macroscopic cross-section 95
macroscopic techniques 337–8, *339*, 340–1
magnetic resonance imaging (MRI) 435
malignancy
  childhood risk 472
  see also cancer therapy; tumour control
mammals/mammalian tissues
  acoustic streaming 396
  bubbles *393, 394*
    formation 391, 392, 395
  cavitation 391–2, *393–4*, 395–6
  non-thermal effects of ultrasound 391–2, *393–4*, 395–6
  standing waves 396

temperature distribution 407
mass, conservation of 4
mast cell degranulation 419
maximum entropy method, autoregressive 314, 318
Maxwell model 102–4
mechanical index (MI) 396–7, 476
mechlorethamine 424
median filtering, velocity guided 279
medium, compressibility 5
Menière's disease 441–2
 calibration of power transducers 83
merocyanine 540 413
metastases 428, 472
micro-massage 408
microbubbles 118–19, 153–5
 attenuation
  coefficient 154–5
  frequency dependence 331
 backscattering 154–5, 280
 bursting 412
 cavitation 280
  in blood vessels 441
 flash-echo phenomenon 280
 human albumin 279
 instability effects 332
 intracellular 461
 non-linear acoustic behaviour 155
 oscillation 331
 resonant vibration 280
 scattering 209
  coefficient 154–5
  frequency dependence 331
 scattering-to-attenuation ratio 153
 spatial resolution enhancement 330
 stabilisation 361
 sugar matrix 279
 temporal resolution enhancement 330
microscopy
 acoustic 192
 see also scanning laser acoustic microscopy
  (SLAM)
misregistration measurement 171
mitochondrial damage 433
mitral valve, M-mode scan 259
modulation transfer function 239, 242–3, 245
 area 242–3, 245
molecular absorption cross-section 96
momentum density 35
 time-averaged flux 36
motes, cavitation 361
motion
 equation of 3–4
 information with real-time two-dimensional
  displays 303
 viscous relative 113
motion detection 304–5
 non-stationary microbubbles 332
 simple continuous wave 304–5
 simple pulsed-wave 305
moving target indicators 34
multielement arrays 25–6
muscle
 absorption 148–9
 anisotropy of sound velocity 233
 attenuation coefficient 353
 heating 355–6, 357
 scattering 210, 211

smooth 464
spasm effects of ultrasound therapy 409
speed of sound 177
mutagenic agents 461
myofibroblasts 419

nerves, heating 356, 357
neurological development 472–3
neuromata, subcutaneous 436–7
neurosurgery, focused beam surgery 436–7
Newtonian liquid, viscosity coefficients 102
noise equivalent quanta 244
noise required modulation 242
non-linear propagation 2
non-linearity 35
nucleic acids
 absorption coefficient 144
 see also DNA
nucleic bases 230
nucleotides 229, 230
Nyquist theorem 318–19

observers, ideal/real 248
obstetric ultrasound, fetal risk 464
ophthalmology, focused beam surgery 437–8
optical diffraction 84–5
optical interferometry 78
optical transfer function 239
organogenesis 471
oscillatory stress 384
oscilloscope 168
 speed of ultrasound measurement 169
 time delay 168
Oseen force 385

pain relief 409
parallel beam-forming 259
parameterisation rates 287
parametric imaging 284
 contrast resolution 285–6
 performance criteria 286
 skin 289
 sound speed 290
 spatial resolution 287
 speed of presentation 287
Parkinson's disease 436, 437
particle acceleration 7
particle displacement 3
 detectors 77–8
 nodes 11
particle pressure
 acoustic pressure/density 113
 amplitude 64
particle velocity 2, 3, 4, 38
 acoustic pressure/density 113
 amplitude 64
 plane wave acoustic field 349
 shock front 115
 thermal vibration 349–50
 vector product 50
path length estimation 172, 174
peptides 230
perception
 of object 248
 quantitative measures 238–9
perfluorochemicals 279

pericoronitis 443
periodontics 443
periosteum 463, 464
phaco-emulsification 442
phase cancellation errors 124, 134, 135–7
phase coherence 71
phase difference spectra 174
phase fluctuation technique 305–20
  aliasing 318–19
  angle dependence 318, *319*
  limitations 318–20
  phase tracking relationship 322, *323*
  signal processing 310–18
  spectral clutter *319*, 320
  velocimetry 305–6
phase quadrature demodulator 317
phase quadrature detection 311–13
phase tracking methods 321–5
  limitations 324–5
  phase fluctuation relationship 322, *323*
  temporal averaging of velocity estimates 325
phonons, thermal 108
phonophoresis 410–11
photodynamic therapy 412–13
physiotherapy 413–15, *416*, 417–22
  applications of ultrasound 417–22
  carrier frequency 414
  contact application 415
  coupling gel 415
  crystal mounting 415, *416*
  equipment 413–15
  exposure levels 414–15
  output characterisation 414
  performance of equipment 414
  pulsed irradiation 414
  radiation balance 414
  soft tissue injuries 417–21
  techniques 413–14, 415, *416*, 417
  timers 414
  transducers 415, 417
  water bath immersion 415
piezoelectric devices 42–6
  acoustic field measurement 70–1
  attenuation measurement 123–4
  diagnostic use 70–1
  electrical impedance 45
  pulsed excitation 45
piezoelectric effect 70
piezoelectric materials
  acoustic mismatch to water/soft tissues 45
  backing 44–5
  composite 45
  hydrophones 71
  properties 43
  quarter-wave matching layers 45
  transducer arrays 58
piezoelectricity 42, 487
planar boundaries, propagation across 26–34
  normal incidence on stationary, sharp
    boundary 26–8
  reflection
    from continuously varying impedance profile
      28–30
    from moving interface 33–4
    from planar interface at oblique incidence 30–3
  transmission through a barrier 30
plane waves 9, 11

plants
  non-thermal cellular effects of ultrasound 390–1
  root subharmonic emissions 391
platelets
  activation 441
  aggregation 390, 441
    around bubbles 387
  damage 465
  motion 390
Pohlmann cell 86
point scatterers 305–8
point spread function 239, 265, *266*
polycrystalline solids 109
polymethacrylate 54
polynucleotides *230*
polysaccharides, absorption coefficient 144
polystyrene, cross-linked 54
porphyrins, acoustic cavitation with 425–6
post-processing 271, 275
potassium, cell content 408
potassium iodide 372
power mode imaging 327–8
  safety 478
pregnancy
  human exposure to ultrasound *462*
  ultrasound exposure safety 478
pressure
  ambient 111
  hydrostatic 182
pressure-dependent velocity 38–9
pressure jump method 184
pressure nodes 11
propagation properties, ultrasonic
  heat-induced tissue coagulation 151–2
  tissue components 152
prostate
  benign disease 438
  cancer treatment 439
  elastogram 294
  focused beam surgery 434, 438
proteins *230*
  absorption coefficient 144, 407
  cross-linking 146
  dehydration 146
  denaturation 146
  fibrillar *230*
  synthesis inhibition 422
  tissue content 224
pseudocavitation 391
pulmonary capillaries, gas bubbles 396
pulse
  arrival time 174
    definition 172–3
  bandwidth 324
  duration 87
  inversion 257
    method 280
  multiple detection sequences 331
  non-Gaussian 126
  propagation 1
  repetition
    frequency 87, 318, 319
    rate 168
  scattering 191
  splitting 16
  superposition method 168
  transit-time 168, 288

ultrasound fields 34
pulse time-of-flight (TOF) 169
pulse time-of-flight (TOF) measurement 168, 171
  reference point 172
  transducer effects 174
pulse-to-pulse correlation 322
pulse transmission systems 121–2
  fixed path 121, 122
  insertion technique 122–3
  reverberation methods 123
  substitution method 122
  variable path 121, 122
pulsed Doppler ultrasound 464
pulsed wave techniques 305, 308
  phase quadrature demodulation 312–13
pulse–echo principle 28, 34, 255
  exposures 88
pulse–echo systems *197*, 256–84
  acoustic output 282
  backscatter 291
  bubble formation imaging 373
  clutter 279
  colour use 278
  contrast media 279–80
  contrast resolution 282
  data acquisition rate 258
  diagnostic 48, 421, 488
    temporal peak source intensity 116
  distributed targets 266–8
  exposure quantification 479
  extended interface targets 268
  fields of application 283
  geometrical conformity 282
  interrogation process 264
  multi-line processing 274
  overlap method 168
  performance assessment 281–3
  performance criteria 284
  point targets 264–5, *266*
  posterior shadowing 288–9
  scanning 258–64
  scattering 192, 198
  sensitive range 282
  signal reconstitution 279
  signal-to-noise ratio
    enhancement 275–9, 280
    lesion 282
  spatial compounding 276–7
  spatial resolution 281–2
  speed of sound 289
  temporal compounding 276–7, *278*
  testing 281–3
  transducer response 199
  transfer function 264–8
  true gain compensation 338
  wave aberration 279

quartz 43–4

radar 488
radiation force 35–6, 380, 381–2
  balance 79, *80*, 81
  gas bubbles 386–8
  measurement 78–9, *80*, 81–3
    large-target methods 79, *80*, 81
    small-target methods 82–3

radiation pressure 380–2
  biological significance 388, 389
radiation stress, blood vessel compression 388
radiation therapy synergy with ultrasound 423–4, 426
radiometer, Cartesian diver 79, *80*
Raman–Nath effect 84
Rayleigh dependence 196
  scattering 208, 213
Rayleigh probability distribution 215
  B-mode image 217
Rayleigh–Plesset equation 364, *366–7*
Rayleigh's integral 13–14, 15, 17
  attenuation 109
  scattering 197
real-time ultrasound 258
receive beam-forming process 282
receive channel-level processing 271
receive channels, individual 271
receiver operating characteristic (ROC) 251
reciprocity 73, 76–7
recognition of object 248
red blood cells
  banding 388, 396
  extravasation 412
  haemolysis 389
reduced variables, method of 110
reference plane reflector 204
reflection 93
  coefficient 27, 28, 213
  from continuously varying impedance profile 28–30
  critical angle 344, 346
  from moving interface 33–4
  from planar interface at oblique incidence 30–3
  specular 268
  at tissue boundaries 131
  total 32, 33
reflectivity
  varying 30
  zero 32
reflector
  specular 32
  velocity 308
reflex transmission imaging (RTI) 126–7, *263*, 289
refracted waves 32–3
refraction 93, 171
  see also Snell's law
refractive deflection 249
refractive index
  fluctuations 192
  optical 84
relaxation 104
  amplitude 97
  frequencies 97–8
  low frequency region 149
  processes
    activation energy 109
    molecular 99–100
    viscothermal/viscoelastic theories 99
  structural 110
  temperature dependence 150
  theory 179
  thermal 99–100, 110
  thermoelastic 108
  time
    distribution 110

relaxation (*Contd*)
  time (*Contd*)
    temperature 109
    velocity dispersion 100
    vibrational 111
    viscoelastic 100
replica pulses 48
retina structure 240
Riemann invariant 39
round-trip transit time 168

saccharides *230*
saline and speed of ultrasound 169
  tests on standard materials 175, 176
saw, ultrasonic 442
scaling, dental 443
scan conversion 271, 275
scanning acoustic microscopy 54, 341
  interference mode 170
scanning acoustic microscopy (SAM) 342–4
  propagation velocities 342–3
scanning laser acoustic microscopy (SLAM) 170,
    341, 344, 346
  acoustic angle of incidence 346
  critical angle for acoustic reflection 344, 346
  dark-field image 346
  interferometric mode 170
scar tissue 408
  elasticity 420
    increase 421
  strength 420–1
scattered wave/scattered wave vector 195
scatterers
  collections 200, 202
  distributed 309
  phase tracking methods 321–2
  point 305–8
  single-point 266
  three-dimensional distribution 266
scattering 1, 93, 191–2, 291–3
  angle 195, 209
  angular 208
  angular dependence 207
  angular distribution 200, *201*
  attenuation
    coefficient measurement 128
    contribution to 146–8
    relationship 207–9
  B-mode image 215–19
  basic equations 193–4
  coefficient 203, 208
    fat 153
    measurement 131, 147
    microbubbles 154–5
  collagen importance 152
  cross-section 202–4
    per unit volume 94
  differential *201*
  discrete model 211–12
  experimental methods 204–7
  forward 128, 131, 212
  frequency dependence 205–7, 209, 331
  gas bubbles 205
  Gaussian model 213
  inhomogeneities 94
  inhomogeneous continuum model 212
  inverse 196

  measurements 204–9, *210*, 211
  models 211–14
  multiple 192
  non-uniform medium 191
  orientation dependence 207
  per inhomogeneity 192
  phantoms 134
  phase cancellation 204
  pressure 203
  pulse 191, 197–9
  pulse–echo imaging 488
  Rayleigh dependence 196
  related phenomena 112–13
  single sphere 199–200
  solid tissues 109
  source terms 6
  sources of error 204–5
  spherical 199, *201*
  temperature dependence 149–50
  theory 191, 192, 193–204
    from tissue 191
  tissue constituents 209
  total cross-section 207–9
  volumes 213
  wave analysis 192
scattering-to-attenuation ratio of microbubbles 153
Schlieren representation 85
sector scanner 26
self-reciprocity 77
semiconductor crystals, photosensitive 86
semiconductors 109
shadowing, posterior 288–9
shear elastic modulus 293
shear elasticity 232
  tissue characterisation 234
shear moduli, soft tissue 224, 225–6
shear stress 102, 383–4
  biological significance 388
  hydrodynamic 464
  non-cavitational sources 389–90
  platelet damage 465
  sinusoidal 100
  waves 262
shear viscosity of liquids 110
shear waves
  heating effect 354–5
  propagation 1–2
  speed of 226
  velocity 232
shock-formation distance 38
shock waves 77
  displacement detector 78
  ultrasound pulses 395–6
  white noise 368
  see also lithotripsy
sidelobe reduction 59
signal processing
  interactive with transducer arrays 58
  minimum entropy 59
  phase tracking 323–4
  sidelobe reduction 59
signal-to-noise ratio
  echo 324
  enhancement 330
  increase 294–5
  lesion 282
  moving soft tissue 320

sing-around system 168, 171
sister chromatid exchange analysis 461, *467*
skin
  grafts 421
  parametric imaging 289
Snell's law 32, 170, 171
soft tissues
  acoustic impedance 228, 234
  attenuation 150
  compressibility determination 228
  elasticity
    estimation 227
    modulus 226, 227
  frequency dependence 149
  hazards 462–3, 464
  incompressibility 225
  injuries 413, 417–21
    oedema reduction 421
  intermolecular interactions 228
  liquid-like media 226
  mechanics 225–8
  semi-solid media 226
  shear elasticity 232
  shear moduli 224, 225–6
  shear wave velocity 232
  speed of sound 177, *178*, 182–3, 228
  temperature dependence 149–50
  thermal index 398, 476, 477
solute–solute interactions 145
solute–solvent interactions 184
Sommerfeld radiation condition 13
sonamacroporation 411
sonochemistry 372–3
sonodynamic therapy 412–13
sonoluminescence 369, 371–2
sonophoresis 410–11
sonoscintigraphy 280
sound velocity *see* speed of sound
sources, circular pulsed 46, 48
spatial resolution 269, 281–2, 287
  contrast resolution 293
speckle
  artefact *267*, 268
  coherent 243, *267*
  decorrelation 263
  distributed targets 267
  image clarity improvement 338
  noise 244, 245, 247
    adaptive filtering 291
    impact on imaging performance 275, *276*
    reduction 274
  reduction methods 258, 276–7, 278–9
  spatial density 281
    of pattern 282
  tracking 256–7, 274–5
spectral analysis techniques 124
spectral broadening 309
spectral estimation 313–15
spectral pulsed Doppler 478
spectroscopy, high frequency 292
speech development 473–4
speed of sound 167, 288–9, *290*
  anisotropy 233
  attenuation coefficient 177
  bone 177, *178*, 179–80
  contrast media non-linearity parameter 185
  crossed beam method 171

finite amplitude propagation 183–5
inhomogeneity in tissues 269
liquid tissue 177, *178*
liver 183
  non-linearity parameter 184
lung 177, *178*
microscopic measurements 170
misregistration measurement 171
muscle 177
non-linearity
  measurement 183–4
  published data 184–5
observation of focusing behaviour 171–2
pressure dependence 182
published data 176–7, *178*, 179–80, *181*, 182–3
pulse–echo systems 289
soft tissue 177, *178*, 182–3, 228
sources of error 184
thermodynamic method 184
tissue components 182–3
speed of ultrasound
  diffraction corrections 173–4
  errors in measuring homogeneous specimens 172–4
  inhomogeneity effects 174
  knowledge of speed in reference medium 172
  measurement in tissues 167–76
    absolute methods 168
    conditions 176
    relative methods 169
  non-linear propagation 173
  path length estimation 172, 174
  phase difference spectra 174
  pulse arrival time 174
    definition 172–3
  techniques 168–72
  temperature dependence 180, *181*, 182
  tests on standard materials 174–6
  transducer effects 174
  in vivo measurement 170–2
springs 102
stabilisation region 116
standing waves 11
  mammalian tissues 396
stimulated acoustic emission 280
Stokes' drag 385
Stokes' formula 110, 359
storage moduli 101
strain estimation, direct/indirect 329
stratum corneum perturbations 411
streaming, ultrasonic 124
streptokinase 411
subharmonic signal emissions 280, 365–7
  plant roots 391
surface tension 361
surgery 428–43
  dentistry 443
  focused beam 428–41
    brain synapse damage 433
    cavitation 434
    cavitation mechanisms 431
    clinical applications 436–41
    endoscopy 430
    exposures 433
    focal depth 428–9
    handheld device for ablation 430
    lesion production 432, *433*, *434*, *437*
    lesion shape/size 430

surgery (*Contd*)
  focused beam (*Contd*)
    lesioning rate parameter 432
    magnetic resonance imaging monitoring 435
    maximum power transmission 429
    mitochondrial damage 433
    neurosurgery 436–7
    ophthalmology 437–8
    optimum frequency 430–1
    principles 428–35, *436*, *437*
    solid angle of irradiation 430
    techniques 428–35, *436*, *437*
    temperature of lesion 431
    thermal ablation 435
    thermal model for lesion development 431
    trans-rectal probes 434
    transducers 429
    tumour ablation 438–40
    urology 438
    vascular occlusion 440–1
  high-intensity focused ultrasound 354
  ultrasonically-driven tools 442
system transfer function 264

target velocity measurement 305, 308
targets, distributed 266–8
television camera, acoustic 338, *339*
temperature
  distribution 60–2
    bone 355
    experimentally determined 355–8
    mammalian tissues 407
  local rate of rise 120
  relaxation time 109
  safety 475–6
  speed of ultrasound
    non-linearity parameter 184
    tests on standard materials 175–6
    tissues 180, *181*, 182
  variations 137
  see also heat
temporal contrast sensitivity 246
tendon
  anisotropy of sound velocity 233
  ultrasound therapy 408, 409
terephthalate acid 372–3
test objects, pulse–echo system performance assessment 282, 283
therapy, ultrasound, physiological basis 407–13
thermal ablation
  surgical 435
  systems 151
thermal conductivity 97, 108, 351
thermal diffusion 60
thermal index (TI) 358, 396, 397–8, 476
thermal pulse decay 121
thermal relaxation 99–100
thermal teratology 467, *468–70*, 471
thermal vibration, particle velocity 349–50
thermocouple dosimetry 83–4
thermodynamic method 184
thermodynamic potential of medium 228–9, *230–1*, 232
thermoelectric potential 84
thrombolysis 411
thyroid *267*, *278*
time delay spectrometry 125

time-gain compensation 268
time-of-flight estimation 289
  changing 305
time-reversal technique 271, 273
tissue impulse response 197, 199, 216
tissue plasminogen activator (t-PA) 411
tissues
  absorption coefficient 146–55
  acoustic attenuation 268
  acoustic properties 223–4
  aspiration 442
  attenuating effect 288
  attenuation coefficient 146–55, 288, 289
    frequency-dependent 245–6
    measurement 139–41, *142*, 143
  bulk acoustic properties 232–3
  bulk modulus 234
  characterisation 233–4, 249
  coagulation
    heat-induced 150–2
    speed of sound 182
  components 152–3
  constituents 209
  cooling 352
  cutting 442
  death effects on attenuation coefficient 141, 143
  elasticity
    imaging 328–9
    phase tracking methods 322
  heat denaturation 182
  heating effects on mobility 408
  homogenisation 441
  movement 217–19
    phase tracking methods 322
  non-thermal effects 390–2, *393–4*, 395–6
    plant systems 390–1
  repair
    phased 419
    stimulation 418
  shear acoustic properties 232–3, 234
  sound speed 131–5
    inhomogeneity 269
  strain rate 329
  temperature distribution 351–3
    experimental determination 355–8
  temperature rise 351, 476
    diagnostic probes 354
  ultrasonic echoes 171
  ultrasound speed measurement 167–76
tissue–ultrasound interactions 94–6
tone-burst signals 204
tools, ultrasonic 442
Toronto hybrid system 59, *60*
tracking
  fast cross-correlation-based algorithms 303
  techniques 305
trans-abdominal pulsed Doppler fetal ultrasound 355
transducer(s)
  annular 48
  diagnostic 70–1
  dosimetry 71
  edge-wave only 48
  electro-mechanical response 271
  energy transmission to tissues 30
  exposimetry 71
  extracorporeal 429–30

focused beam surgery 429
focusing 48–51, *52*, 53–6
    axial dependencies 51, *52*, 53
    radial dependencies 50–1
lens focusing 53, 54–5
measurement use 71
mounting 46
moving head 417
physiotherapy 415, 417
reciprocal 76
stationary head 417
Toronto hybrid system 59, *60*
trans-rectal 429
transmitting 205
vibration 46
see also disk transducer element; hydrophones
transducer arrays
    annular *57*, 58
    beam formation 56–9
    linear 57, 260–1
        curved 58
    non-diffracting design 58
    phased 25, 260–1, 429
    signal processing 58
    signal trains 271, *272*
    sparse 261
    three-dimensional data acquisition 261
    two-dimensional 58–9, 261
transducer fields 15–26
    angular spectrum approach 20–1, *22*
    beam profile/axial pulse description 24–5
    directivity spectrum approach 22–3, *24*
    multielement arrays 25–6
    off-axis field 17–19, *20*
    on-axis field 15–17
transfer heat, transient 352
transmission
    coefficient 27
    plain imaging 337–8, *339*
    reconstruction imaging 288, 338, *340*
travel time variable 29
tropical ulcers, skin graft take 421
tumour-associated antigens 413
tumour control 422–8
    cytotoxic agent synergy with ultrasound 423–6
    cytotoxic effect of ultrasound 423
    dose parameters 426–7
    focused beam surgery 438–40
    hyperthermic therapy 88, 426
    low power ultrasound 428
    metastatic spread potential 428, 472
    radiation therapy synergy with ultrasound 423–4,
        426
    temperature 438
    see also cancer therapy
    tumours, radiosensitivity 424

ultrasonic biophysics 349–50
    non-thermal links 349
    thermal links 349
    thermal mechanisms 350–8
ultrasound devices, output *458*
ultrasound wave scattering 1
ultrasound–tissue interaction 223–34
urokinase 411
urology
    focused beam surgery 438

tumour treatment 439
uterine fibroids 439
uterine leiomyosarcoma 439

van Cittert–Zernicke theorem 282
vascular occlusion 440–1
vascular perfusion 60
vascular tissues 464–7
    see also blood vessels
vasodilatation 409
velocity
    angle-independent motion imaging 326–8
    estimation techniques *306*, 326–8
    gradients
        acoustic streaming 383, 384
        biological significance 388
    potential 8
    resolution enhancement 330
ventricular contractions, premature 466
vertebrae, heating of fetal 357
vertigo 441, 442
viscoelastic model of tissue 106
viscoelastic relaxation 100
viscoelastic theory 101–5
viscoelasticity 100–5
viscosity
    coefficients 102
    temperature dependence 385
vision 240
    machine 247
visual acuity 241–3
visual perception, human 239–48
    features 247
    time factor 246, *247*
Voigt model 102, *103*, 104

water
    absorption of ultrasound 144
    acoustic cavitation 372
    acoustic impedance 369
    equation of state 228
    speed of ultrasound 169
        tests on standard materials 175
water bath immersion 415
wave equation 1
    canonical inhomogeneous of linear acoustics 2–7
        constitutive equation 4–5
        continuity equation 4
        equation of motion 3–4
        harmonic waves 6–7
    homogeneous 6
    wave quantities *10*
    see also acoustic waves
wave-scattering theory 30
Weber ratio 241
white blood cells, threshold shear stress 389
white noise 367–8
Wiener–Kinchin theorem 314, 316, 327
wire, vibrating 389
wounds
    breaking strength 421
    healing 409, 418, 464
    physiotherapeutic ultrasound 415

Young's modulus *225*
Yule–Walker equations 318